GENITOURINARY TRACT
PATHOLOGY

GENITOURINARY TRACT PATHOLOGY

Mark A. Weiss, MD
Director, Surgical Pathology
The Christ Hospital
Professor of Pathology
University of Cincinnati Medical Center
College of MedicineCincinnati, Ohio

Stacey E. Mills, MD
Professor of Pathology
University of Virginia
Health Sciences Center
Charlottesville, Virginia

Gower Medical Publishing
New York ◊ London

Distributed in the USA and Canada by:
Raven Press
1185 Avenue of the Americas
New York, NY 10036
USA

Distributed in Japan by:
Nankodo Company Ltd.
42-6, Hongo 3-Chome
Bunkyo-Ku
Tokyo 113
Japan

Distributed in the rest of the world by:
Gower Medical Publishing
Middlesex House
34-42 Cleveland Street
London W1P 5FB
UK

Library of Congress Cataloging-in-Publication Data
Weiss, Mark A., 1945–
    Genitourinary tract pathology / Mark A. Weiss, Stacey E. Mills.
      p. cm.
    Includes bibliographical references and index.
    ISBN 1-56375-159-3
      1. Genitourinary organs—Diseases. 2. Genitourinary organs—Cancer.
    3. Urogenital system—pathology. I. Mills, Stacey E. II. Title.
      [DNLM: 1. Urogenital diseases—pathology. WJ 100 W431g]
    RC875.W45 1992
    616.6—dc20
                                92-49821

British Library Cataloguing-in-Publication Data
A catalogue record for this book is available from the British Library.

Project Manager: Alison Marek
Designer: Jeffrey S. Brown
Illustrator: Laura Pardi Duprey
Art Director: Kathryn Armstrong
Production Coordinator: Judy Ray
Editorial Assistants: Jean Unger, Sean O'Brien

Printed in Singapore by Imago Productions (FE) PTE Ltd.

10 9 8 7 6 5 4 3 2 1

Preface

Genitourinary Tract Pathology, a condensed, updated version of the *Atlas of Genitourinary Tract Disorders* (1988), is a comprehensive visual reference combined with an integrated text. Redundant images and rare entities have been deleted, as have radiographs and text that were not vital to pathology. Gross and microscopic images have been updated, and several new entities have been added. In addition, we have included a new chapter on adrenal gland neoplasms.

A broad spectrum of disorders involving the upper and lower urinary tract and male genitalia are discussed and illustrated. Although neoplasms are given emphasis, many nonneoplastic disorders are presented, particularly inflammatory lesions. Congenital and developmental anomalies are also included.

A concise definition and information about incidence and epidemiology are given for each entity, followed by current concepts of pathogenesis when appropriate, and a summary of clinical manifestations. Gross and microscopic pathologic features, illustrated in full-color, are presented in detail with emphasis on diagnostic criteria. (Unless special stains are indicated, histologic sections were stained with hematoxylin and eosin.) Every attempt has been made to include "classic" gross specimen images, and to use photomicrographs that reinforce the diagnostic criteria. Cytohisto-logic correlations, electron microscopy, and immuno-cytochemistry, as well as clinical radiographs, are also included when pertinent to the diagnosis. For neoplasms, attention is given to grading and staging, as well as other prognostic features. Illustrations are accompanied by descriptive legends and often supplemented by labeled line drawings.

The selective, up-to-date reading list includes classic papers, major review articles, and textbooks, as well as pertinent references, which can be used for supplemental reading.

It is our goal that *Genitourinary Tract Pathology* will prove invaluable to pathologists and urologists in training and in practice. Many sections should also be helpful to nephrologists, oncologists, and cytotechnologists. In addition, the slide atlas prepared from this volume should be an asset for teaching and course presentation, as well as for individual study and review.

Mark A. Weiss
Stacey E. Mills

Acknowledgments

We would like to acknowledge and formally thank the following friends and colleagues who generously contributed case material to this book: Drs. Shannon Allen, Willie Andersen, Edwin Beckman, Jay Bernstein, Dinyar Bhathena, Philip Cooper, Stewart Cramer, John Crissman, John Eble, Robert Fechner, Philip Feldman, Jackson Fowler Jr., Henry Frierson Jr., Stuart Howards, Howard Levin, Catherine Limas, John Mahoney, Thomas Pope, Denise Ross, Steven Swerdlow, Aleksander Talerman, Anna Walker, Terrence Wesseler, Mark Wick, James Wolfe III, and Robert Young.

Several colleagues made extensive contributions and deserve special recognition. Dr. Edward Ballard kindly contributed case materials used in Chapters 1 and 2. Dr. Sohei Tokunaka provided valuable radiologic, gross, and microscopic photographs of primary obstructive megaureter in Chapter 8. Dr. Bruce Bracken supplied the superb cystoscopic photographs used in Chapters 10 and 12. Dr. Kevin Bove donated material for Chapter 11 from his collection of Wilms' tumor precursor lesions. Dr. Kenneth Greer contributed most of the clinical photographs of external genital lesions in Chapters 18 and 19. Dr. Hugh Hawkins contributed radiologic images used in Sections I, III, and V.

We would also like to thank the staff at Gower, who brought this book to fruition. Special thanks to Jeff Brown for his excellent design, and to Alison Marek for overseeing the entire project.

Dedication

Much of the research, composition, and illustration of this work took place in evenings and on weekends, at the expense of time devoted to our families. Without the support and encouragement of our wives (Ann, Linda) and the understanding and patience of our children (Tracy, Elizabeth, Ben, Elizabeth, Anne), this book could not have been completed.

Contents

10 INFLAMMATORY, PROLIFERATIVE, AND METAPLASTIC LESIONS OF THE BLADDER 10.1

V NEOPLASMS OF THE URINARY TRACT

11 NEOPLASMS OF THE KIDNEY, RENAL PELVIS, AND URETER 11.1

12 BLADDER NEOPLASMS 12.1

VI LESIONS OF THE PROSTATE AND SEMINAL VESICLES

13 NONNEOPLASTIC LESIONS OF THE PROSTATE AND SEMINAL VESICLES 13.1

14 NEOPLASTIC LESIONS OF THE PROSTATE AND SEMINAL VESICLES 14.1

VII LESIONS OF THE TESTIS AND ASSOCIATED STRUCTURES

15 NONNEOPLASTIC LESIONS OF THE TESTIS 15.1

16 TESTICULAR NEOPLASMS 16.1

17 LESIONS OF THE TUNICA VAGINALIS, EPIDIDYMIS, VAS DEFERENS, AND SPERMATIC CORD 17.1

VIII LESIONS OF THE PENIS, SCROTUM, AND URETHRA

18 NONNEOPLASTIC LESIONS OF THE PENIS, SCROTUM, AND URETHRA 18.1

19 NEOPLASTIC LESIONS OF THE PENIS, SCROTUM, AND URETHRA

IX LESIONS OF THE ADRENAL GLAND

20 ADRENAL GLAND TUMORS

REFERENCES AND FURTHER READINGS

INDEX

SECTION 1

Cystic and Dysplastic Lesions of the Kidney

CHAPTER 1

Hereditary Cystic Diseases

ADULT POLYCYSTIC KIDNEY DISEASE

Adult polycystic kidney disease (APKD), one of the most common genetic disorders, is transmitted as a simple autosomal-dominant trait with high penetrance and variable expressivity. At the time of diagnosis, 90% of patients are at least 30 years old, although the age at onset varies, and rare cases of infantile presentation have been reported. Among affected individuals, renal failure progresses slowly after the onset of azotemia; renal mortality, generally occurring early in the sixth decade, is 100%. APKD is therefore a major cause of end-stage renal disease requiring dialysis, and accounts for approximately 5% of renal allograft recipients.

PATHOGENESIS APKD is classified as a Potter type III cystic disease. Theories of pathogenesis implicating abnormalities of development include: (l) failure of the ureteric bud branches to unite with the metanephric anlage, which then lacks an organizing influence and may form cysts; and (2) failure of involution as well as eventual cyst formation by the first generation of nephrons. It should be remembered, however, that initially such kidneys are histologically and functionally normal. Other theories have been proposed, including obstruction of nephrons secondary to papillary epithelial proliferation and/or structural defects in tubular basement membranes (TBMs).

CLINICAL MANIFESTATIONS Initial symptoms usually occur between 30 and 50 years of age. Pain in the back, loin, or groin is the most common presenting complaint. Severe pain may reflect peritoneal irritation secondary to cyst rupture. Intense constant pain may signal acute swelling due to intracystic hemorrhage or pyogenic infection, while colicky pain may be due to an obstructing stone or blood clot. Hematuria, which can be microscopic or macroscopic, occurs in approximately 50% of affected individuals. It is frequently a consequence of a ruptured cyst or stone. Flank masses, representing a bilaterally enlarged kidney, are present in about 60% of patients, although only one kidney may be palpable at presentation in up to one third of patients. Hypertension, which appears in 50%–70% of affected individuals, is typically mild and easily controlled by antihypertensive medications.

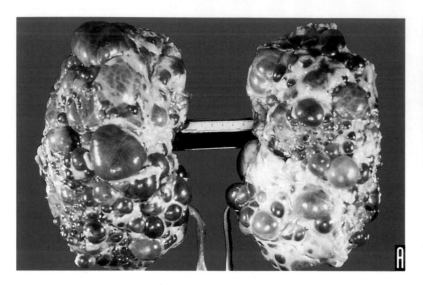
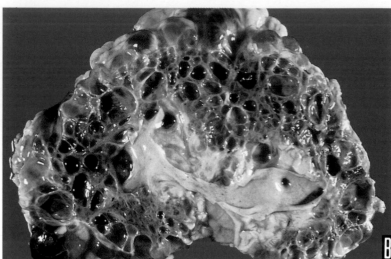

Figure 1.1 A, Bilateral renal enlargement (*right:* 1670 g; *left:* 1520 g) is fairly symmetrical in this case of APKD. A reniform configuration is retained, although the cortical surface is bosselated due to multiple protruding cysts. Cysts have a semilucent capsule and many contain clear, yellow fluid. Those that appear bluish or opaque dark brown have intracystic hemorrhage. Proximity of the cysts to the ureter near the ureteropelvic junction provides a potential mechanism for urinary tract obstruction. **B,** Cut surface of the kidney demonstrates diffuse replacement of cortical and medullary parenchyma by innumerable spherical or round cysts. The pelvicalyceal system, although distorted, is normally formed.

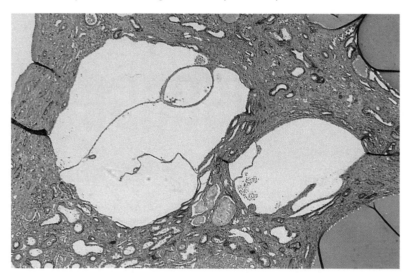
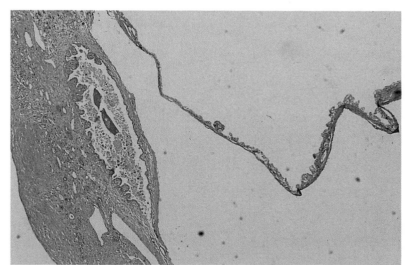

Figure 1.2 Cystic transformation in APKD involves collecting ducts and all parts of the nephron, as well as Bowman's space. Intervening renal parenchyma, which is normally formed, contains dilated convoluted tubules (PAS stain).

Figure 1.3 Cysts in APKD are lined by cuboidal-to-flattened cells. Epithelial proliferation with intracystic polypoid projections formed on fibrovascular stalks is commonly noted (PAS stain).

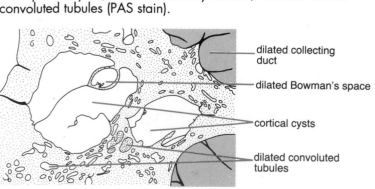

- dilated collecting duct
- dilated Bowman's space
- cortical cysts
- dilated convoluted tubules

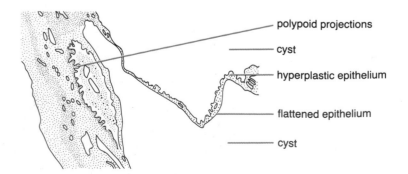

- polypoid projections
- cyst
- hyperplastic epithelium
- flattened epithelium
- cyst

1.2   Cystic and Dysplastic Lesions of the Kidney

MORPHOLOGY In the fully developed disease, the kidneys are bilaterally enlarged but retain a reniform configuration. They may measure over 30 cm in length and weigh 3000–4000 g each. Their contour is markedly distorted, with multiple protruding cysts on the cortical surface producing bosselation (Fig. 1.1A). Ranging from a few millimeters to several centimeters in diameter, the spherical or round cysts are present throughout the cortex and medulla. Their contents, which may be clear yellow, turbid white, opaque dark brown, or gelatinous (secondary to old hemorrhage), are often visible through a semilucent capsule (Fig. 1.1). Calcifications or yellow cholesterol crystals may be evident in the cyst walls.

Microscopically, any part of the nephron, including Bowman's space, may be involved, but cysts characteristically reside in collect- ing tubules (Fig. 1.2). The cysts are lined by a layer of cuboidal-to-flattened cells. Epithelial proliferation may produce polypoid projections into the cysts (Fig. 1.3). Hyperplastic smooth muscle may be seen surrounding larger cysts (Fig. 1.4). The intervening parenchyma shows the changes of evolving end-stage renal disease—i.e., fibrosis, chronic inflammation, tubular atrophy, and vascular sclerosis. With advanced cyst formation, the parenchyma becomes compressed and fibrotic. Foci of intracystic or parenchymal hemorrhage, as well as calcification, are common (Fig. 1.5).

ASSOCIATED ANOMALIES AND COMPLICATIONS Liver cysts occur in about 30% of patients with APKD. Nearly 45% of all hepatic cysts occur in APKD patients. These cysts, which arise from bile ducts (Fig. 1.6), are generally asymptomatic and incidental

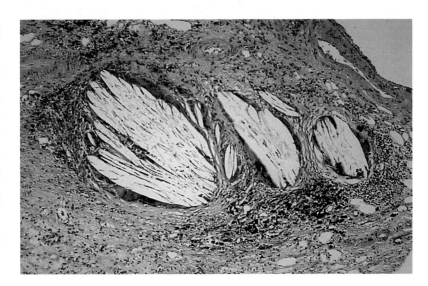

Figure 1.4 Masson's trichrome stain reveals the hyperplastic smooth muscle that may occasionally be identified around larger cysts in APKD.

Figure 1.5 Interstitial hemosiderin and foreign body giant cell reaction surrounding cholesterol clefts with chronic inflammation are seen in areas of organizing parenchymal hemorrhage secondary to cyst rupture.

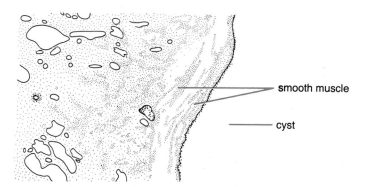

- smooth muscle
- cyst

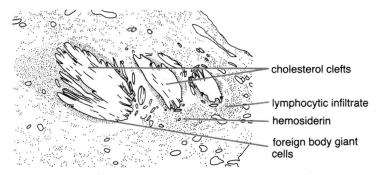

- cholesterol clefts
- lymphocytic infiltrate
- hemosiderin
- foreign body giant cells

Figure 1.6 Microscopically, hepatic cysts in APKD arise from dilated bile ducts. Ductal proliferation and mild portal fibrosis may be present.

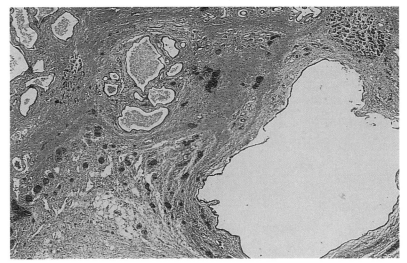

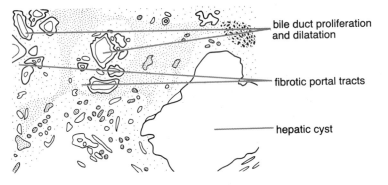

- bile duct proliferation and dilatation
- fibrotic portal tracts
- hepatic cyst

findings at autopsy, but occasionally hepatic involvement is impressive (Fig. 1.7).

Cysts in the spleen (5% of APKD patients), pancreas (10%), thyroid, lungs (5%), testicles, epididymis, and ovary have been reported. In addition, approximately 15% of patients have cerebral berry aneurysms. Subarachnoid hemorrhage is a frequent cause of death. Pyelonephritis develops at some point in one third of patients. Other complications include urolithiasis or nephrocalcinosis and malignant change, particularly renal cell carcinoma (RCC).

INFANTILE POLYCYSTIC KIDNEY DISEASE— CONGENITAL HEPATIC FIBROSIS

The hepatorenal lesions encountered in this complex, which are inherited as an autosomal-recessive trait, are seen predominantly in infancy and childhood. The clinicopathologic spectrum ranges from infants with massive polycystic kidneys and clinically silent hepatic lesions to children with marked hepatic fibrosis and portal hypertension with asymptomatic renal cysts. Classic (early) infan-

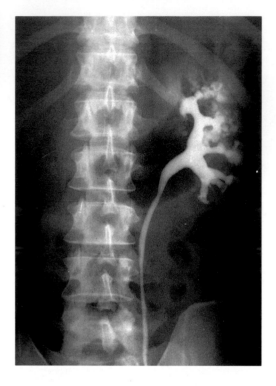

Figure 1.8 IVP in a case of CHF shows medullary tubular ectasia with accumulation of contrast medium in dilated collecting ducts. (Courtesy of H. Hawkins, MD, Cincinnati, Ohio)

Figure 1.7 Hepatic enlargement was clinically evident in this patient with APKD. The liver shows marked cystic change.

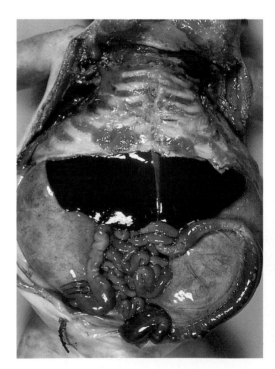

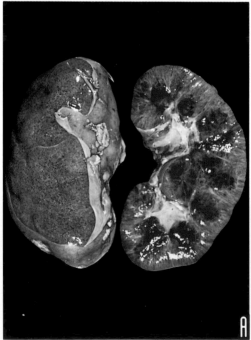

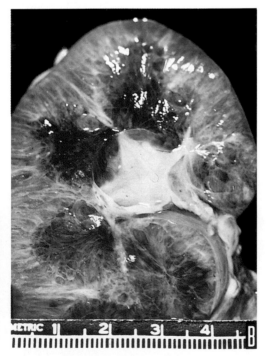

Figure 1.9 In early IPKD, massively and symmetrically enlarged kidneys have caused a protuberant abdomen with displacement of viscera.

Figure 1.10 A, In IPKD the kidneys retain a reniform configuration and have a smooth capsular surface. The pelvicalyceal system is normally formed. **B,** Closer inspection reveals replacement of parenchyma by radially oriented cysts.

tile polycystic kidney disease (IPKD) results in renal failure and is usually fatal shortly after birth. Cases discovered beyond the newborn period constitute an intermediate group that combines clinicopathologic features of both IPKD and congenital hepatic fibrosis (CHF). It would appear then that IPKD-CHF is a spectrum of age-related abnormalities and constitutes a single disease process, although the issue of genetic heterogeneity remains unresolved.

PATHOGENESIS Renal cysts in IPKD, which are thought to be secondary to dilatation and hyperplasia of interstitial portions of collecting ducts, are classified as Potter type I lesions. Hepatic cysts involve the ducts of Hering as well as the adjacent interlobular ducts and, like renal lesions, affect the level of the duct system into which the functioning parenchymal units, i.e., canaliculi, enter. The renal and hepatic lesions may be secondary to an inherited metabolic abnormality that affects epithelial protein or involves the supporting structures.

CLINICAL MANIFESTATIONS Cases of early IPKD typically present with abdominal distention secondary to massive symmetric enlargement of the kidneys with oligohydramnios, Potter's facies, respiratory distress, and anuria or oliguria. Death usually occurs in the first weeks or months, although some patients have been kept alive into puberty. Renal failure is an inconstant finding, and renal enlargement is less apparent in late IPKD. Clinical findings related

to portal hypertension become more prominent secondary to portal fibrosis. Thus, the clinicopathologic findings in IPKD merge with those in CHF.

Medullary ductal ectasia occurring with CHF may be asymptomatic. CHF generally presents after two years of age with symptoms of portal hypertension, ascites, splenomegaly, and evidence of abnormal venous collateral circulation, particularly esophageal varices.

The prominent renal medullary ectasia seen in children and young adults with "mild" IPKD and CHF can be demonstrated radiographically and must be differentiated from medullary sponge kidney (see Chapter 2). IVP in such cases shows cystic dilatation of collecting tubules, which have been described as "bare branches of a leafless bush" (Fig. 1.8).

MORPHOLOGY The kidneys in early IPKD are bilaterally and symmetrically enlarged, weighing up to 10 times more than normal (Fig. 1.9). A reniform shape is preserved and the capsular surface is smooth (Fig. 1.10). The parenchyma appears to be replaced by 1–8 mm cysts, which are radially oriented (i.e., perpendicular to the capsule), particularly in the cortex along medullary rays, and obscure the corticomedullary junctions (Fig. 1.11). In the cortex, the cysts are cylindrical or fusiform, while in the medulla they are spherical (Fig. 1.12).

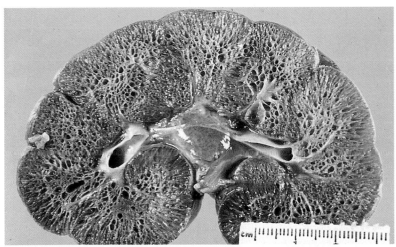

Figure 1.11 In this fixed specimen from a patient with IPKD, diffuse parenchymal involvement is more obvious, and the corticomedullary junctions are obscured.

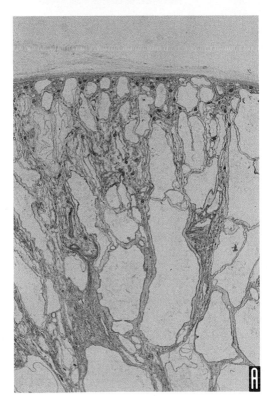
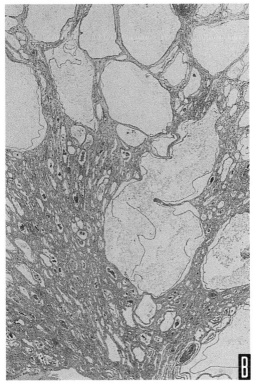
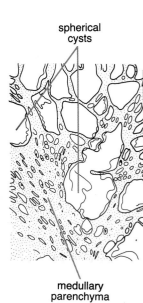

Figure 1.12 **A,** Within the cortex of the infantile polycystic kidney, cylindrical cysts are perpendicular to the capsular surface. Note the scant intervening parenchyma (PAS stain). **B,** Medullary cysts appear spherical (PAS stain). (**B:** Courtesy of E. Ballard, MD, Cincinnati, Ohio)

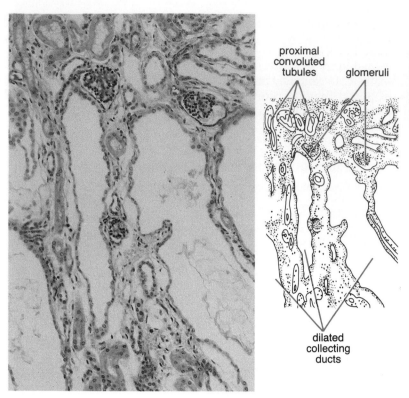

Figure 1.13 In early IPKD, cortical cysts representing dilated collecting ducts are lined by cuboidal epithelium. Immature glomeruli and normally formed convoluted tubules are present (PAS stain).

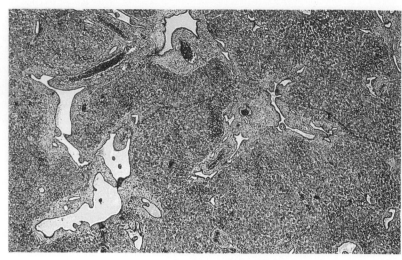

Figure 1.14 Microscopically, the liver in early IPKD has fibrotic, widened portal tracts that contain dilated bile ducts with proliferations of angulated and branched bile ductules.

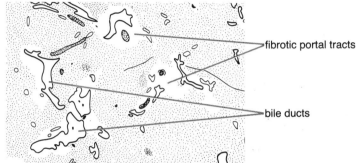

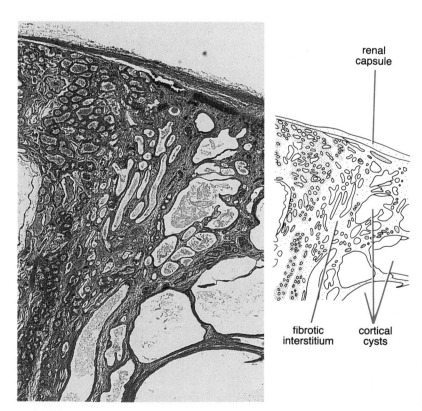

Figure 1.15 In this case of late IPKD, cortical cysts, separated by fibrous tissue, are less numerous than those seen in early IPKD, and become more rounded or irregular in shape with loss of radial orientation (Masson's trichrome stain).

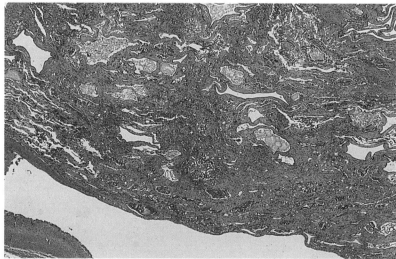

Figure 1.16 Diffuse ectasia of renal medullary collecting ducts is the most prominent feature in CHF and explains the radiographic findings seen in Figure 1.8.

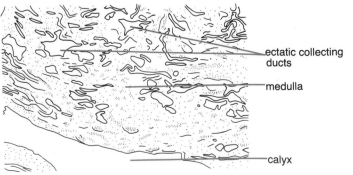

Microscopically, nephrons are generally normal. Collecting tubules are cystic and lined by cuboidal-to-columnar epithelium, which may be hyperplastic (Fig. 1.13). The interstitial connective tissue may be increased. Occasionally, nodules of immature-appearing stroma reminiscent of dysplasia are seen.

Hepatic lesions in early IPKD, although invariably asymptomatic, are always present. Portal areas are fibrotic and widened. Interlobular ducts are dilated, with bizarre proliferations of angulated or dilated ductules of Hering (Myenburg complexes) (Fig. 1.14). Gross cysts are rare.

In the later, or milder, forms of IPKD, the number of renal cysts appears to diminish with age. The kidneys are not as large as in early IPKD, and radial orientation of the cysts is lost. In addition, cortical involvement is less obvious; the cysts, ranging from 2 mm to 2 cm in diameter, bulge from the cortical surface and are rounder, with no particular orientation (Fig. 1.15). Medullary cysts are more prominent. Microscopically, they are lined by cuboidal-to-columnar epithelium, separated by fibrous tissue or renal parenchyma. Hepatic portal fibrosis in children with later IPKD is increased and approaches the hepatic lesions in CHF associated with portal hypertension.

In CHF, renal cortical cysts are inconspicuous, and the kidneys show predominantly medullary tubular ectasia (Fig. 1.16). Corticomedullary cysts are characterized by fusiform enlargement of collecting ducts or clusters of small cysts. The liver shows moderate-to-marked portal fibrosis without inflammatory infiltrate, as well as bridging between portal tracts. Bile duct proliferation in CHF is less prominent than in IPKD. Hepatic lobules are intact and there is no bile stasis (Fig. 1.17).

MEDULLARY CYSTIC DISEASE— FAMILIAL JUVENILE NEPHRONOPHTHISIS COMPLEX

Medullary cystic disease (MCD) and familial juvenile nephronophthisis (FJN) are progressive forms of renal disease that share clinicopathologic features. Clinical variants include hereditary and sporadic forms. Hereditary MCD, which is an autosomal-dominant trait, comprises approximately 15%–20% of cases and typically presents in young adults (mean age, 30 years). About 15% of reported cases are nonfamilial. These sporadic cases are thought to represent an acquired defect. FJN, the autosomal-recessive form of the disease, is more common, accounting for two thirds of cases. Onset occurs in childhood and adolescence (mean age, 12 years). It has a more consistent familial distribution and is frequently associated with parental consanguinity. FJN is one of the most common causes of renal failure in adolescents. An autosomal-recessive variant associated with retinal disease, and termed the renal–retinal syndrome, is included in the MCD–FJN complex.

PATHOGENESIS The renal parenchymal alterations observed in the MCD–FJN complex are not developmental in origin. In addition, although medullary cysts are characteristically observed, they may be totally absent in 25% of cases, particularly in FJN. It is postulated that the basic lesion is a tubulointerstitial nephropathy related to a heritable, nephrotoxic metabolic abnormality. Cysts are not necessary for development of the clinical state or for progression of disease. Microdissection studies suggest that the "cysts" are actually dilatations or diverticula originating from distal tubules and collecting ducts.

CLINICAL MANIFESTATIONS Patients usually present with an insidious, refractory anemia and azotemia. A salt-wasting nephropathy may be prominent. Patients are typically normotensive, although terminal hypertension may develop. The urine sediment is generally normal. Inability to concentrate urine suggests a distal tubular lesion. Inconstant features include glycosuria, aminoaciduria, and impaired acidification. The cystic kidneys have an increased susceptibility to infection.

MORPHOLOGY Grossly, the kidneys in MCD–FJN complex tend to be contracted and granular, with spherical medullary cysts ranging from pinpoint size to 1 cm in diameter throughout the corticomedullary regions. The configuration and organization of the renal parenchyma and pelvicalyceal system are preserved. Minute cortical cysts may be present (Fig. 1.18). The distribution of clustered cysts at the corticomedullary junction is sufficiently characteristic to

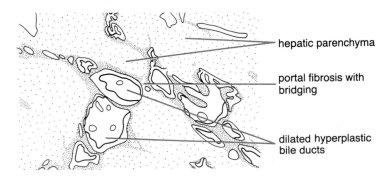

Figure 1.17 The liver in CHF shows ductal dilatation with bridging fibrosis. Bile duct proliferation is less prominent. There is no bile stasis or portal inflammation, and lobules are intact (Masson's trichrome stain).

hepatic parenchyma

portal fibrosis with bridging

dilated hyperplastic bile ducts

permit differentiation from other diseases with medullary cysts, particularly late IPKD–CHF and medullary sponge kidney.

Microscopically, the cysts are lined by a flattened or cuboidal epithelium and surrounded by collagen. Cortical tubulointerstitial changes with tubular damage out of proportion to glomerular alterations are in keeping with the basic disease process, which is a tubulointerstitial nephritis (Fig. 1.19A). The most striking change is marked TBM thickening, particularly involving distal convoluted tubules (Fig. 1.19B). TBMs frequently appear split or reduplicated in association with fibroblastic proliferation and collagen deposition. Interstitial and periglomerular fibrosis is present along with a variable, but often scant, nonspecific lymphohistiocytic infiltrate. With advanced disease, glomerular ischemia and obsolescence occur.

MISCELLANEOUS HEREDITARY CYSTIC DISORDERS
TUBEROUS SCLEROSIS

Renal parenchymal involvement in the tuberous sclerosis complex occurs as angiomyolipomas in 40%–50% of cases. Less commonly, renal cysts may be the first clue to the correct diagnosis. The cysts compress adjacent parenchyma and, when multiple, may cause moderate functional impairment. Their histologic appearance is characterized by a hyperplastic lining composed of granular eosinophilic cells resembling proximal convoluted tubular epithelium (Fig. 1.20).

LINDAU'S DISEASE

Lindau's complex is a familial systemic angiomatous disorder, which in some cases appears to be inherited as an autosomal-dominant trait with 80%–90% penetrance. Clinical onset occurs in early-to-middle adulthood. It has been postulated that Lindau's complex represents a hereditary, persistent abnormality that leads to lack of integration between blood vessels and their field supply, resulting in fetal cysts and adult neoplasms. It is characterized by central nervous system angiomatosis (e.g., cerebellar hemangioblastoma) and visceral cystic lesions. In 20% of cases, retinal angiomas (von Hippel's disease) occur. Pancreatic cysts are present in approximately one half of cases, whereas renal cysts are found in approximately two thirds. The renal cysts have a causal relationship to the development of renal neoplasms, which generally behave as adenomas, although RCC with metastases has been reported.

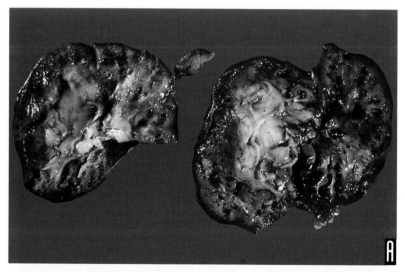

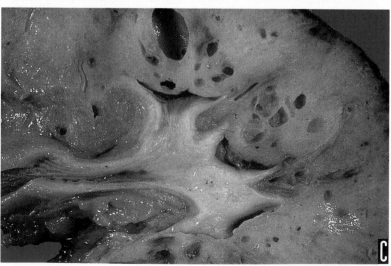

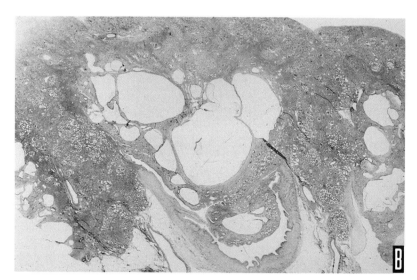

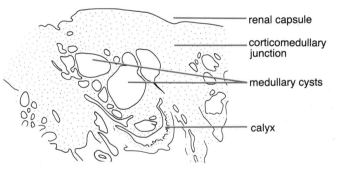

renal capsule
corticomedullary junction
medullary cysts
calyx

Figure 1.18 A, In this 14-year-old patient with MCD, many corticomedullary regions contain cysts. The kidneys are bilaterally contracted, and the cortices are irregularly thinned. **B,** Whole mount section of the same kidney reveals the characteristic clustering of cysts at the corticomedullary junction in MCD. **C,** Close inspection of the kidney from a 15-year-old MCD patient shows 1–6 mm spherical medullary cysts and a few 1–2 mm cortical cysts. The pyramids are not deformed, and the pelvicalyceal system is normally configured. (**C:** Courtesy of E. Ballard, MD, Cincinnati, Ohio)

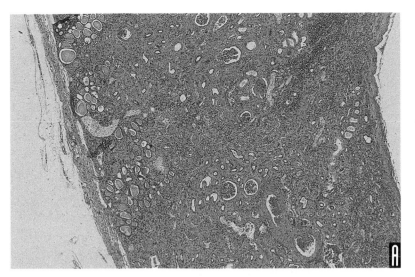

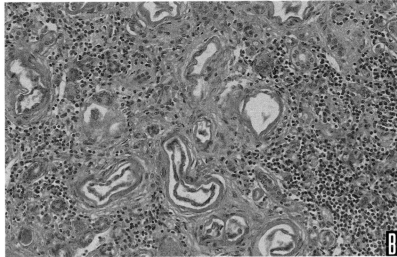

Figure 1.19 A, In the MCD–FJN complex, the cortex overlying a cyst shows marked tubulointerstitial changes with interstitial fibrosis and patchy chronic inflammation. Atrophic tubules and dilated convoluted tubules are present. The presence of scattered preserved glomeruli is in keeping with a chronic interstitial nephritis. **B,** A characteristic,

striking change in the cortex is marked thickening of TBMs, which may also appear reduplicated. This finding in a renal biopsy may provide a clue to the diagnosis. An associated chronic inflammatory infiltrate is consistent with an interstitial nephritis.

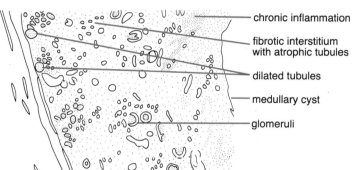

chronic inflammation

fibrotic interstitium with atrophic tubules

dilated tubules

medullary cyst

glomeruli

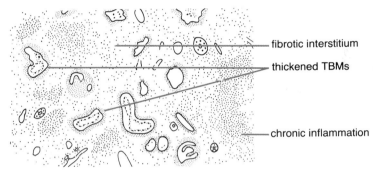

fibrotic interstitium

thickened TBMs

chronic inflammation

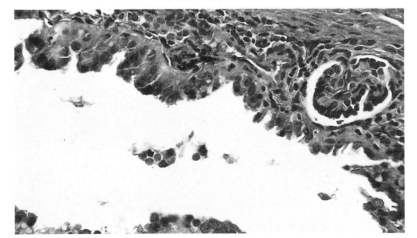

Figure 1.20 In tuberous sclerosis, cysts are lined by a hyperplastic epithelium composed of cuboidal cells that form papillary and polypoid projections. The epithelium's distinctive, markedly granular, eosionophilic cytoplasm may provide a valuable diagnostic aid. (Courtesy of J. Bernstein, MD, Royal Oak, Michigan)

CHAPTER 2

Developmental Cystic Diseases

RENAL DYSPLASIA

Renal dysplasia is defined as disturbed differentiation of nephrogenic tissue with persistence of structures inappropriate to gestational age. Most congenitally small kidneys are dysplastic. Abnormal metanephric development during organogenesis may cause cysts to form, thus dysplastic kidneys are often cystic. Indeed, most cystic kidneys in childhood are also dysplastic. Unilateral dysplasia is the most common cystic disorder in the newborn and young individuals and the most frequently encountered abnormal abdominal mass palpable in the newborn.

The majority of renal dysplasias are sporadic (nonheritable) malformations resulting from urinary tract obstruction, and in 90% of cases they are associated with other anomalies of the urinary tract. A small minority of cases are familial (hereditary) or may be associated with syndromes of multiple congenital malformations.

PATHOGENESIS Microdissection studies have suggested that dysplasia results from: (1) inhibition of ureteral ampullary activity with cessation of branching, and/or (2) expression of some limited, inherent histogenic potency by metanephrogenic tissue not subjected to the organizing influence of the ureteric system. It is classified as a Potter type II cystic disease.

CLINICAL MANIFESTATIONS The degree of dysplasia, and therefore the clinical manifestations, are generally related to the nature and severity of the associated obstruction. A spectrum of clinical forms and pathologic patterns may be encountered. Unilateral ureteral obstruction, for example, results in ipsilateral dysplasia, while lower urinary tract obstruction gives rise to bilateral renal dysplasia. The dysplasia may be total or partial, focal or segmental, and cortical and/or medullary; the kidneys may be of any size or shape, externally normal or misshapen, functioning or nonfunctioning.

PATHOLOGIC CRITERIA   As renal dysplasia may grossly resemble the hypoplastic kidney and various forms of renal cystic disease, criteria for diagnosis are histologic. Microscopically, dysplasia is recognized by the presence of disorganized epithelial structures with a fetal, undifferentiated, or primitive appearance, surrounded by abundant fibrous tissue with islands of cartilage (Fig. 2.1). Nests of metaplastic cartilage, derived from metanephric blastema, are principally cortical. Primitive ducts, frequently present in the medulla and representing altered metanephric ducts, are lined by relatively tall, columnar, often ciliated epithelium and surrounded by fibromuscular collars (Fig. 2.2). Findings that are usually present but not diagnostic include primitive glomeruli, tubules, and ductules, which may represent retrogressive transformation of previously normal nephrons secondary to injury. Primitive glomeruli have capillary tufts covered by cuboidal epithelium; they are often hypoplastic and undergo hyalinization and sclerosis. Primitive tubules are lined by crowded columnar

epithelium; primitive ductules are surrounded by narrow collars of lamellated connective tissue. Glomerular, tubular, or ductular cysts may or may not be present.

CLINICOPATHOLOGIC FORMS

MULTICYSTIC AND APLASTIC DYSPLASIAS   Aplastic dysplasia refers to severe hypoplasia with microscopic features of dysplasia. In both the multicystic and aplastic forms, the kidney is nonfunctional.

BILATERAL TOTAL RENAL DYSPLASIA   This form of dysplasia presents a clinical picture similar to bilateral renal agenesis. Infants are usually stillborn, although some may survive a few days postpartum. Maternal oligohydramnios is present in three fourths of cases. Nodules of squamous epithelium (amnion nodosum) stud the placenta's amniotic surface. Potter's facies (see Chapter 4), characterized by wide-set eyes, receding chin, low-set ears, and deficient auricular cartilage, is apparent. Derivatives of the urogenital sinus (rectum, bladder, urethra) are often severely malformed. Other associated anomalies include esophageal atresia, interventricular septal defect, and pulmonary hypoplasia. Renal calyces and pelves are typically absent, and the ureters are absent or atretic. The medulla may contain primitive ducts radiating from a central area, while the peripheral metanephric cap may contain only cartilage.

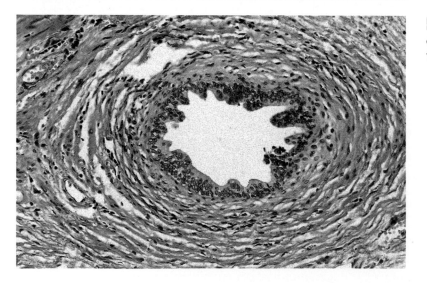

Figure 2.1 Renal dysplasia is histologically characterized by the presence of primitive epithelial structures and islands of cartilage. Renal parenchyma is frequently fibrotic.

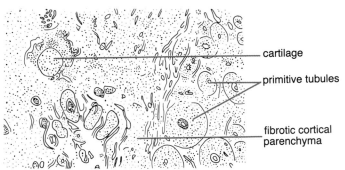

cartilage

primitive tubules

fibrotic cortical parenchyma

Figure 2.2 In renal dysplasia, primitive collecting ducts are lined by columnar epithelium and surrounded by a mantle of fibromuscular tissue.

UNILATERAL TOTAL RENAL DYSPLASIA The amount of metanephric tissue appears to correlate with the stage of altered differentiation in this dysplasia. The early stage produces little parenchyma, while in the late stage parenchyma is abundant. The aplastic variant may be clinically silent or associated with recurrent infections or hypertension. The contralateral, hypertrophied kidney seems to be susceptible to hydronephrosis, pyelonephritis, and lithiasis. Ureteral atresia is often present, sometimes limited to the upper one third. Alternately, the ureter may be patent or may be a megaureter.

The multicystic dysplastic kidney (Fig. 2.3), which predominates in males, is rarely associated with hypertension. Ureteral atresia and pelvic occlusion are invariably present. There is loss of the reniform configuration, with the kidney resembling a "bunch of grapes."

Histologically, corticomedullary dysplasia is characterized by severe disorganization of normal architecture. Large and small cysts and tubules are cuffed by primitive mesenchymal tissue, with intervening areas showing expanses of vascular-collagenous stroma and islands of cartilage. Glomeruli, with or without convoluted tubules, are widely scattered. An essentially complete lobule may be present with a recognizable metanephric cap overlying a medulla that contains unexpanded ducts.

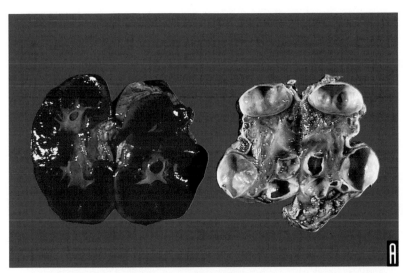

Figure 2.3 A, The multicystic dysplastic kidney loses its reniform configuration and resembles a bunch of grapes. Although frequently palpable, the dysplastic kidney (right) may not be enlarged in comparison with the normal infant kidney. Note the absence of a pelvicalyceal system. **B,** Severe architectural disorganization can be seen. Scattered primitive ducts surrounded by fibromuscular collars are present within the fibrotic medulla (PAS stain). **C,** Despite marked corticomedullary dysplasia, a lobular architecture can be recognized. Note the cystic metanephric cap overlying the medulla, which contains partially expanded ducts (PAS stain).

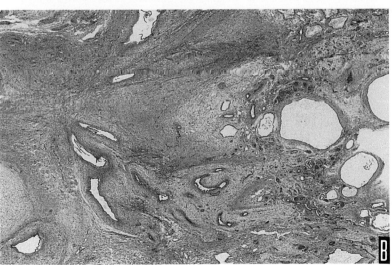

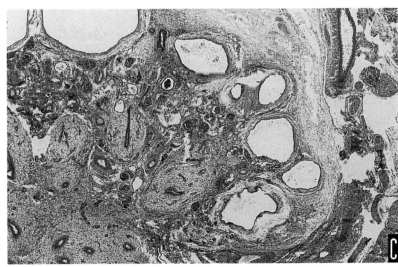

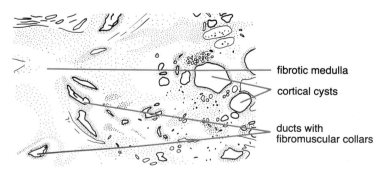

fibrotic medulla

cortical cysts

ducts with fibromuscular collars

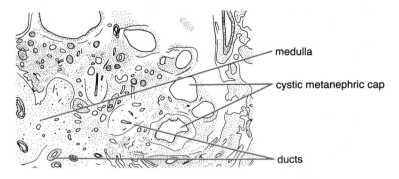

medulla

cystic metanephric cap

ducts

GENERAL AND SEGMENTAL DYSPLASIAS Encompassing degrees of malformation less severe than those in aplastic dysplasia, general and segmental dysplasias retain some semblance of normal renal architecture (Fig. 2.4). A variable degree of renal function is also preserved. The symptoms associated with unilateral forms of general dysplasia include pain due to infection (two thirds of cases) and lithiasis (one third), with associated hypertension in 20%–25% of affected individuals. Bilateral forms of general dysplasia, which are observed in infants with multiple congenital malformations, may grossly resemble IPKD but can be distinguished from IPKD microscopically, as well as by differing associated malformations, including alimentary and cardiac (especially coarctation) anomalies. Combined corticomedullary dysplasia is less severe in general renal dysplasia than in aplastic dysplasia. Cysts are frequently subcapsular and located along interlobular fissures. The kidney is hypoplastic, containing fewer lobes than normal. Segmental dysplasia may be associated with obstruction of the pelvic infundibulum.

FOCAL RENAL DYSPLASIA A very rare variant, it is characterized by single or multiple microscopic dysplastic foci. It is usually found in truly hypoplastic kidneys.

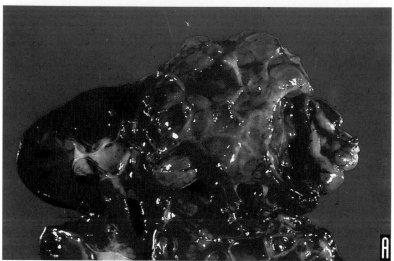

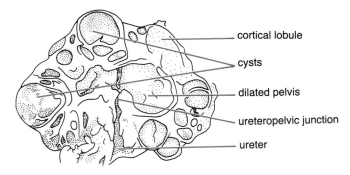

Figure 2.4 A, Segmental multicystic dysplasia in this kidney is not associated with lower urinary tract obstruction or pelviureteral duplication; it may be due to infundibular obstruction. The opposite pole and pelvicalyceal system are normally formed. B, This kidney from a seven-year-old male with clinical and pathologic evidence of chronic pyelonephritis shows general dysplasia. There are multiple 5 mm to 2 cm cysts with only a few solid cortical lobules. The pelvicalyceal cavity is dilated and has probe patency with the ureter. The calyceal mucosa appears fibrotic and does not communicate with the cysts. (B: Courtesy of E. Ballard, MD, Cincinnati, Ohio)

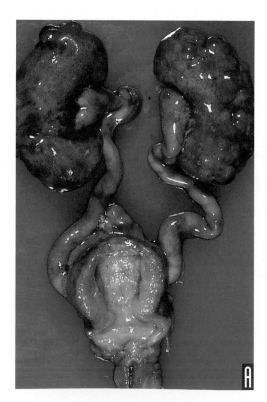

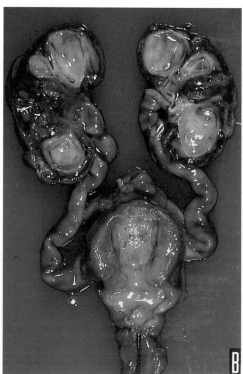

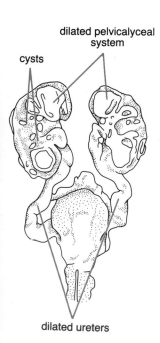

Figure 2.5 Specimen from a newborn male of 37 weeks' gestation who had obstructive posterior urethral valves with bilateral hydroureters. A, Both kidneys have a reniform shape with fetal lobulations. Numerous cortical cysts can be seen. B, Bilateral hydronephrosis is present with multiple parenchymal cysts and obscured corticomedullary demarcations.

DYSPLASIA ASSOCIATED WITH LOWER URINARY TRACT OBSTRUCTION
A consequence of the effects of hydroureter and hydronephrosis, this form of dysplasia is most common in infant boys with obstructive posterior urethral valves; it results in a bilateral multicystic dysplasia, classified as Potter type IV (Fig. 2.5). The renal pelvis is generally formed and dilated. Two patterns are seen: (1) cystic dysplasia of the peripheral cortex, and (2) medullary dysplasia in the form of a deltalike medulla. If urethral obstruction occurs later in development, cortical dysplasia is the sole result. With less severe obstruction, renal manifestations appear later in childhood as hydronephrosis without dysplasia. Segmental dysplasia typically occurs in the upper pole of the kidney in association with pelviureteral duplication and ectopic ureterocele (Fig. 2.6). Severe corticomedullary dysplasia is frequently present (Fig. 2.7).

FAMILIAL AND HEREDITARY DYSPLASIAS These rare dysplasias are most frequently encountered in syndromes of multiple malformations, e.g., Meckel's, Jeune's, and Zellweger's syndromes. Approximately 20% of patients with Meckel's syndrome have hepatic abnormalities, including ductular dysgenesis, intrahepatic cysts, and portal fibrosis. In Jeune's asphyxiating thoracic dystrophy (osteochondrodysplasia), hepatic alterations resemble those of IPKD, and include portal fibrosis with an excess of proliferating, tortuous, often dilated bile ducts. Classification may be further complicated because a spectrum of renal abnormalities may be encountered, including diffuse (poly)cystic disease, multiple peripheral cortical microcysts, and bilateral cystic dysplasia. Morphologic differences may reflect genetic heterogeneity or injury to the kidney at different times in renal development. This spectrum of renal abnormalities is best considered with the syndromes of multiple malformations. When dysplastic renal elements are identified, the possibility of heredofamilial dysplasia should be recognized.

MEDULLARY SPONGE KIDNEY

Although of unknown etiology, medullary sponge kidney (MSK) is included here because it is considered a congenital, nonhereditary developmental anomaly, the vast majority of cases being sporadic. However, MSK is associated with congenital hemihypertrophy and other hereditary diseases, and is familial in rare instances, which suggests that hereditary factors play a role. MSK should be distinguished from other conditions, loosely termed "sponge kidney," in which medullary cysts are found. These conditions, which have been detailed in Chapter 1, include IPKD, CHF with renal tubular ectasia, and the MCD complex.

PATHOGENESIS The pathogenesis of MSK has not been determined. Microdissection studies have demonstrated uniform or segmental enlargement of collecting ducts, which give rise to and are in communication with the medullary cysts. These fusiform or globular dilatations involve only the first two generations of branching of the collecting ducts. Attached nephrons are normal, unless secondary obstruction has occurred.

CLINICAL MANIFESTATIONS MSK, which may be an incidental finding on IVP or at autopsy, has a peak age incidence in

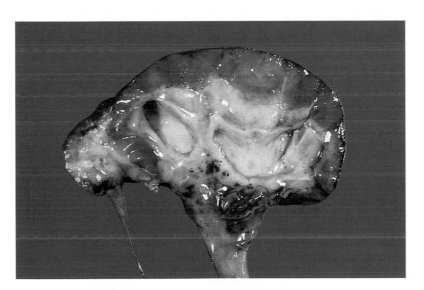

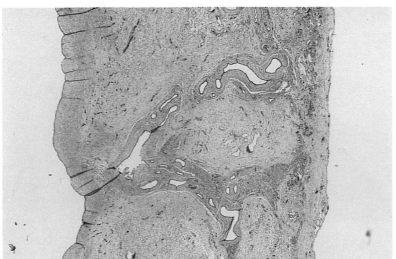

Figure 2.6 This double kidney has a hypoplastic dysplastic upper pole (left) and pelviureteral duplication, with a hypoplastic, ectopic upper-pole ureter and a ureterocele. The lower pole shows hydronephrosis, hydroureter, and chronic pyelonephritis.

Figure 2.7 In segmental dysplasia associated with lower urinary tract obstruction, renal parenchyma in the upper pole is thinned and fibrotic. Lobular architecture is lost secondary to severe combined corticomedullary dysplasia. The medulla has a deltalike appearance, with primitive ducts surrounded by primitive mesenchymal tissue. (Courtesy of E. Ballard, MD, Cincinnati, Ohio)

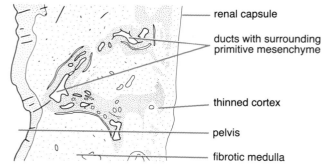

renal capsule
ducts with surrounding primitive mesenchyme
thinned cortex
pelvis
fibrotic medulla

the mid-to-late decades of life. In the absence of complications, it is not a progressive lesion. When symptomatic, patients typically present in their third decade. Although there is no sex predilection, women are more frequently symptomatic. Approximately 50% of patients present with symptoms related to recurrent urinary tract infection, renal colic secondary to passage of renal stones, or hematuria. Hypercalciuria has been reported in up to 50% of affected individuals.

In the majority of cases, MSK is diagnosed radiologically. The presence on IVP of a "pyramidal blush," which may represent the earliest stage of the disease, is suggestive but not specific. A diagnostic IVP demonstrates ductal ectasia with grapelike clusters of retained contrast medium within the medullary papillae (Fig. 2.8).

MORPHOLOGY Grossly, MSK is characterized by multiple, 1–2 mm cysts within the papillae; the cysts may be round, oval,

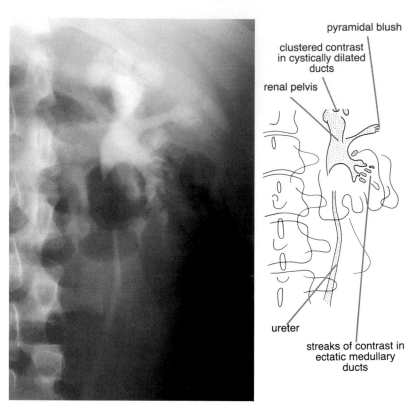

pyramidal blush

clustered contrast in cystically dilated ducts

renal pelvis

ureter

streaks of contrast in ectatic medullary ducts

Figure 2.8 IVP in a case of MSK shows a pyramidal blush and elongated streaks or rounded clusters of retained contrast medium in ectatic medullary ducts. (Courtesy of H. Hawkins, MD, Cincinnati, Ohio)

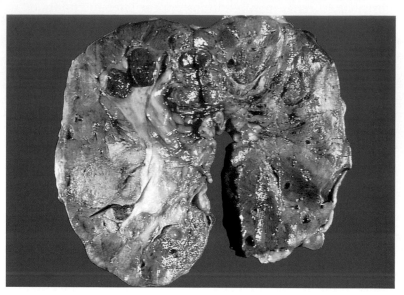

Figure 2.9 MSK in this asymptomatic elderly male was unilateral. The papillae contain single and multiple round cysts. The cortical cysts, which are not a component of MSK, are unrelated findings in this patient, representing acquired cysts.

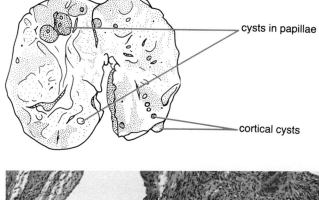

cysts in papillae

cortical cysts

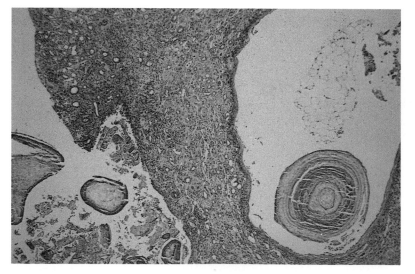

Figure 2.10 These cysts in a patient with MSK are located in the papillary tip and contain noncalcified concretions (stone matrix); they are also focally eroded.

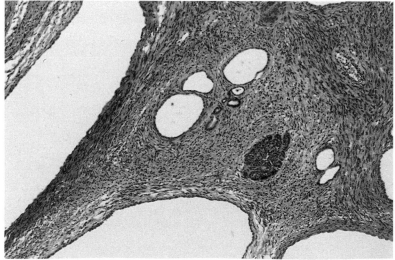

Figure 2.11 Although grossly and microscopically similar to the multilocular cyst, the cystic partially-differentiated Wilms' tumor contains primitive metanephric tissue and clusters of fetal-like tubules.

2.6 Cystic and Dysplastic Lesions of the Kidney

pyramidal, or irregular in shape. Although they may be unilateral and limited to a few papillae (Fig. 2.9), in the majority of cases both kidneys and most or all of the renal pyramids are involved. Macroscopic cortical cysts are usually absent. Calculi may be present in the calyces or pelves.

Microscopically, the cysts are lined by cuboidal, columnar, or transitional epithelium. Those containing calcific material (sand or concretions) may show squamous metaplasia and partial erosion (Fig. 2.10). Nonspecific chronic interstitial inflammation is common, and changes secondary to chronic pyelonephritis may lead to cortical scarring. Obstruction related to calculi or parenchymal concretions may also produce microscopic dilatation of cortical tubules and enlargement of Bowman's space.

Multilocular Cyst

The multilocular cyst is an uncommon, nonfamilial lesion. It is presented here not only because it should be included in the differential diagnosis of renal cysts but because it must be distinguished from true cystic and dysplastic diseases of the kidney.

PATHOGENESIS The pathogenesis of the multilocular cyst is unknown. The possibility that it represents a form of dysplasia or a cystic metanephric hamartoma of developmental origin has been suggested. However, in all likelihood it is a benign neoplasm related to the cystic partially differentiated Wilms' tumor (nephroblastoma) (see Chapter 11). The alternative terms, multilocular cystic nephroma or differentiated nephroblastoma, may be more appropriate to its origin.

CLINICAL MANIFESTATIONS Although the age at diagnosis ranges from newborn to 70 years, approximately 50% of multilocular cyst cases occur in young children; the disorder is rarely reported in adolescents or young adults. A multilocular cyst may present as an abdominal or renal mass on routine physical examination, or produce symptoms secondary to ureteropelvic obstruction.

MORPHOLOGY The criteria for diagnosis include the following gross and microscopic features: (1) unilateral renal involvement, (2) a solitary and multilocular cyst, (3) no communication with the renal pelvis or between locules, (4) an epithelial lining, and (5) absence of differentiated renal elements. Cysts with these features occasionally contain primitive metanephric tissue, a fact that further supports a relationship with Wilms' tumor (Fig. 2.11). The multilocular cyst is a benign lesion, however, and nephrectomy is curative.

Grossly, the multilocular cyst is a bulky, sharply circumscribed mass, ranging from 5–10 cm in diameter. As its size increases, it tends to protrude or herniate into the pelvis and ureter or into the perirenal fat. The dense pseudocapsule and the thin, delicate trabeculae separating the locules are gray-white and fibrous (Fig. 2.12). The locules range from several millimeters to 4 cm in diameter and contain clear, colorless, or bluish fluid. Calcification, hemorrhage, and necrosis are absent.

Microscopically, the locules are separated by variably cellular connective tissue, and frequently contain proteinaceous colloidlike material (Fig. 2.13A). The cysts are lined by cuboidal or flattened epithelium, which may have a "hobnail" appearance (Fig. 2.13B). The connective tissue may be focally hyalinized, but in many areas it is composed of proliferating plump spindle cells resembling fibroblasts. In addition, very cellular areas resemble primitive mesenchymal tissue. Scattered throughout the stroma are small tubules lined by clear, cuboidal cells (Fig. 2.13C). Although smooth muscle differentiation is not present, the external fibrous capsule may contain fascicles of smooth muscle and, rarely, dysontogenetic cartilage.

Pyelocalyceal Cyst

Although the pathogenesis of the pyelocalyceal cyst is uncertain, a developmental or embryologic origin seems likely. More common in adults aged 20–62 years, pyelocalyceal cyst has also been reported in neonates. It is generally regarded as a congenital calyceal diverticulum or the result of congenital stenosis of a minor calyx. Proponents of an acquired origin have suggested that calyceal achalasia results in chronic ineffectual emptying with progressive dilatation behind the sphincter.

CLINICAL MANIFESTATIONS Symptoms arise when recurrent pyelonephritis or calculi develop, and pain is a common complaint. Single or multiple small calculi are present in approximately 50% of cases.

A presumptive diagnosis can be made radiographically, if a saccular structure communicating with a calyx via a narrow channel is demonstrated by IVP or retrograde pyelography. Pyelocalyceal cyst should be distinguished from hydrocalyx, an acquired dilatation secondary to localized infundibular pathology, including calculi or inflammatory reactions.

MORPHOLOGY Grossly, the cyst varies from 1–5 cm in diameter, is spherical and smooth-walled (Fig. 2.14A). It lies adjacent to and communicates with a minor calyx via a narrow channel and may contain calculi, cloudy fluid, or pus.

Microscopically, the cyst is lined by a transitional epithelium and surrounded by smooth muscle (Fig. 2.14B). Variable degrees of chronic inflammation in the cyst wall as well as the adjacent renal parenchyma are common, and may be marked if pyelonephritis is superimposed.

Figure 2.12 The bulky multilocular cyst is sharply circumscribed by a dense pseudocapsule. The locules are separated by distinct fibrous trabeculae. The cystic mass protrudes from the cortical surface of the kidney and has herniated into but does not communicate with the renal pelvis.

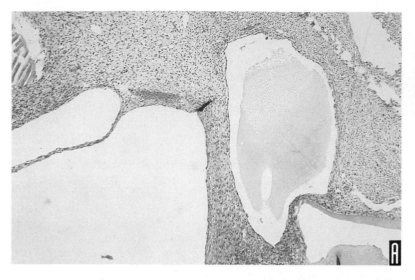

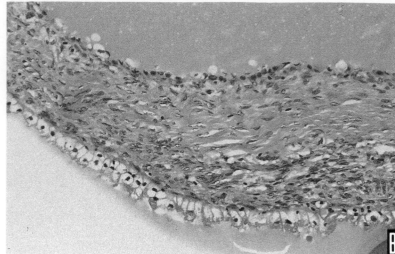

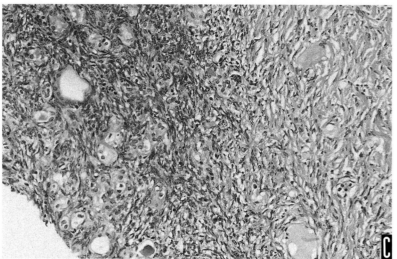

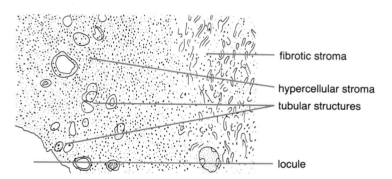

fibrotic stroma

hypercellular stroma

tubular structures

locule

Figure 2.13 A, Multilocular cyst. Locules separated by variably cellular connective tissue do not communicate with each other. Eosinophilic, colloidlike material is focally present within the locules. **B,** Although showing variability among locules, a cuboidal epithelium can frequently be identified. The fibrous trabecula is moderately cellular.

C, The connective tissue stroma is focally hypercellular, resembling primitive mesenchymal tissue. Small tubular structures lined by clear, cuboidal cells are present. Differentiated renal elements, however, are absent.

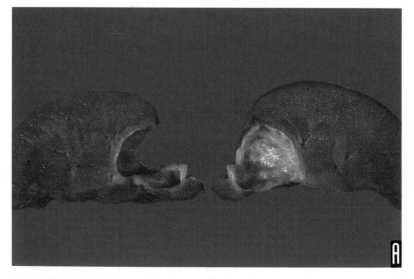

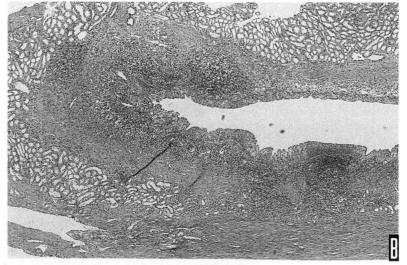

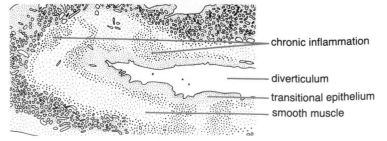

chronic inflammation

diverticulum

transitional epithelium

smooth muscle

Figure 2.14 A, Specimen of a pyelocalyceal cyst shows its relatively smooth, slightly opaque, and thickened wall. Located within the medulla, it is sharply demarcated from the parenchyma. Communication with the minor calyx is not evident. **B,** Transitional epithelium lines the same cyst. The wall is chronically inflamed and contains smooth muscle.

SECTION II

Anomalies of the Urinary Tract

CHAPTER 3

Acquired Cystic Diseases

SIMPLE CYSTS

Simple cysts develop in mature, previously normal kidneys. They may be cortical or medullary, single or multiple, ranging from a few millimeters to several centimeters in diameter (Figs. 3.1–3.3). When multiple, they are usually finite in number, irregularly distributed, and separated by zones of uninvolved renal parenchyma. Multiple renal cysts cannot always be clearly distinguished from evolving adult polycystic kidney disease (APKD) (see Chapter 1). In equivocal cases suggesting early manifestations of APKD, the absence of a family history and of hepatic cysts may indicate acquired multicystic kidney, although 25% of APKD patients also lack a positive family history.

PATHOGENESIS Of unknown pathogenesis, simple cysts are generally attributed to intrarenal obstruction secondary to acquired renal disease with or without ischemia. Minute cysts, commonly referred to as retention cysts, are frequently associated with chronic vascular disease, glomerulonephritis, or pyelonephritis.

CLINICAL MANIFESTATIONS Approximately one half of individuals over 50 years of age have one or more simple cysts. These acquired cysts are often incidental findings at nephrectomy or autopsy, or they may give rise to symptoms secondary to rupture, hemorrhage, infection, or ureteral obstruction. Occasionally, a large pedunculated cyst may undergo torsion. Large simple cysts may present as a renal mass and must be distinguished from renal neoplasms, particularly cystic renal cell carcinoma (RCC). Approximately one third of hemorrhagic cysts are RCCs. Carcinoma arising in a solitary simple cyst has a reported incidence of 2.9%, whereas coexistence of a benign cyst and RCC has been found in 2%–7% of all surgically explored renal cysts.

MORPHOLOGY Grossly, the cyst walls are yellow-white and semitransparent. Cysts typically contain clear, straw-colored fluid resembling a transudate (Fig. 3.4). If intracystic hemorrhage has occurred, the contents become rust-colored or puttylike. The inner surface of the cyst is smooth or trabeculated by partial septa.

Microscopically, the cysts are lined by a cuboidal or flattened epithelium (Fig. 3.5). Focal papillary folds may be present and are sometimes prominent enough to suggest a diagnosis of papillary cystadenoma (Fig. 3.6). The cyst capsule, consisting of variable layers of collagenized fibrous tissue, may contain hemosiderin or calcium. The surrounding parenchyma, which is typically compressed, contains obsolescent glomeruli and atrophic nephrons.

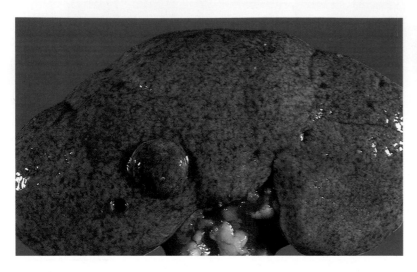

Figure 3.1 A minute simple cyst is evident on the capsular surface of the kidney. It has a transparent capsule and contains clear, colorless fluid. These retention cysts are common incidental findings at autopsy. The larger nodule to the right is a cortical adenoma.

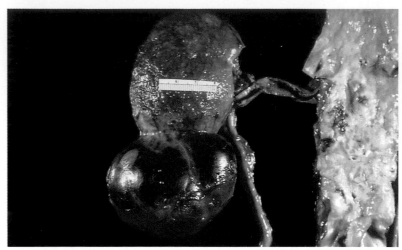

Figure 3.2 Large simple cysts located in the superficial cortex commonly bulge from the cortical surface. This lower-pole cyst appears dark-red secondary to hemorrhage. It was proven histologically to be benign.

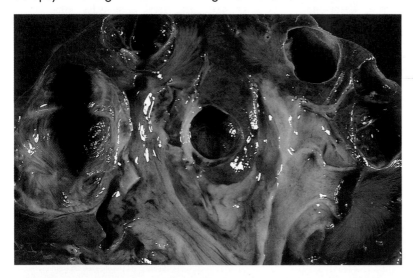

Figure 3.3 Multiple large parenchymal cysts can be distinguished from hydronephrosis by lack of communication with the pelvicalyceal system. Close inspection of this kidney reveals that the cysts are cortical in location and displace the medullae. Several cysts are partially septated.

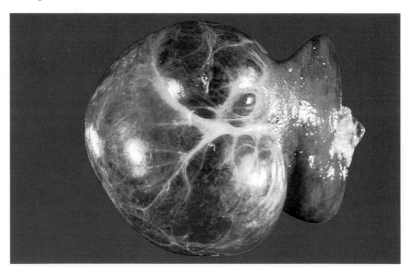

Figure 3.4 A large simple cyst, attached by a relatively narrow pedicle, protrudes from the renal cortex. Pedunculated cysts are more susceptible to rupture or torsion. Straw-colored fluid can be seen through the transparent capsule, which has attenuated trabeculae.

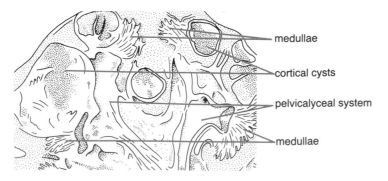

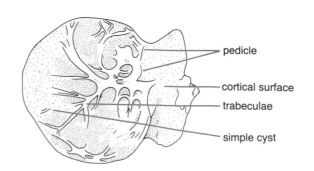

CLINICAL EVALUATION When renal cysts are large enough to appear as a mass on routine urography, further radiographic studies in conjunction with fine-needle aspiration (FNA) biopsy should be performed to establish the diagnosis of a benign cyst. Simple cysts are shown to be avascular by angiography, and ultrasound can confirm an echo-free mass with regular, sharply demarcated margins. The borders may be slightly irregular if the cyst wall is partially septated (Figs. 3.7, 3.8). Therapeutic evacuation using FNA

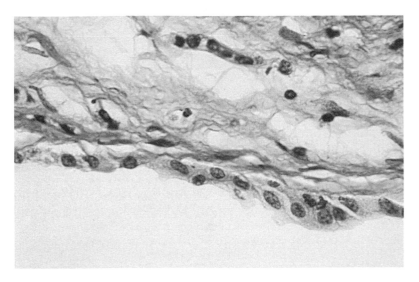

Figure 3.5 The lining of this simple cyst is cuboidal, resembling proximal convoluted tubular epithelium.

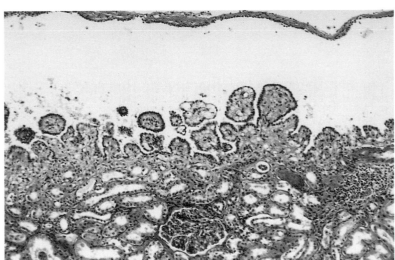

Figure 3.6 Focal polypoid projections within this superficial cortical cyst are lined by a single layer of histologically benign, cuboidal epithelium.

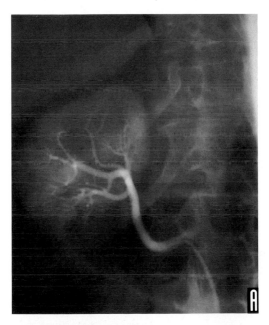
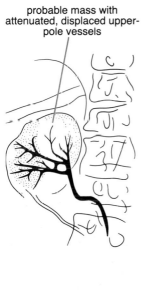

probable mass with attenuated, displaced upper-pole vessels

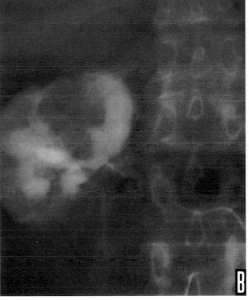
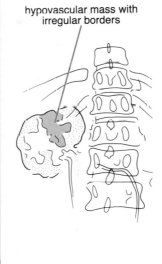

hypovascular mass with irregular borders

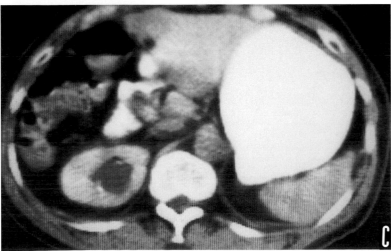

Figure 3.7 Radiographic findings in a benign simple cyst. **A,** Renal angiogram shows attenuated, slightly displaced upper-pole vessels on the arterial phase, suggesting a hypovascular mass. **B,** Venous phase of the angiogram delineates a hypovascular mass with irregular borders. **C,** CT scan confirms the presence of a mass with sharply demarcated but irregular borders. Ultrasonography (not shown) erroneously suggested internal echogenicity suspicious for RCC. Nephrectomy was performed without preoperative FNA biopsy (see Fig. 3.8). (Courtesy of H. Hawkins, MD, Cincinnati, Ohio)

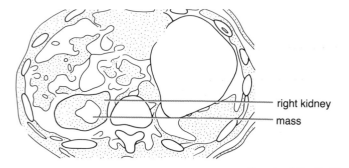

right kidney
mass

yields clear, colorless, or pale-yellow fluid; cloudy or bloody fluid should be regarded as suspicious for a cystic RCC.

Microscopic examination of a benign simple cyst's contents typically reveals a relatively acellular specimen with a clean background and few erythrocytes and histiocytes. The number of proximal convoluted tubular (PCT) cells, individually or in sheets, will vary. PCT cells are round to polygonal in shape with abundant granular cytoplasm and eccentric, small nuclei with distinct nucleoli (Fig. 3.9).

ACQUIRED RENAL CYSTIC DISEASE OF DIALYSIS

Long-term intermittent maintenance hemodialysis for end-stage renal disease has resulted in a spectrum of clinicopathologic complications. These include acquired renal cystic disease (ARCD), atypical cysts, and an increase of tumors derived from tubular epithelium.

PATHOGENESIS The pathogenesis of ARCD is unknown. It has been postulated that cystic transformation may be related to intrarenal tubular obstruction caused by interstitial fibrosis or deposition of oxalate crystals within collecting ducts.

CLINICAL MANIFESTATIONS ARCD is defined as the appearance of multiple, bilateral cysts in the previously noncystic native kidneys of patients on chronic dialysis. Mean length of hemodialysis is approximately 3½ years. It has an overall prevalence of 36% in patients undergoing hemodialysis, although studies have documented ARCD in 75% of patients after three years and 92% after eight or more years of chronic hemodialysis. The condition should be suspected when there is renal enlargement or recurrent hematuria. Ultrasonography is the screening technique currently recommended. CT scan can also detect cysts as small as 3–5 mm in diameter.

ASSOCIATED COMPLICATIONS It has been postulated that cystic transformation of the kidneys is accompanied by a stimulus for neoplastic growth, with renal "adenomas" occurring at a younger age (41–48 years) than in control populations. In necropsy and nephrectomy studies, the incidence of adenomas in end-stage kidney dialysis has been reported to be between 14% and 20%. Tumors were single or multiple, solid or cystic. In up to 30% of the kidneys studied, tumors were accompanied by atypical hyperplastic cysts. Metastatic RCC has also been reported. The incidence of RCC in ARCD has been estimated to be 30 times greater than that predicted for the general population and six times greater than that

Figure 3.8 This kidney contains a typical benign, partially septated simple cyst deep within the parenchyma.

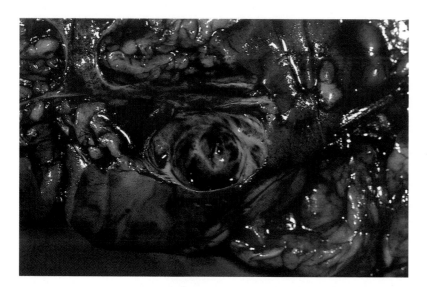

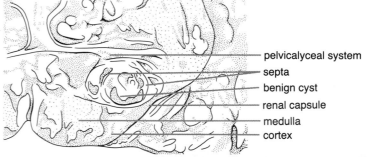

pelvicalyceal system
septa
benign cyst
renal capsule
medulla
cortex

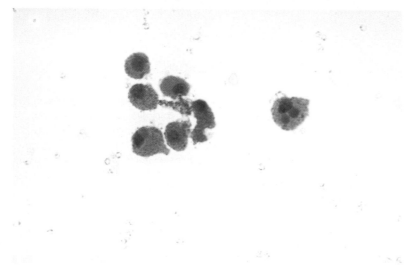

Figure 3.9 FNA biopsy of a benign simple cyst shows a clean background with few erythrocytes. There is a uniform population of individual PCT cells characterized by their round-to-polygonal shape, eccentric, small round nuclei, and abundant granular cytoplasm containing eosinophilic lysosomal droplets (Papanicolaou stain).

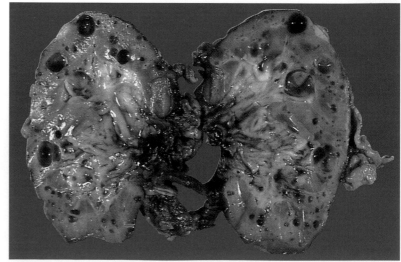

Figure 3.10 Numerous, variable-sized cysts are randomly distributed throughout the cortex and medulla of this kidney with ARCD. Unlike the adult polycystic kidney, this kidney is reduced in size (48 g) and has large zones of uninvolved parenchyma.

found among dialysis patients without ARCD. If ARCD is documented by ultrasonography, angiography and/or CT scan should be performed to detect possible tumors.

MORPHOLOGY Grossly, ARCD generally affects both kidneys equally. Unlike the adult polycystic kidney, however, the kidneys are reduced in size and weight, and the intervening cortex is contracted and granular. Cysts are variable in number, distribution, and size; some measure up to 2.5 cm in diameter but most are less than 5 mm (Fig. 3.10). Medullary cysts may occur adjacent to the pelvis or at the corticomedullary junction. Small adenomas may also be visible.

Microscopically, the interstitium surrounding the cysts is fibrotic, and may contain hemosiderin-laden macrophages or foci of calcification. Oxalate crystals are frequently prominent within the cyst cavities or walls (Fig. 3.11). Simple cysts, which are lined by a single layer of flattened-to-cuboidal epithelium, should be distinguished from atypical cysts. The latter are barely macroscopic or, more frequently, are microscopic cysts located in the renal cortex. Unlike simple cysts, atypical cysts (Fig. 3.12) are lined by finely to coarsely granular, columnar cells. The epithelial lining, which becomes hyperplastic and multilayered, frequently forms papillae and may show nuclear anaplasia. Fibromyxoid stroma surrounding the cysts may contain increased elastic tissue and collagen.

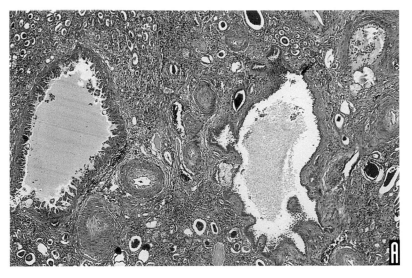

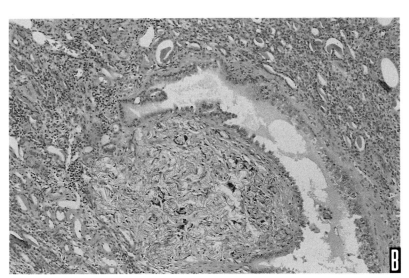

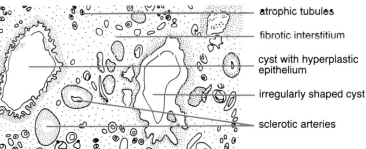

atrophic tubules

fibrotic interstitium

cyst with hyperplastic epithelium

irregularly shaped cyst

sclerotic arteries

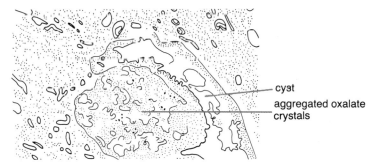

cyst

aggregated oxalate crystals

Figure 3.11 A, Renal parenchyma in ARCD shows changes typical of end-stage renal disease, with interstitial fibrosis, tubular atrophy, glomerular obsolescence, and vascular sclerosis. Cysts frequently are irregularly shaped and show varying degrees of epithelial hyperplasia (Masson's trichrome stain). **B,** Adjacent to this cyst is a nodular accumulation of focally calcified oxalate crystals.

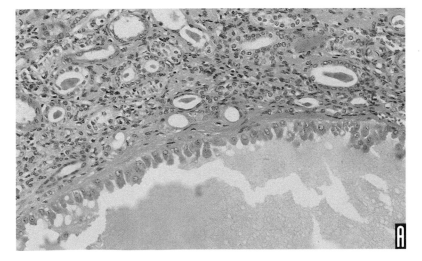

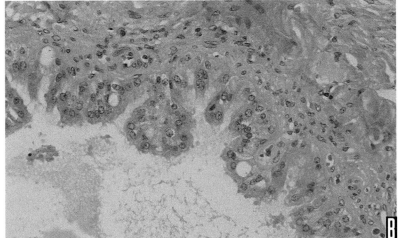

Figure 3.12 A, The atypical cyst in ARCD is lined by columnar cells that have coarsely granular eosinophilic cytoplasm. The basal lamina appears thickened. **B,** Epithelial hyperplasia has produced papillary projections. Nuclei are enlarged and slightly irregular with cleared chromatin and nucleolar prominence.

CHAPTER 4

Anomalies of the Kidney

RENAL AGENESIS

BILATERAL RENAL AGENESIS

Bilateral renal agenesis, the most severe of all renal anomalies, is always fatal. Almost half of affected infants are stillborn, and the remainder usually die within several days. The incidence estimated by Potter in her extensive studies was approximately 1 in 4800 births, with a 3:1 male predominance.

PATHOGENESIS Maternal factors such as age, infection, or other complications of pregnancy have not been associated with this disease. Very rare cases have been described in siblings, possibly representing chance occurrences. The penetrance rate of any genetic predisposition would be extremely low, because identical twins in which only one had renal agenesis have been reported.

The normal development of the kidney requires the presence of a nephrogenic ridge and a ureteral bud. Multiple defects in either component may lead to failure of renal development. This is supported by variable findings in the remaining portions of the urinary and genital systems. The frequent absence of the vas deferens in males, for instance, suggests a wolffian-duct defect, as both the vas deferens and ureteral bud are derived from this structure.

CLINICAL MANIFESTATIONS These infants typically have low birth weights and oligohydramnios, often with amnion nodosum, which are keratinized nodules on the amniotic membrane. The diagnosis is usually made based on anuria without bladder distention and associated abnormalities, particularly of the facies. The facial features are highly characteristic, if not diagnostic (Fig. 4.2). Potter described a prominent fold of skin that begins over each eye, swings down in a semicircle past the inner canthus, and extends onto the cheek. The nose is blunted, and there is a depression between the lower lip and chin. The ears appear low-set and drawn forward. The legs are often bowed, the skin is loose and dry, and the hands are abnormally large. A decrease in amniotic fluid due to compromised renal output probably causes mechanical effects that result in these external characteristics.

Because amniotic fluid is also important for normal pulmonary development, pulmonary hypoplasia is common in these newborns. The associated hypoxia is immediately obvious at birth, often directing attention away from the renal agenesis. Death during the first 24 hours is usually due to respiratory insufficiency, rather than renal failure.

MORPHOLOGY   By definition, both kidneys are completely absent (Fig. 4.3). No renal arteries are present. Rarely, there are small condensations of tissue in the region normally occupied by the kidney; these may contain abortive glomerular structures. The ureter may be apparently normal, but more often it is partially or

Figure 4.1
Anomalies of the Kidney

I. Anomalies in Number
   A. Agenesis
      1. Bilateral
      2. Unilateral
   B. Supernumerary kidney

II. Anomalies of Volume and Structure
   A. Hypoplasia
      1. Diffuse
      2. Oligomeganephronic
      3. Segmental
   B. Cystic and dysplastic lesions (see Section I)

III. Anomalies in Ascent
   A. Abdominal ectopia
   B. Thoracic kidney

IV. Anomalies of Form and Fusion
   A. Crossed ectopia with and without fusion
      1. Unilateral fused kidney (inferior ectopia)
      2. S-shaped kidney
      3. Lump kidney
      4. L-shaped kidney
      5. Disk kidney
      6. Unilateral fused kidney (superior ectopia)
   B. Horseshoe kidney

V. Anomalies of Rotation
   A. Incomplete
   B. Excessive
   C. Reverse

VI. Anomalies of Renal Vasculature
   A. Aberrant, accessory, or multiple vessels
   B. Renal artery aneurysms
   C. Arteriovenous fistula

Modified from Perlmutter et al. (1986)

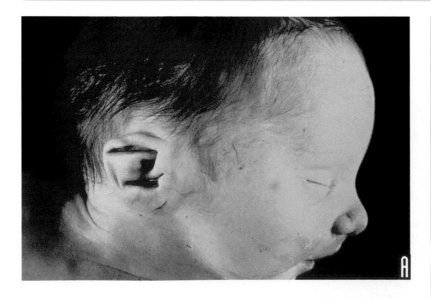

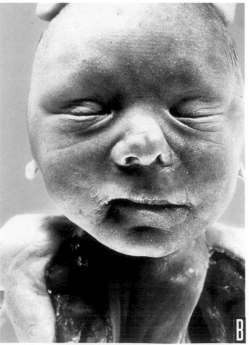

Figure 4.2 A, This mature fetus illustrates the ill-formed, low-set ears seen in bilateral renal agenesis. **B,** The skin fold that begins in the region of the inner canthus and extends in a semicircular shape onto each cheek is highly characteristic of bilateral renal agenesis, as are the blunted nose and cleft between the lower lip and chin.

completely absent. A poorly formed trigone may be present at the distal junction of the ureters. The bladder is missing in about half of cases and hypoplastic in the remainder, while the adrenal glands are almost invariably normal in location and appearance.

ASSOCIATED ANOMALIES Cardiovascular and gastrointestinal anomalies are found in about 50% of cases. In males, about 33% have undescended testes and 10% have testicular agenesis. As noted above, the vas deferens is commonly absent. In females, the incidence of associated genital abnormalities is even higher, with many having hypoplastic or absent ovaries, a rudimentary uterus, and a short or absent vagina.

UNILATERAL RENAL AGENESIS

Unilateral renal agenesis is two to four times more common than the bilateral form. As with bilateral agenesis, unilateral agenesis is more common in males, but the predominance is not as pronounced (1.8:1). There is a familial tendency in some instances.

PATHOGENESIS The embryologic considerations are identical to those for bilateral agenesis. The usual presence of a normal ipsilat-eral gonad formed from tissue in close approximation to the nephrogenic ridge suggests that most cases of unilateral agenesis are caused by defects in ureteral bud formation rather than an anomaly of the nephrogenic ridge. There is also a high frequency of associated abnormalities in structures that, like the ureteral bud, are derived from the mesonephric duct.

CLINICAL MANIFESTATIONS Renal absence occurs slightly more frequently on the left side. Unilateral renal agenesis is completely asymptomatic and, in the absence of external physical abnormalities, is likely to go undetected for many years. There is no evidence that the single kidney is at increased risk for acquired disease.

MORPHOLOGY A nonvisualized kidney on intravenous pyelography (IVP) is most often due to the presence of a diseased, nonfunctioning kidney, rather than renal agenesis. In either situation, the contralateral kidney may show compensatory enlargement (Fig. 4.4). Otherwise, the contralateral kidney in unilateral agenesis is usually normal. Renal arteriography can distinguish agenesis from nonfunction by demonstrating the absence of a renal artery in renal agenesis (Fig. 4.4B). Cystoscopy and retrograde contrast studies are also diagnostic, as the ureter is invariably abnormal (i.e.,

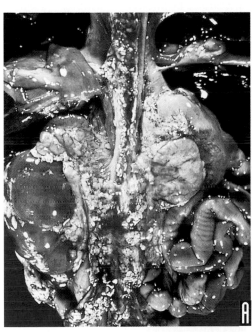
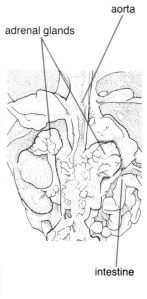
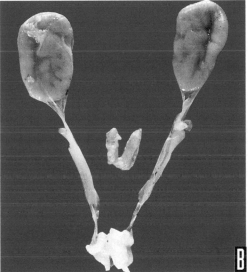
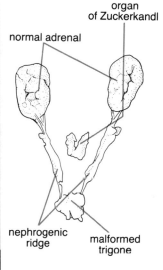

Figure 4.3 A, In this posterior view of an organ block removed at autopsy, both adrenal glands are clearly present, without associated kidneys. **B,** Removal of the genitourinary system from a fetus with bilateral renal agenesis demonstrates well formed adrenal glands, undeveloped nephrogenic ridges, and a malformed trigone. The central U-shaped structure is the organ of Zuckerkandl.

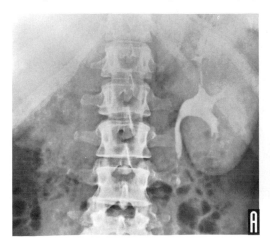
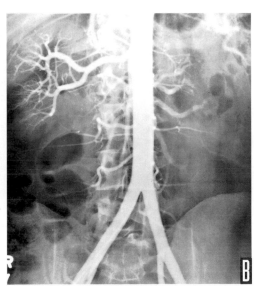

Figure 4.4 A, This IVP demonstrates the absence of functional renal tissue on the right side, with compensatory enlargement of the left kidney. An atrophic, endstage kidney cannot be excluded. **B,** On arteriogram, the complete absence of a left renal artery is compatible with renal agenesis. In renal nonfunction due to arterial occlusion, a small arterial stump is usually identifiable.

absent or partially formed) on the agenetic side. The trigone is also typically malformed or asymmetric.

ASSOCIATED ANOMALIES The adrenal gland on the affected side is absent in about 10% of autopsied cases. Genital abnormalities are the most common defects associated with unilateral renal agenesis. In males, the ipsilateral testis is usually normal, but the proximal ductal structures, including the vas deferens, seminal vesicles, and ejaculatory ducts, are absent or malformed in 10%–15% of cases. The contralateral testis and ducts are always normal.

Genital abnormalities are even more common in females, seen in up to 50% of patients. Most are due to defects in the formation of müllerian duct-derived structures. A unicornuate uterus with absence of the uterine horn or fallopian tube on the affected side is most common. Other anomalies are due to midline fusion defects and include double or septate uterus, double or septate vagina, atretic vagina, and, rarely, double cervix.

Extragenital defects are also encountered, including septal or valvular lesions of the heart, esophageal and anal atresias, as well as abnormal vertebrae and phalanges. Unilateral renal agenesis is sometimes found in patients with Turner's syndrome.

SUPERNUMARY KIDNEY

These are rare, accessory masses of discrete, encapsulated renal parenchyma. As defined by Geisinger, they may be closely related to the normal kidney but should be attached to it by no more than a loose fibrous connective tissue. More often, there is no connection at all. This definition distinguishes supernumerary kidneys from fused masses of renal tissue drained by bifid or duplicated ureters.

CLINICAL MANIFESTATIONS Supernumerary kidneys may be discovered incidentally during radiographic studies, at surgery, or at autopsy. They may also be symptomatic due to secondary changes, including infection, obstruction, or neoplasia. There is no evidence that supernumerary kidneys are more prone to the development of carcinoma than their normal counterparts.

MORPHOLOGY The ectopic kidney, which is usually smaller than normal, is typically located below its normal counterpart, with a predilection for the left side. About two thirds of supernumerary kidneys are attached to the normal kidney on the same side by a bifid ureter. The remaining one third exhibit complete ureteral duplications.

RENAL HYPOPLASIA
DIFFUSE HYPOPLASIA

True (congenital) renal hypoplasia is extremely rare. It must be distinguished from far more common acquired lesions that result in loss of renal parenchyma (Fig. 4.5) and from congenital dysplastic kidneys of small size.

CLINICAL MANIFESTATIONS The presentation depends on the degree of renal function. Most examples of renal hypoplasia are bilateral, although well documented unilateral cases have been reported. If the renal parenchyma is grossly deficient, signs of renal failure manifest in early infancy. If marginal function is available, life may be sustained until normally trivial acquired deficits cause renal failure in later childhood. Published examples of renal hypoplasia in adults, particularly those who are middle-aged and older, usually do not exclude acquired disease. Both unilateral and bilateral hypoplasia may lead to hypertension.

MORPHOLOGY Hypoplastic kidneys are small, histologically normal organs. Parenchymal or vascular changes suggesting inflammatory, infectious, or hypertensive disease imply that the diminutive kidney is probably an acquired defect. The best method for distinguishing congenital hypoplasia from an acquired process is by assessing the renal lobules. True hypoplastic kidneys have five or fewer calyces, in contrast to the normal ten or more (Fig. 4.6). Hypoplastic kidneys containing a single calyx have been described. External examination does not allow this evaluation; a frontal section of the kidney through the renal pelvis must be made.

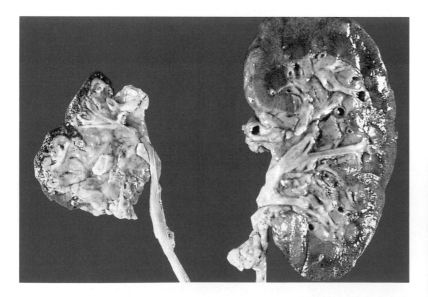

Figure 4.5 The marked thinning of the cortex and medulla in the smaller kidney indicates that this is an atrophic, rather than congenital hypoplastic, kidney.

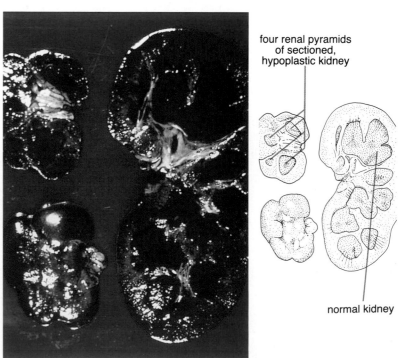

four renal pyramids of sectioned, hypoplastic kidney

normal kidney

Figure 4.6 True hypoplastic kidneys have decreased numbers of renal lobules. Five or fewer calyces are typical. Note that the hypoplastic kidney, sectioned at the upper left, has four lobules.

OLIGOMEGANEPHRONIC HYPOPLASIA

This is a rare, clinically and morphologically distinctive variant of bilateral renal hypoplasia. The pathogenesis is unknown. There is no evidence of a familial tendency, and associated anomalies have not been described.

CLINICAL MANIFESTATIONS Infants with this disorder develop signs of defective urine concentration during the first few weeks or months of life. Vomiting, polydipsia, polyuria, and dehydration are common. Growth retardation, renal osteodystrophy, anemia, and uremia develop somewhat later. Death due to renal failure occurs in childhood. Hypertension is not a feature.

MORPHOLOGY The kidneys are quite small and have the gross features of bilateral hypoplasia. Total renal weight may be as low as 20–40 g. As in typical hypoplasia, the number of calyces is reduced. The characteristic microscopic feature is a reduction in the total number of nephrons, which are markedly hypertrophied. Glomeruli may be two- to threefold larger than normal. Tubules are also markedly dilated and have been shown by microdissection to be increased in length. As the disease progresses, the glomeruli become sclerotic, the tubules atrophy, and interstitial fibrosis supervenes.

SEGMENTAL HYPOPLASIA

Also known as Ask-Upmark kidney, segmental hypoplasia is a rare, usually unilateral variant of renal hypoplasia. There is some controversy regarding whether or not the hypoplastic segment is congenital or acquired, but the former interpretation is favored. About 200 cases have been reported and were summarized by Arant and colleagues.

CLINICAL MANIFESTATIONS The most common clinical presentation—hypertension—is often severe in adolescents. Segmental hypoplasia is the predominant cause of hypertension in this age group. Presentation in childhood or later adult life is also possible. There is a 2:1 female predominance. Nephrectomy may not be effective in controlling the hypertension if secondary vascular-induced changes have produced significant glomerulosclerosis in the nonhypoplastic renal parenchyma.

MORPHOLOGY The kidney in segmental hypoplasia is small and has a reduced number of pyramids. A transverse groove on the capsular surface indicates the thin, hypoplastic segment. Sectioning

the kidney through the collecting system better demonstrates the hypoplastic portion of the parenchyma that overlies an elongated, calyxlike recess of the renal pelvis. A medullary pyramid is absent in the region of hypoplasia.

Microscopically, the hypoplastic segment contains few or no glomeruli; those glomeruli present are typically hyalinized. The tubules are dilated and filled with eosinophilic material. Interstitial fibrosis, a chronic inflammatory cell infiltrate, and thick-walled blood vessels complete the image (Fig. 4.7). The adjacent, microscopically normal renal cortex and medulla are sharply demarcated on each side of the hypoplastic segment. In extremely rare cases, multiple segments of the same kidney may be affected, or there may be bilateral disease.

RENAL ECTOPIA

Renal ectopia is a congenitally malpositioned kidney. Simple ectopia describes an affected kidney that remains lateralized to its proper side. Crossed ectopia, in contrast, is an ectopic kidney that is located on the contralateral side, as evidenced by its attached ureter, which crosses the midline and enters the bladder on the side from which the kidney was embryologically derived. Ectopia may be further subdivided into fused and nonfused forms. Because horseshoe kidneys are typically ectopic in position, they are also included in this section.

SIMPLE ECTOPIA

PATHOGENESIS The mechanism or mechanisms interfering with normal renal ascent are unknown. Proposed etiologies include ureteral bud maldevelopment, defective metanephric tissue, maternal illness, teratogens, genetic abnormalities, and vascular defects. Thoracic kidneys may be due to a delayed closure of the diaphragmatic membrane.

CLINICAL MANIFESTATIONS Simple renal ectopia is present at autopsy in approximately 1 in 900 cases. The left side is involved slightly more often, and there is no sexual predilection. Bilateral simple ectopia occurs in not more than 10% of cases. Rarely, the patient may have a solitary kidney that is ectopically located. Renal ectopia should be distinguished from renal ptosis, in which a normally positioned kidney sinks in the abdominal cavity due to increased mobility. The latter condition most commonly occurs in obese individuals following rapid weight loss.

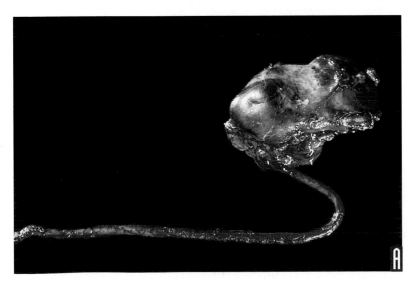

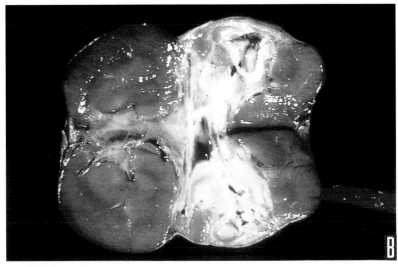

Figure 4.7 **A,** In this specimen demonstrating segmental hypoplasia (Ask-Upmark kidney), the kidney is small and has a characteristic, transversely oriented, depressed scar. **B,** In a section through the collecting system, the number of renal pyramids is seen to be reduced. The renal pelvis extends into the area of scarring.

Simple renal ectopias are classified according to the location of the aberrant kidney (Fig. 4.8). The vast majority represent incomplete ascents. Low-lumbar, iliac, and pelvic forms may be seen. Rarely, the kidney may ascend cephalad to the normal position and be located infradiaphragmatically or even within the thoracic cavity. Thoracic kidneys probably represent intrauterine acquired ectopias of initially normal-positioned organs.

Ectopic kidneys are asymptomatic unless affected by a secondary process. Acquired or congenital renal disease may involve an ectopic kidney. With the exception of pyelonephritis and stone formation, there is no evidence that ectopic kidneys are prone to renal disease or neoplasia. The former associations are probably related to the shortened ureter and inefficient urine drainage caused by a frequently malrotated ectopic kidney with a superiorly located renal pelvis. Rarely, a pelvic kidney may interfere with childbirth.

MORPHOLOGY Ectopic kidneys often lack a typical reniform configuration and appear disk-shaped. They may be below normal in size and frequently have persistent fetal lobulations. Some degree of malrotation is common, with the renal pelvis often oriented anteriorly (Fig. 4.9). The pelvis may also be tilted upward, with the kidney tending to assume a horizontal position. The short, only slightly tortuous ureter and an anomalous vascular supply distinguish ectopia from renal ptosis, which has a redundant ureter of normal length and a normal vascular supply.

ASSOCIATED ANOMALIES Genital anomalies, which are seen in 20%–60% of females, include bicornuate or unicornuate uterus, rudimentary or absent uterus, atresia of the proximal vagina, and duplication of the vagina. Anomalies that are seen in 10%–20% of males include undescended testes, duplications of the urethra, and hypospadias. The adrenal gland, which is only rarely affected, may be malpositioned or absent.

CROSSED ECTOPIA

When an ectopic kidney is located on the opposite side of the midline from its ureteral insertion into the bladder, it is referred to as a crossed renal ectopia.

PATHOGENESIS As with other congenital renal anomalies, the exact cause of crossed ectopia remains unclear. One theory proposes that the ureteral bud "wanders" across the midline to make contact with the contralateral nephrogenic blastema. Another suggests that the embryo becomes abnormally twisted so that the migrating kidney, though following a straight line, crosses to the other side.

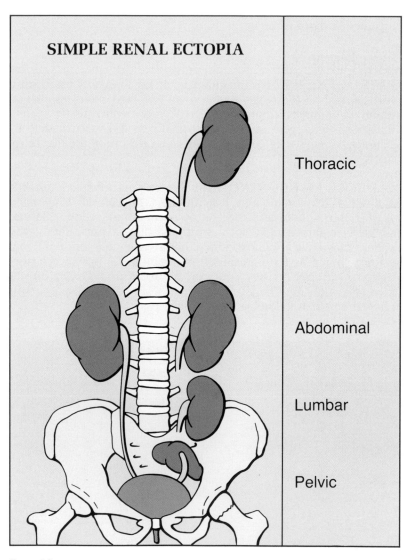

SIMPLE RENAL ECTOPIA

Thoracic

Abdominal

Lumbar

Pelvic

Figure 4.8 Simple renal ectopias are classified according to the anatomic location of the aberrant kidney. Lumbar and pelvic forms are the most common. Thoracic kidneys are rare and probably represent herniations through diaphragmatic defects. (Adapted from Gray and Skandalakis, 1972)

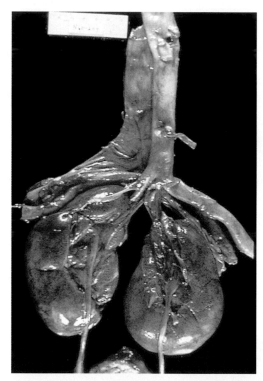

Figure 4.9 In this anterior view of a bilateral pelvic ectopia, the anomalous vascular supply from the aortic bifurcation is easily seen. The abnormal anterior orientation of the renal pelvis is typical of this condition.

Teratogenic and genetic factors have also been evoked, the latter based on occasional familial cases.

CLINICAL MANIFESTATIONS Approximately 90% of crossed ectopias are fused to the contralateral kidney. The resulting single renal mass may assume a variety of shapes, as described below. Crossed ectopias are twice as common in males as in females, and migration from left to right is three times more frequent than the reverse. Because crossed ectopias are typically asymptomatic unless the kidney is affected by a secondary process, the exact frequency of this anomaly is unclear, but has been said to be as high as 1 per 1000 individuals. There is an increased susceptibility to pyelonephritis and renal stone formation, due to incomplete urine drainage. About one third of patients with crossed renal ectopia present with an asymptomatic abdominal mass.

MORPHOLOGY The crossed kidney usually lies below the ipsilateral kidney and, as mentioned above, is fused to it in about 90% of cases. The caudal location probably represents lost cephalic migration during crossover. In about 5% of cases, however, the ectopic kidney is superior. When the two kidneys are not fused, the uncrossed kidney usually occupies its normal location and is properly oriented. The crossed kidney is typically oriented diagonally or horizontally with an anterior pelvis. Another uncommon, nonfused variant is the solitary crossed ectopic kidney, also known as unilateral renal agenesis with crossed ectopia. Rarely, there also may be bilateral crossed ectopias in which a properly positioned and oriented kidney is present in each renal fossa, but the ureters cross in the midline (Fig. 4.10).

Fused, crossed ectopias may assume numerous appearances best appreciated radiographically (Fig. 4.11). Most common is the inferi-

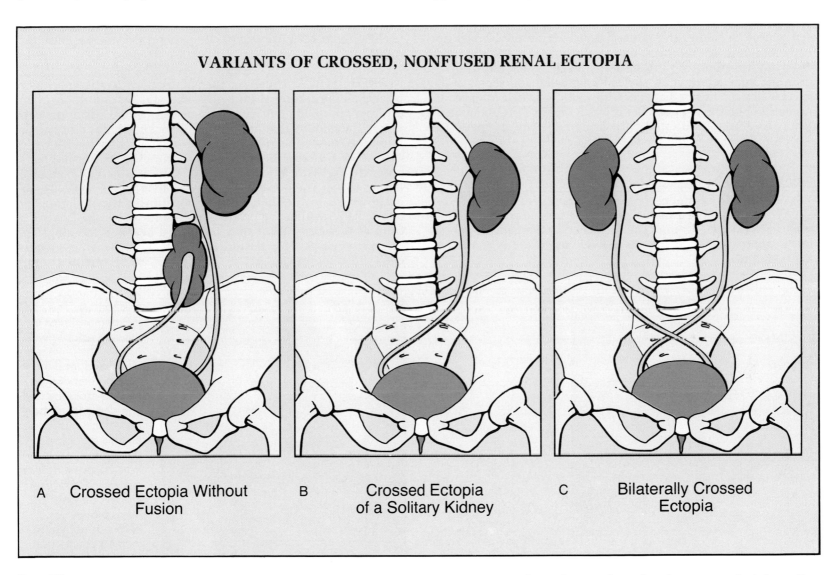

VARIANTS OF CROSSED, NONFUSED RENAL ECTOPIA

A Crossed Ectopia Without Fusion

B Crossed Ectopia of a Solitary Kidney

C Bilaterally Crossed Ectopia

Figure 4.10 **A,** In crossed ectopia without fusion, the ectopic kidney typically lies below the normal kidney and has an anteriorly oriented renal pelvis. **B,** Unilateral renal agenesis may occasionally be associated with a crossed ectopia of a solitary kidney. **C,** Probably the least common form of crossed, nonfused ectopia is the bilaterally crossed variant. The kidneys are normally positioned and oriented, but the ureters cross the midline. (Adapted from Perlmutter et al., 1986)

or ectopia in which the kidneys retain their general outlines, but the superior portion of the crossed ectopic kidney is fused to the inferior portion of the cephalad, noncrossed kidney. Both renal pelves face anteriorly. It is extremely rare for the crossed ectopic kidney to be superior to its normally positioned counterpart. The sigmoid, or S-shaped, fused kidney is the next most frequent pattern. As in inferior ectopia, the general renal outlines are preserved and the same mode of fusion is seen. However, both renal pelves are oriented as if each kidney were normally positioned. Thus the pelvis of the inferior, crossed kidney faces laterally. Other patterns of fusion have also been described, including lump kidney, L-shaped kidney, and disk kidney (Figs. 4.12, 4.13). These subclassifications, reflecting differing embryologic aberrations, have little or no clinical utility.

ASSOCIATED ANOMALIES If two distinct ureters are present, whether or not the renal masses are fused, the incidence of associated anomalies is low. The ureteral orifices enter the bladder normally in almost all instances, and cystoscopy does not suggest an abnormality. About 4% of patients have associated findings, including imperforate anus, skeletal anomalies, and septal cardiovascular defects. In rare patients with solitary crossed ectopias, the incidence of nonrenal anomalies is much higher. This undoubtedly relates to defects associated with unilateral renal agenesis (see above), rather than to the crossed ectopia.

Horseshoe Kidney

One of the most common congenital renal anomalies, horseshoe kidney may be viewed in the present terminology as a bilateral simple ectopia with fusion. The incidence in the general population is approximately 1 in 400 individuals. There is a 2:1 male predominance.

PATHOGENESIS Horseshoe kidney presumably results from a fusion of the bilateral nephrogenic blastema prior to its ascent from the pelvis. Over 95% of the time, the fusion is at the lower poles, which inhibits normal renal rotation.

CLINICAL MANIFESTATIONS About one third of cases are totally asymptomatic and discovered incidentally. The remainder have a palpable abdominal mass or symptoms due to secondary infection, hydronephrosis, or renal stone formation, the latter usually in the form of vague abdominal pains, with or without gastrointestinal symptoms. Retrograde cystoscopy, IVP, or arteriography delineate the renal mass.

Although horseshoe kidney is commonly associated with other anomalies, some of which may be serious or fatal, patients without accompanying defects usually live a normal life. About two thirds with incidentally discovered horseshoe kidneys remain free of disease. The remainder may experience one or more episodes of pyelonephritis or renal calculi. There is no evidence of increased mortality.

MORPHOLOGY There are many variations to the gross morphologic appearance of horseshoe kidney. By definition, there are two approximately vertical masses of renal tissue on each side of the midline that are connected by an isthmus crossing the midline. The connection is at the lower pole in over 95% of cases. Most often, the isthmus is composed of normal renal parenchyma with its own blood supply, but it may consist of fibrous tissue. The horseshoe kidney is invariably ectopic, usually occupying a lower-than-normal position in the abdomen or, occasionally, within the pelvis. The isthmus most often passes in front of the aorta, but it may be located between the aorta and inferior vena cava or posterior to both vessels. An associated defect in rotation causes the renal pelves to be oriented some-

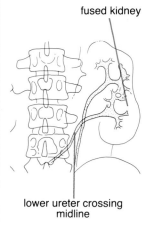

fused kidney

lower ureter crossing midline

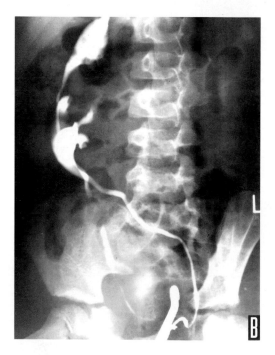

Figure 4.11 A, This IVP demonstrates a crossed ectopia with fusion. The ureters are visualized, and the lower ureter can be seen to cross the midline at the lower portion of the illustration. **B,** This retrograde pyelogram also illustrates a crossed, fused ectopia. The crossed kidney, as identified by its ureter, lies below its normally located counterpart.

VARIANTS OF CROSSED, FUSED RENAL ECTOPIA

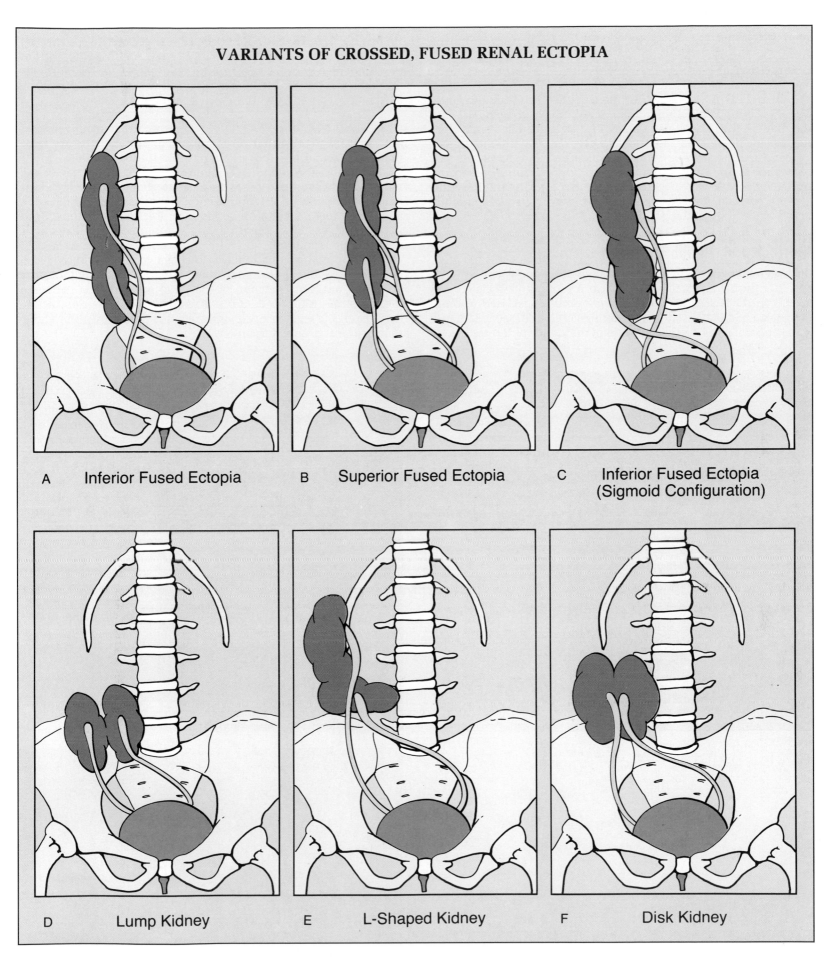

A — Inferior Fused Ectopia

B — Superior Fused Ectopia

C — Inferior Fused Ectopia (Sigmoid Configuration)

D — Lump Kidney

E — L-Shaped Kidney

F — Disk Kidney

Figure 4.12 **A,** In inferior fused ectopia, the ectopic kidney is inferior to its noncrossed counterpart. Both pelves are rotated anteriorly and the fusion is pole to pole. **B,** Superior fused ectopia is extremely rare. The crossed kidney is superior and fused pole to pole to its noncrossed counterpart. Note the anteriorly rotated pelves. **C,** Inferior fused ectopia may also assume a sigmoid configuration to the orientation of the renal pelves. **D,** In the so-called lump kidney variant, the ectopic kidney is located medial to its counterpart, with both renal pelves facing anteriorly. **E,** In the L-shaped variant, the ectopic kidney is rotated 90° and is located inferior to its counterpart. **F,** The disk kidney is a variant of the lump kidney, in which the renal pelves are rotated toward each other. (Adapted from Perlmutter et al., 1986)

what anteriorly (Fig. 4.14). Renal calyces are present in normal numbers. The vascular supply is highly variable and frequently asymmetric.

ASSOCIATED ANOMALIES Frequency is much higher in autopsies of stillborn and young infants with multiple congenital anomalies than in the general population. This suggests that a sizable percentage of horseshoe kidneys are associated with major malformations incompatible with sustained life. Among adults with horseshoe kidneys, Boatman and coworkers found associated anomalies in one third. Included were hypospadias, undescended testis, bicornuate uterus, vaginal septation, and ureteral duplication.

Anomalies of Renal Rotation

During embryogenesis the kidney ascends and undergoes a 90° rotation. Congenital anomalies in rotation are usually associated with defects in renal ascent, but they may occur as isolated findings. Congenital malrotation should be distinguished from secondary rotational abnormalities due to distortion of the kidney by a mass lesion.

PATHOGENESIS/EMBRYOLOGY The exact cause of renal malrotation is unknown. Prior to its ascent from the pelvis, the kidney is oriented with the renal hilum pointing anteriorly. Normally, the kidney rotates medially during its ascent, eventually reaching its adult configuration with the pelvis facing the midline.

CLINICAL MANIFESTATIONS Since malrotation unaccompanied by other congenital or acquired abnormalities is asymptomatic, the actual frequency is impossible to discern. Radiographic studies of the abdomen detect malrotation in approximately 1 in 500 patients (Fig. 4.15). As with most congenital urologic defects, malrotation shows a 2:1 predilection for males, but unlike other anomalies, there is not a predominance of left-sided lesions. Renal malrotation has been reported as a common finding in patients with Turner's syndrome.

The abnormal orientation of a malrotated kidney may lead to problems with blood flow and urine drainage. Impairment of urine flow may result in dilatation of the renal pelvis during periods of high-volume urine production. This is perceived as dull, aching flank pain. Incomplete urine drainage also predisposes the kidney to infection and stone formation.

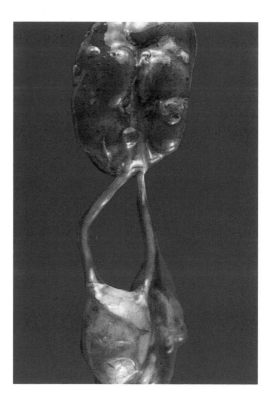

Figure 4.13 This autopsy specimen from a crossed, fused ectopia of the disk type demonstrates the medially oriented and fused renal hila illustrated in Figure 4.12F.

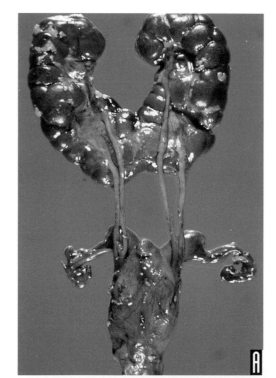

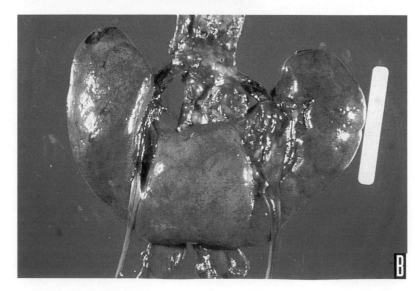

Figure 4.14
A, Horseshoe kidneys may be associated with other minor or major genitourinary anomalies. In this example from a newborn female, there are bilateral double ureters. **B,** The relationship between a horseshoe kidney and the nearby major blood vessels varies. Most often, as in this instance, the kidney is anterior to the aorta.

MORPHOLOGY Anomalies may be described according to the orientation of the renal pelvis or the presumed defect in rotation (Fig. 4.16). The most common variant is the ventral hilum or nonrotated kidney. Also frequent is the ventromedial or incompletely rotated kidney. A dorsally oriented hilum, representing a hyperrotation of 180°, is the rarest form of rotational anomaly. A laterally oriented renal hilum may arise in two ways: The kidney may hyperrotate 270°, in which case the renal vasculature passes over the posterior surface of the kidney; alternately, it may have reverse-rotated 90°, with the renal vessels passing over the kidney's anterior surface.

Malrotation defects are usually associated with other gross anomalies of renal form. The kidney may be disk-shaped, flattened, elongated, or triangular. Fetal lobulations are accentuated, fibrous tissue may encase the renal hilum or surround the kidney, and vasculature is often aberrant.

Vascular Anomalies
Renal Artery Aneurysm

Renal artery aneurysms were once considered to be extremely rare. The advent of selective renal artery angiography has led to the increased detection of small forms, many of which are incidental findings.

PATHOGENESIS Aneurysmal dilatations of the renal artery may be congenital or acquired. Acquired lesions typically result from prolonged hypertension, trauma, or localized infection. In a detailed study, Abeshouse subclassified renal aneurysms morphologically as saccular (Fig. 4.17), fusiform, dissecting, and arteriovenous variants. The last is discussed below.

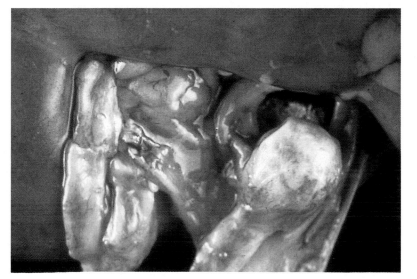

Figure 4.15 A malrotated, slightly ectopic kidney was incidentally discovered on the right side of this IVP. The renal hilum is laterally oriented and may represent a hyperrotated or reverse-rotated kidney. Orientation of the vessels with respect to the kidney allows distinction (see Figure 4.16).

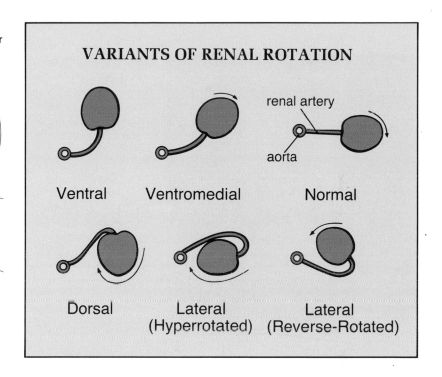

Figure 4.16 Variants of renal malrotation are subclassified according to the orientation of the renal hilum. (Adapted from Gray and Skandalakis, 1972)

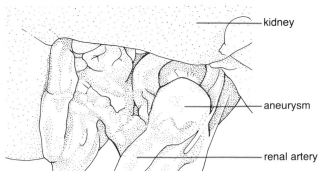

Figure 4.17 This small, saccular renal artery aneurysm was discovered incidentally at autopsy.

CLINICAL MANIFESTATIONS Most renal aneurysms are asymptomatic, although larger lesions may produce pain, hematuria, or hypertension due to associated perfusion defects. A palpable, pulsatile mass indicates a large aneurysm, but even small lesions may produce detectable bruits. Renal artery angiography is diagnostic.

Small aneurysms may be safely followed without intervention. However, lesions greater than 2.5 cm, lesions with a documented increase in size, aneurysms in women who may become pregnant, or aneurysms associated with arteriovenous fistulas have a significant frequency of rupture and should be resected.

ARTERIOVENOUS MALFORMATIONS

Arteriovenous malformations are uncommon, with fewer than 100 reported cases. Although occasionally discovered incidentally, many are symptomatic and require therapy.

PATHOGENESIS About one fourth of renal vascular malformations are believed to be congenital; the remainder represent acquired lesions. Penetrating vascular trauma is the leading cause of acquired lesions and is a recognized, albeit rare, complication of needle biopsy.

CLINICAL MANIFESTATIONS Arteriovenous malformations, even the presumably congenital forms, are often not discovered until adulthood. There is a strong female predilection (3:1). Symptoms are related to the size of the lesion and the associated amount of vascular shunting. A loud bruit is commonly heard over the back or abdomen; hypertension secondary to decreased renal blood flow is also common. Large lesions lead to left ventricular hypertrophy and high-output cardiac failure.

IVP may show a hilar filling defect if the malformation involves this portion of the kidney, but frequently this procedure is not valuable. Renal artery angiography, with digital subtraction for smaller lesions, is the diagnostic procedure of choice (Fig. 4.18).

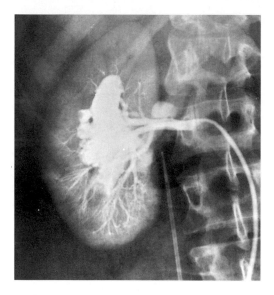

Figure 4.18 A large arteriovenous malformation is outlined by contrast injection into the renal artery on this selective angiogram. Note that the renal vein is filling, due to shunting, while the renal parenchyma is still in the arterial phase of injection.

CHAPTER 5

Ureteral and Bladder Anomalies

URETERAL ANOMALIES

URETERAL DUPLICATION

Duplications of the ureter are a common developmental anomaly not typically associated with clinical symptoms. In partial duplication, also known as a bifid ureter, double ureters fuse prior to entering the bladder through a single orifice. Complete duplication of the ureter results in separate ureteral orifices, one of which is usually ectopically located in the bladder or, rarely, drains into another segment of the genitourinary tract.

PATHOGENESIS Normally, the ureter begins as a single bud from the mesonephric duct. The majority of complete duplications appear to result from the formation of a second ureteral bud. By convention, the ureter draining the lower pole is said to have arisen from the "normal" ureteral bud, and the ureter draining the upper pole is considered ectopic or accessory. As discussed below, completely duplicated ureters maintain an orientation defined by the Weigert–Meyer law. Rare exceptions to this rule probably represent complete duplications arising from a single ureteral bud that bifurcated very early in its development. Partial duplications of the ureter apparently develop due to a "late" bifurcation of a single ureteral bud.

CLINICAL MANIFESTATIONS   Because ureteral duplications are frequently asymptomatic, incidence rates are best obtained from large, unselected autopsy series. Based on such series, partial or complete duplication of the ureter exists in about 0.8% of the population, with the two forms seeming to occur with approximately equal frequency. Autopsy studies suggest little if any sex predilection. In contrast, duplicated ureters are detected clinically twice as often in women as in men, probably due to the increased frequency of abdominal radiographic studies in women (Fig. 5.1). Ureteral duplications develop with equal frequency on both sides of the abdomen. Bilateral duplication of the ureter is about one sixth as common as unilateral disease.

Ureteral duplications are found with increased frequency in patients with urinary tract infections. In children with such infections, the incidence of ureteral duplication is approximately 8%–12%, or more than 10 times the incidence in the general population. It thus seems clear that duplications predispose a minority of individuals to infection, probably due to urinary stasis or reflux.

MORPHOLOGY   Grossly, partial and complete ureteral duplications have an identical appearance at their proximal (renal) attachments. Partial duplications of the ureter are Y-shaped and converge distally to enter the bladder through a common orifice. Occasionally, one limb of a partial ureteral duplication (bifid ureter) does not make contact with the kidney and ends blindly (Figs. 5.2, 5.3). This phenomenon occurs twice as often on the right side of the body. Blind-ending ureters with complete duplications are rare. Typically, the blind segments are completely asymptomatic, but there may be pain due to urinary stasis with dilatation. Very short blind ureteral duplications are often labeled as congenital ureteral diverticula (see below). Partial triplications of the ureter are almost never encountered.

Complete ureteral duplications have two intravesicular openings that tend to be reversed in comparison with their orientation at the renal pelvis (see Fig. 5.2). Thus the "ectopic" ureter draining the

upper portion of the kidney enters the bladder inferior (and medial) to the ureter draining the lower portion of the kidney. This nearly constant orientation is referred to as the Weigert–Meyer law. In complete duplication, the upper or ectopic ureter typically drains about one third of the renal calyces, with the lower ureter accounting for the bulk of renal drainage. Hydronephrosis, particularly involving the lower pole, is a common finding secondary to urinary reflux.

The rarest form of complete ureteral duplication is the inverted-Y configuration (see Fig. 5.2). In this variant, a single ureter draining the kidney bifurcates distally to enter the bladder as two distinct ureters with separate orifices. Embryologically, this process probably represents the initial development of two ureteral buds that subsequently fused before merging with the metanephros to form the embryologic kidney.

URETEROCELE

A ureterocele is a cystic enlargement of the ureter at its junction with the urinary bladder. It may occur with otherwise normal, single ureters, in association with ectopically placed, duplicated ureters, or, rarely, with solitary ectopic ureters. Several systems have been devised for categorizing ureteroceles, the most straightforward of which divides them into simple or orthotopic ureteroceles and ectopic ureteroceles.

PATHOGENESIS   Although the embryologic defect responsible for ureterocele formation is not entirely clear, the most popular theory ascribes simple ureterocele to delayed rupture of Chwalle's membrane, which separates the embryologic ureter from the urogenital sinus. This delay presumably leads to enlargement of the terminal ureter with a stenotic ureterovesicular orifice. Ectopic ureteroceles may be due to defective ureteral bud formation with a deficit in ureteral musculature or abnormal insertion of the ureter into the bladder wall. Another theory suggests that the ureteral orifice fails to expand.

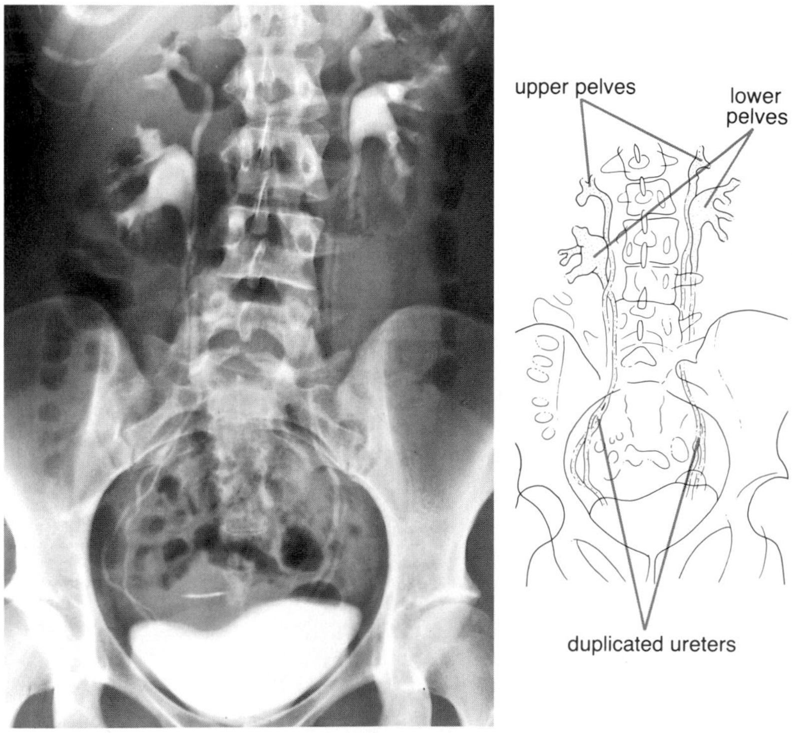

upper pelves

lower pelves

duplicated ureters

Figure 5.1 In this example of bilateral, complete duplication of the collecting systems, the bulk of renal drainage feeds into the lower system.

VARIANTS OF URETERAL DUPLICATION

kidney

bladder

| A | Partial Duplication | B | Blind-Ending Bifurcation | C | Complete Duplication | D | Inverted-Y Formation |

Figure 5.2 A, In partial duplication, the two ureters converge somewhere along their course before entering the bladder. **B,** The blind-ending bifurcation is a rare variant in which one segment of a partially duplicated ureter ends blindly. Short bifurcations of this type may be diagnosed as ureteral diverticula. **C,** Complete ureteral duplications are common anomalies. The ureters tend to cross, with the segment draining the upper portion of the kidney entering the bladder ectopically. **D,** The inverted-Y formation is the rarest variant of ureteral duplication. The kidney is drained by a single ureter that diverges to enter the bladder through two separate orifices.

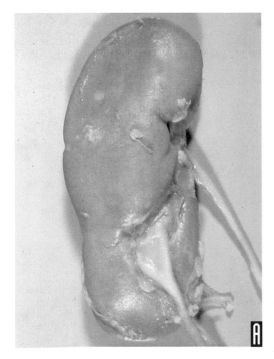

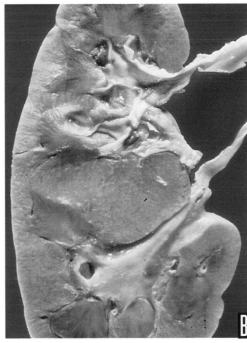

Figure 5.3 A, In this specimen of a complete ureteral duplication, the lower portion of the kidney is malrotated—an unusual variant. **B,** This section through a partially duplicated collecting system clearly demonstrates the separate pelves and renal pyramids drained by each ureter.

CLINICAL MANIFESTATIONS Simple ureteroceles arising from normally placed, single ureters are most commonly detected in adulthood (Fig. 5.4). Longstanding partial obstruction usually leads to hydroureter, some degree of hydronephrosis, and pyelonephritis. Stones may form in the ureterocele or more proximally in the urinary tract.

Ectopic ureteroceles tend to be larger lesions, almost always associated with ureteral duplication (Fig. 5.5). They usually present in childhood with signs and symptoms of infection or obstruction. Ectopic ureteroceles are far more common in girls, even though ureteral duplications do not show an obvious sex predilection. Occasionally, large ectopic ureteroceles may occlude the urethral orifice, producing acute urinary obstruction.

Small ureteroceles with little or no associated reflux do not require therapy, but reimplantation of the ureter is necessary for larger lesions. Before undertaking such procedures, renal status should be evaluated to ascertain that functional parenchyma remains. If the kidney has been severely damaged by infection, nephroureterectomy may be required. Transurethral resection of ureteroceles, once a common practice, is no longer favored because of the invariable development of reflux.

MORPHOLOGY Cystoscopic examination of a ureterocele demonstrates a cystic, translucent mass of variable size. Smaller lesions may be only small bulges at the ureteral orifice, and larger lesions may fill the entire bladder. The outer surface of the ureterocele is covered with normal transitional epithelium in continuity with the bladder mucosa, and the inner surface is lined by similar epithelium as a direct extension of the ureter. Between the two layers is a zone of scattered muscle fibers and fibrous tissue.

Simple ureteroceles, by definition, are confined to the urinary bladder and originate from a normally positioned ureteral orifice. As noted above, they tend to be small, often asymptomatic lesions

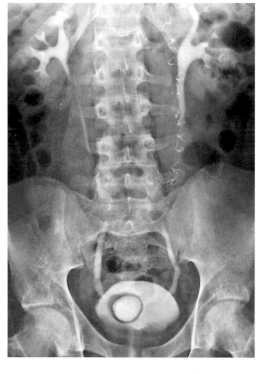

Figure 5.4 In the simple ureterocele shown in this IVP, the markedly dilated distal end of the right ureter produces a filling defect at its point of entrance into the urinary bladder.

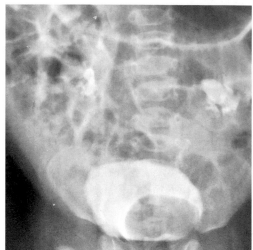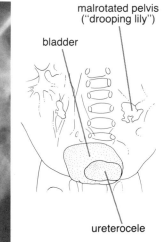

malrotated pelvis ("drooping lily")

bladder

ureterocele

Figure 5.5 In this IVP from a child with a complete duplication of the left-sided collecting system, the lower collecting system on the left is angled upward, creating a characteristic "drooping lily" appearance. The upper collecting system is not visualized, but its ureter enters the bladder ectopically. The associated large ureterocele produces the filling defect seen here.

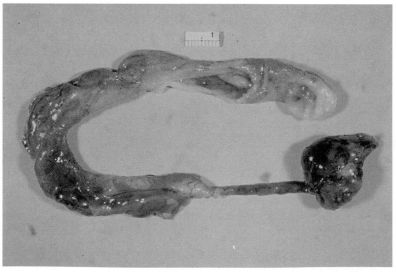

Figure 5.6 The hypoplastic and dysplastic kidney in this specimen had a dilated distal ureter that formed a large ureterocele.

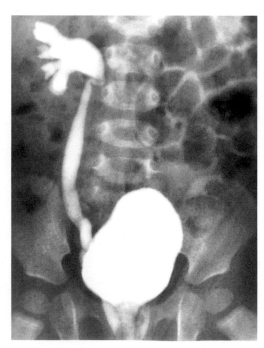

Figure 5.7 In this cystogram, injection of contrast material into the bladder lumen demonstrates reflux into the right collecting system. The ureter and renal pelvis are dilated (grade 3 reflux).

(Fig. 5.6). Ectopic ureteroceles originate from a malpositioned ureteral orifice and may extend into the bladder neck or urethra. They are almost always associated with complete ureteral duplication and, under this circumstance, invariably arise from the ectopically placed ureteral segment draining the upper pole of the kidney. An ectopic ureterocele from a solitary ureter is extremely rare.

VESICOURETERAL REFLUX

In humans, the normal course of the ureter through the bladder wall with extension beneath the submucosa of the trigone creates a flap valve that prevents urinary reflux. Congenital or acquired anomalies of this delicate valvular structure result in retrograde urinary flow. Therapy depends upon the degree of reflux and attendant renal compromise.

PATHOGENESIS Vesicoureteral reflux (VUR) may be divided into two general categories. Primary or congenital reflux is due to an intrinsic defect in the ureterovesicular junction. Secondary or acquired reflux is the sequela of one or more typically chronic vesicular processes, including persistently elevated intravesicular pressure, infection, and weakness of the bladder musculature.

In primary reflux, the intravesicular ureteral orifice is more lateral than normal, with a corresponding decrease in the length of the submucosal segment. The probability of reflux is inversely correlated with the length of this segment. As discussed in the section on ureteral duplication, the ureter arises as a bud from the mesonephric duct. Eventually, the site of origin is incorporated into the developing trigone and forms the ureteral orifice. Embryologic studies suggest that ureteral buds originating closer than normal to the urogenital sinus are displaced laterally in the trigone, with consequent shortening of the intramucosal segment and increased frequency of reflux.

A predisposition to primary reflux appears to be an inherited trait. Familial clustering has been repeatedly demonstrated. While in the overall population the incidence is at least 1 per 1000 individuals, the rate of asymptomatic reflux in the subgroup of children who have siblings with reflux is as high as 25%. First-degree relatives of patients with reflux are affected at a rate many times greater than that of the general population.

CLINICAL MANIFESTATIONS VUR is a dynamic process that may be documented by numerous techniques of varying sophistication. Simply demonstrating the presence of reflux is of little value in determining the best mode of therapy. Additional factors to be considered include the degree of reflux, the status of the affected kidney, the anatomy and cystoscopic morphology of the ureteral orifice, the patient's age, the frequency of urinary infection, and the presence of potentially confounding factors.

Reflux can be confirmed cystoscopically by filling the bladder with a nontoxic dye such as methylene blue, waiting for several minutes, draining and refilling the bladder with clear, sterile water, and then noting the color of fluid emerging from the ureteral openings. Radiographic techniques are the mainstay of reflux evaluation. Cystography (filling the bladder with radiopaque fluid) is the primary mode of evaluation (Fig. 5.7) and may be accompanied by voiding cineradiography. Radionuclide scans and ultrasonographic studies have also been employed.

A scale for grading cystographically documented reflux was devised by Dwoskin and Perlmutter:

Grade 1   Only the lower portion of the ureter fills with contrast material.
Grade 2A The entire ureter and pelvicalyceal region fill without dilatation or evidence of renal abnormality.
Grade 2B The same features as in grade 2A are present, but there is also mild calyceal blunting.
Grade 3   The entire ureter and pelvicalyceal region fill; there is calyceal clubbing and pelvic dilatation without tortuosity.
Grade 4   The ureter exhibits massive dilatation and tortuosity.

MORPHOLOGY The changes seen radiographically are paralleled by gross abnormalities that range from mild distal ureteral dilatation to severe hydronephrosis (Fig. 5.8).

THERAPY Mild degrees of reflux may be safely followed without intervention. More severe cases require surgical reimplantation of the ureter, using one of several techniques to produce a competent ureterovesicular valve.

Several factors must be evaluated to determine optimal therapy for ureteral reflux. The radiographic subclassification described

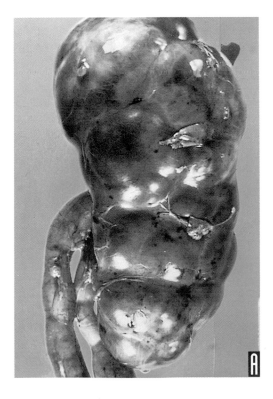
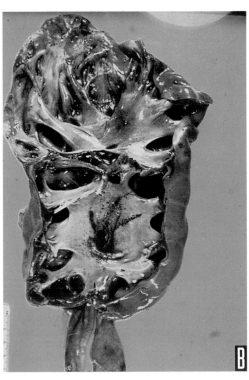

Figure 5.8 A, In this kidney from a patient with a duplicated collecting system, ureteral reflux, perhaps with a component of obstruction, has led to hydronephrosis. **B,** Section through the kidney more clearly shows the dilatation of the renal pelvis and corresponding loss of renal parenchyma.

above and the morphology of the ureteral orifice should be considered. Lyon and colleagues described four patterns of orifice configuration seen at cystoscopy. The normal orifice is volcano-shaped. The least severe deformity is the "stadium" orifice, which is an enlarged ellipse, usually with slight lateral displacement. "Stadium" orifice may be competent or associated with mild reflux. The "horseshoe" orifice is parabolic and is associated with a short intramucosal segment; reflux is usually but not invariably present. The most severe deformity is the "golf hole" orifice, which is circular, laterally located, with little or no intramucosal component; reflux is present and often persistent.

The laterality of the ureteral orifice and the length of the intramucosal segment are factors that tend to correlate with the Lyon orifice morphology but may be independently evaluated. This is best done by inserting a ureteral catheter, thereby estimating the length of the intramucosal, elevated segment. The diameter of the ureter must also be estimated, as it is the ratio of length to diameter that determines valvular competence.

Age is another important factor in the evaluation of reflux. In young children, even severe reflux abnormalities may spontaneously resolve during subsequent growth. The status of the affected kidney should also be considered; evidence of pyelonephritis or hydronephrosis (see Fig. 5.8) usually mandates prompt surgical intervention.

In light of the features outlined above, the criteria for surgery are generally accepted to consist of grade 3 to 4 reflux on cystography; lateral orifice with "horseshoe" or "golf hole" configuration, or a short intravesicular ureter; and renal scarring or frequent clinical infections.

Bladder Anomalies

Anomalies of the Urachus

The urachus is a normal embryologic structure representing the progressively narrowing channel connecting the embryonic bladder with the extraembryonic allantois. Anomalies of the urachus are invariably due to failures of regression rather than defects in formation. Such failures may result in a patent urachus with periumbilical drainage of urine, urachal cysts, urachal sinuses, and urachal diverticula. Urachal anomalies are more common in males than females by a ratio of about 5:2.

PATHOGENESIS During embryogenesis, the cloaca is divided by the urorectal septum and its anterior portion becomes the bladder. Early in its development, the bladder maintains a connection to the extraembryonic allantois. As the caudal portion of the anterior cloaca expands to form the bladder, the cranial portion does not contribute to bladder development and is drawn into a narrowing tubular structure—the fetal urachus—that remains in continuity with the allantois in the umbilical region. Progressive descent of the bladder after birth results in further narrowing of the urachus and, normally, conversion to a cordlike structure. The adult urachus is a fibromuscular tube (median umbilical ligament) lying in the anterior abdominal wall's space of Retzius. In up to half of adults, a tiny, epithelium-lined canal is present within the urachus in apparent continuity with the bladder lumen. In the rest of the population, the urachal lumen is absent or obstructed at its connection to the bladder by an intact layer of mucosa.

CLINICAL MANIFESTATIONS/MORPHOLOGY
PERSISTENT PATENT URACHUS As noted above, the adult urachus may contain a tiny lumen in or out of continuity with the bladder lumen. This does not indicate urachal patency, a term reserved for urachal ducts demonstrating drainage of urine. Patent urachus is a rare condition, easily diagnosed in the newborn by observing urine drainage from the region of the umbilical cord or umbilicus (Fig. 5.9). The opening may be quite small and the urine output may be intermittent. Diagnosis is usually verified by cystography or by filling the bladder with a visible, nontoxic dye and documenting drainage in the umbilical region.

"ACQUIRED" PATENT URACHUS Adults with urinary outflow obstruction and chronically increased intravesicular pressures may develop urine drainage in the periumbilical region. In some instances this represents pressure-induced, acquired patency of a luminal urachus. In other cases it seems more likely that urinary

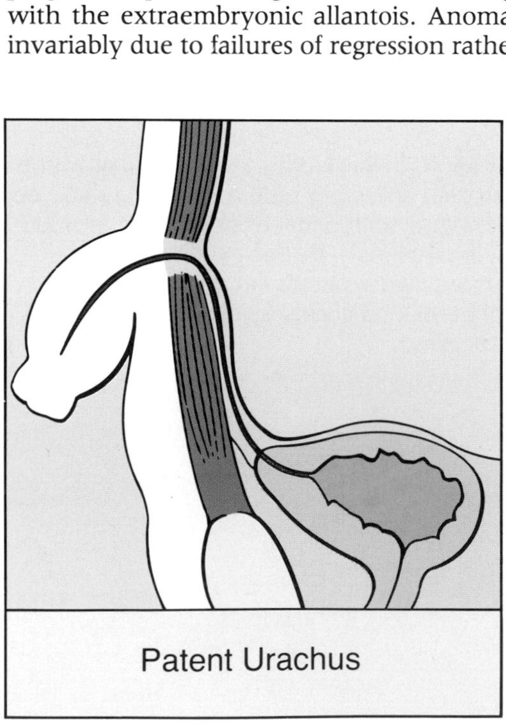

Figure 5.9 Patent urachus is usually detected at birth when urine is noted to be dripping from an enlarged and edematous umbilical stump. An acquired form may occur in patients with elevated intravesicular pressure. (Adapted from Perlmutter et al., 1986)

Patent Urachus

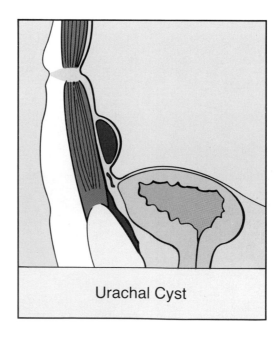

Figure 5.10 In urachal cyst, a portion of the urachus, isolated from both the bladder and the umbilicus, enlarges due to the accumulation of fluid and cellular debris. (Adapted from Perlmutter et al., 1986)

Urachal Cyst

leakage in the region of the bladder dome occurs with the development of a vesicoumbilical fistula, which does not require a urachal remnant for its formation.

URACHAL CYST If the urachus contains an epithelium-lined lumen, cellular debris and mucin may accumulate, expanding the lumen to cystic proportions in a manner analogous to that of epidermal inclusion cysts (Fig. 5.10). A tiny connection to the bladder may permit bacterial infection of the cyst, with resultant tenderness in the midline suprapubic region. The cyst may remain loculated or may drain to the bladder or overlying umbilicus.

URACHAL SINUS When a urachus that contains a lumen is isolated from the bladder lumen but retains continuity with the umbilicus, an external urachal sinus results (Fig. 5.11). These typically remain asymptomatic until they become infected, causing pain, swelling, and discharge. An omphalomesenteric duct remnant may present an identical clinical picture; careful probing of the sinus usually allows distinction. Urachal sinuses curve sharply caudad toward the bladder, whereas omphalomesenteric duct remnants extend directly into the abdominal cavity. Urachal sinuses may also be acquired anomalies caused by rupture of an untreated urachal cyst.

URACHAL DIVERTICULUM If the urachus retains patency with the bladder lumen but ends blindly without continuity with the umbilicus, a urachal diverticulum is formed (Fig. 5.12). These are usually incidental findings at cystography. While therapy is not required if the diverticulum is small and normally contractile, large diverticula or diverticula that expand during voiding should be resected.

Urachal diverticula, like the embryologic urachus, may be partly lined by glandular epithelium. Adenocarcinomas rarely arise in these diverticula and presumably originate from this glandular mucosa. Most adenocarcinomas of the bladder probably develop in areas of glandular metaplasia, however, and may also occur in the dome region. Adenocarcinomas of the bladder and their occasional association with the urachus are discussed in more detail in Chapter 12.

THERAPY As with other congenital sinuslike lesions, such as branchial cleft sinuses, adequate surgical therapy usually requires removal of the entire urachal tract. This should be accomplished without removing the umbilicus.

EXSTROPHY OF THE BLADDER

Exstrophy of the urinary bladder is a rare congenital defect seen in about 1 out of 40,000–50,000 births. No convincing evidence supports a genetic predisposition. In one study, siblings of children with exstrophy had an increased risk over the general population, but the frequency was still only 1 in 200. Marshall and Muecke reported on 26 mothers with exstrophy who gave birth to a total of 33 children, none of whom had this condition.

PATHOGENESIS An abnormally large and persistent cloacal membrane during early embryogenesis probably accounts for the constellation of findings in exstrophy. The persistent cloaca lies beneath the umbilicus on the anterior abdominal wall, where it prevents the convergence of normal wall musculature. If it extends inferiorly, development of external genitalia is also affected. This results in epispadias, accompanied by some degree of penile malformation in the male, and a bifid clitoris with other defects in the female. Later in embryonic development, the cloacal membrane breaks down and the underlying bladder mucosa everts onto the abdominal wall.

CLINICAL MANIFESTATIONS Exstrophy has a definite male predominance, estimated at 5:1. It is a complex developmental defect that involves more than the eversion of the bladder mucosa onto the abdominal wall. Associated anomalies of the abdominal musculature, pelvic girdle, and external genitalia are almost always present. Abnormalities of the lower gastrointestinal tract may also occur.

Exstrophy of the bladder is invariably accompanied by radiographic abnormalities in the pelvic bones. Widening of the pubic symphysis, due to outward rotation of the innominate bones, is most common, often accompanied by lateral displacement (Fig. 5.13).

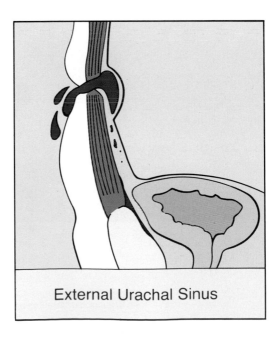

Figure 5.11 In external urachal sinus, a portion of the urachus maintains contact with the umbilicus but is isolated from the bladder. Secondary infection usually leads to symptoms. (Adapted from Perlmutter et al., 1986)

External Urachal Sinus

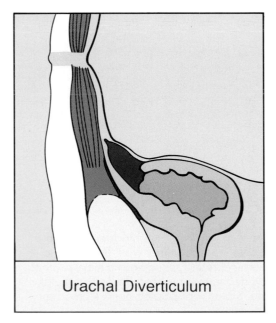

Figure 5.12 In urachal diverticulum, a segment of the urachus remains patent and maintains continuity with the bladder lumen. These are typically small, incidental findings. (Adapted from Perlmutter et al., 1986)

Urachal Diverticulum

MORPHOLOGY In the classic form of the anomaly, the bladder lies everted on the lower abdominal wall with its erythematous, moist mucosa exposed (Fig. 5.14). Ureteral orifices may be easily visible. The pubic bones are separated. A fibrous band connecting the pubic symphysis may be palpated. In males, the penis is epispadiac and deformed to some degree (Fig. 5.14B; also see Fig. 18.23). Typically, it is short and broad with abnormally separated corpora. In severe forms, the corpora may be completely detached. In females, the bladder location is identical to that in males. The labia are separated superiorly, and the clitoris may be bifid. Below the everted bladder mucosa lies an epispadiac urethra. Vaginal anomalies are common and include stenosis, absence, septation, as well as abnormal angulation. The uterus may be bicornuate or duplicated with two separate cervices.

SECONDARY CHANGES The ureters and kidneys are normal at the time of birth, but obstruction at the ureteral orifices may develop secondary to chronic inflammation and infection. This leads to hydronephrosis, often accompanied by pyelonephritis in older children and adults with untreated disease. The anal canal is normally formed in these children, but it lacks proper support due to the widened pelvis. Anal prolapse may occur at birth or may develop later in life.

A serious complication is the development of carcinoma in the exstrophic mucosa. Engel and Wilkinson documented this change in 7.5% of 42 patients with exstrophy. Adenocarcinomas are by far the most common form, although a few patients develop squamous cell carcinomas. The neoplasms presumably arise in zones of glandular or squamous metaplasia that occur secondary to long-

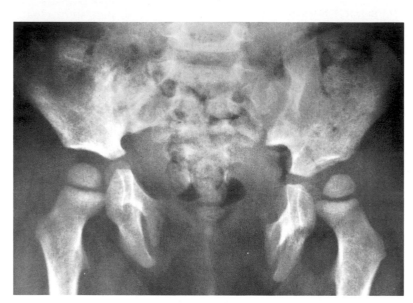

Figure 5.13 Marked widening of the pubic symphysis is highly characteristic of exstrophy of the bladder. This radiographic anomaly may also be seen with less severe defects of the genitourinary system.

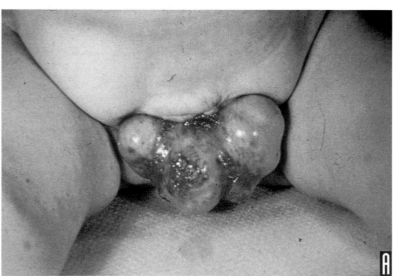

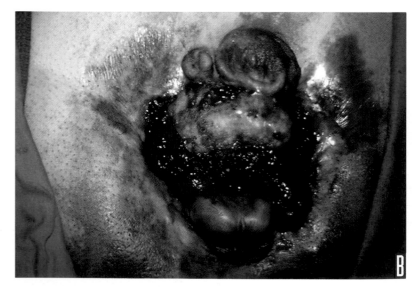

Figure 5.14 **A,** This example of exstrophy of the bladder shows the bladder mucosa everted onto the abdominal wall. **B,** In this adult male about to undergo surgical repair, squamous metaplasia has occurred in part of the everted mucosa, giving it a less vascular appearance. Note the malformed, epispadiac penis located at the lower portion of the exstrophy.

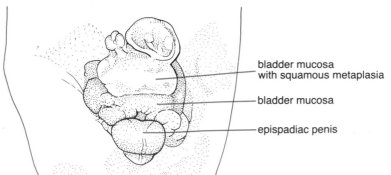

bladder mucosa with squamous metaplasia

bladder mucosa

epispadiac penis

standing inflammation (see Chapter 10). Patients tend to be younger than individuals with carcinomas of the bladder unassociated with exstrophy.

THERAPY Children with exstrophy should be carefully evaluated for primary surgical closure and repair or urinary diversion with ureterosigmoidostomy. The preferred treatment is primary closure and repair, but it requires adequate bladder size, functional detrusor muscle, and an absence of other contraindicating anomalies. Even very small reconstructed bladders will grow with the patient and function properly if the bladder musculature is intact. Primary closure, accompanied by closure of the associated pelvic ring defect, is best performed on newborns. Subsequent surgical procedures at a later date may be directed at correcting urinary incontinence and ureteral reflux, followed by repair of genital anomalies.

CLOACAL EXSTROPHY

This extremely rare anomaly is estimated to occur in approximately 1 in 200,000 live births. As with bladder exstrophy, there is no obvious genetic predisposition. Unlike the former, however, cloacal exstrophy affects both sexes with equal frequency.

PATHOGENESIS Cloacal exstrophy results from an abnormally large cloacal membrane. The membrane ruptures before the urogenital septum has formed, resulting in an exstrophic mass that contains both vesicular and intestinal elements.

CLINICAL MANIFESTATIONS The anomalies associated with cloacal exstrophy are similar to those of bladder exstrophy, except that they are much more severe. In addition, the everted mass contains both urinary and intestinal elements, and there are other, often severe intestinal malformations.

MORPHOLOGY A complex exstrophic mass is present below the umbilicus. Two hemibladders are separated by a zone of colonic mucosa, apparently representing the cecum. The ileum enters the latter structure. A caudal colonic pouch is in continuity with the intestinal mucosa inferiorly, extending to end blindly in an imperforate anus. In males, the corpora are usually widely separated as two small masses of erectile tissue. Less commonly, an intact epispadiac penis may be formed. In females, an absent or bifid clitoris is common, as is an absent or duplicated vagina. Associated anomalies include duplication of the vena cava, pelvic bone deformities such as spina bifida, myelomeningocele, hydrocephalus, cardiopulmonary malformations, and midgut defects, including a short ileal segment with malabsorption.

THERAPY This is a severe defect that, if accompanied by other anomalies, may be incompatible with prolonged life. Less severely affected patients are candidates for aggressive surgical intervention with ileostomy, closure of the pelvic bone defect, and anastomosis of the hemibladders. Urinary incontinence may be corrected later. Genital anomalies should be carefully assessed; sex reassignment should be considered for males with severe defects who are unlikely to achieve sexual function.

DIVERTICULUM OF THE BLADDER

Diverticula of the bladder are common lesions of diverse origin. Most are small, asymptomatic, or only mildly symptomatic, and require no therapy. Larger, more symptomatic diverticula or those developing secondary complications require surgical intervention.

PATHOGENESIS Except for those arising from urachal remnants, most diverticula of the bladder are acquired outpouchings secondary to outflow obstruction with increased intravesicular pressure (Fig. 5.15). A few reports of diverticula in children presumably represent congenital lesions, mostly arising from the trigone area.

CLINICAL MANIFESTATIONS Occasionally, large diverticula of the bladder may be discovered incidentally (see Fig. 5.15). Typically, however, patients complain of an abdominal mass. They may also need to void again shortly after emptying the bladder due to paradoxical expansion of the diverticulum during bladder contraction, with subsequent reverse flow into the bladder after urination. Narrow-necked diverticula may develop stasis with secondary infection and/or stone formation (Fig. 5.16).

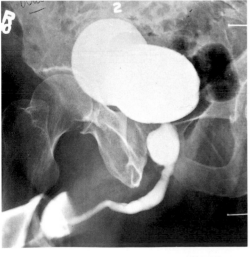

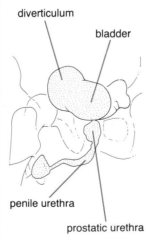

diverticulum

bladder

penile urethra

prostatic urethra

Figure 5.15 The contrast-filled mass arising from the lateral aspect of the bladder and extending superiorly in this voiding cystogram is a large diverticulum. The contrast-filled defect below the bladder represents a prior transurethral resection. Increased intravesicular pressure due to prostatic hyperplasia probably produced the diverticulum seen in this patient.

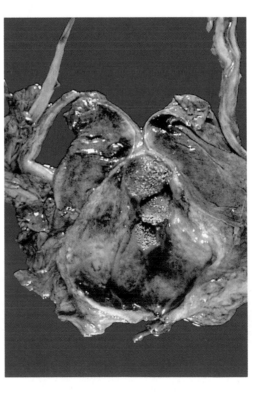

Figure 5.16 This bladder has been opened to demonstrate a large diverticulum containing several stones. They develop due to urinary stasis in diverticula with narrow openings.

MORPHOLOGY Bladder diverticula almost always exhibit microscopic abnormalities. Chronic inflammation is usually present in the mucosa or wall and may be accompanied by zones of squamous metaplasia. Variable numbers of smooth muscle fibers may be present, alternating with stromal fibrosis, but a well formed muscular layer typical of normal bladder wall is absent.

Rarely, carcinomas develop in diverticula, where they may produce filling defects in radiographic studies (Fig. 5.17). Such tumors may be difficult to biopsy cystoscopically. All forms of carcinoma occur, with transitional cell and squamous types predominating (see Chapter 12). Unlike neoplasms arising in urachal diverticula, adenocarcinomas occur infrequently.

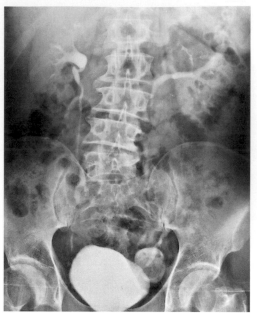 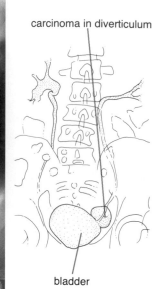

carcinoma in diverticulum

bladder

Figure 5.17 IVP demonstrating a filling defect in a bladder diverticulum that strongly suggests a neoplasm obstructing the lumen. The diverticulum was resected and contained a squamous cell carcinoma.

SECTION III

Obstructive Uropathy

CHAPTER 6

Hydronephrosis and Urolithiasis

HYDRONEPHROSIS

Hydronephrosis refers to pelvicalyceal dilatation and associated renal parenchymal atrophy resulting from urinary tract obstruction (UTO). It may occur with or without bladder dilatation and/or ureteral dilatation (hydroureter), depending on the cause and location of the obstruction. Clinicopathologic findings depend on whether the obstruction is unilateral or bilateral, partial or complete, and intermittent or continuous.

PATHOGENESIS The renal parenchymal atrophy associated with hydronephrosis is produced by transmission of high pelvic pressures back through the collecting ducts into the cortex. Diminished plasma flow in the inner medulla results from compression of the renal medullary vasculature; interference with venous drainage is a major factor in producing parenchymal loss. Glomerular filtration continues for a variable time, even after complete obstruction. The pelvicalyceal system, therefore, becomes dilated. Part of the filtrate diffuses back into the interstitium and perirenal spaces, ultimately returning to the lymphatic and venous systems. A decrease in the glomerular filtration rate follows the initial tubular functional defects. Experimentally, recovery of the glomerular filtration rate rapidly follows relief of up to one hour of complete obstruction but is delayed if obstruction persists for even a few hours.

The pediatric kidney appears to be much more vulnerable than the adult kidney to progression of hydronephrosis and parenchymal damage whenever it is subjected to volume expansion. Experimental data suggest that the larger-capacity adult pelvis requires more volume to become distended and, once overdistended, is subjected to a slower rate of overstretching and pressure increase than the smaller pediatric pelvis. Consequently, more than 50% of adults apparently lack progression of hydronephrosis, but silent progression of hydronephrosis, such as with ureteropelvic junction obstruction (see Chapter 7), is recognized in children.

CLINICAL MANIFESTATIONS Early symptoms may be related to the basic cause of the UTO—for example, bladder symptoms with benign prostatic hyperplasia or renal colic secondary to ureteral calculi. With acute obstruction, distention of the collecting system or renal capsule may result in pain. Early symptoms of bilateral partial obstruction are functional and include nocturia and polyuria secondary to inability to concentrate urine, as well as distal tubular

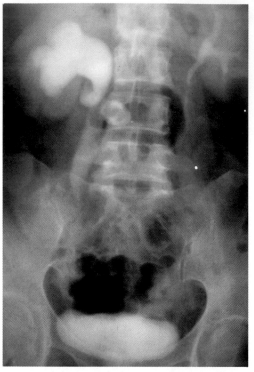
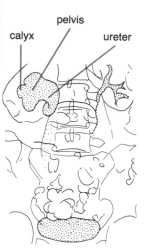

Figure 6.1 On this IVP, the normal left renal collecting system contrasts with the markedly dilated right renal pelvis and upper ureter. The calyces are distended and clubbed. The cortex is minimally involved. This moderate hydronephrosis is due to obstruction by a stricture in the midureter. (Courtesy of H. Hawkins, MD, Cincinnati, Ohio)

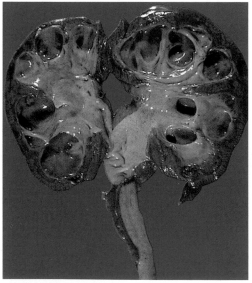
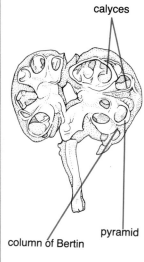

Figure 6.2 Hydronephrosis with progressive cystic dilatation of the calyces has resulted in a cup-shaped appearance of the pyramids. Columns of Bertin are compressed, and there is diffuse cortical thinning. UTO in this child was secondary to stricture of the ureteropelvic junction.

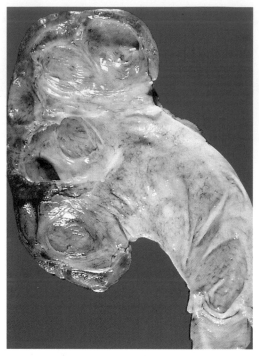

Figure 6.3 At this advanced stage of hydronephrosis, the cystically dilated pelvicalyceal system is surrounded only by a thin rim of renal parenchyma. Pyramids are obliterated, and there is marked cortical atrophy.

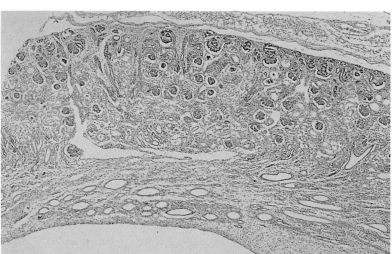

Figure 6.4 Histologic changes secondary to UTO in this 32-week-gestation newborn with ureteropelvic junction obstruction are mild, although marked deformity of the papilla indicates significant hydronephrosis. Collecting ducts are dilated and compressed. The cortex shows orderly nephrogenesis, with more immature glomeruli and tubules at the lobule periphery.

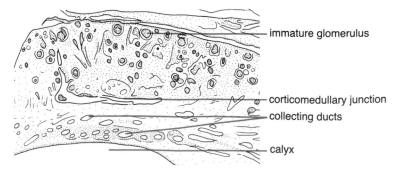

acidosis and renal salt wasting. Hypertension may occur as a late manifestation of hydronephrosis. Unilateral hydronephrosis secondary to complete or partial obstruction may remain clinically silent and be discovered incidentally during intravenous pyelography (Fig. 6.1). Complete bilateral obstruction results in oliguria or anuria. As a general rule, serious, irreversible renal damage occurs after approximately three weeks of complete obstruction or three months of incomplete obstruction. Early treatment, therefore, improves the outcome for patients with obstructive uropathy.

MORPHOLOGY The gross appearance of hydronephrosis can be quite variable. The kidney may be only slightly increased in size or massively enlarged. Early changes are predominantly those of pelvicalyceal dilatation. With bilateral hydronephrosis due to low obstruction, pelvicalyceal dilatation frequently is mild by the time uremia becomes clinically apparent. In addition, when UTO is sudden and complete, renal parenchymal atrophy may occur with only mild pelvicalyceal dilatation. At an intermediate stage, the apices of the

pyramids are progressively blunted until they appear cup-shaped, and the columns of Bertin are compressed (Fig. 6.2). Moderately advanced hydronephrosis may superficially resemble a multicystic kidney. However, free communication between the pelvis and apparent cysts confirms that these are dilated calyces. Pelvic dilatation may be predominantly extrarenal or inward with greater destruction of renal parenchyma. At an advanced stage, the kidney is transformed into a thin-walled cystic structure that has a diameter up to 15–20 cm (Fig. 6.3). Renal parenchyma is markedly atrophic, with extreme cortical thinning and obliteration of the pyramids.

Microscopically, the earliest changes of hydronephrosis are characterized by dilatation of the tubular system, particularly the collecting ducts (Fig. 6.4). Atrophy of proximal convoluted tubules ensues, while glomeruli are spared (Fig. 6.5). Rupture of tubules, particularly near the corticomedullary junction, leads to extravasation of tubular Tamm-Horsfall protein into the interstitium or tubulovenous anastomosis (Fig. 6.6). Tubular rupture evokes a fibroinflammatory response. Cortical interstitial fibrosis is usually

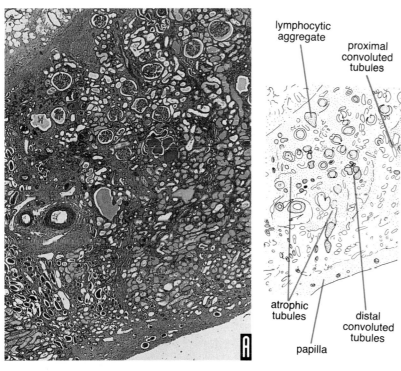

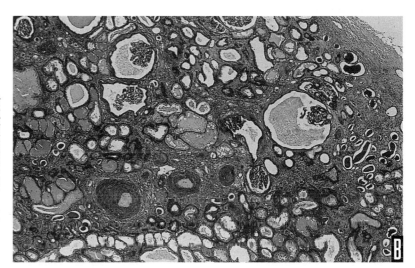

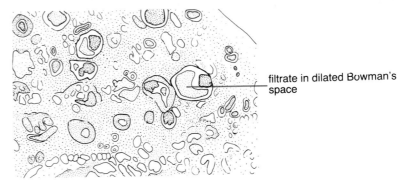

Figure 6.5 Progressive hydronephrosis results in cortical changes. **A,** In this histologic section, glomerular filtrate is present within dilated proximal convoluted tubules, and distal convoluted tubules contain waxy casts. Foci of tubular atrophy and mild lymphocytic interstitial infiltrates are present (PAS stain). **B,** Although glomeruli are preserved at this stage, dilatation of Bowman's space with filtrate accumulation is present.

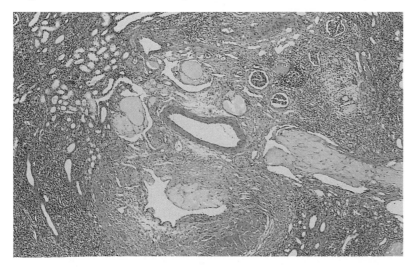

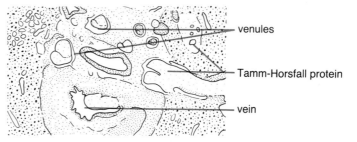

Figure 6.6 Tubular disruption may occur with severe UTO. Large intraluminal and intramural masses of Tamm-Horsfall protein are present within numerous veins and dilated venules at the corticomedullary junction as a result of tubulovenous anastomoses. In response to interstitial extravasation of Tamm-Horsfall protein from ruptured tubules, localized fibroblastic proliferation and marked chronic inflammation are present.

mild. Interstitial inflammation is also generally mild unless pyelonephritis is superimposed. With chronicity, arteries become sclerotic and glomeruli are hyalinized. With advanced hydronephrosis, medullae become fibrotic (Fig. 6.7).

GIANT HYDRONEPHROSIS AND HYDROURETERONEPHROSIS

Giant hydronephrosis describes massive dilatation of the kidney and renal pelvis. In adults, it is defined as a kidney containing one liter or more of fluid in the renal collecting system. In children, it is defined as a kidney containing the equivalent of one day's urinary output or, alternatively, a volume of fluid more than 4% of body weight at birth or more than 2% of body weight at puberty. Giant hydronephrosis is usually produced by a congenital lesion; the most common cause in children is ureteropelvic junction obstruction (Fig. 6.8) (see Chapter 7). Radiologic criteria for the diagnosis include a kidney that occupies the hemiabdomen, a kidney that meets or crosses the midline, or a kidney at least five vertebrae in length.

With giant hydroureteronephrosis, distal obstruction, which is invariably ureteral, causes the ureter to reach massive proportions, completely overshadowing the dilated renal pelvis in size and volume. It has been described secondary to ureteral ectopias, with or without duplication anomalies, and in rare cases of trauma (Fig. 6.9). Partial obstruction of the contralateral ureter may occur, as may traumatic rupture and spontaneous or iatrogenic infection. The frequent lack of superimposed infection, however, allows the ureter to attain massive proportions. Most patients present with an asymptomatic abdominal mass, occasionally with pain and hematuria.

UROLITHIASIS

Urolithiasis, or calculus formation within the urinary tract, may either be a primary cause of UTO or a consequence of the urinary stasis and/or complicating urinary tract infection associated with UTO. UTO increases susceptibility to both infection and stone formation. Indeed, the obstructed kidney is particularly prone to infection (see discussion of pyelonephritis, Chapter 9).

PATHOGENESIS One of the most important factors causing calculus formation is an increased concentration of stone constituents, which may involve an increased production and excretion of stone-forming substances due to a familial or hereditary predisposition. Examples of such inborn errors of metabolism include gout, cystinuria, and primary hyperoxaluria. While 15%–20% of gout cases are complicated by renal calculi, only 6%–14% of urolithiasis cases are due to uric acid stones, and only 25% of uric acid stones are associated with gout. Cystine stones constitute approximately 1%–3% of cases. The vast majority of stones (75%–80%) are radiopaque and contain calcium with oxalate (13%–33% of stones) or phosphate (20% of stones). The causes of hypercalciuria, with or without hypercalcemia, are varied, but when both are present pri-

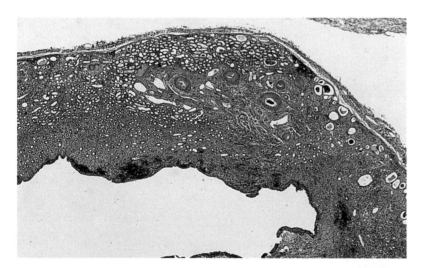

Figure 6.7 This end-stage hydronephrotic kidney has prominent medullary fibrosis and a thinned, atrophic cortex with few residual foci of functioning glomeruli and preserved tubules (Masson's trichrome stain).

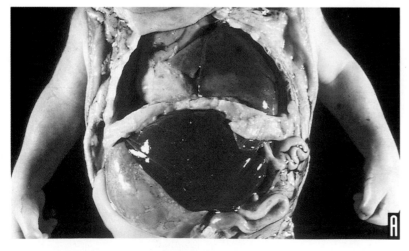

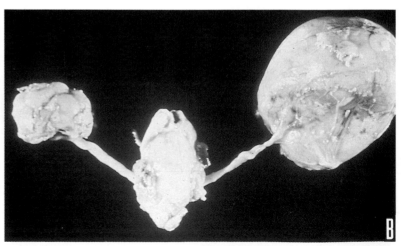

Figure 6.8 A, Giant hydronephrosis in this male neonate with multiple cardiopulmonary anomalies was due to ureteropelvic junction obstruction. The right kidney occupies the hemiabdomen and pushes the liver upward and medially. **B,** The (anatomic) right kidney has been transformed into a fluid-filled mass approximately five times the size of the normal (anatomic) left kidney. (This is the same case as Figure 7.6.)

mary hyperparathyroidism should be considered, particularly since stones occur in approximately 50% of these patients.

Alterations in urinary pH may also predispose to stone formation. For example, excretion of an acidic urine (pH < 5.5) favors the formation of radiolucent uric acid stones and radiopaque cystine stones. Certain bacterial urinary tract infections, such as those associated with the urea-splitting organism *Proteus*, increase the urinary concentration of ammonia; the resulting alkaline urine leads to precipitation of magnesium ammonium phosphate. These so-called triple stones account for approximately 15% of cases and are often some of the largest stones.

All calculi contain a mucoprotein, mucopolysaccharide matrix. Changes in the urinary concentration of this stone matrix may also predispose to stone formation. Urinary colloidal substances probably play a major role in holding crystalloids in solution. Defective urine glycoprotein crystallization inhibitors have been identified as an important reason for calcium renal stones. For example, deficiency of gamma carboxyglutamic acid from an acidic urinary glycoprotein inhibitor that is functionally and immunologically different from Tamm-Horsfall protein allows growth of calcium oxalate crystals.

A final factor involved in precipitation of calculi is the existence of a nucleus of crystallization. This nidus may be a crystalloid or a foreign body such as an indwelling catheter, a bacterial mass, cellular detritus, blood coagula, or fibrin.

Bladder calculi may be either primary or secondary, representing passage of a renal or ureteral stone. The pathogenesis and chemical composition of intravesical stones is similar to that of renal calculi.

For example, bladder infection with urea-splitting bacteria produces an alkaline urine, which favors the precipitation of magnesium or calcium ammonium phosphate.

CLINICAL MANIFESTATIONS In the general population, urolithiasis occurs with an incidence of 0.1%–6%, with a greater frequency in males; most patients are over 30 years of age. Urolithiasis is unilateral in 80% of cases. Favored sites of stone formation are the renal pelves/calyces (nephrolithiasis) or the bladder. Bladder calculi usually occur in patients over 40 years of age. They are most often asymptomatic but may cause symptoms related to chronic irritation, including dysuria, pyuria, and hematuria, or frequency and urgency related to bladder neck obstruction.

MORPHOLOGY In the majority of cases of nephrolithiasis, stones are small (2–3 mm), smooth, or irreglar masses of spicules and are often multiple. Phosphate stones are gray, either hard or soft, crumbly, often irregularly shaped, and may be large (staghorn calculi). The central core may be oxalate or urate. Calcium oxalate stones are hard, have a dark surface, and are smooth or nodular. Uric acid stones are hard, yellow-brown, smooth, and rounded; they are usually multiple, and may be up to 2 cm in diameter (Fig. 6.10). Cystine stones are yellowish and waxy, smooth, rounded, small, and are usually multiple.

Small stones may obstruct the ureteropelvic junction or may pass into the ureter, producing renal colic and ureteral obstruction (Fig. 6.11). Large stones remain in the renal pelvis and may be silent or

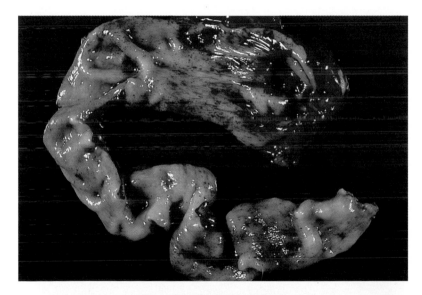

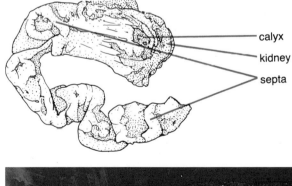

Figure 6.9 This specimen from a two-year-old girl with ureteral ectopia and duplication anomaly shows a giant hydroureter, with the attached focally dysplastic upper pole of the kidney shrunken from chronic pyelonephritis. The massively dilated ureter is tortuous and appears to be kinked, with mucosal septations.

calyx
kidney
septa

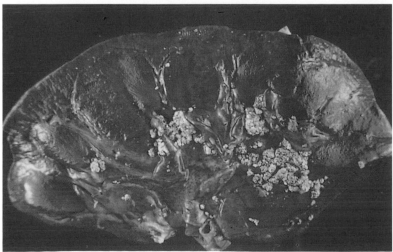

Figure 6.10 The numerous, small, smooth, rounded, hard-appearing yellow-brown calculi present in the renal pelvis and calyces of this patient with nephrolithiasis are typical of uric acid stones.

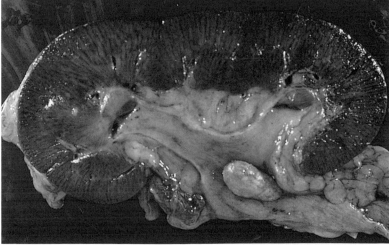

Figure 6.11 Small calculi may produce UTO. In this specimen, obstruction of the ureteropelvic junction has caused early changes of hydronephrosis with blunting of the renal papillary tips.

cause hematuria (Fig. 6.12). Staghorn calculi are large, branched stones that form a cast of the pelvicalyceal system and are usually nonobstructive (Fig. 6.13).

Vesical calculi may be single or multiple and are frequently large, rounded stones that fill the bladder (Fig. 6.14). A nonspecific form of cystitis (see Chapter 10) characterized by precipitation of urinary salts, particularly phosphates, is termed *encrusted cystitis*. Grossly, it appears as focal or diffuse crystalline gray-white precipitates on the bladder mucosa (Fig. 6.15). Microscopically, partially calcified crystals, which may be associated with stone matrix, are present on and within the mucosa (Fig. 6.16).

ASSOCIATED COMPLICATIONS Patients with metabolic disorders may develop tubulointerstitial renal disease. Gouty nephropathy is characterized by tophus formation in the renal medullae (Fig. 6.17). Amorphous or elongated crystals form in collecting tubules, where the urine is more acidic, and cause tubular destruction with foreign body giant cell reaction, chronic inflammation, and fibrosis (Fig. 6.18). Primary hyperoxaluria manifests clinically in early childhood. Oxalates form calcium oxalate stones; they also deposit within tubules, causing dilatation, damage, and atrophy (Fig. 6.19).

Hypercalcemia, particularly when due to primary hyperparathyroidism, may also result in nephrocalcinosis. Radiologic nephrocal-

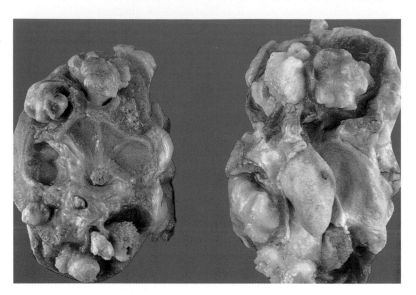

Figure 6.12 These large renal calculi were nonobstructive, forming as a consequence of clinically silent, unilateral UTO. The kidney shows end-stage hydronephrosis.

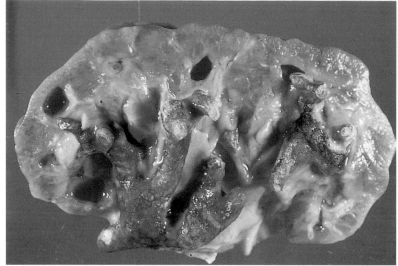

Figure 6.13 The staghorn calculus in this kidney is somewhat fragmented but conforms to the configuration of the pelvis and calyces.

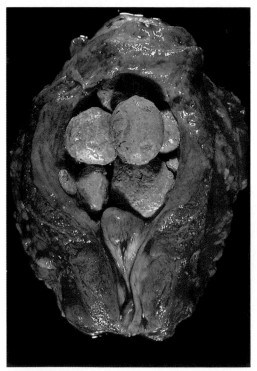

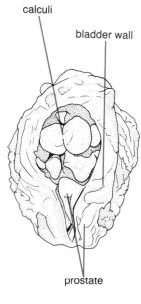

calculi

bladder wall

prostate

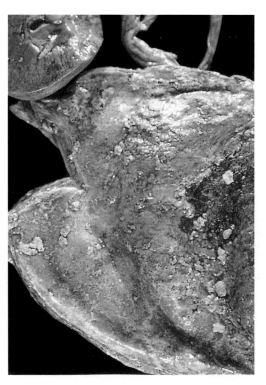

Figure 6.15 In encrusted cystitis, urinary salts crystallize without forming calculi. In this case, the bladder mucosa is diffusely coated with gray-white precipitates.

Figure 6.14 Multiple, large, rounded calculi fill the bladder. The patient had chronic urinary stasis with bladder infections secondary to marked benign prostatic hyperplasia. The muscular wall of the bladder is hypertrophied secondary to the chronic outlet obstruction.

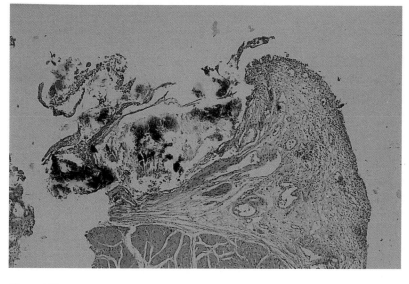

Figure 6.16 Microscopically, partially calcified crystals in encrusted cystitis adhere to the urothelium and are embedded within the edematous, chronically inflamed lamina propria.

Figure 6.17 The grossly visible yellow-white flecks and streaks in the medulla are deposits of urate crystals. The nodular accumulation is a tophus.

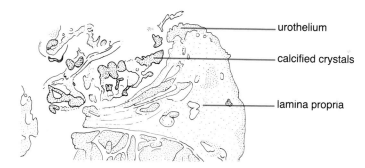

urothelium
calcified crystals
lamina propria

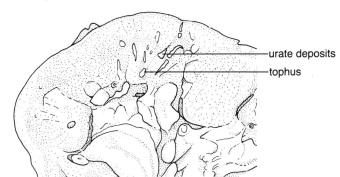

urate deposits
tophus

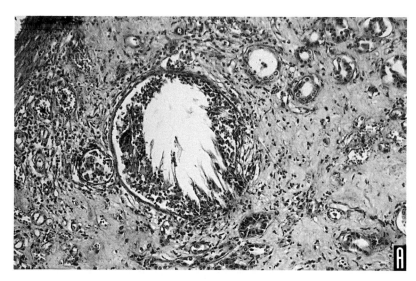

Figure 6.18 A, In gouty nephropathy, needlelike spaces within a dilated, partially disrupted collecting duct represent urate crystals that have dissolved out from this formalin-fixed, routinely processed tissue. Acute inflammation and a foreign body giant cell are present.

B, Progressive accumulation of urate crystals and destruction of collecting ducts lead to parenchymal tophus formation. Interstitial crystalline deposits are surrounded by numerous foreign body giant cells; marked acute and chronic inflammation occurs.

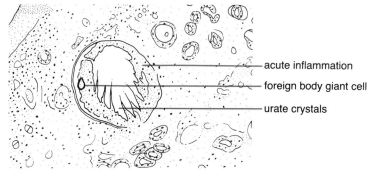

acute inflammation
foreign body giant cell
urate crystals

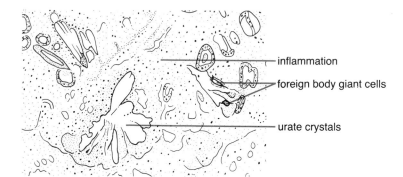

inflammation
foreign body giant cells
urate crystals

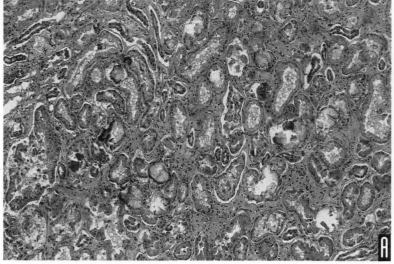

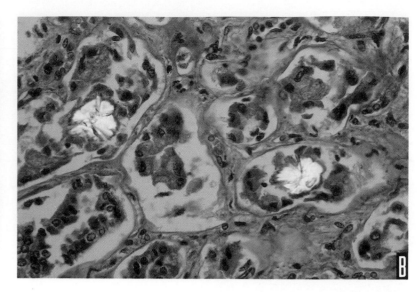

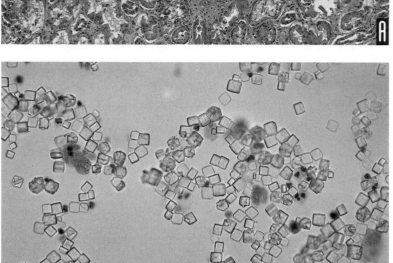

Figure 6.19 A, Large numbers of oxalate crystals deposit in proximal convoluted tubules in primary hyperoxaluria. Variable amounts can also be observed in acute tubular necrosis of diverse etiologies, including ethylene glycol poisoning and methoxyfluorane exposure. **B,** Polarized light facilitates recognition and quantitation of the birefringent oxalate crystals. **C,** Calcium oxalate crystals present in the Papanicolaou-stained urine sediment have a characteristic centrally located "X" formation. The anucleate cells with granular cytoplasm are necrotic proximal convoluted tubular epithelial cells and indicate renal parenchymal damage.

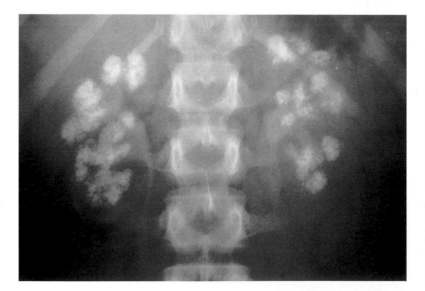

Figure 6.20 Linear calicifications radiating from the papillary tips on a plain film of the abdomen characterize this classic and striking example of nephrocalcinosis. The cortex is spared and the collecting system is normal. Calcification may be sloughed and form urinary stones.

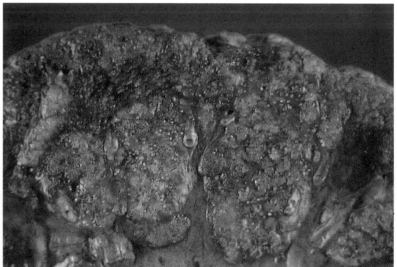

Figure 6.21 In cases of primary hyperparathyroidism, severe nephrocalcinosis may occur and be visible both grossly and radiologically. The cut surface of this kidney has diffuse granular and nodular yellow-tan calcium deposits in the cortex and medulla.

cinosis (Fig. 6.20) is rare, whereas histologic evidence is present in 15%–20% of adults and 8% of children at autopsy. This parenchymal deposition of calcium may cause azotemia and tubular dysfunction or may be clinically silent (Fig. 6.21). Microscopically, the tubular basement membranes (particularly proximal convoluted segments), Bowman's capsule, hyalinized glomeruli, peritubular interstitium, and arterial walls calcify, and intraluminal concretions occur, especially in collecting ducts (Fig. 6.22). There is associated tubular atrophy, interstitial fibrosis, as well as chronic inflammation. Clinical and experimental data also indicate that hypercalcemia can depress renal function, particularly tubular

concentrating ability, leading to azotemia without permanent structural change.

Secondary hyperparathyroidism, in which serum calcium levels are below normal or normal, may also produce striking nephrocalcinosis. Conditions that may cause significant renal parenchymal calcification, with or without stones, and that may or may not produce hypercalcemia include: (1) increased absorption of calcium (sarcoidosis, milk-alkali syndrome, vitamin D intoxication), (2) deossification of skeleton (multiple myeloma, osseous metastases), (3) dystrophic calcification, and (4) miscellaneous disorders (renal tubular acidosis, hypochloremic alkalosis) (Fig.6.23).

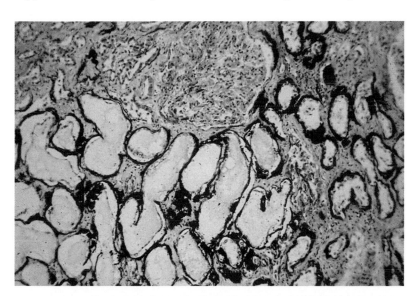

Figure 6.22 In this H&E stained section, basement membranes of proximal convoluted tubules and Bowman's capsule appear blue and markedly thickened due to heavy calcium deposition.

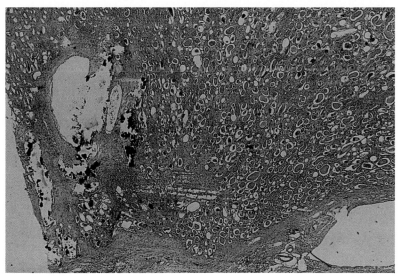

Figure 6.23 Large calcium deposits are present within the lumina of dilated medullary collecting ducts of this hydronephrotic kidney. Microscopic parenchymal calcifications are a common incidental finding that can result from a variety of clinical conditions. Papillary nephrocalcinosis, however, is frequently related to hypercalciuric states.

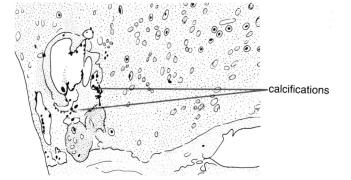

CHAPTER 7

Ureteropelvic Junction Obstruction

Ureteropelvic junction obstruction (UPJO) commonly afflicts the pediatric population and is the predominant form of urinary tract obstruction (UTO) in children. In most cases it is congenital and appears spontaneously. A hereditary as well as familial incidence, however, has been reported in humans, and genetic transmission has been demonstrated in animal models.

In general, 20% of UPJO cases are bilateral, although among infants bilaterality increases to approximately 30%. An asynchronous presentation may occur. UPJO is the most common cause of neonatal hydronephrosis; after the newborn period UPJO with hydronephrosis supplants multicystic dysplastic kidney as the cause of a flank mass.

PATHOGENESIS Although most cases are considered congenital in origin, the etiology of UPJO is frequently unknown. Reported causes of congenital UPJO include intrinsic or functional abnormalities of the ureteropelvic junction (UPJ), mucosal folds, extrapelvic adhesions or extrinsic bands, an abnormally situated junction between the pelvis and ureter, and aberrant vessels to the lower pole of the kidney. Also offered as possible pathogenetic mechanisms are ischemic hypoplasia, localized developmental arrest secondary to in-utero compression by fetal vessels, incomplete recanalization of the proximal ureter, and increased collagen or disordered muscle at the UPJ. On the basis of operative findings in children, causes of UPJO have been divided into intrinsic abormalities of the UPJ (70%), extrinsic bands (10%), and extrinsic vessels (20%). However, some studies have shown that at least one third of UPJO cases in infants and children have accompanying aberrant vessels. In comparison, up to 50% of adults with UPJO have an associated lower-pole vessel.

The pathogenetic role played by aberrant renal vessels remains controversial. Multiple renal arteries have been found in 28% and aberrant renal arteries in as many as 25% of autopsies (Fig. 7.1). Lower-pole renal arteries originating from the aorta or renal artery occur in approximately 6% of all kidneys, although the incidence in association with UPJO is approximately 45%. In cases where the lower-pole vessels are the primary cause of UPJO, division or transposition of the vessels without pyeloplasty is curative.

In most instances, aberrant vessels are not the primary cause of hydronephrosis, but are felt to aggravate the obstruction. Normally, the kidney ascends posterior to the renal arteries, and the pelvis rotates from an anterior to a medial position. UPJO due to an intrinsic/functional blockage that interferes with transmission of peristaltic waves from the pelvis to the ureter, results in pelvic distention and renal rotation with subsequent anterior lie of the pelvis. In the presence of "aberrant" lower-pole vessels, the UPJ becomes angulated. Defects of the medial rotation of the renal pelvis, which may be permanent (congenital) or transient (acquired), make the UPJ vulnerable to obstruction. In this form of ureterovascular hydronephrosis associated with polar, rather than hilar, insertion of the lower-pole artery, the renal pelvis and UPJ protrude anteriorly between the middle and lower segmental vessels, bulging over the lower anterior segmental vessels instead of under, as in other forms of hydronephrosis. The anterior segmental branch may not be aberrant in all cases.

In patients with acquired UPJO, a malignant cause, such as transitional cell carcinoma (see Chapter 11) or metastatic carcinoma (see Chapter 8), should be ruled out. Benign causes of acquired UPJO are uncommon. These have included vesicoureteral reflux with chronic periureteritis and tortuosity of the pyeloureteral junction as well as renal ptosis associated with "innocent" aberrant renal vessels. Inflammatory lesions (see Chapter 9), such as xanthogranulomatous pyelonephritis and eosinophilic ureteritis, have been reported as a cause of UPJO. Etiologic anatomic abnormalities have included large renal cysts (see Chapter 3) and aortic aneurysms that cause ureteral compression, renal rotation, or perianeurysmal fibrosis (see Chapter 8).

CLINICAL MANIFESTATIONS   In children, UPJO is slightly more common in males (1.7:1) and most frequently involves the left side. Among newborns, 75% present with an asymptomatic abdominal mass. If recognition is delayed, bleeding and urinary tract infection (UTI) become more common presenting features. Abdominal pain is present in 35%–58% of patients. UTI is more common in females. Approximately 60% of patients between the ages of one month and six years present with UTI, with or without gross painless hematuria. After six years of age, however, flank or upper abdominal pain, which is frequently accompanied by UTI, is present in approximately 70% of patients. The pain is frequently intermittent and may be associated with nausea and vomiting. Most patients presenting with hematuria are between 4 and 12 years of age. Occasionally, UPJO manifests as failure to thrive.

UPJO in adults occurs with equal frequency in males and females. Patients may range from 18–65 years of age (71% are younger than 32 years) at the time of diagnosis. Flank pain, UTI, hematuria, and hypertension are usual clinical manifestations. A history of urolithiasis is common. Diagnosis is often delayed, reportedly averaging almost four years from the onset of symptoms. Approximately 10% of cases in adults are an incidental finding.

The intravenous pyelogram (IVP) may demonstrate the typical box-shaped, dilated renal pelvis and narrow UPJ or may reveal nonvisualization (Fig. 7.2). Calyceal crescents, a reliable sign of upper UTO, require preserved renal concentrating ability and indicate that some function is recoverable. For equivocal cases, a diuretic renogram with furosemide should be performed. The resulting increase in urine flow produces pain and increases the hydronephrosis. Intravenous digital angiography may reveal an associated accessory lower-pole vessel (Fig. 7.3).

MORPHOLOGY   The stenotic UPJ is typically probe patent (Fig. 7.4). Extrarenal dilatation of the pelvis is also characteristic, frequently producing a large, bulbous, saccular structure (Fig. 7.5). In most cases, hydronephrosis has progressed to an advanced stage (Fig. 7.6).

The normal adult renal pelvic and ureteral muscle bundles are similarly arranged in two crude coats that are often not clearly defined: an inner coat of longitudinal fibers and bundles with a spi-

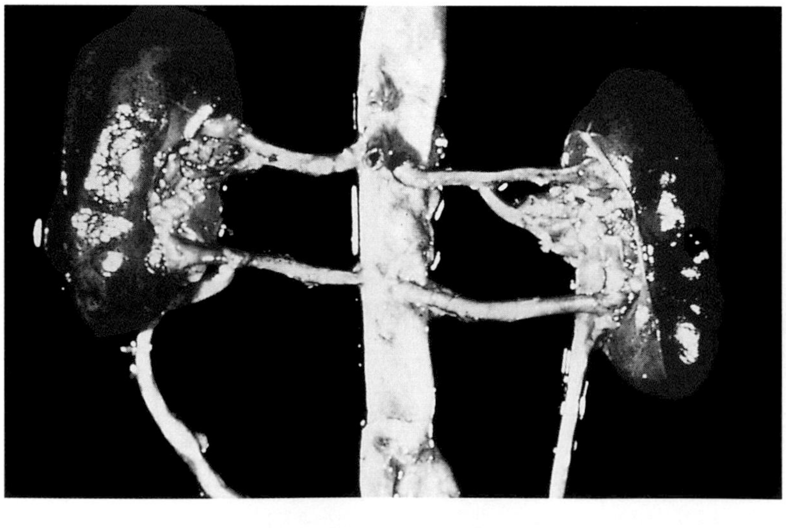

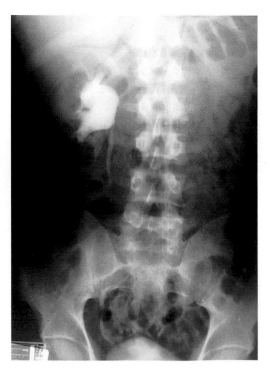

Figure 7.2 In this patient with UPJO, IVP demonstrates a square, dilated pelvis. Instead of the normal funnel-shaped, inferior ureteropelvic region, the UPJ is narrow and located high on the pelvis.

Figure 7.1 Multiple, frequently aberrant renal arteries are a common incidental autopsy finding. This patient had bilateral double renal arteries originating from the aorta, with anomalous branching of the right upper artery. The right renal pelvis has a normal medial position. Although the lower renal artery crosses the ureter posteriorly, there is no evidence of UPJO.

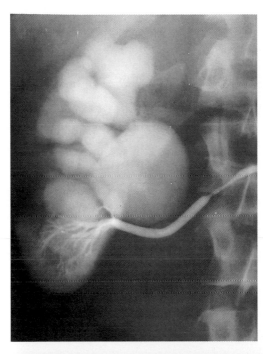

Figure 7.3 Selective angiogram in a patient with UPJO shows a lower-pole renal artery traversing the inferior aspect of the contrast-filled pelvis. IVP showed a narrow UPJ with extrinsic compression corresponding to the crossing vessel.

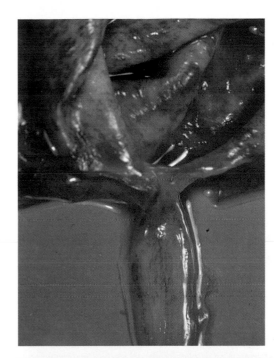

Figure 7.4 Probe patency of the UPJ is typically demonstrable grossly. In this case, the stenotic lumen at the UPJ is continuous with the normal ureter (below) and markedly dilated renal pelvis (above).

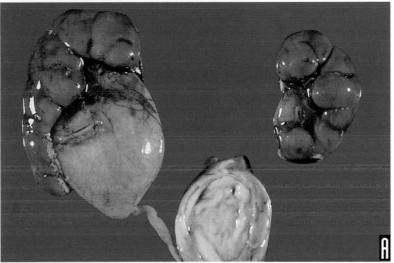

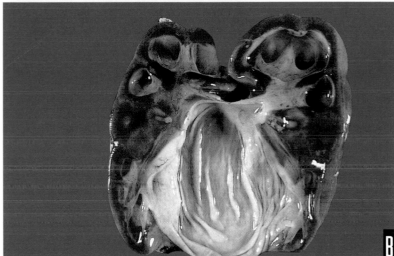

Figure 7.5 A, In this specimen from a female neonate, obstructive changes due to stenosis of the UPJ are asymmetric. In contrast to the right kidney, which has marked hydronephrosis, the left kidney has only mild dilatation of the renal pelvis. **B,** The bivalved right kidney shows extrarenal saccular dilatation of the pelvis as well as caliectasis and parenchymal changes of hydronephrosis.

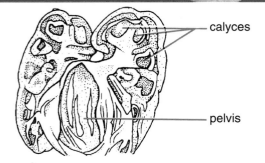

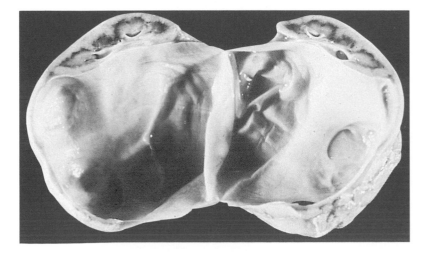

Figure 7.6 Unilateral UPJO in this newborn male has produced severe hydronephrosis. A thin rim of renal parenchyma surrounds the massively enlarged, bulbous-appearing pelvis. (This is the same case as Figure 6.8.)

ral course and an outer coat with a circular pattern (Fig. 7.7). At the UPJ there is a localized increase of muscle bulk but no significant anatomic definition, and tangential sections show the normal complex, spiral, basket-weave pattern (Fig. 7.8).

A variety of microscopic changes have been reported in cases of congenital UPJO. These have included: (l) opening and elongation of spiral muscle bundles, with an excess of longitudinal muscle resulting in muscular incoordination; (2) decreased pelviureteric muscle, which is associated with a crossing accessory renal blood vessel in 35% of cases; (3) excess submucosal fibrous tissue; (4) muscular hypertrophy with submucosal fibrosis; and (5) abnor-

mally distinct inner and outer muscular coats without the normal interwoven pattern.

From a light-microscopic and ultrastructural study of congenital UPJO in children, it was concluded that the obstruction represents a congenital stricture resulting from an inelastic collar of collagen that impedes urine flow. The majority of cases showed diminished, and frequently maloriented, UPJ muscle with increased collagen between and around muscle cells (Figs. 7.9, 7.10). A spectrum of light-microscopic changes was noted, however, including variable inflammation and adventitial abnormalities. In addition, some cases showed no definite light-microscopic changes. However, electron

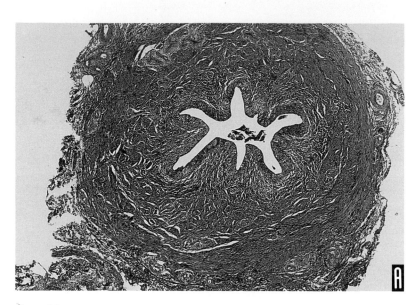

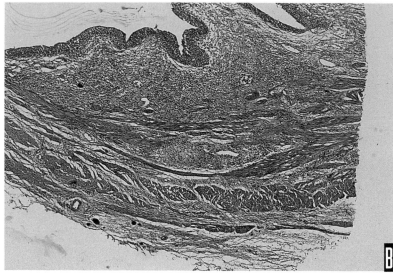

Figure 7.7 A, Muscle bundles in the normal ureter are arranged in a circular outer coat and a longitudinal inner coat, which is less clearly defined because of its usual spiral orientation. This section is taken distal to an obstructed UPJ occurring in a l9-year-old female.

B, In this tangentially cut section of renal pelvis, the inner coat has a normal interdigitating pattern due to the spiral arrangement of muscle bundles. **(A,B:** Masson's trichrome stain)

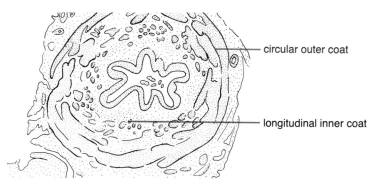

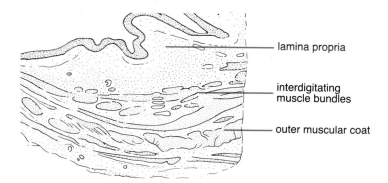

Figure 7.8 The UPJ normally has an increase in muscle bulk. Tangential section of this grossly stenotic UPJ in a 16-year-old female accentuates the normal complex basket-weave pattern. Thickness of the muscular wall cannot be evaluated (Masson's trichrome stain).

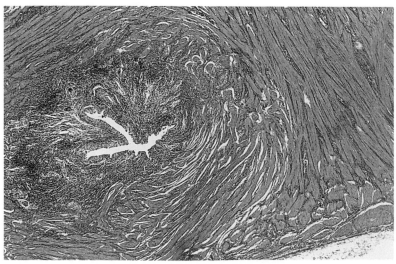

microscopy consistently confirmed the presence of increased collagen between muscle cells of the UPJ. Above the UPJ muscle atrophy, ruptured or attenuated nexuses, and increased collagen and ground substances were found; hypertrophied pelvic wall muscle occasionally was present.

ASSOCIATED RENAL ANOMALIES A variety of congenital anomalies (see Chapter 4) are associated with UPJO. Partial or complete ipsilateral ureteral duplication is typically associated with lower-pole UPJO. Renal agenesis, contralateral malrotation, ipsilateral ectopia, and renal fusion have been reported. The horseshoe kidney may have a high ureteral insertion with primary UPJO, and hydronephrosis secondary to UPJ or upper ureteral obstruction is the most common mode of presentation. Ectopic pelvic kidneys often have malrotated pelves and some degree of pyelocaliectasis, which may be mistaken for UPJO.

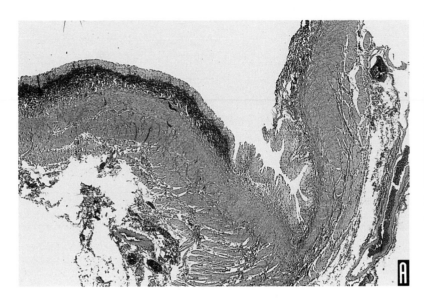
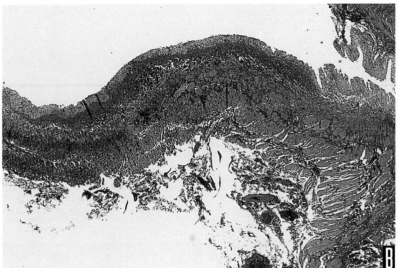

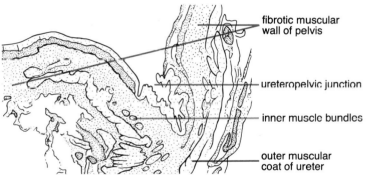

fibrotic muscular wall of pelvis

ureteropelvic junction

inner muscle bundles

outer muscular coat of ureter

Figure 7.9 These longitudinal sections were taken from the stenotic UPJ of a 26-year-old man with end-stage hydronephrosis. **A,** Trichrome stain shows decreased muscle (red) with increased collagen (green) in the lamina propria and surrounding the inner muscle bundles. Immediately proximal to the UPJ, the atrophic muscular wall is replaced with fibrous tissue. **B,** In the area of muscle loss and transmural fibrosis (left), elastic tissue (black) is abnormally increased and condensed. Compare with the muscle wall of the UPJ on the right (Verhoef–van Gieson stain).

Figure 7.10 Histologic sections of the UPJ that are optimum for evaluating the orientation and thickness of the muscular coats are difficult to obtain. This tangential cut of the stenotic UPJ in a 21-year-old male shows collagen surrounding muscle bundles that appear diminished in amount and size (compare with Fig. 7.8).

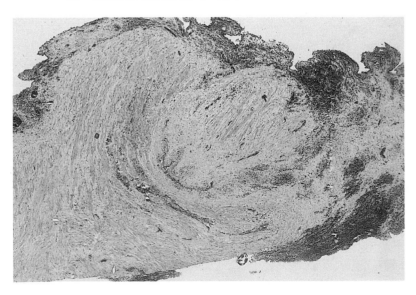

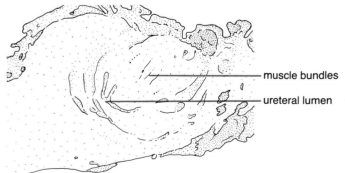

muscle bundles

ureteral lumen

CHAPTER 8

Urinary Tract Obstruction

A broad spectrum of intrinsic and extrinsic lesions may produce obstructive uropathy. Except for lesions such as ureteropelvic junction obstruction (see Chapter 7) and primary obstructive megaureter, a specific etiology can be determined in most cases. Obstructing lesions may be congenital, inflammatory, or neoplastic in origin, or may be secondary to mechanical obstruction from intraluminal ureteral masses derived from the kidney or renal pelvis, such as necrotic renal papillae, blood clots, and stones (see Chapter 6).

Obstructive uropathy due to infravesical, bladder, and most ureteral lesions is generally accompanied by hydroureter, which may be severe. Megaureter is a nonspecific term that refers to a widely dilated and tortuous ureter. Although it is usually congenital, megaureter may be produced by a wide variety of acquired structural and functional abnormalities. Megaureter can be categorized as: (1) refluxing; (2) nonrefluxing, nonobstructed; or (3) obstructed (Fig. 8.1).

INTRINSIC URINARY TRACT OBSTRUCTION

POSTERIOR URETHRAL VALVES

Posterior urethral valves are one of the most important causes of urinary tract obstruction (UTO) in boys and the most common abnormality affecting both kidneys. Approximately 30% of patients with this congenital anomaly present in the first months of life, and 50% are seen within the first year; mean age of presentation is 2^1_2 years.

CLINICAL MANIFESTATIONS Urinary tract infection (UTI), which is the most common presenting manifestation, occurs in approximately two thirds of patients up to five years of age and 50% of patients over five years old. Renal failure is most pronounced in those with superimposed UTI. Renal function is often more severely compromised in younger patients. The overall mortality rate is approximately 15%, compared with 41% for those presenting in the first three months of life.

Other symptoms are, in part, related to age. In patients less than one year of age, urinary dribbling, failure to thrive, and respiratory distress may occur. Patients aged one to five may manifest urinary dribbling, poor stream, and acute retention of urine. An additional symptom occurring in patients older than five years is enuresis, frequently with daytime wetting. There is a high incidence of urinary incontinence, which usually disappears following valve ablation. Incontinence is seen in patients with persistent ureteral dilatation and noncompliant bladders, or it may be a postoperative complication following bladder neck surgery.

Vesicoureteral reflux (VUR) affects approximately 50% of infants presenting in the first year of life but is uncommon in older children. VUR in association with posterior urethral valves implies a worse prognosis for the associated kidney. At presentation, approximately one third of patients have bilateral VUR, one third have unilateral VUR, and one third show no evidence of VUR. Mortality

Figure 8.1
Classification of Megaureter

I. Refluxing
  A. Primary (incompetence of ureterovesical junction)
  B. Secondary
    1. Infravesical obstruction (urethral valves, bladder neck contracture)
    2. Neurogenic bladder

II. Nonrefluxing, Nonobstructed
  A. Primary (prune-belly syndrome, dysmorphic ureter)
  B. Secondary
    1. Metabolic or toxic (decompensated Bartter's syndrome, endotoxin aperistalsis)
    2. Postoperative

III. Obstructed
  A. Primary
    1. Mechanical factors (ureteral strictures, ureterocele, tumor)
    2. Functional defects (adynamic ureteral segment)
  B. Secondary
    1. Intrinsic (urethral valves or stricture, bladder neck stenosis, neurogenic bladder)
    2. Extrinsic ureteral compression (tumor, fibrosis, vessels)

(Modified from Lockhart et al., 1979)

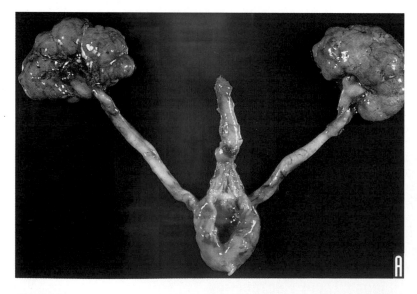 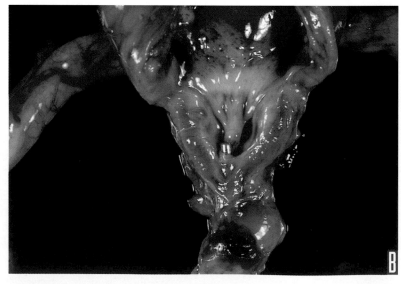

Figure 8.2 A, Posterior urethral valves in this newborn male resulted in bilateral multicystic dysplasia. Ureteral dilatation and bladder wall hypertrophy are indicative of infravesical obstruction. **B,** Dilatation of the posterior urethra provides further diagnostic evidence of valves. Although urine flow is severely obstructed, a probe can be easily passed retrograde through the urethra.

rates have been reported to be 57%, 17.4%, and 9.1%, respectively. Unilateral reflux is most often left-sided, associated with a nonfunctioning or poorly functioning kidney, and is persistent. When reflux is right-sided, it is usually associated with a functioning kidney and resolves following valve ablation. A nonfunctioning kidney in a patient with valves and reflux is indicative of renal dysplasia (see Chapter 2).

MORPHOLOGY The normal male urethra has small, distinct, bilateral folds (plicae colliculi) that may simulate valves. These folds arise at the lateral side of a midline ridge (crista urethralis) located at the distal end of the verumontanum and run distally for a short distance to attach to the lateral walls of the urethra.

Three forms of posterior urethral valves have been described. The most common type is characterized by a bicuspid valve originating just distal to the verumontanum on the floor of the posterior urethra. It diverges distally in an anterolateral orientation to fuse anteriorly in the midline (Figs. 8.2, 8.3). The anterior flow of urine is obstructed as the margins of the cusps blow out and appose each other in the midline. Posterior urethral dilatation provides diagnostic evidence of obstructive valves. The second form of valves, which is nonobstructive, consists of folds that run between the verumontanum and bladder neck (Fig. 8.4). A rare, third form of valves occurs just distal to the verumontanum and has more of a diaphragmlike appearance, with a small posterior opening (Fig. 8.5).

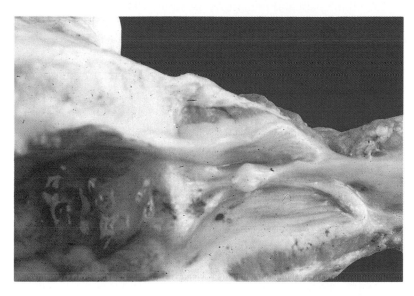

Figure 8.3 Type I valves are bicuspid, originate from the floor of the urethra just distal to the verumontanum, and diverge distally in an anterolateral orientation. In this specimen from a six-year-old boy, the right cusp is larger than the left, producing an asymmetric appearance.

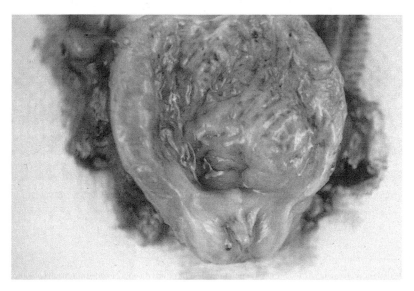

Figure 8.4 In this specimen from a male neonate, two or three membranous folds that join the enlarged verumontanum and the bladder neck resemble type II nonobstructive valves. A prominent horizontal muscular bar in the trigone is also present.

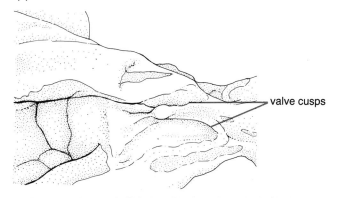

valve cusps

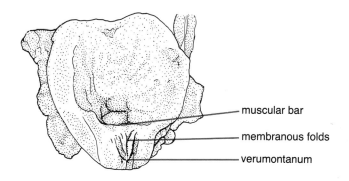

muscular bar
membranous folds
verumontanum

Figure 8.5 This specimen illustrates the rare type III valve that occurs distal to the verumontanum and appears diaphragmlike. The saccular outpouching distal to the valve is a urethral diverticulum.

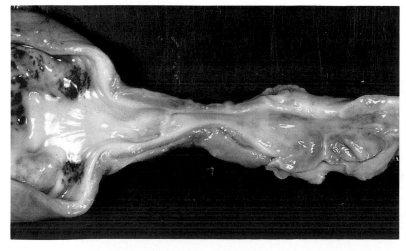

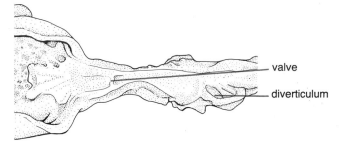

valve
diverticulum

Primary Obstructive Megaureter

Primary obstructive megaureter (POM) is produced by an adynamic ureteral segment, which results in functional (nonocclusive) ureteral obstruction. It must be distinguished from secondary obstructed megaureter. The latter is usually associated with severe infravesical obstruction with bladder hypertrophy and may give rise to fibrotic, adynamic transmural ureteral segments. The majority of secondary obstructed megaureters are caused by urethral valves. Extrinsic causes of ureteral obstruction should also be excluded, as should causes of congenital ureteral obstruction, such as atresia and valves. Differentiation from a dysmorphic ureter, which produces a nonrefluxing, nonobstructed megaureter, may be difficult. POM is not associated with reflux. Congenital massive primary reflux with a large-capacity, thin-walled bladder describes the radiologic appearance of the megaureter–megacystis syndrome.

PATHOGENESIS The etiology of POM is obscure, but the condition is generally considered congenital. Proposed causes for the adynamic segment have included achalasia, with decreased numbers of sympathetic ganglia, and aberrations of muscle and collagen. Embryologic explanations have been proposed, including embryonal arrest of differentiation and faulty interaction between the ureteric bud (epithelial elements) and mesenchymal cells (mesodermal elements). During the 37th to 41st days of gestation, the normal ureteral lumen is secondarily obstructed. Recanalization starts in the midsection, and after the 41st to 42nd days, the ureter is completely recanalized. If this process is disturbed, there may be partial or complete stenosis of the prevesical segment. Delayed recanalization may result in dilatation of the proximal segment. Alternatively, there may be interference with the lengthening process of a localized segment in the juxtavesical ureter.

CLINICAL MANIFESTATIONS POM has a marked male preponderance in children, and the left side is involved more often than the right. Clinical symptoms are seen mainly in early childhood. Children frequently present with pyelonephritis; symptoms include flank pain and hematuria. In adults, POM is commonly discovered on routine investigation, with patients ranging from 18–80 years of age. Progressive ureteral dilatation or deterioration of renal function is not expected in this age group.

The grade of ureteral dilatation correlates with progressive renal functional deterioration; if renal function is impaired at the time of surgery, improvement cannot be expected. Various systems have been devised for clinically grading the extent of the adynamic segment and the degree of ureteral dilatation. Children, particularly boys with bilateral megaureter, tend to have high-grade lesions.

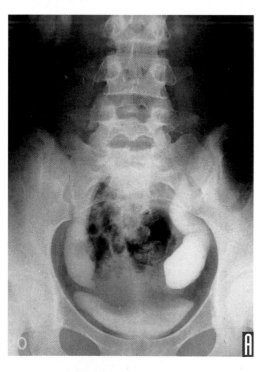
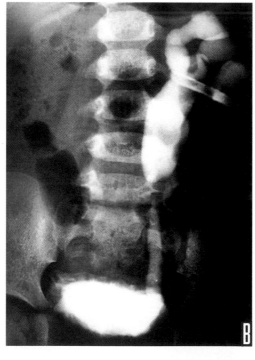

Figure 8.6 **A,** Delayed IVP in a 17-year-old woman with bilateral POM (group I) shows ureteral dilatation along the entire length of the ureter except the ureterovesical junction. **B,** Left antegrade pyeloureterography in this five-year-old girl with POM (group II) shows segmental ureteral dilatation from the upper half of the ureter to the kidney, which was dysmorphic. (Reproduced with permission of the authors and publisher from Tokunaka and Koyanagi, 1982)

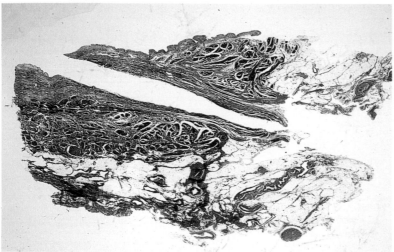

Figure 8.7 Longitudinal section of the normal ureterovesical junction shows the intravesical ureter, which consists of pure longitudinal muscle bundles. The deep periureteral sheath, which envelops the intravesical ureter, and the superficial periureteral sheath are separated by Waldeyer's space (trichrome stain). (Reproduced with permission of the authors and publisher from Tokunaka et al., 1982)

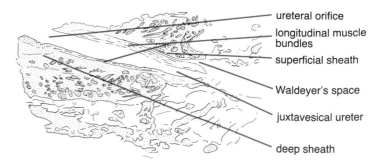

ureteral orifice
longitudinal muscle bundles
superficial sheath
Waldeyer's space
juxtavesical ureter
deep sheath

Delayed IVP and antegrade or retrograde pyeloureterography are useful for evaluating POM and demonstrate the location and extent of the narrowed segment (Fig. 8.6). The degree of ureteral dilatation and hydronephrosis can also be assessed.

MORPHOLOGY The normal juxtavesical and intramural segments of ureter are surrounded by decussating dual ureteral sheaths separated by Waldeyer's space: a deep sheath originating in the deep trigonal muscle and a superficial sheath originating in the superficial detrusor muscle of the bladder (Fig. 8.7). Intrinsic ureteral muscle has a purely longitudinal orientation and fans out to form the superficial trigone. Therefore, no spirally arranged smooth muscle bundles are present in the intrinsic terminal ureteral end.

In most cases of POM, the ureter is dilated throughout its length except for the terminal (0.5–4 cm) segment (Fig. 8.8). The prevesical segment appears narrowed but is usually normal in caliber.

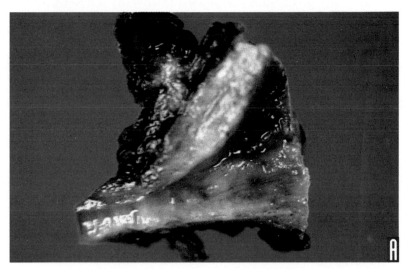

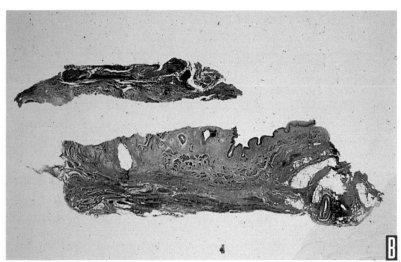

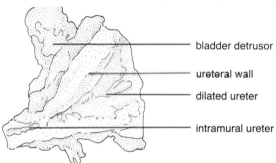

bladder detrusor

ureteral wall

dilated ureter

intramural ureter

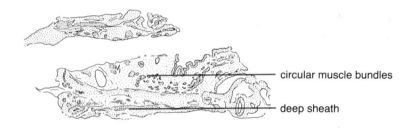

circular muscle bundles

deep sheath

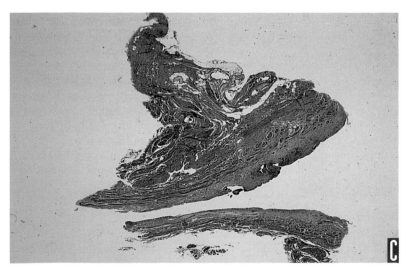

Figure 8.8 POM (group 1) longitudinal sections. **A,** In the formalin-fixed distal ureteral end from a 37-year-old woman, the dilated ureter abruptly narrows at its intramural portion. **B,** Distal ureteral end. A predominantly circular muscle arrangement is seen with in-creased connective tissue between muscle bundles in the intravesical ureter. The deep periureteral sheath is more developed than normal. **C,** Distal ureteral end from the patient in **A** displays almost normal structure of the intravesical ureter. Longitudinal muscular arrangement is almost pure, with only a slight increase of connective tissue between muscle bundles. The deep periureteral sheath is larger than normal (**B,C:** trichrome stain). (**A:** Courtesy of S. Tokunaka, MD, Asahikawa, Japan. **B,C:** Reproduced with permission of the authors

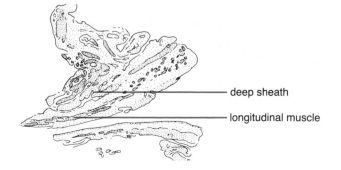

deep sheath

longitudinal muscle

A variety of histologic changes have been reported in the non-dilated ureteral segment in POM: circular orientation of smooth muscle without longitudinally oriented fibers, muscular hyperplasia or hypoplasia, and complete fibrosis or increased collagen fibers, as well as a normal wall. Marked circular hypertrophy has been reported immediately proximal to the narrow adynamic segment. In one light- and electron microscopic study, however, the changes in the obstructed segment and dilated portion were similar to those in ureteropelvic junction obstruction (see Chapter 7).

The role of the ureteral sheaths and ureteral dysplasia has been demonstrated by Tokunaka and colleagues in detailed morphologic studies of primary nonreflux megaureter. Two groups have been identified. In group I, which has the larger number of cases, the narrowed segment is entirely intra- or juxtavesical, and ureteral dilatation extends the whole length proximal to it. Microscopically, the periureteral sheaths are extensively developed and prevent free distention (Fig. 8.8B,C). The dilated segment is normal. In group II, the narrowed segment is long and extravesical, and is often associated with dysmorphism of the adjoining kidney and pelvis (dysplasia and hypoplasia). Microscopically, the muscle and interstitial tissue are normal in the nondilated (narrowed) segment; in the dysplastic dilated segment, small muscle cells are scattered within

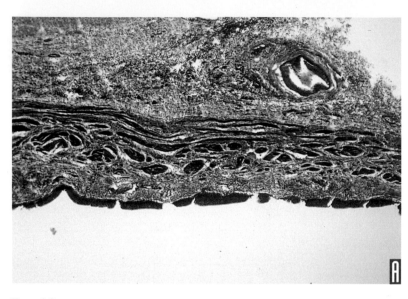
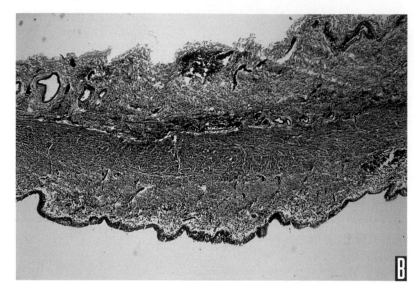

Figure 8.9 A, Longitudinal section of the nondilated portion of ureter in a four-year-old boy with POM (group II) shows many muscle bundles with a minimal amount of connective tissue. **B,** In contrast, the dilated portion of ureter has a thin muscle layer interposed between large amounts of connective tissue (**A,B:** trichrome stain). (Courtesy of S. Tokunaka, MD, Asahikawa, Japan)

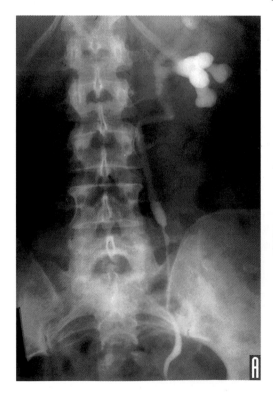
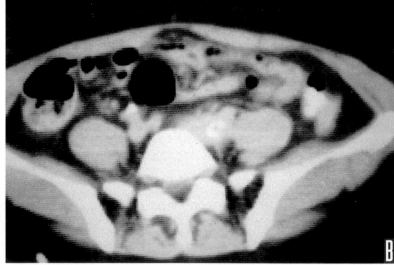

Figure 8.10 A, The focal midureteral narrowing did not change during urography and is associated with hydronephrosis. **B,** CT scan reveals that the segment is encased by retroperitoneal fibrosis, which does not extend across the midline to involve the opposite ureter. (Courtesy of H. Hawkins, MD, Cincinnati, Ohio)

right ureter

fibrosis

left ureter

psoas

increased connective tissue without formation of muscle bundles (Fig. 8.9). Ultrastructurally, although nerves exist, nexuses are attenuated and muscle cells, which are deficient in myosin, lack almost all thick myofilaments. Group I is distinguished from primary reflux (see Chapter 5), where the ureteral sheaths are poorly developed. Changes in group II are similar to the prune-belly syndrome and are designated *ureteral muscle dysplasia*.

Ureteral Valves

Congenital ureteral valves are a rare lesion, usually diagnosed preoperatively as a ureteral stricture or primary megaureter. The diagnosis requires proximal obstructive changes such as hydroureter and hydronephrosis with a normal ureter distally, no other causes of obstruction, and no history of prior trauma or infection as possible etiologies of ureteral strictures.

PATHOGENESIS Up to 5% of newborns have vestigial transverse mucosal folds in the distal ureter, which normally disappear. It is postulated that ureteral valves represent persistence of these folds, although no definite etiology is known.

CLINICAL MANIFESTATIONS Ureteral valves may present at any age, and there is no sex predilection. They are usually unilateral and are present in the distal ureter in approximately 50% of cases.

MORPHOLOGY Grossly, ureteral valves appear as filamentous webs across the ureteral lumen. Microscopically, these true valves consist of transverse folds of transitional epithelium containing smooth muscle bundles.

Extrinsic Urinary Tract Obstruction
Idiopathic Retroperitoneal Fibrosis

Idiopathic retroperitoneal fibrosis (IRF), first described in the English literature in 1948, is an uncommon fibrosing, inflammatory process, which causes renal failure by extrinsic ureteric obstruction. It constitutes 40%–70% of cases of retroperitoneal fibrosis. Specific etiologies, such as retroperitoneal injury due to hemorrhage, urinary extravasation, surgery, or radiotherapy, should be excluded, and IRF must be distinguished from malignant retroperitoneal fibrosis due to primary retroperitoneal sarcomas or lymphoma and metastatic carcinoma.

PATHOGENESIS The pathogenesis of IRF is unknown, although hypersensitivity and autoimmune disease have been postulated. There is a well documented association with certain drugs, particularly methysergide. Other etiologies that have been suggested include vasculitis or phlebitis, lymphatic obstruction, vitamin E deficiency, trauma, and infection.

CLINICAL MANIFESTATIONS IRF occurs twice as often in men as in women and most commonly occurs in the fifth or sixth decade of life, although patients have ranged from the teens to 83 years of age. The disease is progressive but its course is variable. It may be unilateral and later become bilateral. In two thirds of patients symptoms do not exceed eight weeks' duration. Patients with rapid progression present with acute obstruction, whereas slow progression produces ill health with chronic obstructive uropathy and renal atrophy. The ability to pass a number 5 or 6 ureteral catheter suggests that obstruction is functional—due to loss of peristalsis—rather than mechanical. With acute obstruction, retrograde catheterization localizes the level of obstruction and may lead to prompt flow of urine and resolution of renal failure. Ureterolysis is also more likely to result in postoperative recovery of renal function if obstruction is acute.

Symptoms are generally nonspecific. Pain is the most common complaint, occurring in approximately 90% of patients, and may be poorly localized to the back, flank, or abdomen. Testicular pain and swelling due to a hydrocele, renovascular hypertension, and phlebothrombosis with pulmonary emboli may also be present. Symptoms are related to entrapment of retroperitoneal structures—ureters, vena cava, gonadal veins, and the aorta and its branches. Patients may experience anorexia, weight loss, and vomiting or other nonspecific gastrointestinal complaints. However, a minority (approximately 10%) present with genitourinary symptoms, such as nocturia, frequency, or anuria. The presence of uremia with a normal urinalysis is a diagnostic aid. Patients typically have a markedly elevated sedimentation rate, and positive antinuclear and smooth muscle antibodies have been reported.

The association of IRF with mediastinal fibrosis, sclerosing cholangitis, Riedel's thyroiditis, and pseudotumor of the orbit has led to the concept that it is one component of a broader disease complex termed *systemic idiopathic fibrosis*. Additional systemic findings have included pericarditis, Raynaud's phenomenon, and arthritis.

A normal IVP has been reported in 2.5%–7% of cases at presentation and corresponds to the early inflammatory stage of the disease. Intravenous or retrograde pyelogram may show the pathognomonic triad of ureteral narrowing at L-5, medial deviation of the ureter(s), and caliectasis or hydronephrosis and ureterectasis proximal to the obstruction. Medial deviation of one or both ureters, however, is an unreliable sign since the ureters may be in a normal position.

Computed tomography (CT) scan has replaced ultrasonography as the best noninvasive diagnostic modality because it provides more detail. CT can determine the distribution and geometric shape of the retroperitoneum and absence of normal tissue planes about the inferior vena cava and aorta, as well as furnish evidence of ureteral involvement (Fig. 8.10).

MORPHOLOGY A thick mass of gray-white fibrous tissue is centered around the aorta in the retroperitoneal space and spreads out from the midline to envelop a variety of structures. The ureters are frequently drawn toward the aorta and may be encircled or compressed by the dense sclerotic plaque of fibrous tissue (Fig. 8.11). The fibrosis, which is almost cartilaginous in consistency, may vary from 2–6 cm in thickness. The fibrotic mass usually covers the sacral promontory at the L4-5 level, and the margins are discrete but variable in extent. Fibrosis may extend from the midrenal hilus

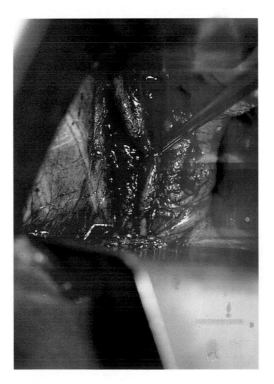

Figure 8.11 Grossly, IRF causes ureteral entrapment by dense fibrous tissue. In this patient, the sclerotic plaque was localized to the sacral promontory at the L4-5 level. The ureter is drawn medially and shows proximal dilatation. (This is the same case as Figure 8.10.)

or ureteropelvic junction superiorly to the pelvic brim inferiorly and follow the aortic bifurcation and iliac vessels. While extension into the pelvis or above the renal vessels is rare, the mass can extend laterally beyond the psoas muscle margins.

Microscopically, nonspecific chronic inflammation and fibrosis are present. The fibrocollagenous stroma may show active fibroblastic proliferation or may be densely hyalinized with entrapped lipoid aggregates (Fig. 8.12). In early lesions, polymorphous inflammatory infiltrates consist predominantly of lymphocytes with variable polymorphonuclear leukocytes, plasma cells, eosinophils, and mast cells. Adjacent skeletal muscle and adipose tissue are frequently infiltrated by lymphocytes (Fig. 8.13). Vasculitis and necrosis are not present. At a chronic stage, the fibrosis is acellular, avascular, frequently calcified, and is not inflamed.

Aortic Aneurysm with Perianeurysmal Fibrosis

Urologic manifestations constitute the presenting symptoms in approximately 10% of patients with aortic aneurysms and include renal colic, abnormal micturition, sexual disturbances, and anuria.

Because of the cushioning effect of the soft tissues, ureteric obstruction is not common with aortic aneurysms, whereas aneurysms of the iliac arteries may cause compression of the ureters against the pelvic brim.

PATHOGENESIS The perianeurysmal fibrosis may be secondary to inflammatory changes in the wall of the aneurysm, which extends into the adventitia or perivascular tissues, or may result from minute perforations with escape of blood into the soft tissues, evoking a chronic inflammatory reaction.

CLINICAL MANIFESTATIONS Ureteric obstruction secondary to perianeurysmal fibrosis, which is an uncommon complication of aortic aneurysms, has been observed more commonly in males than in females. Presenting symptoms are typically those of abdominal, flank, or back pain, which may radiate to the groin or leg. An abdominal mass is frequently palpable.

MORPHOLOGY Perianeurysmal fibrosis may be grossly indistinguishable from IRF. A hard, woody, glistening white mass surrounds the aneurysm and ureters, often extending around the

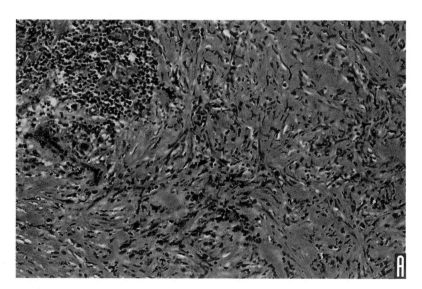

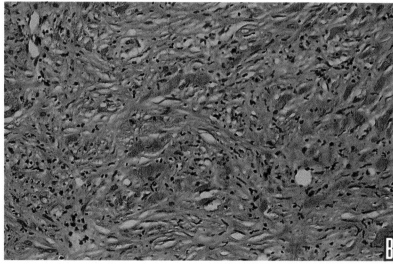

Figure 8.12 **A,** Microscopically, the retroperitoneal fibrous plaque typically contains a lymphocyte-rich inflammatory infiltrate with active fibroblastic proliferation. **B,** With chronicity, inflammation is less

and the fibrocollagenous stroma becomes avascular, acellular, and densely hyalinized.

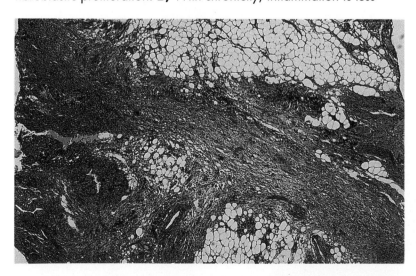

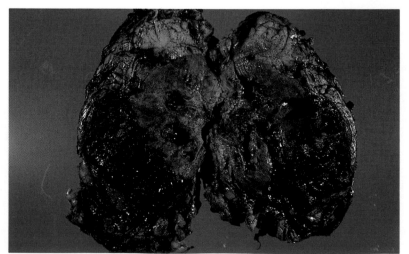

Figure 8.13 Although grossly discrete, IRF has ill-defined borders microscopically and shows irregular extension of the fibroinflammatory process to envelop retroperitoneal structures. Lymphocytic infiltrates are present within entrapped lobules of adipose tissue.

Figure 8.14 Grossly, a massive lower-pole perinephric hematoma is largely contained by the renal (Gerota's) fascia. It occurred spontaneously in a patient receiving prophylactic anticoagulants who had UTO with multifocal ureteral and pelvicalyceal papillary transitional cell carcinomas.

inferior vena cava and bowel. Microscopically, dense fibrous tissue contains a nonspecific chronic inflammatory infiltrate with variable hemosiderin-laden macrophages.

PERIRENAL URINIFEROUS PSEUDOCYST

Perirenal pseudocysts are relatively rare lesions since most extravasations of urine or blood are sterile, are absorbed, and cease within a short period of time. The perirenal uriniferous pseudocyst, or *urinoma*, is an encapsulated collection of urine secondary to chronic extravasation into the extraperitoneal tissues around the kidney and upper ureter, and is usually associated with hydronephrosis. It forms within and is bounded by the lower reflections of the renal (Gerota's) fascia.

Perinephric extravasation of urine should be clinically and pathologically distinguished from perinephric hematoma (Fig. 8.14), which may be related to trauma or occur spontaneously secondary to ruptured aneurysm, vascular erosion by carcinomas or tuberculosis, periarteritis, or hemorrhagic diathesis.

PATHOGENESIS Uriniferous pseudocysts, with few exceptions, are a complication of injury to the pelvicalyceal system or ureter, which may be accidental or iatrogenic—for example, following pyeloplasty, pyelolithotomy, or ureterolithotomy for calculi and diagnostic ureterocystoscopy complicated by perforation. Perforation of the renal pelvis by a calculus has also been reported as an etiology.

Three factors, together with trauma, must be present in order to produce the uriniferous pseudocyst: (1) complete tear of a collecting system (calyx, renal pelvis, or ureter) or a wide separation of cortical fragments; (2) failure of the defect to seal off; and (3) the presence of an obstructed ureter below the site of injury, which causes persistent efflux. Extravasation of urine into the perirenal fat causes rapid lipolysis and initiates an inflammatory reaction. The resultant ureteral compression sets up a vicious cycle leading to UTO. Hydronephrosis results from fibrotic changes about the ureter at the junction of its upper and middle thirds.

CLINICAL MANIFESTATIONS Uriniferous pseudocysts are rarely asymptomatic. Clinically, progression may be slow, and the latent period between the traumatic episode and appearance of symptoms, although usually one to four months, can be as long as two years. Patients complain of mild abdominal discomfort or flank pain, which may occasionally radiate to the testis. Physical exam reveals a firm, nontender flank mass filling one side of the abdomen to the level of the iliac crest.

The characteristic radiologic complex consists of: (1) a lucent defect or soft-tissue mass that obscures the psoas shadow; (2) superior displacement of the kidney with lateral displacement of the inferior pole and medial deviation of the ureter, which occasionally crosses the midline; and (3) extravasation of contrast medium into the perirenal space at the point of leakage or gross communication with the collecting system (Fig. 8.15).

MORPHOLOGY Grossly, the axis of the pseudocyst conforms to the distended core of the renal fascia and is therefore elliptical and obliquely oriented inferomedially. The wall is derived from the perirenal fat and renal fascia, as the anterior and posterior fibroelastic layers fuse and loosely blend with the iliac fascia inferiorly and the periureteric connective tissue medially. The ureter becomes embedded in fibrous tissue. The pseudocyst contains cloudy yellow fluid with fatty or oily debris. In chronic cases, the pseudocyst may be loculated or calcified. A demonstrable fistula between the hydronephrotic and perinephric cavities helps to confirm the diagnosis but may only be possible very early in the process.

Microscopically, absence of an epithelial lining confirms the diagnosis of pseudocyst. Foci of recent hemorrhage, focal aggregates of chronic inflammatory cells, and organizing granulation tissue are present. Hyalinizing scar tissue extends into the fat.

ENDOMETRIOSIS

Symptomatic involvement of the urinary tract in endometriosis is rare. The relative frequency of bladder, ureter, and kidney involvement is 25:3:1. Ureteral involvement in endometriosis is uncommon and seldom extensive. It may be extrinsic (due to extension of pelvic endometriosis) or intrinsic (implants of endometrium invade the ureteral wall and less commonly the mucosa). Ureteric obstruction is caused by the fibrous and inflammatory reaction.

PATHOGENESIS Theories regarding the pathogenesis of endometriosis include embryonic rests, implantation following retrograde tubal menstruation, vascular or lymphatic dissemination, and metaplasia of coelomic epithelium.

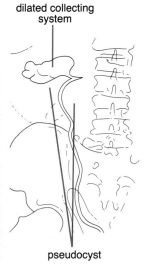

Figure 8.15 Retrograde pyelogram shows the lower pole of the kidney displaced laterally and upward by a perirenal uriniferous pseudocyst around which the ureter courses. The extrinsic pressure on the ureter has resulted in hydronephrosis. Other retroperitoneal masses and fluid accumulations could cause the same appearance. (Courtesy of H. Hawkins, MD, Cincinnati, Ohio)

dilated collecting system

pseudocyst

CLINICAL MANIFESTATIONS Patients generally have symptoms of pelvic endometriosis, including dyspareunia, menstrual irregularities, backache, and infertility, each of which may be associated with a pelvic mass. Symptoms of ureteral involvement include flank or abdominal pain, urinary frequency, dysuria, and gross hematuria.

MORPHOLOGY Implants of endometriosis may appear hemorrhagic and cystic or become fibrotic (Fig. 8.16). Microscopically, the diagnosis requires the identification of at least two of the following:

benign endometrial glands, endometrial stroma, or hemorrhage, which may be acute or chronic with accumulation of hemosiderin-laden macrophages (Fig. 8.17).

MALIGNANT NEOPLASMS

Renal functional impairment may be due to a wide variety of complications related to direct or indirect involvement of the urinary tract by malignant neoplasms; UTO with hydronephrosis is

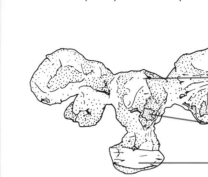

Figure 8.16 In this specimen with endometriosis, numerous variable-sized hemorrhagic and cystic foci are present in the serosa of the uterus and adnexal structures. Tubo-ovarian adhesions have resulted from the associated fibroinflammatory reaction. (Courtesy of T. Wesseler, MD, Cincinnati, Ohio)

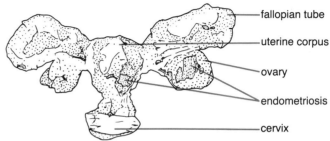

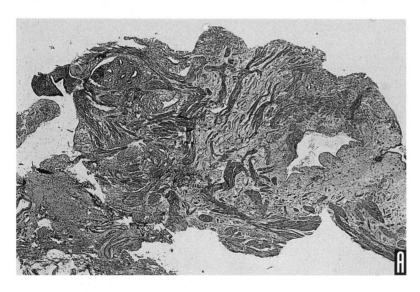

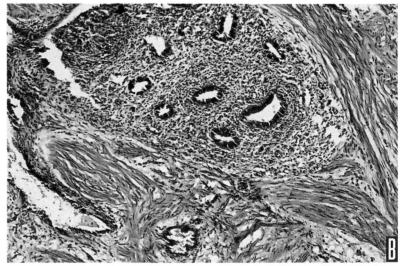

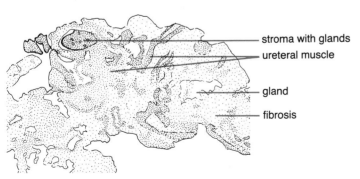

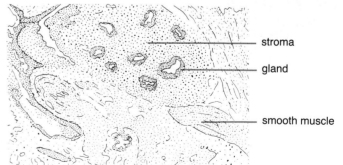

Figure 8.17 A, Tangential section of an obstructed ureter with intrinsic endometriosis shows variable-sized glands that are focally associated with a densely cellular stroma. The ureteral smooth muscle bundles

are separated by edema and fibrosis. **B,** At higher magnification, the presence of benign endometrial-type glands with accompanying stroma confirms the diagnosis of endometriosis.

just one of the many manifestations (Fig. 8.18). UTO may be the result of localized extension of a pelvic genitourinary malignancy, ureteral or periureteral metastases, or malignant retroperitoneal fibrosis.

CLINICAL MANIFESTATIONS Malignant neoplasms secondarily involving the urinary tract may produce unilateral or bilateral UTO with decreased renal function or anuria. In up to 50% of cases, the cancer may be clinically unsuspected. Malignant neoplasms are approximately three times more frequent as a cause of bilateral ureteric obstruction with acute renal failure than benign causes such as IRF or stones.

Bilateral ureteral occlusion usually takes place at the level of the bladder, and obstruction is due to localized extension of a pelvic malignancy in approximately 75% of cases. Carcinomas of the cervix and prostate are most common, although ovarian, bladder, and colonic cancers may also produce lower UTO. Obstructive nephropathy accounts for 60%–80% of deaths due to cervical carcinoma. Nonspecific signs and symptoms include oliguria, weakness, and abdominal or lower back pain.

Ureteral and periureteral metastases may also cause UTO. Obstructing lesions close to the kidney generally cause more severe anatomic renal changes. The most common cancers, in order of frequency, are stomach, prostate, kidney, breast, lung (Fig. 8.19),

Figure 8.18
Renal Complications of Neoplasms

I. Glomerular Lesions (nephrotic syndrome)

II. Obstructive Nephropathy
   A. Tubular precipitation syndromes
      1. Uric acid and hypercalcemic nephropathy
      2. Paraproteinuric syndromes (multiple myeloma, monoclonal gammopathy)
   B. Obstruction of urethra, bladder, ureters

III. Direct Invasion (primary or metastatic renal tumors)

IV. Treatment-Related Nephropathies (radiation, drug nephrotoxicity)

V. Miscellaneous (disseminated intravascular coagulation, amyloidosis)

(Modified from Fer et al., 1981)

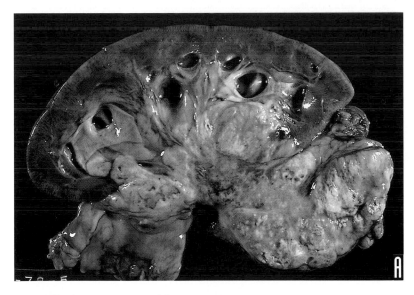
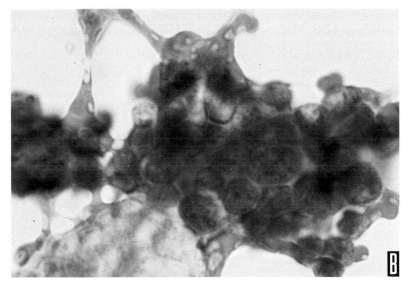

Figure 8.19 **A,** Ureteral and periureteral, as well as renal, metastases are commonly observed with lung cancers, and UTO is a frequent complication. In this specimen, metastatic small cell undifferentiated carcinoma of the lung extensively infiltrates the renal hilum, producing moderate hydronephrosis. **B,** Fine-needle aspiration biopsy specimen from the same kidney contains loose aggregates of small, malignant cells with the cytologic characteristics typical of oat-cell carcinoma—nuclei with moderately granular chromatin, small, inconspicuous nucleoli, scant cytoplasm, and prominent nuclear molding. Fine-needle aspiration is a useful diagnostic procedure for differentiating metastatic tumors from primary urinary tract malignancies (Papanicolaou stain).

colon, uterus/cervix, bladder, and skin (i.e., melanoma) (Figs. 8.20, 8.21). The incidence of secondary ureteral involvement by lymphoma is low.

Approximately 8% of cases of retroperitoneal fibrosis are due to malignancy; in 50% of cases retroperitoneal fibrosis is the first indication of malignant disease. Clinical features of malignant retroperitoneal fibrosis are identical to those of idiopathic cases, and patients typically experience pain. Ureteral obstruction may be unilateral or bilateral. Malignant retroperitoneal fibrosis is most often due to primary retroperitoneal tumors, such as pancreatic carcinomas, sarcomas (Figs. 8.22, 8.23), neuroblastoma, and lymphoma.

MALIGNANT LYMPHOMAS

Sclerosing variants of follicular center cell lymphomas constitute approximately 20% of lymph-node–based lymphomas and 75% of retroperitoneal non-Hodgkin's lymphomas. Although typically presenting in the retroperitoneum or inguinal area, they also occur in the mediastinum.

CLINICAL MANIFESTATIONS Patients most commonly are middle-aged to elderly and present with a palpable mass and abdominal pain. Fever and weight loss may also be present.

MORPHOLOGY Typical autopsy findings in extrinsic UTO secondary to nonsclerosing lymphomas consist of ureteral compression or encasement by retroperitoneal lymphadenopathy or bulky tumor (Fig. 8.24).

Primary sclerosing retroperitoneal lymphomas grossly mimic IRF. Microscopically, extensive perinodal lymphomatous infiltrate is associated with marked sclerosis of a distinctive pattern; compartmentalizing collagenous band formation imparts an epithelioid appearance to the infiltrate (Fig. 8.25). Focal or regional hyalinization of the bands may occur, as may foci of lymphoid depletion

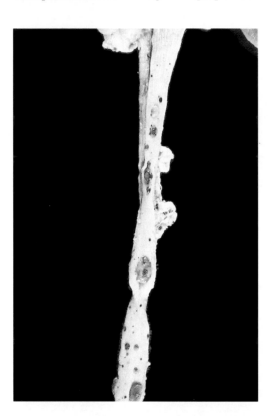

Figure 8.20 This ureter contains multiple brown-to-black nodules typical of metastatic melanoma. Extensive mucosal involvement of the urinary tract is common in widely disseminated melanoma.

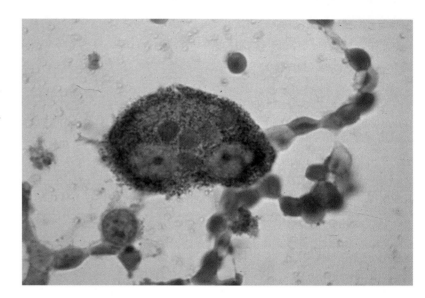

Figure 8.21 In this photomicrograph, the cytoplasm of a malignant binucleate cell is heavily laden with finely granular, as well as globular, brown melanin pigment diagnostic of malignant melanoma. Metastatic adenocarcinoma and squamous cell carcinomas, as well as amelanotic melanoma, may also appear in the urine sediment and are difficult to distinguish from primary urinary tract malignancies (Papanicolaou stain). (Courtesy of T. Wesseler, MD, Cincinnati, Ohio)

Figure 8.22 The hilum of this bivalved kidney contains a large, lobulated, fatty tumor that displaces the lower pole and has compressed the proximal ureter, producing hydronephrosis. Although clinically and grossly suspected of being malignant, the tumor was histologically composed of mature adipose tissue typical of a benign lipoma.

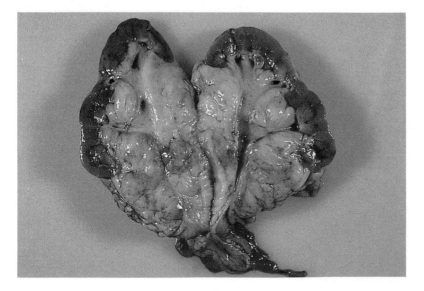

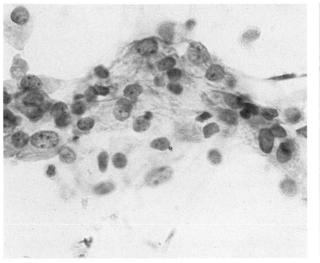
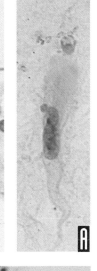
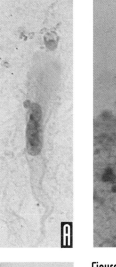
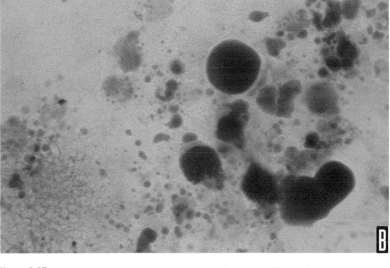

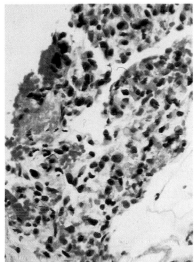
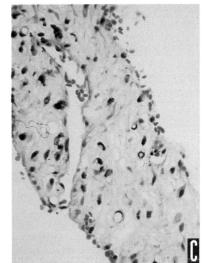

Figure 8.23 A, *Left:* Fine-needle aspiration biopsy of an obstructing perirenal mass in a 55-year-old man contains sheets of malignant cells with round-to-oval, variable-sized nuclei that have finely granular chromatin and nucleoli. Cytoplasm is finely vacuolated and cell borders are indistinct. *Right:* The few individual, large, pleomorphic spindle cells with finely vacuolated cytoplasm are typical of a sarcoma (Papanicolaou stain). **B,** Oil red O stain demonstrates intracytoplasmic vacuoles containing lipid (red). Nuclear displacement by large lipid vacuoles is typical of lipoblasts seen in liposarcoma. **C,** *Left:* Open biopsy of the mass contains small, primitive mesenchymal cells with eccentric, hyperchromatic, polygonal or elongated nuclei. *Right:* Lipoblasts, as well as the large spindle cells with hyperchromatic nuclei, are diagnostic of liposarcoma.

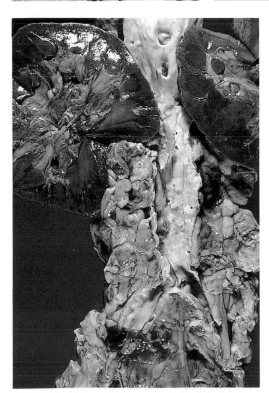

Figure 8.24 Malignant lymphoma has caused massive, confluent retroperitoneal lymphadenopathy, with encasement and compression of the ureters bilaterally by pink-tan, fleshy tumor.

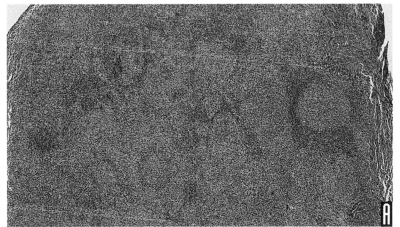
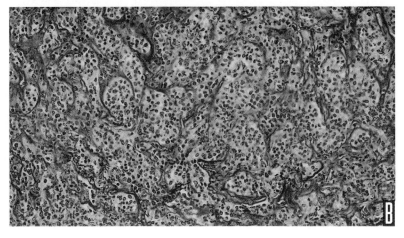

Figure 8.25 A, Histologically, the nodal portion of a retroperitoneal lymphoma shows a nodular growth pattern characteristic of a B-cell lymphoma. An area of perinodal sclerosis is on the right. **B,** Distinctive compartmentalizing collagenous bands within the extranodal infiltrate give an epithelioid appearance to this sclerosing small cleaved follicular center cell lymphoma (Rappaport—diffuse poorly differentiated lymphocytic).

with broad birefringent bands (Fig. 8.26). These follicular center cell lymphomas, which may be small cleaved cell, large cleaved cell, or large noncleaved cell, have a diffuse extranodal pattern. They can be differentiated from IRF, which has a polymorphous infiltrate with predominantly mature lymphocytes in a bland, collagenous stroma with small foci of fibroblastic proliferation. They must also be distinguished from nodular sclerosing and lymphocyte-depleted Hodgkin's disease, node-based T-cell lymphomas, and retroperitoneal sarcomas such as malignant fibrous histiocytoma.

Exogenous Intraluminal Masses

Intraluminal ureteral masses derived from the kidney and renal pelvis include calculi (see Chapter 6) blood clots, and necrotic renal papillae.

Renal Papillary Necrosis

In the United States, papillary necrosis has an incidence of less than 1% in the general autopsy population, whereas in some countries (e.g., Australia, where large analgesic consumption is common) the incidence has been reported to be 3.7%–9.5%. In addition to analgesic abuse, predisposing factors include UTO and diabetes mellitus (approximately 50% of cases); pyelonephritis is a frequent complication (see Chapter 9). Papillary necrosis has also been associated with use of nonsteroidal anti-inflammatory drugs.

PATHOGENESIS Papillary necrosis is thought to be ischemic or toxic in origin. UTO causes compression of thin-walled blood vessels and obstruction of the renal vein by the hydronephrotic pelvis, which compromises the papillary blood supply and results in ischemic necrosis. Therefore, the kidney in diabetes or with chronic pyelonephritis, both of which have arteriosclerosis, is more prone to papillary necrosis, particularly in the presence of UTO, with or without acute infection.

Phenacetin, the noxious agent in analgesic nephropathy, is usually taken as a mixture, and the role of aspirin and caffein is unclear. The mechanism of injury is thought to be either interference with the papillary blood supply or a toxic effect that poisons papillary constituents. Chronic dehydration predisposes to papillary necrosis by further increasing the medullary concentration of the toxic agent.

CLINICAL MANIFESTATIONS Almost 90% of patients are over 40 years of age, and more than 50% are older than 60. In nondiabetic, nonobstructed patients, however, most are less than 50 years old. Females are more commonly affected in cases associated with diabetes mellitus and analgesic abuse. The obstructive form is more common in males.

In the obstructive form or in cases with diabetes, patients typically present with fever, chills, flank or abdominal pain, and oliguria with rapid progression to acute renal failure and uremia. Patients may have a less dramatic onset characterized by anorexia, nausea, vomiting, abdominal pain, or headache secondary to uremia. Colicky pain and hematuria are related to passage of necrotic

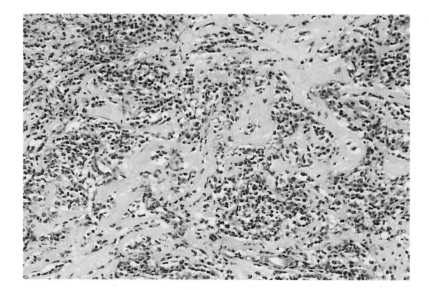

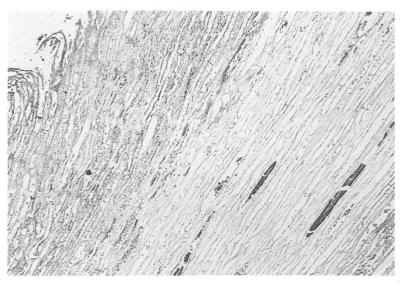

Figure 8.26 Compartmentalizing bands are hyalinized in this sclerosing retroperitoneal lymphoma.

Figure 8.27 Sloughed necrotic papillae in the urine sediment should be recognized as renal tissue fragments by the presence of preserved outlines of collecting duct structures, which frequently contain casts and necrotic ("ghost") cells. The papillary tip characteristically will be devoid of surface urothelium.

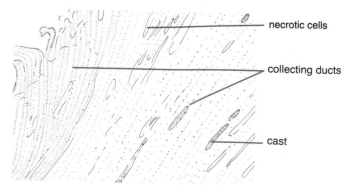

necrotic cells

collecting ducts

cast

papillae down the ureter. The sloughed papillae may cause uretero-pelvic or ureteral obstruction or may be voided in the urine (Fig. 8.27). The prognosis is generally poor.

Patients with papillary necrosis secondary to analgesic abuse frequently have recurrent UTI and hypertension. Acute renal failure may be secondary to obstruction or septicemia, and uremic symptoms may be present. Renal colic is secondary to ureteral passage of stones or sequestered papillae. Urine sediment exam shows pyuria, which may be sterile; hematuria and necrotic papillae may be present. Prognosis is variable since not all papillae are affected to the same degree. Two thirds of patients show improvement or stabilization of renal function.

MORPHOLOGY In the obstructive form, papillary necrosis is usually bilateral. Necrotic papillae appear as sharply defined, yellow or gray-red, lanceolate or box-shaped areas in the distal two thirds of the medullae and may have a congested border (Fig. 8.28). Changes of acute pyelonephritis with pyelocalyceal exudate and cortical abscesses may be present. Old necrotic papillae may be gritty secondary to calcification, and sloughing produces a ragged surface.

With analgesic nephropathy, the kidney may be small or normal in size. With total papillary necrosis, the cortical surface has alternating, depressed, atrophic areas and raised, hypertrophied nodules, which overlie necrotic papillae and columns of Bertin, respec-

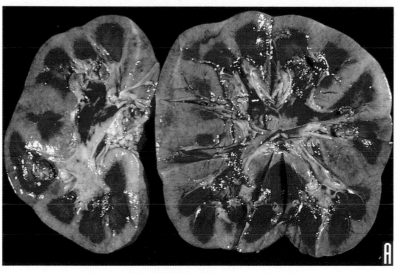

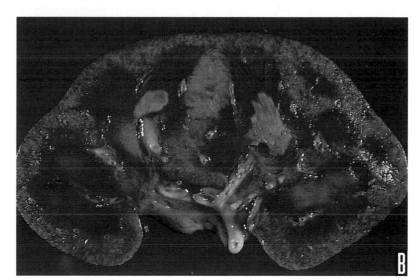

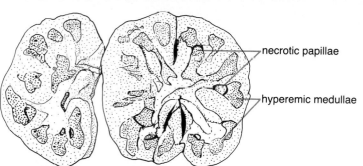

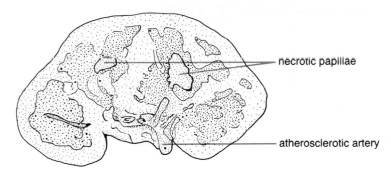

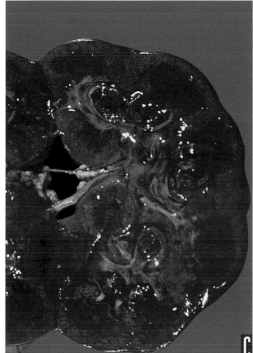

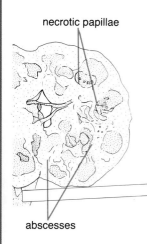

Figure 8.28 A, Both kidneys contain multiple necrotic papillae, which appear pale, dull, and granular in comparison to the hyperemic medullae. The obstructive form of renal papillary necrosis is frequently bilateral and, as in this case, a cause of acute renal failure. **B,** This diabetic kidney contains two necrotic papillae, which appear gray and are sharply demarcated from the proximal one third of the medulla. The renal arterial branches show luminal narrowing secondary to atherosclerosis. (Microscopy is shown in Figures 8.30A, 8.31.) **C,** The multiple necrotic papillae in this kidney have a congested border. Yellow mottling is secondary to acute pyelonephritis with abscess formation.

tively (Fig. 8.29). Papillae appear shrunken and pale or darkened, and may become calcified. Sequestered papillae may lie free in the renal pelvis.

Microscopically, the necrotic papillae appear structureless (Fig. 8.30). Typical of coagulative (ischemic) necrosis, ghosts of tubular structures and nuclear debris are present without inflammatory cells. Papillary urothelium is denuded. Sloughing of the papilla produces a raw, ragged surface with numerous dilated, frequently thrombosed blood vessels, which is eventually covered by a new urothelial lining. Calcification and occasionally bone formation are more common in late stages of analgesic abuse.

In obstructive forms of papillary necrosis, there is a dense zone of polymorphonuclear leukocytes at the border of the necrotic tissue (Fig. 8.31). In analgesic nephropathy, this zone of demarcation is absent and there is barely perceptible merging with the less severely involved fibrotic proximal part of the pyramid (Fig. 8.32). Periodic acid–Schiff (PAS)-positive medullary interstitial fibrosis is more prominent in analgesic nephropathy, and necrotic loops of Henle can be identified in early and intermediate forms, as well as overlying totally necrotic papillae.

Cortical changes are not present in early and intermediate forms of papillary necrosis associated with analgesic abuse. At an advanced stage of analgesic nephropathy, the histologic appearance resembles chronic interstitial nephritis: loss and atrophy of convoluted tubules, interstitial fibrosis, and chronic inflammation, with or without glomerular obsolescence (Fig. 8.33). These nonspecific changes are not indicative of chronic infection or ischemia, and probably represent obstructive atrophy. In nonanalgesic cases, the cortex may also show obstructive changes as well as acute or chronic pyelonephritis (see Chapter 9) and diabetic glomerulosclerosis.

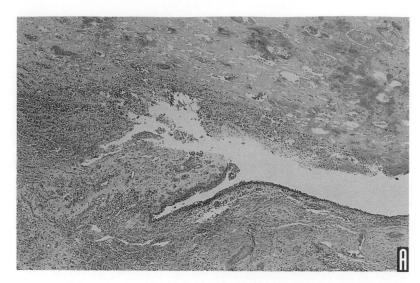

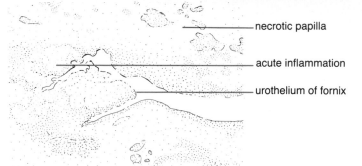

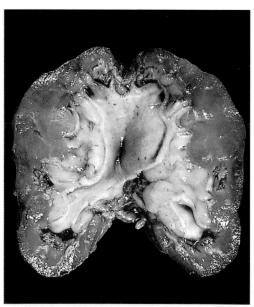

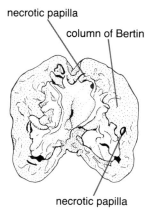

Figure 8.29 Total papillary necrosis is present in this specimen from a patient with analgesic nephropathy. Cortical depressions overlying the pale, shrunken, granular necrotic papillae reflect cortical atrophy. In contrast, cortex overlying columns of Bertin is preserved and appears raised. (Microscopy is shown in Figure 8.30B.)

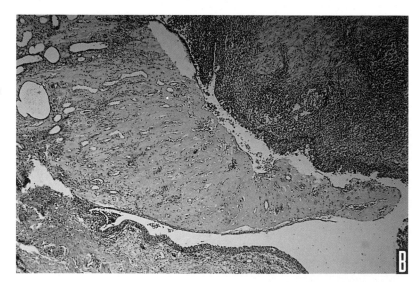

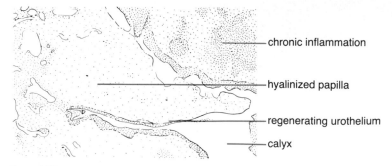

Figure 8.30 A, Urothelium is denuded from the necrotic acellular papilla, and acute inflammation is present at the site of partial detachment from the fornix. (This is the same case as Figures 8.28B, 8.31.) **B,** At this healing stage of papillary necrosis associated with analgesic abuse, the deformed, incompletely sloughed papilla, which protrudes into the calyx, is hyalinized and partially covered by an attenuated layer of regenerating urothelium. Chronic inflammation with lymphoid nodules is present in the adjacent mucosa. (This is the same case as Figure 8.29.)

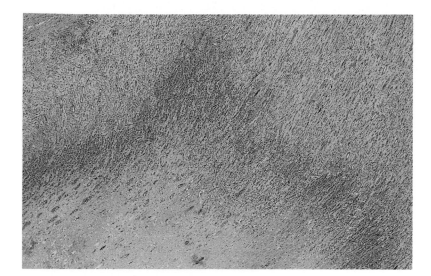

Figure 8.31 A dense zone of acute inflammation with capillary conges-tion demarcates the necrotic papilla (below) in this diabetic patient. Fewer polymorphonuclear leukocytes and white blood cell casts are present in the overlying viable medulla. (This is the same case as Figures 8.28B, 8.30A.)

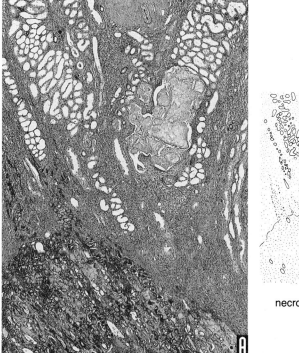

disrupted tubules

necrotic papilla

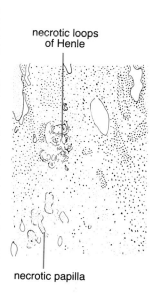

necrotic loops of Henle

necrotic papilla

Figure 8.32 **A,** In papillary necrosis secondary to analgesic abuse, a bordering zone of inflammation is typically absent. The dilated, focally disrupted tubules in the overlying medulla are the result of the intrarenal obstruction. Tubular outlines can still be identified at this

late stage of papillary necrosis (PAS stain). **B,** At higher magnifica-tion, the necrotic papilla imperceptibly merges with the more proxi-mal medulla, which contains necrotic loops of Henle. (These are from the same case as Figure 8.33.)

Figure 8.33 With chronic analgesic nephropathy, the depressed zones of cortical thinning show marked histologic changes. Crowding of preserved glomeruli with shrinkage of tubules is characteristic of cor-tical atrophy. Patches of dense interstitial lymphocytic infiltrates may resemble a chronic interstitial nephritis.

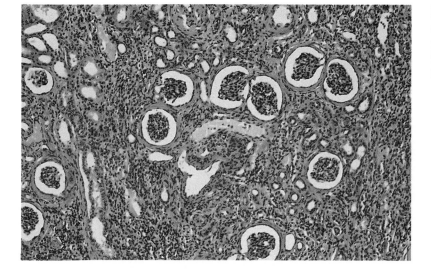

SECTION IV

Urinary Tract Infection and Inflammatory Lesions

CHAPTER 9

Pyelonephritis and Inflammatory Lesions of the Kidney

Urinary tract infection (UTI), which may be acute, recurrent, or chronic, is characterized by large numbers of bacteria and leukocytes in the urine. The significance of UTI must be interpreted with respect to its origin and nature, its localization to different levels of the urinary tract, its effects on the kidneys, and its long-term prognosis.

Gram-negative bacilli—normal inhabitants of the gastrointestinal tract—account for 80%–95% of cases of uncomplicated bacterial UTI and represent a form of endogenous infection. In more than 95% of UTI cases, a single bacterial species is cultured. *Escherichia coli* is responsible for 80% of cases, with a smaller percentage caused by *Proteus*, *Klebsiella* and *Enterobacter* species; the remainder is produced by *Pseudomonas*, *Staphylococcus*, and *Streptococcus faecalis*. In cases of chronic or recurrent pyuria, one or more of these organisms may be encountered. Less common enteric organisms cause infections in special circumstances, such as following antimicrobial therapy, urinary tract instrumentation (especially catheterization), or septicemia.

Pyelonephritis

Acute Pyelonephritis

Acute pyelonephritis (APN) is a specific bacteriologic and anatomic entity. It is defined as a combination of renal parenchymal, calyceal, and pelvic inflammation, and is usually caused by bacterial infection.

The incidence of APN is related to age and sex. In the first year of life and with increasing frequency after the age of 40, UTI is most common in males. Bacteriuria is often associated with congenital anomalies and occurs in approximately 1% of neonates, with a male preponderance. After infancy, UTI is predominantly a female disease; between the ages of 15 and 40 years, the incidence in females outnumbers that in males by 8:1.

Predisposing conditions associated with UTI and APN include congenital or acquired urinary tract obstruction (UTO) (see Section III), urinary tract instrumentation, preexisting renal lesions that cause intrarenal scarring and obstruction, vesicoureteral reflux (VUR) (see Chapter 4), and pregnancy. Renal transplant recipients and diabetics, particularly those who are hospitalized, also have a greater risk of developing infection.

PATHOGENESIS The development of APN is related to the type of organism, the route of infection, and predisposing factors.

As mentioned above, *E. coli*, particularly type O4 and O6 serogroups, are the most common urinary tract pathogens. These bacteria possess virulence factors, including O and K antigens and P-fimbriae–mediated adherence to urothelial cells. Adhesion is a characteristic of more than 90% of pyelonephritogenic *E. coli*. These fimbriae, or pili, are proteinaceous, filamentous organelles that recognize specific receptors on host urothelial cells. Both host receptor density and the nonsecretor state are responsible for susceptibility to UTI. In addition, endotoxins may inhibit ureteral peristalsis, thus favoring upper UTI.

More than 95% of UTIs, including most bacterial UTIs, occur via the ascending route up the column of urine from the bladder. The source of infection in females is the urethral mucosa and vestibule; in males the chronic sources of infection are the prostate and urethra. The hematogenous route is most often a complication of septicemia or endocarditis (for example, staphylococcal). Hematogenous seeding is also more common with *Salmonella* species and *Pseudomonas aeruginosa*. The bloodstream or lymphatics are the mechanisms of involvement in renal tuberculosis. The kidney is a favored site for both miliary and progressive isolated organ tuberculosis, which leads to lower urinary tract involvement via the urine. Fungi and *Actinomyces* species may also infect the kidney via the bloodstream.

Several important predisposing factors are involved in the pathogenesis of APN. Renal tissue, particularly the medulla, is susceptible to infection because it is deficient in reticuloendothelial tissue, the granulocytes in the medulla are not actively mobilized, and the bactericidal power of serum is inhibited by renal anticomplementary activity. Local physiochemical factors, such as hypertonicity and the high tissue concentration of ammonium and urea, increase the likelihood of infection. Abnormalities in the urinary tract, such as VUR (see Chapter 4), malformations, and lithiasis also play a major role in the development of APN. With renal injury such as that due to UTO, both hematogenous and ascending infections are more common. Anomalous urinary tracts are infected 20 times more frequently than normal tracts. Finally, general factors such as altered immune response are also implicated. Normally, serum and renal antibodies are produced in response to renal infection. With *E. coli* infection, O antibodies are initially of the IgM class; later, in recurrent infection, they are of the IgG class.

The reasons for the female preponderance of UTI after infancy include: (1) a shorter urethra, (2) absence of prostatic fluid's antibacterial properties, (3) hormonal changes that affect bacterial adherence to mucosa, and (4) urethral trauma secondary to intercourse (so-called honeymoon cystitis).

Bacteria in the urine does not indicate sustained bacteriuria or symptomatic infection, as long as bladder clearance mechanisms are intact. These include complete emptying with constant replacement of urine; bacteriostatic substances in urine, such as hydrogen ion, urea, ammonia, lysozyme, and immunoglobulins; and inherent antibacterial properties of urothelium. All of these natural defense mechanisms depend on the absence of foreign bodies. Individuals susceptible to UTI, however, have receptors on urothelial cells that avidly bind *E. coli.*

CLINICAL MANIFESTATIONS APN is typically manifested by the sudden onset of symptoms. Patients frequently present with fever, chills, sweats, and general symptoms of bacteremia; they may also have gastrointestinal upsets. Abdominal, loin, or costovertebral angle pain and renal tenderness may be present. Rarely, a swollen kidney is palpable. Pain during micturition indicates reflux. Symptoms of bladder and urethral irritation include dysuria, frequency, and urgency. Symptoms in the pediatric population depend on age. The neonate may have only transient or lasting icterus, respiratory distress, or neurologic signs, while the young infant may be febrile with anorexia, vomiting, and weight loss.

Urine sediment and renal function changes can be expected with APN. Urinalysis will show macro- or microhematuria, with pyuria and white blood cell casts, which are typical of renal parenchymal infection. Urine cultures grow more than 10^3–10^5 bacteria/mL. With more than 10^5 bacteria/mL in a clean, voided midstream urine specimen, particularly of a single gram-negative species, there is an association with true UTI in more than 90% of cases. However, as many as 30% of bacterial UTIs have fewer organisms. Sterile pyuria is common with renal tuberculosis as well as with calculous disease. Laboratory findings reflecting renal dysfunction include diminished concentrating ability, hyperchloremic acidosis, decreased glomerular filtration rate with increased blood urea nitrogen (BUN) and serum creatinine, and tubular proteinuria of more than 1 g per 24 hours (moderate albuminuria and triple globulinuria).

To summarize, in the presence of acute UTI, the diagnosis of APN is favored if there is heavy tubular proteinuria, renal tubular dysfunction, and hemagglutinating antibodies to O antigens of *E. coli* in the urine. Malformations and stones make the diagnosis probable, while VUR only suggests the possibility. Relapse of APN (persistence of the same infection) is characterized by the presence of hemagglutinating antibody. With the occurrence of a totally new infection, precipitating antibody appears; in some series up to 30% of patients develop recurrent infections with a new serotype of *E. coli*.

COMPLICATIONS APN associated with diabetes mellitus or UTO may be complicated by *papillary necrosis* (see Chapter 6). Other complications of APN include pyonephrosis, emphysematous pyelonephritis, and perinephric abscess.

With total or almost complete UTO, particularly when it occurs high within the collecting system in the renal pelvis or upper ureter, *pyonephrosis* may result. Stones are the source of obstruction in more than 50% of cases. Gram-negative bacteria are usually the infecting organism. Pyonephrosis ranges in severity from infected hydronephrosis with excellent renal function to xanthogranulomatous pyelonephritis (XGP) with destroyed renal function.

Emphysematous pyelonephritis is a rare suppurative renal parenchymal and perirenal infection characterized by the presence of intra- and perirenal gas. It occurs mainly in diabetics and is frequently associated with UTO. It is caused by gas-producing, gram-negative enteric organisms, with *E. coli* encountered in approximately 70% of cases and mixed cultures (*Klebsiella, Aerobacter,* and *Proteus*) in approximately 20%. It has also been reported secondary to pyelonephritis caused by *Candida tropicalis* in association with papillary necrosis and pyeloureteral fungus balls. Gas is produced by two major factors: severe necrotizing infection in association with impaired vascular supply and fermentation of glucose by microorganisms. Clinically, emphysematous pyelonephritis may present abruptly or have an indolent course. Symptoms are those of severe APN, although emphysematous pyelonephritis may present as a fever of unknown origin or result in shock and coma. In a diabetic, the presence of subcutaneous emphysema and fever with costovertebral angle tenderness and an abdominal mass should suggest the diagnosis. The majority of patients, however, have no physical findings.

Staphylococcal renal infection may result in renal abscess or carbuncle leading to secondary perinephritis or *perinephric abscess*. Clinical signs include fever, pain, psoas irritation, pyuria, and inflammatory reaction in the neighboring pleura and lung.

MORPHOLOGY Cortical involvement in APN is evident grossly as small (up to several millimeters), raised, yellow-white, rounded nodules with a surrounding narrow hyperemic rim, which represent abscesses (Fig. 9.1A). Foci of confluent suppurative inflammation produce patchy, fan-shaped, white areas in the cortex, extending to the subcapsular surface; this patchy distribution is characteristic of APN. Healthy zones of tissue alternate with infected zones that are often arranged in a roughly triangular or wedge shape, with the base situated under the renal capsule and the apex reaching the mucosa of the renal pelvis. Collecting ducts that drain sites of cortical infection become filled with polymorphonuclear leukocytes and appear as yellow streaks in the papillae. Ducts of Bellini, which permit intrarenal reflux in compound papillae of the upper and lower poles, are more commonly involved. The pelvicalyceal mucosa is hyperemic, dull, and granular (Fig. 9.1B).

With APN associated with obstruction, the kidney is enlarged and has a bulging cut surface. The parenchyma may be diffusely thinned, and papillae may be blunted (see Chapter 6). Calyces are

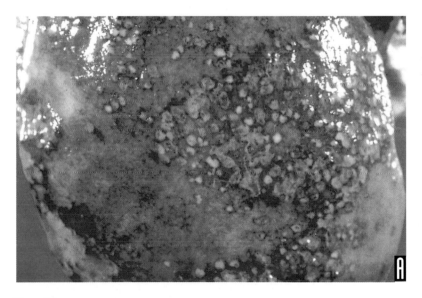

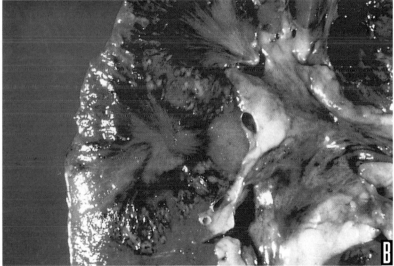

Figure 9.1 A, Cortical abscesses in APN produce discrete or confluent, raised, yellow-white, rounded nodules with surrounding hyperemia. **B,** The cut surface also contains abscesses; there are straight yellow streaks and hyperemia in the medullae. Pelvic mucosa is congested, granular, and dull.

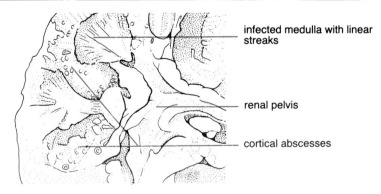

infected medulla with linear streaks

renal pelvis

cortical abscesses

dilated, and the pelvic wall is thickened. Pus may simply be present in the dilated collecting system, or in severe pyonephrosis the kidney may be converted into a pus-filled sac (Fig. 9.2).

Renal involvement in miliary tuberculosis appears as small, yellow-white, barely visible lesions resembling millet seeds. These lesions may heal and calcify. Progressive renal tuberculosis pro-duces large, confluent areas of caseation, which may ulcerate into the calyx. Secondary ureteral involvement causes scarring and stenosis; the resulting UTO may convert the kidney into a hydro-nephrotic sac filled with cheesy material (Fig. 9.3).

Microscopically, APN results in acute inflammatory destruction of the parenchyma, especially in the cortex, with abscess formation

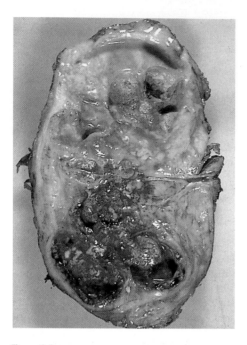
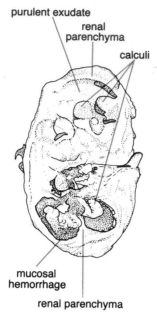

Figure 9.2 Severe pyonephrosis converts the kidney into a pus-filled sac with little identifiable renal parenchyma. The collecting system of this kidney is focally hemorrhagic and covered by creamy exudate; it contains several calculi.

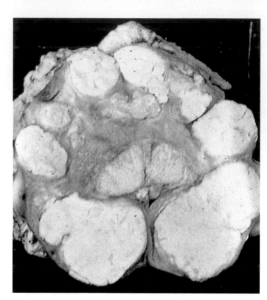

Figure 9.3 Renal tuberculosis, which secondarily involves the ureter, may result in UTO. The hydronephrotic kidney may then fill with cheesy material, forming so-called chalk kidney, as in this specimen.

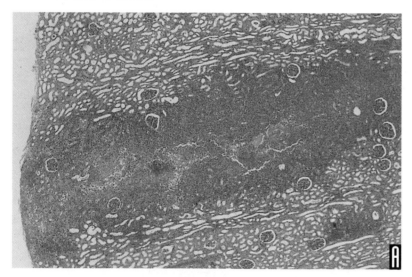
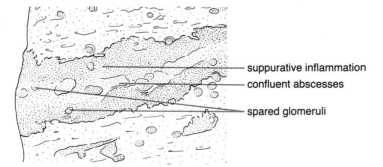
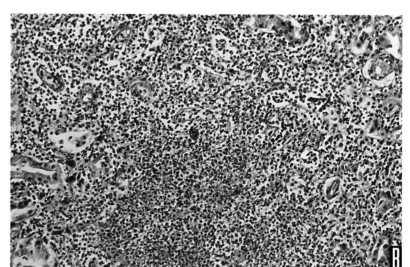

Figure 9.4 A, APN is characterized by patchy, suppurative inflammation extending to the capsular surface (left). Multiple confluent microabscesses are present. Note the sparing of glomeruli. B, At higher magnification, the marked cortical interstitial infiltrate of polymorphonuclear leukocytes is evident. Tubular destruction with parenchymal liquefactive necrosis (lower center) indicates early abscess formation.

(Fig. 9.4). Striking numbers of polymorphonuclear leukocytes infiltrate the interstitium and penetrate the tubules. Chronic inflammatory cells, particularly plasma cells, as well as lymphocytes and eosinophils, appear after several days. Abscesses may also occur in the outer medulla, while the inner medulla contains intratubular polymorphonuclear leukocytes and white blood cell casts (Fig. 9.5). The papillary tip and congested pelvicalyceal mucosa are infiltrated by polymorphonuclear leukocytes.

Usually, the acute inflammation and parenchymal destruction associated with APN leave arteries and arterioles intact. Glomeruli are generally resistant to bacterial infection, although they may be secondarily infiltrated by inflammatory cells.

In comparison with ascending APN, cortical abscesses are even more prominent in blood-borne infections and may be centered around glomeruli. In hematogenous infection with *Staphylococcus aureus,* suppurative inflammation may extend through the renal capsule into the perirenal tissue, resulting in collections of pus outside the renal parenchyma that form a carbuncle or perinephric abscess.

Pathologic findings encountered in cases of emphysematous pyelonephritis, in addition to severe acute (and chronic) pyelonephritis, include multiple cortical abscesses, papillary necrosis, intrarenal vascular thrombi, infarcts (Fig. 9.6), and total renal necrosis.

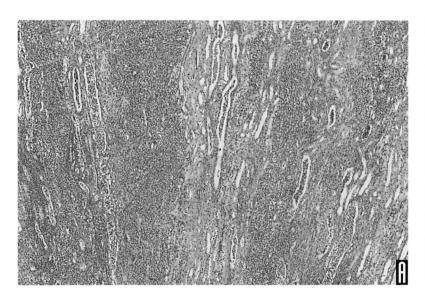

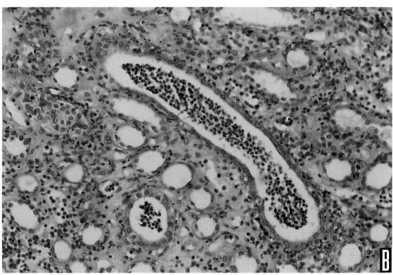

Figure 9.5 A, The medullary inflammatory infiltrate of APN has a typical linear distribution. Collecting ducts are filled with polymorphonu- clear leukocytes. **B,** At higher magnification, white blood cell casts are readily identified.

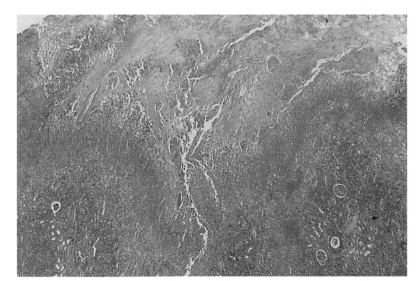

Figure 9.6 Cases of emphysematous pyelonephritis typically show changes of severe acute (and chronic) pyelonephritis. Cortical infarcts, which occur secondary to thrombosis of intrarenal vessels, are triangular areas of coagulation necrosis demarcated by a zone of hemorrhage and intense inflammation.

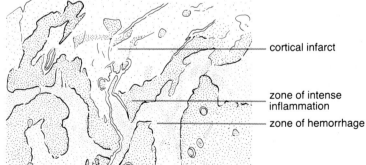

cortical infarct

zone of intense inflammation

zone of hemorrhage

Progressive renal tuberculosis produces numerous discrete and confluent caseating granulomas with parenchymal destruction (Fig. 9.7). Broad zones of tubular atrophy with lymphocytic infiltrates and interstitial fibrosis are present. Granulomas may be difficult to identify in the scarred ureter.

Fungal Pyelonephritis

Systemic fungal infection is a frequent complication in immunologically compromised patients. As many as 75% of these infections are due to *Candida albicans*, with the kidney most susceptible to

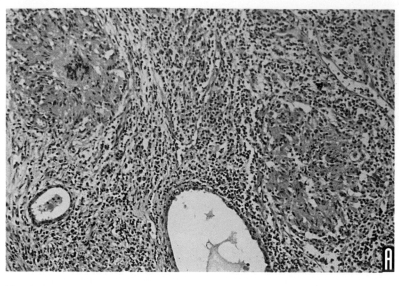

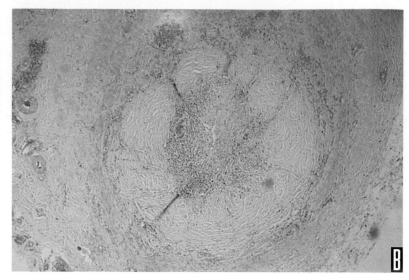

caseating granuloma with multinucleated giant cell

interstitial lymphocytic infiltrate

granuloma composed of epithelioid histiocytes

tubule

periureteral fibrosis

hyalinized nodules

Langhans' giant cells

fibrotic muscular wall

chronically inflamed, fibrotic lamina propria

Figure 9.7 A, Microscopically, renal tuberculosis is characterized by caseating granulomas composed of epithelioid histiocytes and multinucleated giant cells. The surrounding parenchyma has a dense lymphocytic infiltrate with loss of tubules and interstitial fibrosis. **B,** With

secondary ureteral involvement, transmural and periureteral fibrosis cause lumenal stenosis. This inflamed lamina propria contains several Langhans' giant cells and hyalinized nodules, which are markers of the granulomatous inflammation.

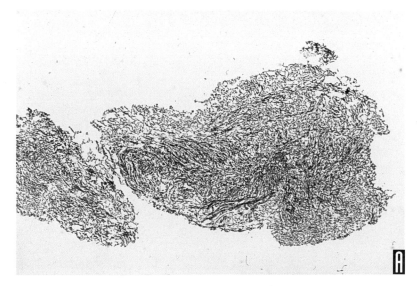

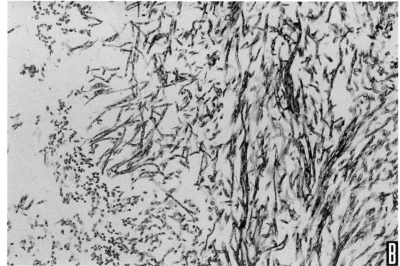

Figure 9.8 Fungus balls may be passed in the urine and be mistaken for amorphous debris. **A,** Silver or PAS stains highlight the tangled mass of hyphae (Grocott's stain). **B,** At higher magnification, branched

septate hyphae are easily identified. Urine cultures from this elderly diabetic grew *Aspergillus flavus* (PAS stain).

infection. Renal candidiasis complicates systemic infection more frequently than infection that follows ascending UTI. An increased frequency of systemic candidiasis occurs in premature newborns who require intensive care and life-sustaining invasive instrumentation such as hyperalimentation and intravascular catheterization. Renal candidiasis in children is rare, affecting mainly newborns and young infants with hereditary immune disorders or those receiving antibiotic therapy.

Infections due to *Cryptococcus neoformans,* which have an incidence in transplant centers of 0.8%–5.8% and a treated mortality of 36%–59%, are of increased concern in renal transplant patients. An autopsy study showed renal involvement in 26%–45% of patients with systemic cryptococcosis.

PATHOGENESIS In experimental renal candidiasis, organisms localize within glomerular and peritubular capillaries in the cortex. Infection is mediated through an adherence mechanism involving surface fibrils. Replicating yeast penetrate endothelium and epithelium by forming germ tubes, thus allowing access to tubules and providing a temporal advantage for the replication of organisms.

CLINICAL MANIFESTATIONS Candidal pyelonephritis has been reported as a cause of oliguric acute renal failure in a premature newborn secondary to obstructing fungus balls. Renal failure, however, is a rare complication from isolated renal candidiasis or as part of systemic infection. In systemic candidiasis with renal involvement, cultures of urine and arterial blood are more frequently positive than those of venous blood. With cryptococcal infection, encapsulated yeast can be demonstrated in the urine by india-ink staining. Fungus balls may form in the urine in cases of renal aspergillosis (Fig. 9.8).

MORPHOLOGY Grossly, abscesses may be diffusely scattered throughout the cortex (Fig. 9.9A). Microscopically, they are com-

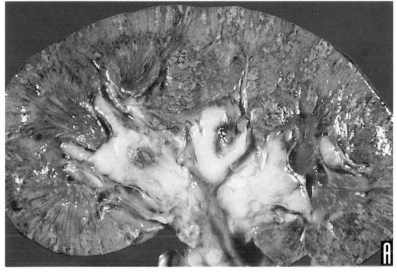

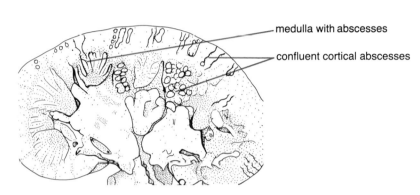

medulla with abscesses

confluent cortical abscesses

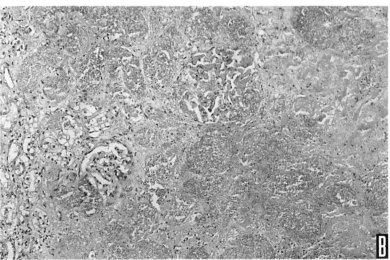

Figure 9.9 Candidal septicopyemia is a serious complication in immunocompromised hosts. **A,** This kidney is from a patient treated for leukemia with radiation and chemotherapy. The cut surface contains large, confluent corticomedullary fungal abscesses.

B, Microscopic examination of the same kidney shows a large zone of necrotic cortex with parenchymal hemorrhage. There is a striking lack of inflammation. **C,** With Grocott's stain, large numbers of *Candida* yeast, which occasionally form germ tubes, can be identified.

monly centered around glomeruli (Fig. 9.10). In both hematogenous and ascending infections, inflammation may be conspicuously absent in the immunocompromised host (Fig. 9.9B,C). Cryptococcal organisms, which may be demonstrated in glomerular capillaries (Fig. 9.11), may also be found within corticomedullary abscesses in association with granulomas, caseation necrosis, interstitial inflammation, fibrosis, and papillary necrosis.

CHRONIC PYELONEPHRITIS

Chronic pyelonephritis (CPN) refers to a chronic tubulointerstitial disorder in which renal scarring is associated with involvement of the calyces and pelvis. The diagnosis of CPN requires clinical, laboratory, urographic, and morphologic evidence, as well as definite proof of infection.

The wide disparity in the frequency of CPN (0.2%–33%) reported in older autopsy studies is in large part related to the variable criteria utilized for diagnosis. Recent autopsy studies indicate an incidence of 1.5%–2%. When strict morphologic criteria were applied, Farmer and Heptinstall reported a frequency of 0.23% when obstruction and diabetes were absent and 1.4% with associated obstruction. Cotran reported a frequency of 1.85% when cases with and without obstruction were included.

CPN remains an important cause of chronic renal failure and is found in 11%–25% of patients (approximately 19% of children) requiring dialysis or transplantation. In pathologic studies of pretransplant nephrectomies, CPN has been reported in 9.5%–15% of cases.

PATHOGENESIS In both adults and children, UTI by itself does not lead to significant long-term renal injury. Although UTIs can seriously impair renal function, renal damage from pyelonephritis sufficient to cause end-stage renal disease only occurs in the presence of associated complicating factors.

Although controversial, bacterial infection plays a dominant role in the pathogenesis of CPN. Potential complicating factors that may cause progressive renal damage in CPN include obstruction, hypertension, and VUR (with focal segmental hyalinosis). Indeed, bacterial infection superimposed on obstruction or VUR plays a role in most cases of CPN, and it is widely believed that renal function is not lost unless there is some anatomic abnormality in addition to UTI. Diabetes mellitus and analgesic abuse are other predisposing factors.

Chronic nonobstructive pyelonephritis, which has been equated with reflux nephropathy, remains controversial. It has not been proven that sterile reflux causes scarring, although high-pressure pyelotubular backflow or intrarenal reflux may result in scarring secondary to leakage of urine and Tamm-Horsfall protein into the interstitium. Most renal damage caused by UTI develops in childhood and is caused by both infection and an anatomic abnormality, most commonly VUR. In one study of children less than 13 years old with UTI, 35% had VUR, 15% had urinary tract abnormalities such as a calculus or ureteral duplication, and 12% had CPN. It is clear that children with reflux have an approximately 30% risk of developing CPN. Twenty to thirty percent of children with significant bacteriuria have VUR, and 20%–25% of these children have renal scars by age five. Scars induced by intrarenal bacterial reflux play a primary role in the development of hypertension. It should be noted, however, that in younger children normal maturation of the ureterovesical junction often leads to disappearance of VUR. The probability of disappearance is related to the severity of reflux (79% with mild versus 24% with severe) (see Chapter 4).

Epidemiologic data suggest that clinical pyelonephritis and renal scarring usually occur without demonstrable VUR; in one study reflux was absent in up to two-thirds of children who developed renal scarring following acute clinical pyelonephritis. It has been hypothesized that functional obstruction of urinary excretion may occur with infection by P-fimbriated E. coli as a result of endotoxin or ureteritis with structural damage and paralysis.

There is little evidence to support immunologic mechanisms in CPN, such as cell-mediated immunity to bacterial antigens or autoimmune processes involving antitubular basement membrane (TBM) antibodies and immune complexes.

Pathogenesis of the focal, segmental sclerosis and hyalinosis-type lesion associated with reflux nephropathy remains unknown. Postulated mechanisms include adaptive hemodynamic changes

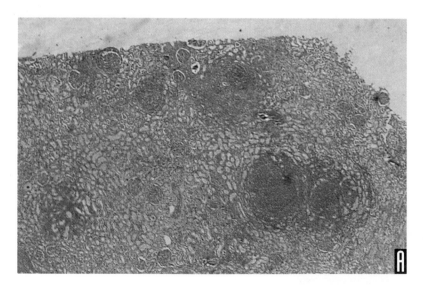

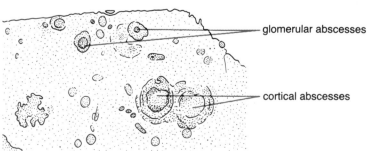

glomerular abscesses

cortical abscesses

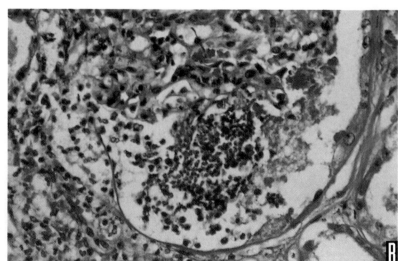

Figure 9.10 **A,** Microscopically, many abscesses in fungal pyelonephritis surround and destroy glomeruli. **B,** *Candida* yeast can usually be identified within glomerular, as well as peritubular, capillaries.

such as increased nephron glomerular filtration rate, increased transcapillary flux of macromolecules, or altered mesangial function.

CLINICAL MANIFESTATIONS The clinical presentation depends on whether CPN is bilateral or unilateral and whether there are associated urinary tract abnormalities. Bilateral CPN may be divided into four clinical groups: (1) bilateral CPN with urinary tract malformation and/or lithiasis, which includes the majority of cases; (2) bilateral CPN with isolated VUR; (3) chronic bacterial pyelonephritis without uropathy, lithiasis, or reflux, which is extremely rare in children; and (4) CPN without urinary infection ("abacterial pyelonephritis"), which has been hypothesized to occur either as a result of a single or asymptomatic infection or secondary to an immune process resulting from persistence of bacterial antigen.

In general, patients with bilateral CPN develop slowly progressive renal insufficiency. The clinical course in patients with chronic obstructive pyelonephritis may be insidious or punctuated by recurrent attacks of APN with back pain, fever, pyuria, and bacteriuria. Sixty to seventy percent of patients with associated urinary tract abnormalities have significant urologic symptoms. Nonobstructive forms of CPN, including those with reflux, may have a silent, insidious onset of renal failure with hypertension manifested only by pyuria with bacteriuria. Bacteriuria may be absent in late stages of CPN.

Renal insufficiency principally affects tubular function, resulting in decreased concentrating power, nocturia, polyuria, tubular acidosis, and, rarely, a salt- or potassium-losing syndrome. Blood urea nitrogen (BUN) and phosphate levels are elevated. Mild to moderate proteinuria may occur in the absence of continued infection, VUR, or hypertension.

The presence of proteinuria can help assess the prognosis in patients with VUR and chronic atrophic pyelonephritis (reflux nephropathy). Proteinuria in the presence of focal segmental sclerosis and hyalinosis is a poor prognostic sign that is almost invariably associated with progressive deterioration of renal function. Antireflux surgery may not alter the course of the glomerulopathy in spite of the absence of continued VUR, infection, or hypertension.

Terminal uremia is often associated with hypertension. In older series, hypertension occurred in 65%–75% of CPN cases. Patients with bilateral CPN have hypertension more frequently than those with unilateral scarring. CPN has been reported in 15%–30% of all hypertensive patients and in 15%–20% of patients dying from malignant hypertension. It has been reported to be the most frequent cause of childhood hypertension, accounting for approximately 30% of cases; reflux is also reported as a common cause.

Unilateral chronic bacterial pyelonephritis may also be secondary to lithiasis or urinary tract malformation. A single pole may be affected, especially in the presence of renal duplication. Unilateral CPN is not a common cause of pediatric hypertension.

MORPHOLOGY CPN reduces renal size and causes irregular scarring, which is asymmetric in bilateral disease (Fig. 9.12). With the capsule stripped, coarse, depressed scars are evident on the cor-

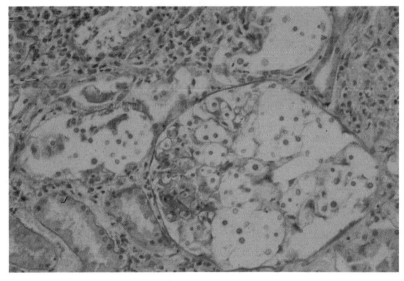

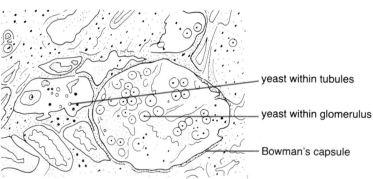

Figure 9.11 Renal involvement in systemic cryptococcosis is common, particularly in renal transplant recipients. In this photomicrograph, yeast can be identified in glomeruli and tubules and are separated by clear halos corresponding to their thick capsule.

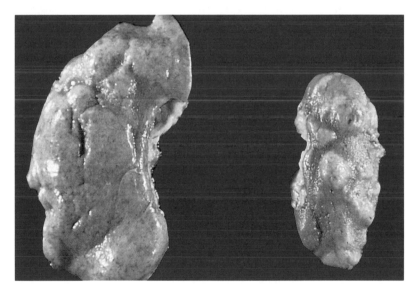

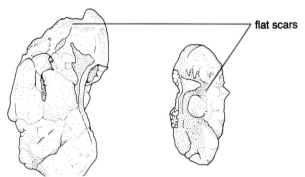

Figure 9.12 Bilateral CPN is typically asymmetric. Although both kidneys in this example have irregular, large, flat scars, the right kidney is more severely involved and shows greater reduction in size. The finely granular appearance of the intervening cortex is secondary to hypertensive nephrosclerosis.

tical surface (Fig. 9.13). These scars are larger and flatter than those seen with infarction. They may vary in number but tend to be more prominent and more common in the upper and lower poles, where there are compound papillae draining two to three lobes and reflux is more frequent. Intervening parenchyma is either smooth or granular if hypertensive nephrosclerosis is present. The characteristic morphologic changes of CPN, which are evident on cut section of the kidney, consist of a coarse, discrete corticomedullary scar overlying a blunted or deformed calyx (Fig. 9.14). Pelvic mucosa is generally thickened and finely granular and may be hemorrhagic or covered by exudate. Pyelitis cystica or ureteritis cystica may be present (see Fig. 9.16 and Chapter 10).

In nonobstructive CPN, there is no pelvic dilatation, but one or more calyces are dilated, particularly at the poles (Fig. 9.15). Obstruction is accompanied by varying degrees of pelvicalyceal dilatation and parenchymal thinning (see Chapter 6).

In advanced stages of CPN, the kidneys are markedly contracted. The renal capsule is typically thickened, fibrotic, and difficult to strip from the capsular surface. In rare cases, chronically inflamed hilar and perirenal fat becomes fibrotic and merges with the scarred renal parenchyma, leading to an appearance of diffuse or segmental fibrolipomatous replacement (Fig. 9.16).

Microscopically, the changes are predominantly tubulointerstitial. The degree of chronic interstitial inflammation varies and is often

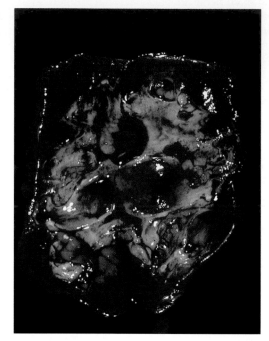

Figure 9.13 As seen in this specimen, CPN produces irregular, coarse, depressed scars on the cortical surface that are easily appreciated with the capsule stripped. Uninvolved parenchyma appears raised and nodular.

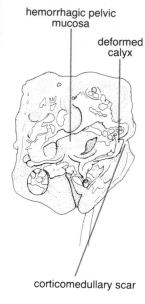

Figure 9.14 This bivalved kidney with CPN shows the characteristic corticomedullary scars overlying deformed calyces. The pelvic mucosa is hemorrhagic.

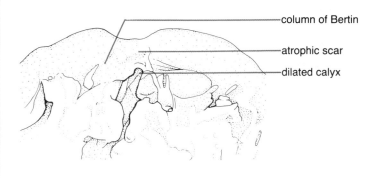

Figure 9.15 The coarse renal scar in this patient with VUR is surrounded by bulging parenchyma, and the pale, atrophic parenchyma overlies a dilated calyx. Reflux-associated scars may show disproportionate centrilobar atrophy with relative sparing of the laterally situated parenchyma and columns of Bertin. End-stage pyelonephritic scars characteristically involve the whole renal lobe. (Courtesy of D. Bhathena, MD, Detroit, Michigan)

inconspicuous. In areas of preserved parenchyma, an infiltrate of lymphocytes, plasma cells, and occasional eosinophils is more likely to be prominent (Fig. 9.17). Peritubular polypoid projections of lymphoid cells in the cortex are a useful indicator of infection. With terminal infection, intratubular polymorphonuclear leukocytes, as well as cellular debris and cholesterol, are evident. Cortical interstitial fibrosis may vary from fine to dense. There is a marked loss of

tubular mass or prominence of atrophic tubules with flattened epithelium and thickened TBMs. Zones of atrophic tubules, which may be dilated, frequently contain waxy casts and have been called "thyroidization." These changes extend to the outer medulla, which generally has fine fibrosis.

As noted grossly, the cortical scar overlies a destroyed papilla and dilated, deformed calyx, which microscopically is chronically

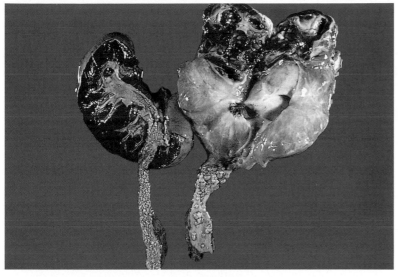

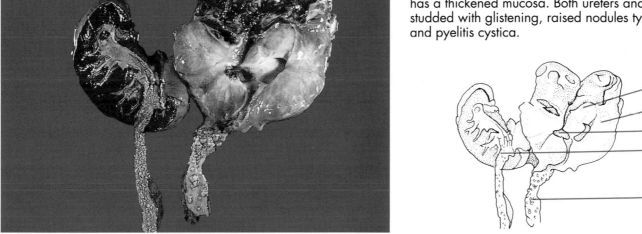

Figure 9.16 The right bivalved kidney shows fibrolipomatous replacement of the lower pole. The dilated pelvis, which contains a calculus, has a thickened mucosa. Both ureters and the left renal pelvis are studded with glistening, raised nodules typical of ureteritis cystica and pyelitis cystica.

- renal pelvis
- fibrolipomatous replacement
- calculus
- pyelitis cystica
- ureteritis cystica

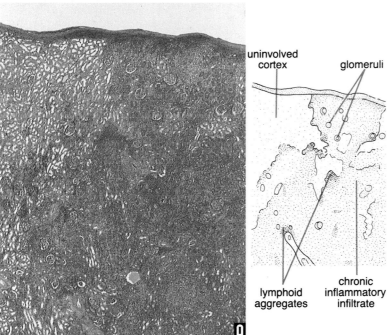

uninvolved cortex — glomeruli

lymphoid aggregates — chronic inflammatory infiltrate

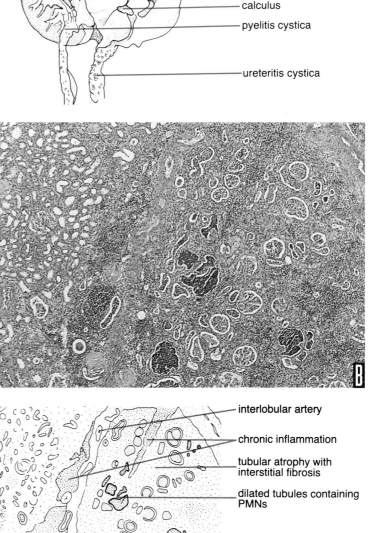

- interlobular artery
- chronic inflammation
- tubular atrophy with interstitial fibrosis
- dilated tubules containing PMNs
- obsolescent glomeruli

Figure 9.17 A, This photomicrograph shows zones of relatively preserved cortical parenchyma, in which CPN is characterized by an intense interstitial chronic inflammatory infiltrate, occasionally with nodular lymphoid aggregates. As expected with a primary tubulo-interstitial process, glomeruli are spared at this stage. **B,** Tubular atrophy and interstitial fibrosis reflect chronicity. Medial thickening of interlobular arteries with focal glomerular obsolescence is common, particularly with superimposed hypertension. These cortical changes by themselves are not diagnostic of CPN. However, the presence of dilated tubules with intraluminal polymorphonuclear leukocytes and nuclear debris is supportive of pyelonephritis with terminal infection.

inflamed and fibrotic (Fig. 9.18). Pelvic mucosa is also thickened and fibrotic, with a chronic inflammatory infiltrate occasionally associated with lymphoid follicles, polymorphonuclear leukocytes, or hemorrhage. Giant cells, foam cells, and pyelitis cystica or pyelitis glandularis may also be present.

Arteries within scarred zones may be normal or may show medial thickening and intimal fibrosis. The vascular fibrosis may be fine or coarse, cellular or fibrous, and concentric with or without elastic reduplication (see Figs. 9.17, 9.18). Arteriolar thickening and hyalinization may be present. The vascular changes are more prominent in cases complicated by hypertension.

Glomeruli within pyelonephritic scars may show variable changes. Thickening of Bowman's capsule with concentric periglomerular fibrosis is common. Regional ischemia causes collapse and solidification with collagen internal to Bowman's capsule. Other glomeruli may show global hyalinization merging into the surrounding interstitium. Focal segmental sclerosis and hyalinosis, which may also be present, is the most common glomerular lesion in proteinuric patients with reflux (Fig. 9.19). Glomerular proliferative changes and necrosis occur secondary to malignant hypertension.

Cortical parenchyma abutting the scar may be completely normal. In hypertensive patients, there are changes of nephrosclerosis with glomerular ischemic obsolescence, tubular atrophy, and interstitial fibrosis, as well as arteriosclerosis and hyaline arteriolosclerosis.

The cortical tubulointerstitial changes are not diagnostic of CPN; a wide variety of factors, including ischemia, simple obstruction, drug reactions, irradiation, and changes secondary to papillary necrosis, can result in a similar histologic picture.

Discrete, coarse, single or multiple corticopapillary scars may also have differing causes. Those due to CPN must be microscopically distinguished from those due to segmental dysplasia, a developmental anomaly, and segmental hypoplasia, which may be related to renal lobar growth failure secondary to VUR (see Chapter 4).

INFLAMMATORY PSEUDOTUMORS

Inflammatory pseudotumors comprise a diverse group of lesions that clinically mimic malignant neoplasms and pathologically may be mistaken for renal cell carcinoma, lymphoma or leukemia, and sarcoma. They have been associated with localized infection and trauma or previous surgery, and a small number remain idiopathic (Fig. 9.20). The postoperative pseudosarcomatous spindle cell nodules have thus far been reported only in the lower urinary tract (see Chapter 13).

With the exception of primary localized amyloidosis of the urinary tract, idiopathic inflammatory pseudotumors are characterized by a polymorphic histologic appearance. Confusing terminology has been used for analogous lesions in the lung, which have been referred to as xanthoma, xanthogranuloma, fibroxanthoma, mast cell tumor, fibrous histiocytoma, and sclerosing hemangioma. Features common to this group of lesions include: (1) rapid growth, (2) sharp circumscription, (3) mixed inflammatory cell infiltrate, (4) proliferation of pleomorphic mesenchymal cells that may form a storiform or fascicular pattern, and (5) prominent microvasculature resembling granulation tissue.

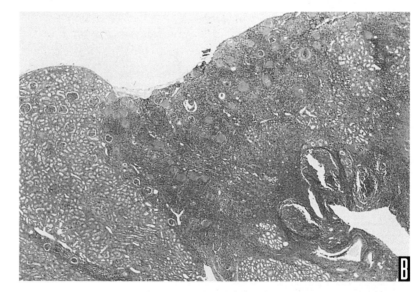

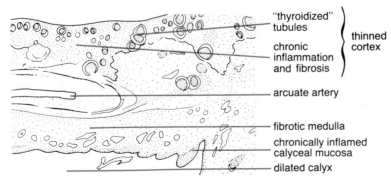

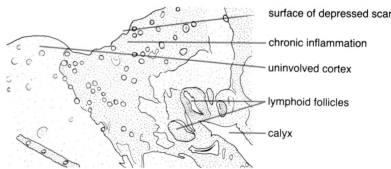

Figure 9.18 A, The diagnostic appearance of CPN is seen in this low-power view. The thinned, chronically inflamed cortex has variable interstitial fibrosis with prominent "thyroidized" tubules; the medulla is also fibrotic. This corticomedullary scar overlies a dilated calyx, with a chronically inflamed mucosa. **B,** As observed grossly, the depressed scar characteristic of CPN is flat and often sharply demarcated from the uninvolved, normal-appearing cortical parenchyma. In this advanced scar, marked interstitial chronic inflammation persists, and lymphoid follicles surround the deformed upper pole calyx.

Xanthogranulomatous Pyelonephritis

Xanthogranulomatous pyelonephritis (XGP) is a rare complication of chronic pyelonephritis, occurring in fewer than 1% of cases. It is more frequent in females and generally occurs in the fourth to sixth decades of life (mean, 47 years). Although it may occur at any age (11 months to 82 years), it is rarer in children than in adults. XGP may be diffuse or localized to one pole and is very rarely bilateral. It is a great imitator and may be erroneously diagnosed as renal cell carcinoma or tuberculosis.

PATHOGENESIS The most common bacterial organisms present in urine or renal cultures are *Proteus* (more than 60% of cases) and *Klebsiella* species, as well as *E. coli.* In more than 50% of cases, however, bladder urine is sterile. The pathologic appearance of XGP is probably related to poor drainage from the collecting system; in massive tissue necrosis, liberated lipids are phagocytosed by macrophages.

CLINICAL MANIFESTATIONS A history of obstructive uropathy or urologic procedures may be present, and 20%–70% of cases are associated with nephrolithiasis, particularly staghorn calculi. Duration of symptoms may range from two weeks to five years (mean, 10 months) and most commonly include flank pain, recurrent low-grade fever, weight loss, colic, chills, malaise, anorexia, hematuria, and cystitis. A palpable, occasionally draining flank mass may be present. Hepatomegaly is present in 30% of cases. Hepatic dysfunction, found in 40% of cases, is thought to be due to necrosis of renal parenchyma. Adult symptoms are frequently absent in pediatric patients, who may have only disturbances of micturition and discoloration of urine, with pyuria, mild proteinuria, hypochromic anemia, and leukocytosis.

MORPHOLOGY Grossly, XGP may be categorized into one of three stages, reflecting the severity and extent of involvement. In stage I, the process is confined to the kidney (nephric). Stage II indicates perinephric extension with involvement of Gerota's fas-

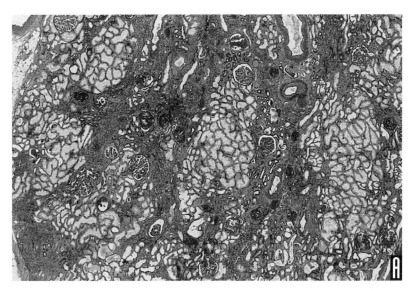

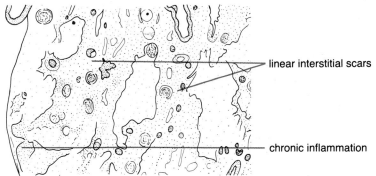

linear interstitial scars

chronic inflammation

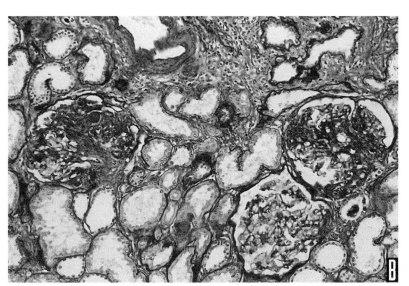

Figure 9.19 **A,** Cortex from the upper pole of a kidney with reflux nephropathy contains linear interstitial scars with atrophic tubules and obsolescent glomeruli. Focal chronic inflammation is present (PAS stain). **B,** Glomeruli within preserved parenchyma are enlarged and focally contain sclerotic segments. In glomeruli with sclerosis and hyalinosis, increased mesangial matrix causes segmental tuft obliteration with associated capsular adhesions. Entrapped protein within obliterated loops appears as occasionally vacuolated, globular hyaline masses (PAS stain).

Figure 9.20
Inflammatory Pseudotumors of the Urinary Tract

I. Infectious
    A. Xanthogranulomatous pyelonephritis
    B. Malakoplakia (megalocytic interstitial nephritis)
    C. (Fibro) lipomatous replacement of the kidney

II. Postoperative—proliferative spindle cell nodule

III. Miscellaneous
    A. Amyloid tumor
    B. Hematopoietic tumor (renal hilus)
    C. Plasma cell granuloma
    D. Myxoid inflammatory pseudotumor

cia. Involvement of the perinephric fat may resemble a renal carbuncle. In stage III, there is massive spread of the inflammatory process into the paranephric (retroperitoneal) fat or down the paracolic gutter.

In typical cases, an enlarged hydronephrotic kidney has perirenal fibrosis and often contains a staghorn calculus. The dilated calyces, which contain purulent exudate, are lined by a friable yellow zone, and yellow cortical nodules may be prominent (Fig. 9.21). Cortical abscesses and/or changes of CPN may also be present.

Microscopically, the yellow zone surrounding the necrotic, acutely inflamed pericalyceal parenchyma consists of granulomatous inflammation with numerous large, finely granular, foamy histiocytes containing neutral fat and cholesterol esters (xanthomatous cells) (Fig. 9.22). Smaller, periodic acid–Schiff (PAS)-positive, granular mononuclear cells are also present, as are giant cells and an admixture of plasma cells, polymorphonuclear leukocytes, and fibroblasts. Inflammatory fibrous tissue separates the granulomatous zone from the atrophic cortex.

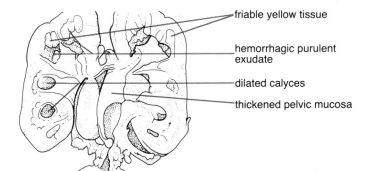

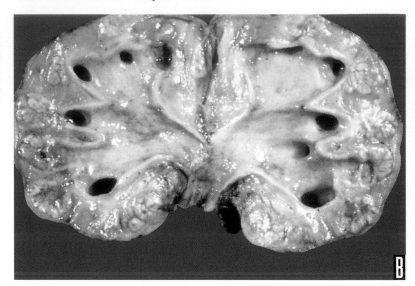

friable yellow tissue

hemorrhagic purulent exudate

dilated calyces

thickened pelvic mucosa

Figure 9.21 A, Milder forms of XGP can be recognized grossly by the friable yellow tissue surrounding the dilated calyces. As in this case, pyonephrosis is frequently present. The pelvic mucosa is thickened, and the dilated calyces contain hemorrhagic purulent exudate. **B,** Other cases of XGP may have multiple, discrete, yellow nodules diffusely scattered throughout the parenchyma. When large and confluent, these yellow masses may be mistaken for renal cell carcinoma.

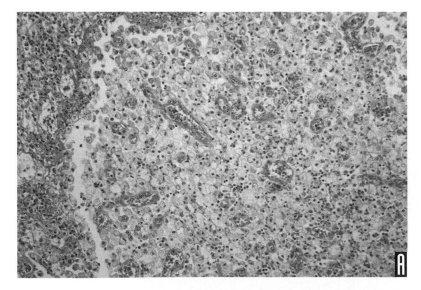

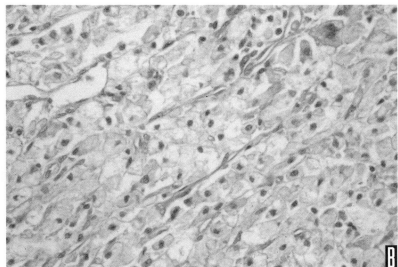

Figure 9.22 A, Adjacent to the acutely inflamed, necrotic pericalyceal parenchyma (left) in this photomicrograph are numerous lipid-laden histiocytes, which are characteristic of XGP and impart the yellow color observed grossly. The capillary pattern in this zone is that of granulation tissue. **B,** Xanthogranulomatous nodules may contain a uniform population of mononucleated histiocytes with abundant clear or finely granular cytoplasm. This monomorphic population of foam cells with a delicate, rich capillary vascularity may resemble the clear cell variant of renal cell carcinoma.

Malakoplakia

Malakoplakia is a complication of chronic bacterial UTI, most frequently with *E. coli*. It usually involves the bladder; the clinicopathologic features and pathogenesis are discussed in Chapter 10. This granulomatous lesion may occur in the renal pelvis and ureters, as well as in the prostate and testis. Females are more commonly affected, and most patients are in their fifth decade of life. When renal involvement occurs, it is usually accompanied by lower urinary tract disease; resultant ureteral stricture may be responsible for urinary tract obstruction.

CLINICAL MANIFESTATIONS Patients typically have a history of UTI with symptoms of flank pain, fever, and chills. A palpable flank mass or signs of a perinephric abscess may be present. Urinalysis reveals variable proteinuria, white blood cells, and, occasionally, red blood cells. Severe bilateral renal involvement may result in renal failure.

MORPHOLOGY Most cases of renal malakoplakia primarily involve medullary zones, and kidneys frequently show changes of obstructive uropathy. Dilated calyces are lined by yellowish tissue, and there may be cortical abscesses, multiple, raised, yellow subcapsular areas, or extensive replacement of renal parenchyma by yellow masses resembling renal cell carcinoma.

Cases with predominant cortical involvement have been termed megalocytic interstitial nephritis. Grossly, these are discrete or confluent variable-sized, firm, slightly bulging, yellow-gray foci.

Microscopically, renal malakoplakia is characterized by sharply demarcated interstitial clusters of polygonal cells with PAS-positive, coarsely granular eosinophilic cytoplasm containing Michaelis–Gutmann bodies (Fig. 9.23). Similar histiocytic cells may be seen within intact tubules and may be observed cytologically in the urine sediment. Extensive destruction and loss of tubules within involved areas is common. Few polymorphonuclear leukocytes, moderate plasma cells, small numbers of lymphocytes, and occasional eosinophils may also be present, as may abscesses and foci of fibrosis.

Primary Localized Amyloidosis

Primary systemic amyloidosis has a 35% incidence of renal involvement in comparison with secondary forms of amyloidosis, which involve the kidney in 100% of cases and commonly lead to death in uremia with nephrotic syndrome. In contrast, the lower urogenital system is involved in approximately 50% of cases of primary systemic amyloidosis and 25% of cases of secondary amyloidosis.

Primary localized (tumefactive) amyloidosis usually involves the bladder (see Chapter 10). In the genitourinary tract, excluding the kidney, microscopic amounts of amyloid are not uncommon and are of no pathologic significance. These deposits are thought to be secondary to aging.

An isolated case of primary amyloidosis of the renal pelvis was reported in a 39-year-old male who had ureteropelvic junction obstruction and presented with flank pain and hematuria. IVP demonstrated irregular infundibular and pelvic constrictions, with linear submucosal calcifications outlining the pelvicalyceal system.

Hematopoietic Tumor of Renal Hilus

Extramedullary hematopoiesis occurs rarely in extraparenchymal sites, and the formation of a mass is uncommon. The usual soft tissue site for a mass of extramedullary hematopoiesis is the paravertebral thorax. The renal hilus is the second most common site. Renal hilar extramedullary hematopoiesis is most often part of a diffuse reactive process with widespread involvement of reticuloendothelial organs. Bilateral or unilateral hilar involvement is rarely limited to the renal hilus without concurrent predisposing diseases.

PATHOGENESIS The pathogenesis of renal hilar hematopoietic tumor is unclear. An embryologic basis has been suggested, as the hilus is normally a site of hematopoiesis in the fetus. A localized hormonal effect from renal erythropoietin production is unlikely.

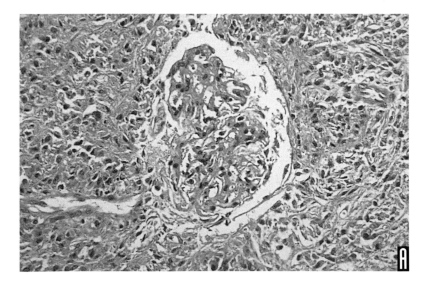

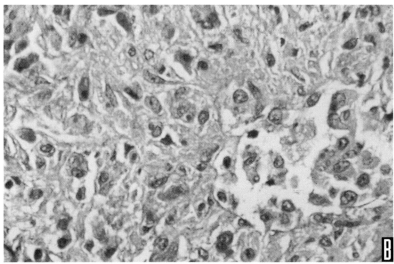

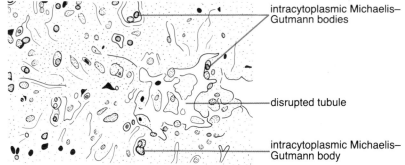

Figure 9.23 **A,** Renal cortical malakoplakia, shown in this photomicrograph, causes inflammatory destruction of tubules. The interstitial infiltrate is composed of histiocytes with granular eosinophilic cytoplasm, which may be mistaken for a granular cell variant of renal cell carcinoma. **B,** Demonstration of Michaelis–Gutmann bodies within the cytoplasm of these histiocytes with the PAS stain is diagnostic of malakoplakia.

intracytoplasmic Michaelis–Gutmann bodies

disrupted tubule

intracytoplasmic Michaelis–Gutmann body

CLINICAL MANIFESTATIONS The typical patient is a severely malnourished, anemic child with infection. The tumor may also be found in patients with agnogenic myeloid metaplasia. In most cases, the hematopoietic tumor is asymptomatic and is an incidental autopsy finding. It has been reported in association with gross, painless hematuria and flank pain.

MORPHOLOGY The pseudotumor is typically a well circumscribed mass located between the renal parenchyma and pelvis (Fig. 9.24A). It is soft and purple-red to red-brown.

Microscopically, the mass is unencapsulated, consisting of islands of hematopoietic cells, including megakaryocytes and normally maturing myeloid and erythroid elements (Fig. 9.24B). Unlike leukemic infiltrates, which commonly involve the renal hilus, the cell population is not monomorphic. The stroma consists of a loose, slightly spindled fibromyxoid matrix with only small amounts of adipose tissue. Occasional lymphoid follicles, scattered lymphocytes, and plasma cells are present. Focal deposits of hemosiderin pigment reflect old hemorrhage.

Plasma Cell Granuloma

Plasma cell granuloma has been reported in the kidney and renal pelvis. Its etiology remains obscure.

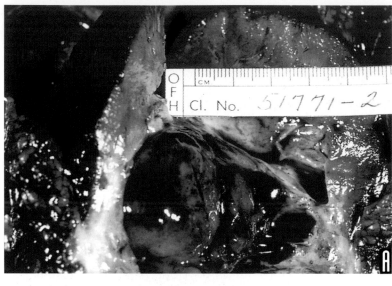

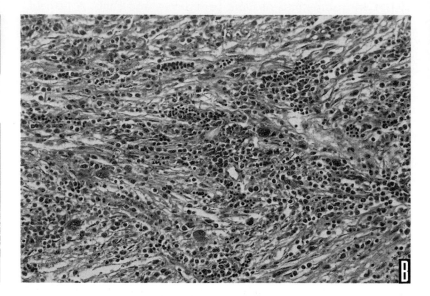

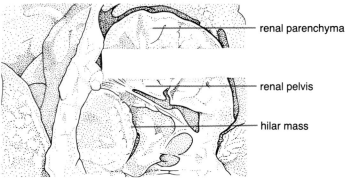

renal parenchyma

renal pelvis

hilar mass

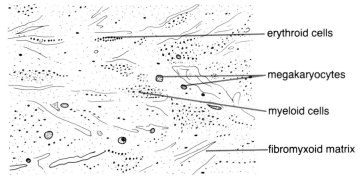

erythroid cells

megakaryocytes

myeloid cells

fibromyxoid matrix

Figure 9.24 A, This hematopoietic tumor of the renal hilus is typically located between the renal parenchyma and pelvis. It is a sharply circumscribed mass with a hemorrhagic, tan, cut surface. **B,** Photomicrograph of the same tumor shows myeloid elements, clusters of erythroid cells, and scattered megakaryocytes in a spindle cell fibromyxoid matrix. This polymorphous population distinguishes the hematopoietic tumor from a leukemic infiltrate. (**A,B:** Courtesy of E. Beckman, MD, New Orleans, Louisiana)

Figure 9.25 Compressing the lower pole of this bivalved kidney is a plasma cell granuloma. It is a sharply circumscribed, yellow-white, solid mass lacking hemorrhage and necrosis. These reactive lesions may be mistaken for a renal tubular neoplasm. (This is the same case as Figure 9.26.)

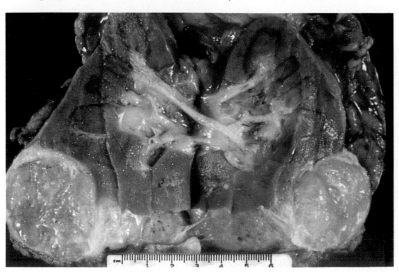

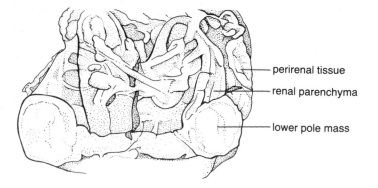

perirenal tissue

renal parenchyma

lower pole mass

CLINICAL MANIFESTATIONS Symptoms have included flank pain, which may be colicky, and recurrent, gross, painless hematuria. There is no associated fever or urinary tract infection.

MORPHOLOGY Grossly, plasma cell granuloma is a solid, yellow-white, sharply demarcated mass. When located in the renal pelvis, it appears as a polypoid tumor. Hemorrhage and necrosis are typically absent (Fig. 9.25).

Microscopically, the mass is composed of abundant collagenous fibrous stroma, which is often hyalinized and resembles paramyloid. Interlacing or whorled masses of fibroblasts may also be present. There is a heavy infiltrate of mature plasma cells with frequent Russell bodies. An admixture of lymphocytes, scattered lymphoid follicles, monocytes, macrophages, eosinophils, and large reticuloendothelial cells may be present (Fig. 9.26). A granulation tissue-type stroma may be seen, as well as myxoid or edematous areas. Thick-walled, medium-sized vessels have also been described. The histologic appearance differs from extramedullary primary solitary plasmacytoma, which is monomorphic and has only scant connective tissue stroma. Ultrastructural studies have confirmed the presence of myofibroblasts in pulmonary plasma cell granulomas.

MYXOID INFLAMMATORY PSEUDOTUMOR

This unusual pseudotumor has been reported to occur in the bladder (see Chapter 10) and shares histologic similarities with the postoperative spindle cell nodule, as well as with nodular fasciitis and similar lesions that occur in the lung.

We have observed one example of myxoid inflammatory pseudotumor of the kidney in an elderly female with painless gross hematuria. Grossly, it was a sharply circumscribed, light-brown, gelatinous

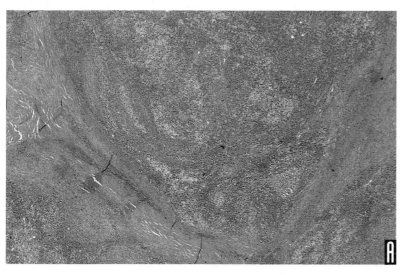

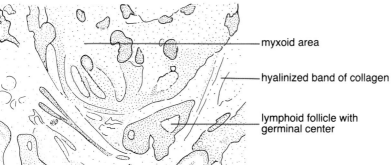

myxoid area

hyalinized band of collagen

lymphoid follicle with germinal center

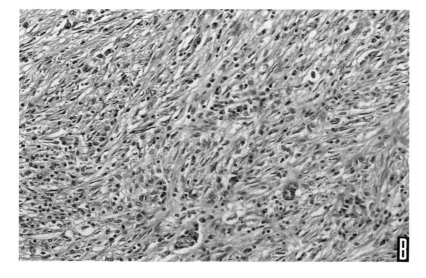

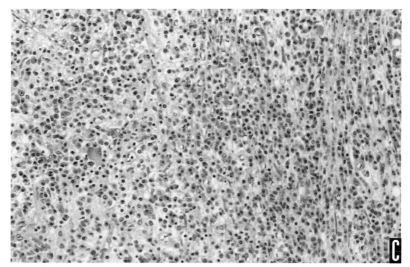

Figure 9.26 A, Plasma cell granuloma typically has abundant, densely hyalinized bands of collagen that focally may resemble paramyloid. Scattered lymphoid follicles with germinal centers and myxoid areas distinguish this inflammatory pseudotumor from lymphoma and plasmacytoma. B, Focally, there may be a more cellular fibroblastic stroma, which forms interlacing or whorled masses. Within this spindle cell stroma is an infiltrate of plasma cells, including occasional binucleated forms, scattered lymphocytes, and occasional large reticuloendothelial cells. C, In the myxoid or edematous area in this photomicrograph, the plasma cell granuloma has a more monomorphic infiltrate of mature plasma cells, with occasional binucleate forms and Russell bodies.

mass with foci of hemorrhage (Fig. 9.27). Histologically, proliferating spindle cells were separated by a myxoid stroma with a prominent arborizing or plexiform capillary vascularity, as well as foci resembling granulation tissue. In cellular foci, a vague fascicular pattern was present, but storiform areas were not seen. Extravasated erythrocytes, acute hemorrhage, and hemosiderin deposits were prominent. Mononucleate and multinucleate giant cells, as well as ganglionlike cells were present (Fig. 9.28). There was a diffusely scattered infiltrate of histiocytes, plasma cells, mast cells, lymphocytes, and eosinophils, with small foci of extramedullary hematopoiesis. On electron microscopy, the stromal cells included undifferentiated mesenchymal cells, fibroblasts, fibrohistiocytic cells, and myofibroblasts.

This pseudotumor may be confused with a sarcoma, particularly myxoid or inflammatory malignant fibrous histiocytoma and myxoid liposarcoma. However, the lack of significant nuclear pleomorphism, hyperchromasia, and atypical mitotic figures are differentiating features. As in nodular fasciitis, the histologic appearance is that of reparative mesenchymal tissue.

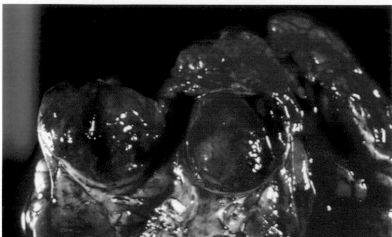

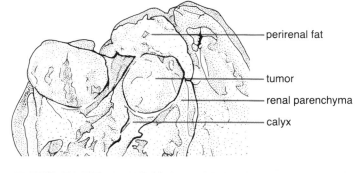

Figure 9.27 The intrarenal inflammatory pseudotumor in this specimen compresses the overlying renal parenchyma and displaces the upper-pole calyx. It is a sharply circumscribed, gelatinous, tan-brown mass with foci of hemorrhage. (This is the same case as Figure 9.28.)

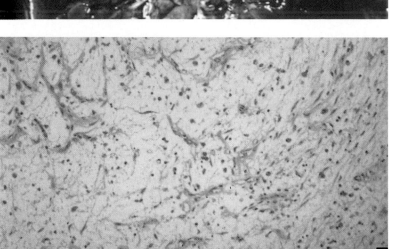

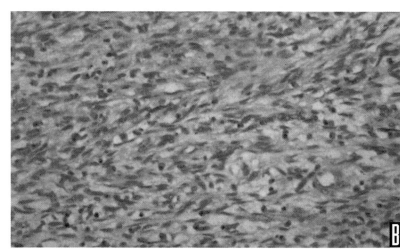

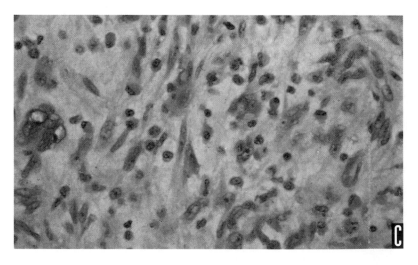

Figure 9.28 A, The majority of the inflammatory pseudotumor has a myxoid stroma with a prominent capillary network. It contains spindle cells and scattered inflammatory cells. **B,** More compact cellular foci containing proliferating spindle cells are also present. In this myxoid variant, the absence of cytologic atypia and abnormal mitoses, as well as the lack of a storiform pattern, exclude a diagnosis of myxoid malignant fibrous histiocytoma. **C,** Plump spindle cells, lymphocytes, plasma cells, mast cells, histiocytes containing hemosiderin pigment, and occasional ganglionlike cells are present.

CHAPTER 10

Inflammatory, Proliferative, and Metaplastic Lesions of the Bladder

Cystitis refers to a variety of lesions, including some that are noninflammatory in origin. Diagnostic terminology is frequently descriptive and employs qualifying adjectives that have no clinicopathologic specificity. A variety of proliferative or metaplastic abnormalities may be associated with the clinical symptoms or pathologic findings of cystitis. Some of the variants of cystitis may have a gross and microscopic appearance suggestive of tumor.

In this chapter, cystitis is divided into acute and chronic nonspecific forms and variants with distinctive morphologies or specific etiologies. Proliferative and metaplastic lesions and miscellaneous pseudotumors or "infiltrative" lesions are also discussed. The pathogenesis of infectious cystitis in the context of bacterial urinary tract infection (UTI) and pyelonephritis is considered in Chapter 9.

CYSTITIS

NONSPECIFIC FORMS OF CYSTITIS

Nonspecific acute and chronic inflammation in the bladder mucosa is observed in the majority of cystitis cases. These inflammatory reactions arise in a variety of clinical settings and may have an infectious or noninfectious etiology.

PATHOGENESIS Inflammatory lesions lacking a distinctive morphologic appearance most commonly occur with bacterial infections. More rarely, nonspecific forms of cystitis may occur with trichomonal, viral (e.g., adenovirus), chlamydial, and mycoplasmal infection. The bladder is a reservoir for a wide variety of potential irritants and toxins. Patients receiving cytotoxic antitumor drugs or radiation therapy may also develop nonspecific inflammatory changes.

CLINICAL MANIFESTATIONS Regardless of etiology, all forms of cystitis characteristically produce three symptoms: urinary frequency, dysuria, and abdominal pain, which may be localized to the bladder or suprapubic region. Gross or microscopic hematuria may be present. Cystitis secondary to a localized bladder infection does not usually induce constitutional symptoms. Systemic signs, such as fever, chills, and malaise, usually indicate upper UTI (see Chapter 9).

MORPHOLOGY

NONSPECIFIC ACUTE CYSTITIS In the early acute stage, the mucosa retains its normal velvety character but becomes hyperemic. In more advanced cases or with more severe inflammatory reactions, the mucosa may have focal or diffuse hemorrhages and precipitation of gray-white to yellow exudate (*suppurative cystitis*). In certain cases, such as adenovirus infection, severe mucosal hemorrhage may be the dominant feature and is termed *hemorrhagic cystitis* (see

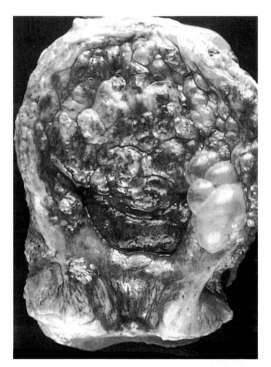

Figure 10.1 The large blebs along the left lower lateral bladder wall of this specimen correspond to gas bubbles of emphysematous cystitis. The mucosa also has diffuse, bullous edema and is dull, granular, and hyperemic with a yellow-gray surface exudate.

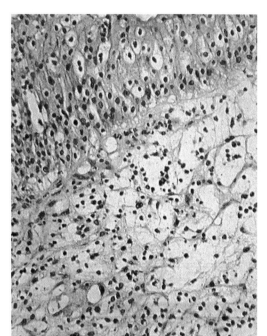

Figure 10.2 In nonspecific acute cystitis, the lamina propria is edematous and contains a heavy infiltrate of neutrophils. Reactive urothelial hyperplasia (upper left) can be seen in this photomicrograph. Neutrophils have migrated into the hyperplastic urothelium and occasionally are contained within cytoplasmic vacuoles. (Reproduced with permission from Schumann and Weiss, 1981).

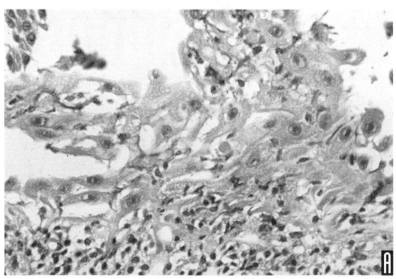

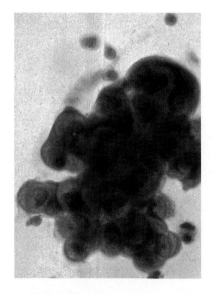

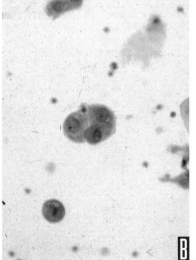

Figure 10.3 Severe acute cystitis causes extensive sloughing of urothelial cells and fragments and may result in extensive mucosal denudation. **A,** The partially detached urothelium in this photomicrograph shows marked reactive changes with characteristically large nucleoli. **B,** Urothelial fragments in a voided urine specimen indicate urinary tract pathology. In acute cystitis, reactive urothelial cells occur in large papillary fragments showing maturation to superficial cells (left panel), or smaller fragments and single cells (right panel). Nuclei are enlarged and have smooth borders, dusty chromatin that is condensed peripherally, and large nucleoli. Cells with eccentric nuclei and cytoplasmic vacuolization are common (Papanicolaou stain).

Fig. 10.24). The granular mucosal surface may become friable and have multifocal shallow ulcerations filled with exudate. Sloughing and ulceration of large mucosal areas typifies *ulcerative cystitis*, whereas *membranous cystitis* is characterized by coagulation of the exudate and necrotic mucosa. Deep ulcers and intramural abscesses may occur, and virulent organisms may produce perivesical abscesses, perforation, sinus tracts, and pelvic peritonitis. When inflammatory edema is severe enough to produce marked ischemia, the mucosal surfaces may appear green-black and necrotic (*gangrenous cystitis*). *Emphysematous cystitis*, which most frequently strikes diabetics, is characterized by gas bubbles in the submucosal connective tissue (Fig. 10.1). Also known as *pneumatosis of the bladder*, it is presumably caused by gas-forming bacteria. It should be distinguished from *bullous cystitis*, which corresponds to marked edema of the lamina propria and produces large mucosal folds (see Figs. 10.19, 10.30).

Microscopically, nonspecific acute cystitis is characterized by an infiltrate of polymorphonuclear leukocytes in the lamina propria and urothelium with variable edema, vascular congestion, and hemorrhage (Fig. 10.2). Reactive and degenerative changes in the urothelium are evident histologically and cytologically, with sloughing and ulceration leading to marked exfoliation of cells (Fig. 10.3). The surface exudate is composed of polymorphonuclear leukocytes, fibrin, blood, and necrotic cells. In emphysematous cystitis, rounded spaces, corresponding to gas bubbles, are surrounded by giant cells.

NONSPECIFIC CHRONIC CYSTITIS   With persistence of bladder infection, the mucosa appears granular, red, and friable, and may be ulcerated. Heaped-up mucosa may form prominent folds, referred to as *papillary* or *polypoid cystitis* (Fig. 10.4). The mucosa may become studded with multiple, small, round, yellow-white elevations or papules, a condition that corresponds to *follicular cystitis* (Fig. 10.5). Precipita-tion of urinary salts on the bladder mucosa characterizes *encrusted cystitis* (see Chapter 6). Chronic cystitis associated with bladder neck obstruction may have prominent trabeculation (Fig. 10.6).

Microscopically, the lamina propria contains a nonspecific mononuclear inflammatory infiltrate composed of variable numbers of lymphocytes and plasma cells (Fig. 10.7). Histiocytes and

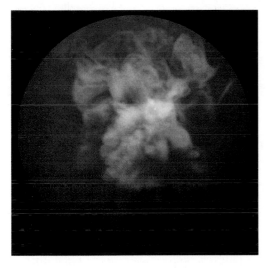

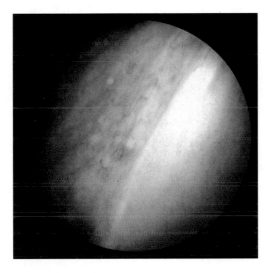

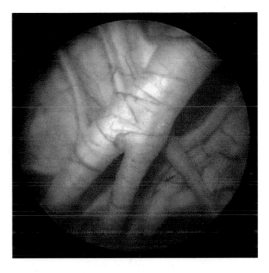

Figure 10.4 Cystoscopically, polypoid cystitis may resemble a papillary transitional cell carcinoma. Clinical history helps differentiate this lesion from a vesical neoplasm. (Courtesy of B. Bracken, MD, Cincinnati, Ohio)

Figure 10.5 Follicular cystitis viewed through the cystoscope appears as yellow, raised nodules that represent large lymphoid aggregates in the lamina propria. (Courtesy of B. Bracken, MD, Cincinnati, Ohio)

Figure 10.6 Bladder trabeculation is due to detrusor muscle hypertrophy and may be prominent cystoscopically in cases of chronic cystitis associated with bladder outlet obstruction. Saccular mucosal outpouchings occur between hypertrophied muscular bands or ridges. (Courtesy of B. Bracken, MD, Cincinnati, Ohio)

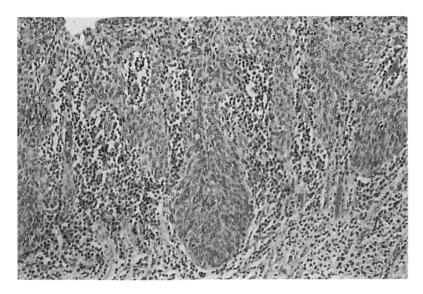

Figure 10.7 Nonspecific chronic cystitis may have a heavy mononuclear infiltrate in the lamina propria. In this photomicrograph, the urothelium shows downward proliferation into the lamina propria with formation of epithelial buds.

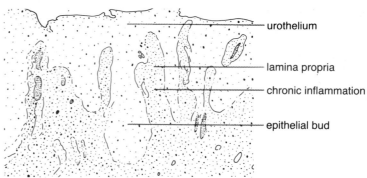

scattered eosinophils may also be present. Persistent edema or fibrous thickening may be present, as well as prominent vascular dilatation. The urothelium, which normally is not more than five to seven cell layers thick, may be variably thinned and contain prominent "umbrella" cells, depending on the degree of bladder distention and prior saline irrigation (Fig. 10.8). The urothelium may also be hyperplastic (more than seven cell layers) and show orderly maturation with preserved polarity (Fig. 10.9). In polypoid cystitis,

there is an outward proliferation of bladder mucosa with thin or broad projections of edematous, congested lamina propria containing a variable, occasionally scant, chronic inflammatory infiltrate (Fig. 10.10). The surface may be ulcerated. As it heals, the urothelium may proliferate to form small villous projections. In follicular cystitis, the lamina propria contains multiple nodular aggregates of lymphocytes that form lymphoid follicles with well developed germinal centers (Fig. 10.11).

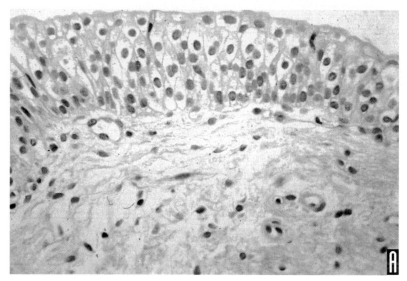
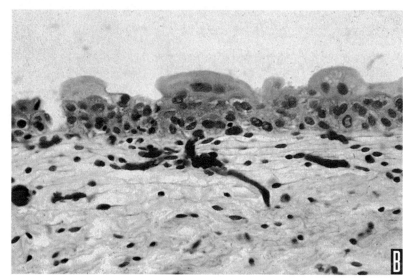

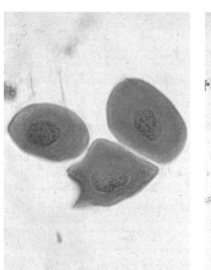
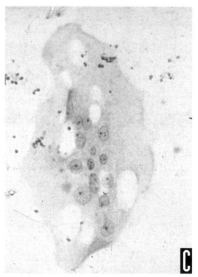

Figure 10.8 Edema of the lamina propria with a relatively scant nonspecific mononuclear inflammatory infiltrate may be seen in some cases of chronic cystitis. Urothelial thickness varies depending on the degree of bladder distention. **A,** In this photomicrograph, urothelium from a nondistended bladder has five to seven cell layers and cuboidal, superficial cells. **B,** Following bladder distention and saline irrigation, prominent, enlarged, multinucleated umbrella cells are visible. **C,** Normal urothelial cells (left panel) have central, round-to-oval single nuclei and densely stained cytoplasm with a pale outer rim. Saline irrigation results in the appearance in the urine sediment of enlarged, multinucleated superficial cells with prominent cytoplasmic vacuolization (right panel) (Papanicolaou stain). (**A–C:** Reproduced with permission from Schumann and Weiss, 1981)

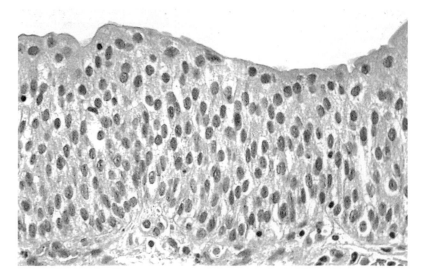

Figure 10.9 Hyperplastic urothelium has more than seven layers. However, polarity is maintained and there is normal maturation with preservation of superficial cells. (Reproduced with permission from Schumann and Weiss, 1981)

Specific Variants of Cystitis

Although a heterogeneous group of inflammatory lesions, these variants of cystitis share distinctive morphologic features and/or specific etiologies, including allergy, infection, and chemotherapy or radiation therapy. They may present as a bladder mass suggestive of neoplasm or are associated with urothelial cytologic changes that must be distinguished from transitional cell carcinoma. Finally, they may require specific modes of therapy.

Eosinophilic Cystitis

Although urinary tract allergy, including allergic cystitis, is frequently referred to in the allergy literature, reported cases of eosinophilic cystitis are uncommon. Patients have strong allergic histories or asthma. Concurrent or previous eosinophilic gastroenteritis has been recorded. Patient age has ranged from 5 days to 76 years (mean, 30 years), with slight female and pediatric predominances. Three quarters of the children with this type of cystitis have been black. Eosinophilic cystitis may mimic other forms of intractable cystitis (e.g., interstitial cystitis and tuberculosis) and is commonly mistaken for a bladder neoplasm.

PATHOGENESIS   Eosinophilic cystitis is generally considered to represent an allergic reaction. Foods, inhalants, medications, and alcohol have been incriminated, as have contact allergens such as microorganisms and topical agents. Attempts to document a parasitic etiology (e.g., schistosomiasis and visceral larva migrans) have been unsuccessful. To date, therefore, the antigenic stimuli and mechanism for tissue eosinophilia remain unknown, although a type I hypersensitivity reaction is favored.

CLINICAL MANIFESTATIONS   Eosinophilic cystitis may be acute or chronic with periods of remission and exacerbation. Resolution is usually spontaneous, and steroids provide only symptomatic relief. Most cases in children are self-limited, require no specific therapy, and resolve rapidly and completely in 2–12 weeks.

Bladder symptoms, which are most commonly irritative, include nocturia, dysuria, urgency, and frequency. Patients may complain of a dull suprapubic ache and may experience abdominal or flank pain. Proteinuria as well as microscopic or gross hematuria are common. Although pyuria may be present, urine cultures are negative; fever and chills are absent. Eosinophiluria, which is present in 10%–30% of all cases of urinary tract allergy, is a variable finding. Blood eosinophilia may be as high as 56%; although characteristic, it has been found in only one-third of patients and is not considered necessary for diagnosis. Eosinophilic cystitis may result in markedly diminished bladder capacity or significant residual urine. Ureteral obstruction secondary to eosinophilic ureteritis is a rare complication.

MORPHOLOGY   Eosinophilic cystitis may be a diffuse or localized lesion. Cystoscopically, it is characterized by 5–10 mm, yellowish, velvety, erythematous plaques. Bullous edema and verrucous or polypoid folds may be noted, as well as trabeculation, ulcerations, and bladder wall thickening.

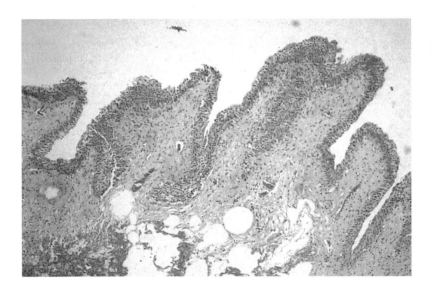

Figure 10.10 Polypoid cystitis is characterized by thin or broad mucosal projections, which should not be misdiagnosed as papillary transitional cell carcinoma. The edematous or fibrotic lamina propria is covered by a variably thick, nondysplastic urothelium.

Figure 10.11 Follicular cystitis has multiple, discrete, nodular lymphoid aggregates in the lamina propria. This example shows large lymphoid follicles with well developed germinal centers.

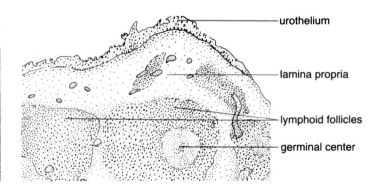

Microscopically, the hallmark is a heavy infiltrate of eosinophils in the lamina propria and muscularis, which may have perivascular prominence (Fig. 10.12). Plasma cells, lymphocytes, and macrophages are present in smaller numbers. Foci of fibrinoid necrosis may be observed, and late stages of healing result in fibrosis.

INTERSTITIAL CYSTITIS

This rare, nonbacterial form of chronic cystitis was originally reported by Hunner in 1915 as a type of deep bladder ulcer that involved the full thickness of the bladder wall. Hunner's ulcers remain a diagnostic hallmark of interstitial cystitis. Ninety percent of patients with this uncommon condition are females. Although reported in children, it has a peak age between 30 and 50 years.

PATHOGENESIS The etiology of interstitial cystitis remains obscure. Absence of urinary bacterial pathogens is a prerequisite for diagnosis. There has been no evidence of viral or fungal agents. Recent findings have suggested an autoimmune mechanism of injury involving IgM antibodies reactive against cytoskeletal intermediate filaments in the urothelium and vascular endothelium. Also supporting an autoimmunity hypothesis is the high incidence of allergies, especially to drugs (26%–70% of cases), a positive antinuclear antibody (ANA) (53%–85%), and an association with other autoimmune diseases, such as systemic lupus erythematosus, rheumatoid arthritis, and autoimmune thyroiditis. It has been suggested that the autoimmune process may have its origin in a urothelial injury that destroys the protective mucin layer and increases mucosal permeability. Mucin breakdown produced by specific microorganisms, such as *Chlamydia*, has been postulated, although ultrastructural studies have shown no significant changes in the surface glycocalyx.

CLINICAL MANIFESTATIONS The diagnosis of interstitial cystitis is based on symptom patterns as well as cystoscopic findings and histology. Symptoms, which are typically severe and disabling, include frequency, urgency, nocturia, dysuria, hematuria that may be gross initial or terminal, and suprapubic, urethral, or perineal pain. Symptoms may be partially relieved by voiding. Onset of symptoms is often acute, mimicking acute UTI; however, this chronic form of cystitis characteristically has a long clinical course with remissions and exacerbations. In men, symptoms are frequently misinterpreted as vesical irritability from an obstructing prostate.

MORPHOLOGY Cystoscopic findings, which are important in establishing the diagnosis of interstitial cystitis, range from linear scarring to erythematous areas that blanch during bladder filling. Ulcerations may occur in any part of the bladder, including the trigone, but are not a prerequisite for diagnosis. Most patients present at a stage when bladder capacity is normal and there are no ulcers. Petechial bleeding or glomerulations occur either during filling or on subsequent decompression and bladder refill (Fig. 10.13). These pinpoint areas of hemorrhage may coalesce and bleed freely. The remainder of patients present with late disease characterized by diminished bladder capacity and classic ulcerations. The ulcers, which may be 1–2 cm in diameter or larger, vary in both consistency and color (from white to brown).

Bladder biopsy is important in excluding conditions that may resemble interstitial cystitis, such as carcinoma in situ, tuberculosis, schistosomiasis, and malakoplakia. Histologic findings are considered nonspecific. The most consistent feature is edema of the lamina propria with vasodilatation. Telangiectatic vessels may be thickened. Nonulcerative forms of disease may show only mucosal ruptures and foci of hemorrhage corresponding to glomerulations. In severe cases, large areas of epithelium are lost. Ulcerations tend to be deeply penetrating and may be wedge-shaped. There are varying degrees of fibrosis of the lamina propria and muscle layer with a variable infiltrate of lymphocytes, plasma cells, eosinophils, and mast cells. Increased numbers of mast cells have been found in both ulcerated areas and apparently normal regions. It has been suggested that mast cell counts in the detrusor muscle are valuable when establishing a diagnosis, with greater than 20/mm^2 of muscle giving a diagnostic specificity of 88% and sensitivity of 95%.

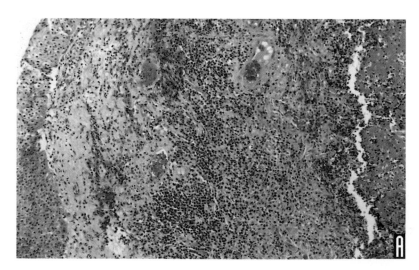

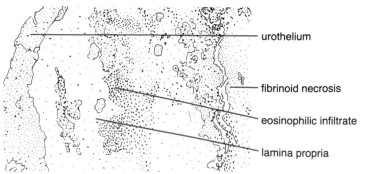

urothelium

fibrinoid necrosis

eosinophilic infiltrate

lamina propria

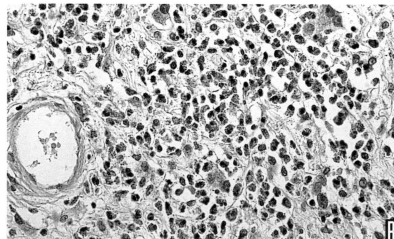

Figure 10.12 A, Eosinophilic cystitis is characterized by a heavy infiltrate of eosinophils in the lamina propria. A focus of fibrinoid necrosis is present in this photomicrograph. **B,** Unlike nonspecific cystitis, eosinophilic cystitis may contain a few histiocytes, but other chronic inflammatory cells, such as lymphocytes and plasma cells, are inconspicuous.

Granulomatous Cystitis

An infectious etiology for bladder granulomas should always be considered, especially when discrete or confluent caseating granulomas typical of tuberculosis are encountered. Tuberculous cystitis is virtually always a component of generalized spread from a pulmonary focus; however, bladder involvement is often clinically misinterpreted as a neoplasm.

Granulomatous cystitis comprises a histologically and etiologically broad group of inflammatory lesions, many of which are noninfectious. They may be characterized by necrobiotic, foreign body, or epithelioid granulomas, as well as diffuse histiocytic inflammation, and may be postsurgical in origin, secondary to intravesical chemotherapy with bacille–Calmette-Guérin (BCG), or related to bacterial infection. As a group, they may mimic bladder cancer or may be encountered in patients treated for cancer.

Postsurgical Granulomas

Bladder granulomas have been reported in 3% of patients who have had bladder biopsy or resection and in approximately 14% of patients who have had at least two prior transurethral bladder resections.

PATHOGENESIS Granulomas occur as a local reaction to tissue necrosis secondary to surgery and/or cautery. The possibility that they are immune in nature and directed against exposed or altered antigens has been suggested.

CLINICAL MANIFESTATIONS Because these granulomas are encountered in patients who have had multiple transurethral resections of bladder tumors, clinical findings are related to the neoplasm or resultant therapy.

MORPHOLOGY Grossly, the bladder mucosa typically has broad irregularities, with areas of hemorrhage and ulceration. Fissuring necrosis sometimes extends deeply into the muscularis propria. Areas of fibrous scarring are sometimes encountered.

Two histologic subtypes of granulomas may be observed (Fig. 10.14). The first, usually seen after about one month, consists of necrotizing, palisading granulomas that resemble necrobiotic rheumatoid nodules. They may be oval, linear, or serpiginous, with a central core of eosinophilic, amorphous necrosis, often containing thick, yellow-orange strands. Fibrin, elastin, collagen, smooth mus-

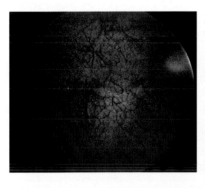
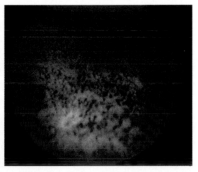

Figure 10.13 Cystoscopy in this woman with severe bladder symptoms showed changes typical for the nonulcerative form of interstitial cystitis. *Left:* The intact bladder mucosa initially showed marked hypervascularity. *Right:* Bladder distention with subsequent decompression and refill resulted in numerous, discrete, pin-point foci of hemorrhage (glomerulations). (Courtesy of R. Shank, MD, Cincinnati, Ohio)

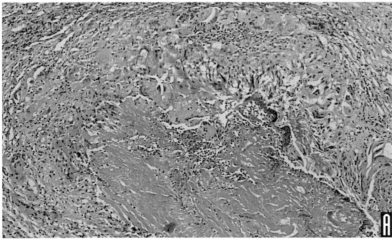
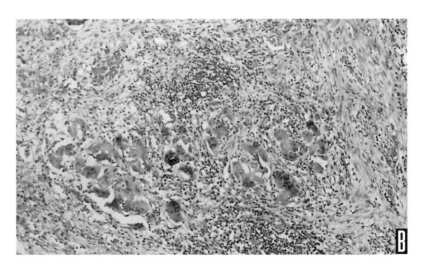
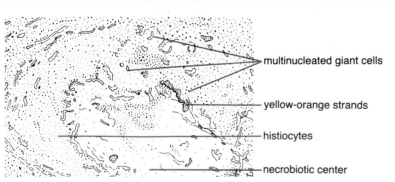

multinucleated giant cells

yellow-orange strands

histiocytes

necrobiotic center

Figure 10.14 A, The postsurgical granuloma in this photomicrograph has a necrobiotic center with a surrounding border of palisading histiocytes and multinucleated giant cells. Thick strands of yellow-orange material are focally present. **B,** The foreign body–type postsurgical granuloma consists of a circumscribed collection of multinucleated giant cells with surrounding chronic inflammation and fibrosis.

cle, and reticulin can be identified in the necrotic centers. The surrounding zone contains spindled, palisading histiocytes and few multinucleated giant cells, including some of Langhans' type. Eosinophils may be prominent in specimens obtained after a recent biopsy. The second type of granuloma, typically occurring at least three months after surgery, is the foreign body–type. It consists of circumscribed collections of multinucleated foreign body–type giant cells and epithelioid cells surrounded by lymphocytes, plasma cells, and eosinophils. Foreign body giant cells may contain thick strands of yellow-orange material representing altered elastin and/or fibrin.

Bacille–Calmette-Guérin (BCG) Granulomatous Cystitis

BCG is an attenuated strain of tubercle bacillus. Several variant strains of freeze-dried living organisms have been used in cancer therapy to stimulate cellular immunity. As a form of immunotherapy, it has been tried orally, by percutaneous administration, and by intravesical installation. Disseminated granulomatous lesions following BCG vaccination occur at a rate of 0.72 per million and have involved skin, bones, lymph nodes, lungs, liver, and salivary glands. It is not surprising, therefore, that intravesical BCG used in the treatment and prevention of superficial bladder cancer results in a granulomatous cystitis.

PATHOGENESIS BCG evokes an immunologic reaction that is central to its activity in the treatment of bladder tumors. Mediators of the immune response—for example, tumor necrosis factor, interleukin I, and other proteolytic enzymes secreted by macrophages—may have a role in local tumor destruction. Although high-viability vaccine more consistently produces a granulomatous reaction in the bladder lamina propria, this response per se shows no definite correlation with tumor recurrence rates. In contrast, systemic sensitization, as measured by conversion to a positive purified protein derivative (PPD) skin test is predictive of tumor response and is more frequently achieved with high-viability vaccine.

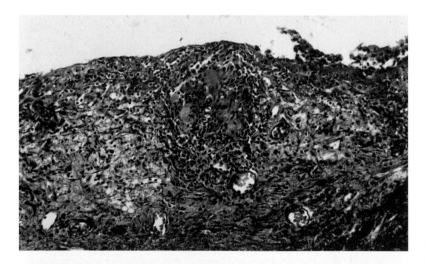

Figure 10.15 The granulomatous response following intravesical BCG therapy may consist only of loosely clustered Langhans'-type giant cells in the lamina propria associated with chronic inflammation. Sloughing and denudation of the urothelium is frequent.

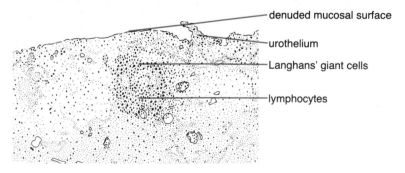

denuded mucosal surface
urothelium
Langhans' giant cells
lymphocytes

CLINICAL MANIFESTATIONS Following intravesical installation of BCG, most patients develop irritative bladder symptoms, including dysuria and frequency. Hematuria is typically insignificant. Fever, nausea, and malaise may also occur. Symptoms typically last only one to two days after treatment but increase with successive treatments. Prolonged or frequent courses are more likely to cause severe irritative symptoms and systemic reactions, such as pneumonitis, hepatitis, arthritis/arthralgia, skin rash, ureteral obstruction, and orchitis. These local and systemic reactions can be minimized or prevented by the use of isoniazid, antihistamines, and nonsteroidal anti-inflammatory agents.

MORPHOLOGY Lage and colleagues reported the early morphologic effects of intravesical BCG in a study of bladder biopsies obtained six weeks after completion of therapy. The majority showed erosion of the superficial urothelium, sloughing and denudation, or frank ulceration. The edematous lamina propria contained proliferating capillaries and a lymphoplasmacytic infiltrate with variable eosinophils and mast cells. The granulomatous response included foreign body and Langhans' giant cells, early granulomas, and mature, noncaseating epithelioid granulomas; acid-fast bacilli were only rarely identified (Fig. 10.15). With severe inflammatory reactions, granulomas occurred between muscle bundles of the bladder wall. Noncaseating granulomas were common in the prostatic urethra.

BCG may cause severe single-cell atypia or atypical hyperplasia that likely represents degenerative and regenerative urothelial changes. Partially denuded urothelium may be lined by fusiform cells with slight nuclear hyperchromasia and decreased cytoplasm showing basophilia. Unlike dysplasia or carcinoma in situ, epithelial maturation is generally preserved, nuclear/cytoplasmic (N/C) ratios are normal, nuclear contours are smooth, and there is no nuclear pleomorphism, cytomegaly, true hyperchromasia, or macronucleoli.

Malakoplakia

This uncommon granulomatous disease caused by bacterial infection was first described by Michaelis and Gutmann in 1902 and termed *malakoplakia* (*malakos*, soft; *plakos*, plaque) by von Hansemann in 1903. It has been reported to occur in all parts of the urinary tract, including the kidney (see Chapter 9), renal pelvis, and ureters, as well as the prostate (see Chapter 13) and testes (see Chapter 15), but it most commonly involves the bladder. It has its highest incidence in the fifth decade of life. It is four times more common in females than in males.

PATHOGENESIS Chronic UTI, most commonly with *Escherichia coli*, leads to malakoplakia in predisposed individuals. The diagnostic granulomatous response is related to defective lysosomal degradation of bacteria that have been phagocytosed by macrophages.

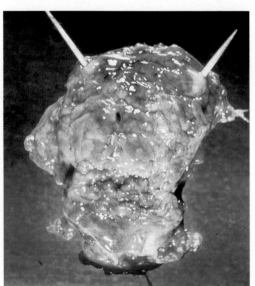

Figure 10.16 In this partial cystectomy specimen from a patient with malakoplakia, the mucosa has multiple, discrete, and confluent, raised, yellow-tan nodules as well as gray plaques. (Reproduced with permission from Schumann and Weiss, 1981)

... and lipoprotein membrane whorls that progressively calcify to form dense crystalline deposits.

CLINICAL MANIFESTATIONS The disease may be asymptomatic; however, bladder involvement typically results in hematuria and symptoms of bladder irritability, such as frequency, urgency...

... with circumferential hyperemia; occasi... ulcerated or hemorrhagic.

Microscopically, the lesions are sha... the muscularis, and usually cover... Lymphoid follicles are frequently see... overlapping histologic phases may be e...

Fig. 10.16). Excrescences may appear yellow-gray to red-brown

quently show artifactual separation fro...

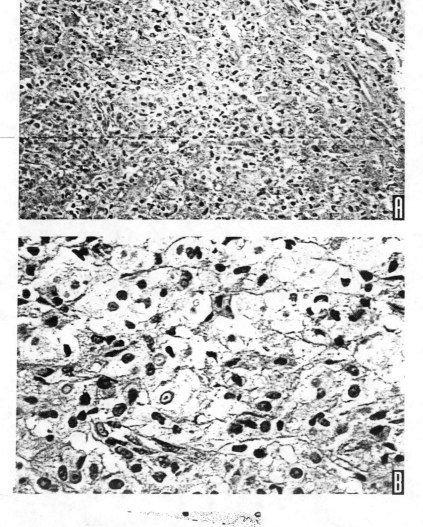

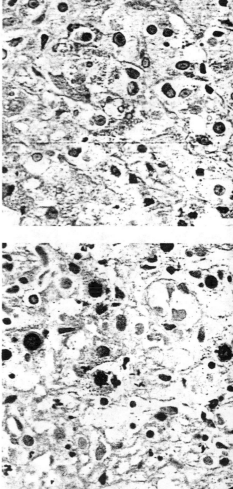

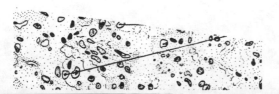

Figure 10.17 A, The soft plaques characteris... composed of confluent sheets of histiocyte... pria, visible here with PAS stain. B, The h... ... abundant foamy to slig...

stalla-
toms,
ignifi-

Michaelis–Gutmann bodies represent large lysosomes containing partially degraded bacteria and li

Michaelis–Gutmann bodies represent large lysosomes containing partially degraded bacteria and lipoprotein membrane whorls that progressively calcify to form dense crystalline deposits.

CLINICAL MANIFESTATIONS The disease may be asymptomatic; however, bladder involvement typically results in hematuria and symptoms of bladder irritability, such as frequency, urgency, dysuria, as well as pain and pyuria. Symptoms may last for weeks to many years (median, six months), and lesions, which are either continuous or recurrent, tend to be persistent. Weight loss and urinary retention may result. With coexistent urinary tract obstruction and pyelonephritis, recurrent pyrexia may develop.

MORPHOLOGY Cystoscopically, malakoplakia may be mistaken for an infiltrative neoplasm. Grossly, the lesions are characterized as multiple, raised, discrete plaques from 1 mm to 3 cm in size, or as firm, thickened, and granular nodules that may become confluent (Fig. 10.16). Excrescences may appear yellow-gray to red-brown

with circumferential hyperemia; occasionally, lesions are centrally ulcerated or hemorrhagic.

Microscopically, the lesions are sharply demarcated, limited by the muscularis, and usually covered by an intact mucosa. Lymphoid follicles are frequently seen at the periphery. Three overlapping histologic phases may be encountered. In the early, or prediagnostic, phase, the edematous, congested lamina propria contains a mixed inflammatory infiltrate composed of lymphocytes, plasma cells, foci of eosinophils, and numerous macrophages with periodic acid–Schiff (PAS)-positive granules (lysosomes). In the classic phase, the lamina propria is packed with large, plump (von Hansemann) histiocytes that have finely vacuolated or granular cytoplasm (Fig. 10.17). Intracellular Michaelis–Gutmann bodies (calcospherules) are recognized as 2–10 μ, concentrically laminated, round or oval bodies that are PAS-positive, iron-positive, and calcium-positive (von Kossa's or alizarin red S stains). Extracellular Michaelis–Gutmann bodies frequently show artifactual separation from the surrounding tissue,

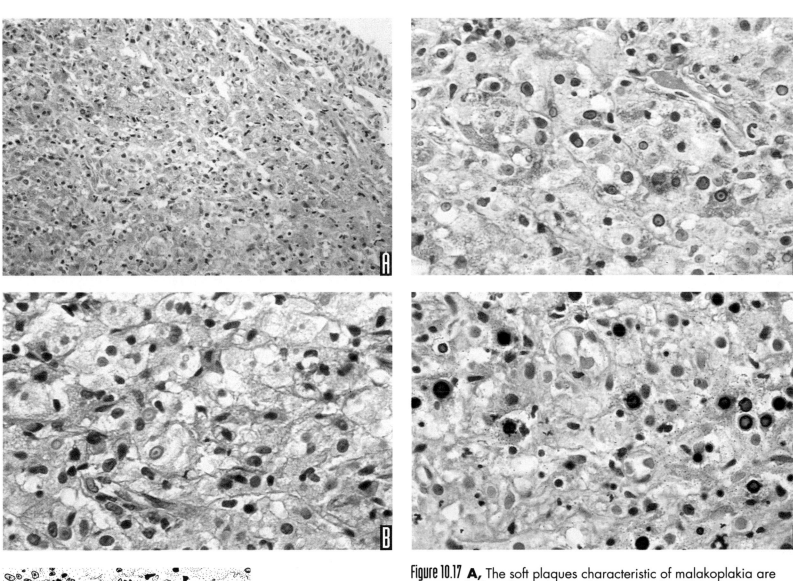

Michaelis–Gutmann bodies

Figure 10.17 A, The soft plaques characteristic of malakoplakia are composed of confluent sheets of histiocytes that fill the lamina propria, visible here with PAS stain. **B,** The histiocytes in this higher-power view have abundant foamy to slightly granular cytoplasm and contain numerous intracytoplasmic round-to-oval Michaelis–Gutmann bodies, which classically are concentrically laminated. **C,** Michaelis–Gutmann bodies can be more easily identified with PAS stain. **D,** With the von Kossa stain, calcified Michaelis–Gutmann bodies appear as discrete, black calcospherules. (**A,C,D:** Reproduced with permission from Schumann and Weiss, 1981)

giving a "bird's-eye" effect. Lymphocytes and plasma cells are focally distributed, and there may be focal hemosiderin deposits. Foreign body and Langhans' giant cells may also be focally identified. In the late, or fibrosing, phase, proliferating fibroblasts and collagen bundles become more prominent within the lesion and peripherally.

Cystitis Secondary to Therapy

Both radiation therapy and systemic chemotherapy can result in severe forms of cystitis that have a high morbidity and are difficult to treat. In addition, intravesical chemotherapy frequently produces a denuding cystitis and marked urothelial atypia, which may complicate subsequent follow-up of patients with transitional cell carcinoma and make the cytohistologic diagnosis of carcinoma in situ more difficult.

Radiation Cystitis

Radiation cystitis includes a variety of bladder lesions associated with diverse symptoms and pathologic findings. These complications may occur early or late and are of variable severity. The overall lower urinary tract complication rate for radiotherapy of female genital tract neoplasms is 1%–4% (approxi-

mately 7% for recurrent cervical cancer), while hemorrhagic cystitis following pelvic irradiation for bladder and cervical carcinomas has a reported incidence of 7%–9%.

PATHOGENESIS Both physical and biologic factors are important variables in the development of radiation cystitis. The most important physical factor is the type of therapeutic regimen—that is, external beam, radium, or radioisotope. Inherent in these techniques are critical dose-time-volume relationships. A single dose of greater than 2000–2500 rads or a complete course of therapy greater than 5000–6000 rads carries a risk of late subacute reactions. Biologic factors include preexisting disease such as infiltrating cancer, associated infection, anatomic variations, previous treatment, and racial differences. Bladder neck obstruction, extensively ulcerated tumors, and surgical procedures performed within three weeks prior to beginning radiation therapy also predispose to complications in the treatment of bladder cancer.

CLINICAL MANIFESTATIONS The clinical course can be divided into three reaction patterns dependent on the onset of symp-

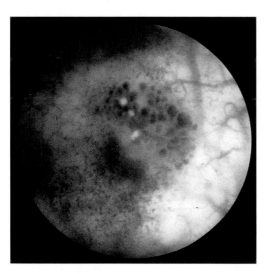

Figure 10.18 Radiation cystitis has many different endoscopic appearances. In this example, ectatic superficial vessels are viewed through an atrophic mucosa. (Courtesy of B. Bracken, MD, Cincinnati, Ohio)

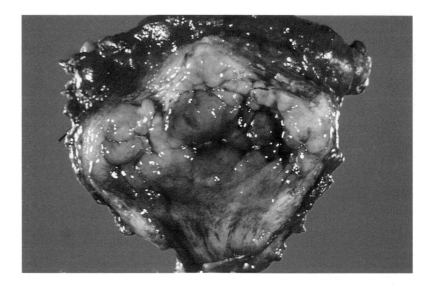

Figure 10.19 In this example of acute radiation damage, there is bullous edema and diffuse marked hyperemia with obscuration of the normal vascular pattern. The mucosal ulcer in the right lateral wall is the site of previous transurethral resection.

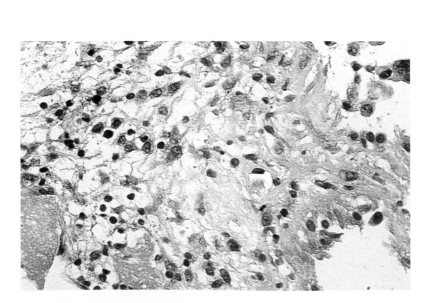

Figure 10.20 In acute radiation cystitis, endothelial damage results in capillary thrombosis and hemorrhage in the lamina propria. Desquamation of the urothelium may be marked. The edematous lamina propria in this high-power view contains lymphocytes, histiocytes

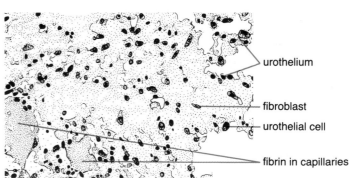

with scant hemosiderin, and reactive fibroblasts. Several capillaries contain fibrin. Desquamating urothelial cells show nuclear enlargement and hyperchromasia with loss of chromatin texture and pyknosis.

toms: acute (less than six months), subacute (six months to two years), and chronic (two to five years).

In the acute clinical period, acute radiation cystitis typically occurs four to six weeks after therapy begins and is marked by the onset of dysuria, urgency, frequency, and nocturia. Diffuse hemorrhage, which is rare, usually develops after external beam radiation doses of 3000 rads or more and occurs in approximately 50% of cases of treated bladder cancer. Symptoms typically subside two to six weeks after therapy is completed. Secondary ureteritis and hydroureter, although rare complications, can develop in the presence of UTI. Bladder perforations and fistulas, which are invariably due to radionecrosis of invasive tumor, may also occur.

During the subacute clinical period, the sudden onset of painless hematuria indicates chronic radiation cystitis with trigonal ulcers. Protracted, life-threatening hemorrhage may occur months to years post-therapy and may be difficult to control. Recurrence and severity of this complication are not necessarily related to the severity of acute symptoms or radiation dose (if less than 7000 rads external beam or 10,000 mg hours radium exposure). Complete healing of the mucosal ulcers may take weeks to months with conservative management. Symptoms of urgency, frequency, and dysuria indicate secondary infection with acute cystitis.

Complications that arise during the chronic clinical period are the result of fibrosis. Symptoms from a contracted bladder include frequency, nocturia, and dribbling, which are not commonly associated with hematuria. Bladder contracture, which has an insidious onset and tends to be progressive, most often occurs in cases with concurrent infection, prior radionecrosis of extensive intramural or perivesical cancer, or surgery performed in conjunction with radiation therapy. Radiation-induced ureteral strictures tend to occur 4–6 cm from the vesical junction and are only rarely due to scarring of the intravesical ureter. Unilateral obstruction, especially at

the vesicoureteral junction, is most often due to carcinomatous invasion. This is particularly true for irradiated cervical cancer, where complications associated with recurrent or persistent tumor occur eight times more frequently than late complications attributable to radiation alone.

MORPHOLOGY   Gross changes are best observed at cystoscopy (Fig. 10.18). In cases of mild-to-moderate acute radiation cystitis, there is diffuse mucosal hyperemia with occasional petechiae that obscure the normal vascular pattern (Fig. 10.19). In severe or advanced cases, partial desquamation, with or without superficial ulcerations, is present. Susceptibility to infection increases with the degree of radiation damage, and encrusted cystitis or stones may develop with growth of urea-splitting organisms. During the subacute period, circumscribed areas of atrophic pale mucosa with central fine telangiectasia, sharply demarcated bleeding ulcers, or bladder wall necrosis with fistulization may be noted. Mucosal blood vessels may also appear tuftlike or tortuous. Bullous edema may persist for months to years. In contracted bladders, mucosal atrophy is frequently prominent.

Microscopically, acute radiation cystitis is characterized by congestion and edema, with damage to the fine vasculature and connective tissue (Fig. 10.20). Endothelial cells show swelling, degeneration, necrosis, and proliferation. Injury to mucosal basal cells is associated with urothelial degeneration and desquamation. Ulceration, which is variable, may be shallow and covered by fibrinopurulent exudate. Large, deep ulcers extending into the muscularis indicate tumor necrosis, and a foreign body giant cell reaction may be prominent. Progressive vascular changes include luminal narrowing and mural thickening secondary to endothelial proliferation and subendothelial/medial fibrosis (Fig. 10.21). Fine vasculature decreases, and telangiectatic vessels appear. With pro-

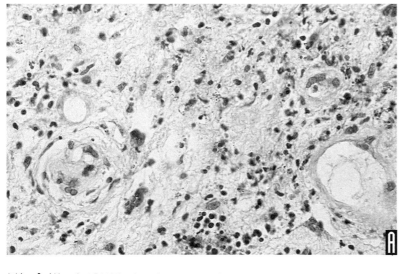

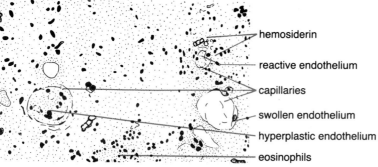

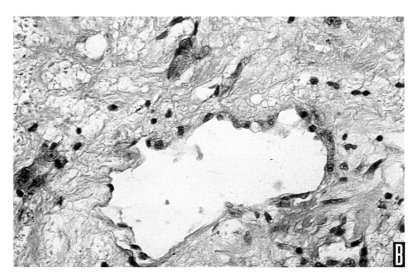

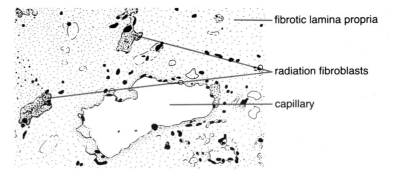

Figure 10.21 A, Severely damaged capillaries in acute radiation cystitis show endothelial swelling and proliferation with luminal narrowing. The edematous lamina propria contains extracellular hemosiderin deposits. Eosinophils and markedly reactive fibroblasts are present. **B,** The swollen endothelium of this ectatic capillary has reactive as

well as pyknotic nuclei. The edematous lamina propria contains increased collagen fibers. Bizarre giant cells are radiation fibroblasts. When these are present in large numbers, the term *giant cell cystitis* has been used. (**B:** Reproduced with permission from Schumann and Weiss, 1981)

gressive changes, connective tissue becomes hyalinized, and fibrosis extends into the muscular wall. Giant or bizarre fibroblasts and occasional multinucleated mesenchymal cells may be noted (*giant cell cystitis*).

During the subacute clinical period, microscopic changes reflect the marked susceptibility to infection and ulceration. Both healing ulcers with epithelial regeneration plus scarring and new ulcers may occur. Irregular areas of mucosal atrophy alternate with normal or hyperplastic urothelium. The lamina propria often has marked edema with accumulation of proteinaceous fluid and variable chronic inflammation, including macrophages and plasma cells.

Histologic changes during the late, chronic period are characterized by slowly progressive deterioration of fine vasculature by endarteritis obliterans, with increasing amounts and density of subepithelial connective tissue (Fig. 10.22). The lamina propria has variable chronic inflammation and edema; persistent, fragile telangiectatic vessels may hemorrhage. Ischemia may result in delayed atrophic ulcers, fissures, or fistulas; delayed mucosal breakdown may occur many years after irradiation.

Cytologic changes may persist in urine sediments for years (Fig. 10.23). Urothelial cells are enlarged with cytoplasmic polychromasia, and they have enlarged, vacuolated nuclei with prominent nucleoli or show nuclear pyknosis.

Cytoxan-Induced Hemorrhagic Cystitis Cyclophosphamide (Cytoxan) is used in the treatment of lymphoproliferative diseases, certain solid tumors, and nonneoplastic disorders, such as nephrotic syndrome and systemic lupus erythematosus. Urologic complications include hemorrhagic cystitis, vesical fibrosis, and urothelial carcinomas (which occur much more commonly in the bladder than in the renal pelvis and ureter). Sterile hemorrhagic cystitis occurs in 2%–40% of treated patients; it may occur in as many as 68% of patients given high doses for allogeneic bone marrow transplant, in which case it is associated with a 4% mortality rate. Ifosfamide, a structural isomer and also a member of the oxazaphosphorine family, has even greater urotoxicity, producing severe and restrictive hemorrhagic cystitis. Although the true incidence of bladder cancer in Cytoxan-treated patients is unknown, there appears to be a ninefold increase.

PATHOGENESIS The antineoplastic metabolite of Cytoxan is phosphoramide mustard. The urotoxic metabolite, acrolein, is an aldehyde and oxidizing agent that kills urothelial cells. It may also play a role in promoting abnormal cellular proliferation and may be carcinogenic. No correlation has been found between the degree of cytologic atypia and total dose of Cytoxan. Ranges of doses associated with urothelial cancer have been 12.8–547 g. The average total dose thought to be carcinogenic lies between 100–150 g.

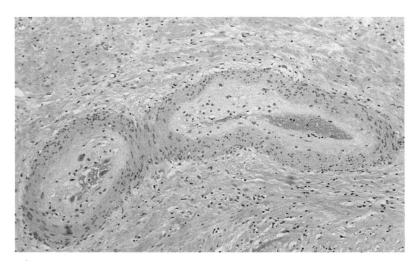

Figure 10.22 Chronic radiation cystitis is associated with marked endarteritis obliterans. In this photomicrograph, large arteries show marked intimal fibrosis with entrapped chronic inflammatory cells, including a few foam cells. The surrounding dense connective tissue is chronically inflamed.

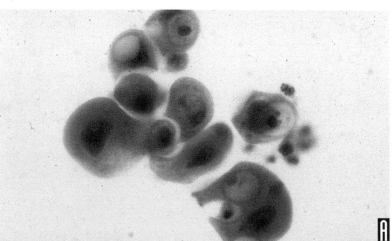

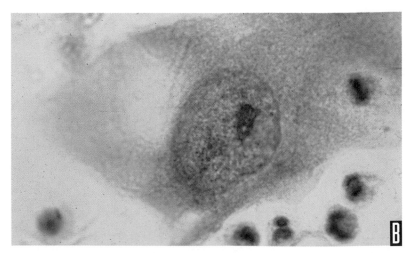

Figure 10.23 **A,** Urothelial cells in this loosely cohesive fragment have enlarged, slightly hyperchromatic nuclei with loss of chromatin texture and cytoplasmic polychromasia (Papanicolaou stain). **B,** This gigantic urothelial cell has both nuclear and cellular enlargement, and the N/C ratio remains low. A macronucleolus is present (Papanicolaou stain). These cytologic changes were observed in the urine sediment two years after radiation therapy. (**A,B:** Reproduced with permission from Schumann and Weiss, 1981)

CLINICAL MANIFESTATIONS Hemorrhagic cystitis may occur three weeks to six months after initiating Cytoxan therapy. Urotoxicity ranges from asymptomatic hematuria to fulminant, ulcerating inflammation with severe, protracted and life-threatening hemorrhage. Effects of Cytoxan are augmented by irradiating the pelvis. Most cases are mild and controlled by withdrawal of Cytoxan and hydration. Prophylactic measures have included intravesical acetylcysteine (Mucomyst) or oral 2-mercaptoethane sodium sulfonate (Mesna). Mesna forms a nontoxic ether with acrolein and, unlike other thiol compounds, does not interfere with tumoricidal properties of Cytoxan. In severe cases, intravesical formalin (1%–10%) has been used; however, with life-threatening hemorrhage, supravesical diversion or cystectomy may be required. Patients with hematuria should have regular cytologic urine evaluation for possible bladder carcinoma.

MORPHOLOGY Severe mucosal hyperemia, telangiectasias, hemorrhage, ulceration, and focal necrosis may be noted grossly (Fig. 10.24). Histologic changes induced by Cytoxan have been shown experimentally to be very rapid. Epithelial necrosis, which begins at 1 hour and is almost complete by 24 hours, is quickly followed by epithelial regeneration and hyperplasia; it progresses to atypical papillary hyperplasia by day 15. Atypical urothelial hyperplasia, which also occurs in humans, may represent an exaggerated healing response. Other histologic changes include vascular ectasia and fibroblastic proliferation. In the more severe intractable forms of hemorrhagic cystitis, fibrous scarring may result in diminished bladder capacity.

Cytoxan produces cytologic alterations in the urothelium that are similar to marked radiation-induced changes. In patients followed one to four months during treatment, urine cytologies have shown a gradual increase in urothelial atypia that either disappeared or significantly decreased when treatment was reduced or discontinued. Cytologic changes include nuclear and cellular enlargement. Cytoplasmic vacuolization is common, as are smudging and break-

down of cell borders. There may be occasional multinucleated cells. Nuclei are frequently eccentric with slightly irregular outlines and may appear hyperchromatic with coarse, evenly distributed chromatin granules ("salt-and-pepper" appearance). One or several nucleoli or large chromocenters may be present. Nuclear pyknosis is a common late effect resulting in large hyperchromatic nuclei with loss of chromatin texture or karyorrhexis. These large degenerated atypical cells with high N/C ratios and smudged nuclear chromatin are characteristic of Cytoxan, but are not specific (Fig. 10.25). When observed in the urine sediment, they should be considered suspicious for malignancy.

Denuding Cystitis Secondary to Thiotepa
Intravesical installation of thiotepa (triethylenethiophosphoramide), a polyfunctional alkylating agent, has been used to treat superficial bladder cancer and prevent recurrence. Most therapeutic success has occurred in patients whose tumors responded to initial treatment; in some cases this is as high as 60%. Overall response rates, however, are 50%–80%, with approximately 30% complete remission. From experimental studies of FANFT-induced murine bladder cancer, thiotepa is ineffective in preventing eventual tumor growth, but appears to delay recurrences and inhibit progression to high-grade and/or high-stage tumors.

PATHOGENESIS The action of thiotepa is unrelated to metabolic inhibition of DNA replication. Instead, it acts as a toxic substance that causes increased exfoliation of urothelial cells with mucosal denudation. The drug, therefore, does not produce radiationlike cytologic atypia that might be confused with carcinoma. The cytologic alterations reflect cellular degeneration and regeneration of normal urothelium.

CLINICAL MANIFESTATIONS Thiotepa causes marked denudation of the bladder mucosa; symptoms of bladder irritability may increase. The "shaving" effect on the urothelium may compli-

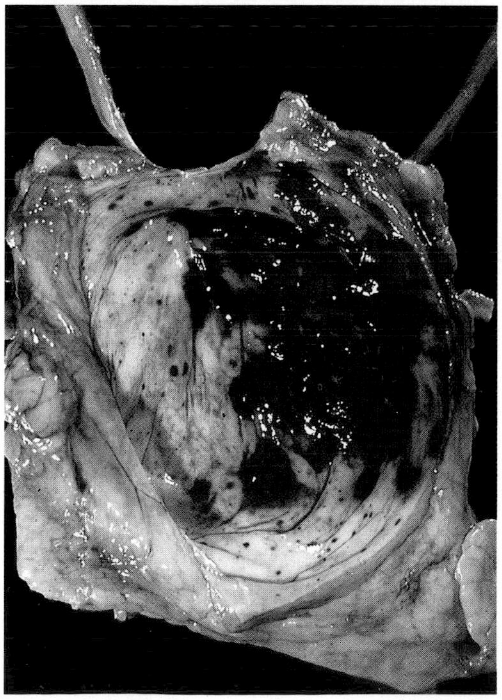

Figure 10.24 In this specimen with Cytoxan-induced hemorrhagic cystitis, confluent areas of mucosal hemorrhage as well as discrete ecchymoses, petechial hemorrhages, and patches of hyperemia are present.

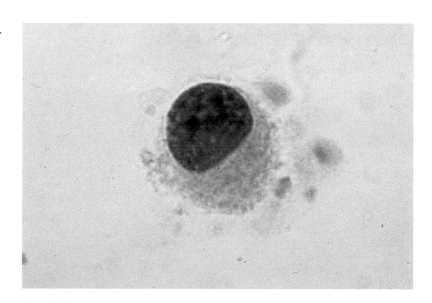

Figure 10.25 Urothelial atypia is frequently observed following Cytoxan therapy. This atypical urothelial cell with frayed borders has an eccentric nucleus that is enlarged and hyperchromatic. It appears dysplastic and should be regarded as suspicious for malignancy (Papanicolaou stain). (Reproduced with permission from Schumann and Weiss, 1981)

cate follow-up cystoscopic evaluation in patients who have received intravesical thiotepa for carcinoma in situ, which also is a cause of denuding cystitis (Fig. 10.26). Similarly, selection of biopsy sites and interpretation of microscopic findings are made more difficult and may yield false-negative results. Because of these pitfalls, urine cytology remains invaluable in follow-up of these patients (see Chapter 12).

MORPHOLOGY Urothelium may show degenerative changes in the superficial cells, denudation, or regeneration (Fig. 10.27). The lamina propria consistently shows inflammation and edema unrelated to the duration of treatment. Although denudation is often extensive, fibrosis is rarely observed, even with long-term treatment.

Cytologic changes occur predominantly in superficial cells, which have convex outer borders and scalloped inner surfaces (Fig. 10.28). Cells show no significant increase in nuclear chromatin, and the slight-to-moderate hyperchromasia is due to degenerative smudging of chromatin with loss of a sharply detailed pattern. Degeneration also leads to cytoplasmic vacuolization and fragmentation of cell borders. Nuclei with slight-to-moderate enlargement are generally round-to-ovoid with smooth, thin chromatin rims. They have multiple, usually small nucleoli, representing reactive or regenerative changes. Multinucleated cells and cells with atypical nuclei are unusual. These changes are not specific for thiotepa and can be seen after catheterization with installation of saline alone.

PROLIFERATIVE AND METAPLASTIC LESIONS OF THE BLADDER

Nonneoplastic proliferative and metaplastic mucosal lesions are commonly associated with inflammation. Lymphocytic infiltrates have been noted in approximately 84% of cases. Lesions are frequently found in combination and associated with nonspecific and specific forms of cystitis. Although commonly observed in cases of bladder cancer, these lesions are generally not considered premalignant.

The bladder has a complex embryologic derivation from the cloaca posteriorly, the wolffian (mesonephric) ducts laterally, and the omphaloallantoic duct anteriorly. At birth the bladder is completely

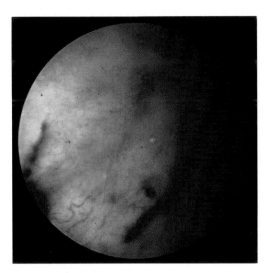

Figure 10.26 Denuding cystitis has a nonspecific cystoscopic appearance. These dull, erythematous patches may occur with carcinoma in situ and various inflammatory conditions. (Courtesy of B. Bracken, MD, Cincinnati, Ohio)

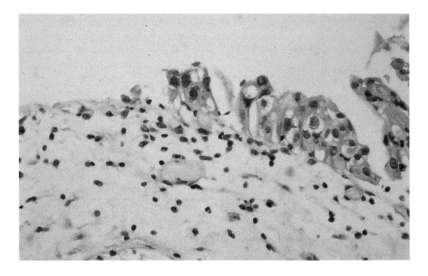

Figure 10.27 Thiotepa causes denudation of urothelium (left). Attached urothelial cells are degenerated with pyknotic, darkly stained nuclei.

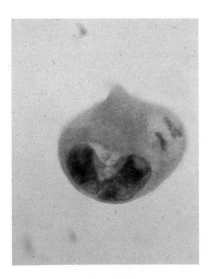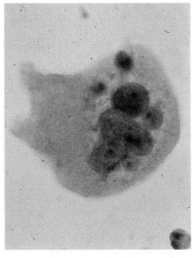

Figure 10.28 Degenerated superficial cells are recognized by their convex outer borders and scalloped inner surface. *Left panel:* The binucleate cell has moderate nuclear hyperchromasia due to smudging of chromatin. *Right panel:* Multinucleation is seen only occasionally (Papanicolaou stain). (This is the same case as Figure 10.27.)

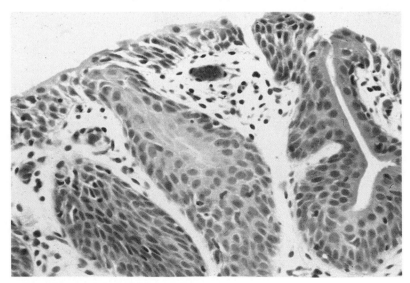

Figure 10.29 Brunn's nests, visible in this photomicrograph, are finger-like projections of urothelial cells into the lamina propria that form solid nests or have a central ductlike lumen. The nests lie adjacent to or attached to the normal urothelium. (Reproduced with permission from Schumann and Weiss, 1981)

lined by transitional epithelium of endodermal origin. Embryonic rests have been suggested as an explanation for finding squamous, mucus-producing, columnar, or cuboidal epithelium lining the mucosal surface or intramural cysts. These variants, however, represent the biologic potential to undergo metaplastic change that is retained by the bladder epithelium and is also reflected in urothelial neoplasms.

PROLIFERATIVE CYSTITIS

Proliferative cystitis refers to a spectrum of lesions and has traditionally included Brunn's nests, cystitis cystica, and cystitis glandularis.

CLINICAL MANIFESTATIONS In autopsy studies, Brunn's nests are seen in approximately 85% of cases. They are most common in the trigone (91%) and anterior (80%) walls. Depending on the patient's age, they occur in 60%–100% of cases with no sex differences; 30% of patients have been less than 20 years old. Inflammation was absent in approximately 50%–80% of cases. These data suggest that Brunn's nests represent a normal variant of bladder urothelium. However, they are also the simplest form of proliferative cystitis and are considered to be a reactive proliferative abnormality in response to inflammation that is the precursor lesion for *cystitis cystica* and *cystitis glandularis*.

Depending on age, cystitis cystica and cystitis glandularis are found in 40%–93% of autopsy cases, with peak incidence in the eighth decade. They occur in 87% of males and 93% of females, and have a predilection for the trigone (84%) and anterior (50%) walls. Lymphocytic infiltrates have been absent in approximately 80% of cases. Cystitis cystica and cystitis glandularis are often found incidentally in biopsies obtained for other reasons. They are seen in association with chronic or recurrent infection, lithiasis, bladder outlet obstruction, chronic irritation secondary to foreign bodies, and neoplasms. In one study, at least one such risk factor was present in 95% of adults. Presenting symptoms, therefore, can relate to any one of the multiple responsible factors. However, in some series a combination of dysuria, hematuria, and infection occurred in approximately 90% of patients.

Cystitis cystica occurs in approximately 2.4% of children from birth to 16 years of age (mean, 7–8 years). In a study of 3- to 12-year-old girls (mean, 7.5 years) with UTI, it was diagnosed in 22% and was observed after a 3½ year average time lapse from first UTI.

Cystitis cystica may produce a localized, solid-appearing, intravesical soft-tissue mass in the trigone that simulates transitional cell carcinoma. In rare cases, there is marked bladder wall thickening secondary to edema and inflammation that extends into the perivesical fat to produce a retrovesicular mass. Eighty percent of patients with pelvic lipomatosis have cystitis glandularis. Approximately two thirds of patients with exstrophic bladders have cystitis cystica and/or cystitis glandularis; these patients have a 200-fold increase in the incidence of bladder cancer, with 87% being adenocarcinomas.

MORPHOLOGY Brunn's nests are recognized microscopically as a nodular thickening of urothelium that results in nests of cells in the lamina propria adjacent to or in direct continuity with the surface epithelium. The latter may show squamous metaplasia. The nests are either solid or have a central ductlike lumen containing colloid material (Fig. 10.29).

Grossly, cystitis cystica is characterized by cysts that are regular and rounded, 1–5 mm in diameter, translucent, pearly or yellowish, and covered by a thin layer of mucosa (Fig. 10.30). In florid cases, which may also be observed in the ureter (ureteritis cystica), numerous large, occasionally confluent cysts produce a characteristic cobblestone appearance (Fig. 10.31).

In cases diagnosed cystoscopically as cystitis cystica, the full spectrum of proliferative cystitis, as well as follicular cystitis, is commonly seen microscopically. Cystitis cystica forms by dilatation of Brunn's nests. The cysts, which are located in the lamina propria, are lined by a flattened or stratified transitional-type epithelium and contain luminal secretions. With transition to cystitis glandu-

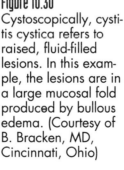

Figure 10.30 Cystoscopically, cystitis cystica refers to raised, fluid-filled lesions. In this example, the lesions are in a large mucosal fold produced by bullous edema. (Courtesy of B. Bracken, MD, Cincinnati, Ohio)

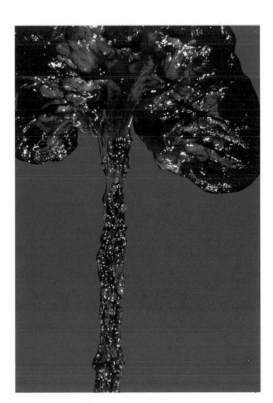

Figure 10.31 In this florid example of ureteritis cystica, the cysts are numerous, large, and occasionally confluent; the mucosa has a characteristic cobblestone appearance.

laris, columnar cells line the inner surface of the cysts (Fig. 10.32) and may exfoliate into the urine as glandular cells and fragments. Cysts may also be lined by a nonstratified layer of cuboidal, columnar, or colonic-type epithelium.

SQUAMOUS METAPLASIA

Squamous metaplasia refers to replacement of urothelium by mature squamous epithelium. Two subtypes of squamous metaplasia should be clinically and pathologically distinguished, as their frequency, sex predilection, and, possibly, their malignant potential are different.

The first type, *nonkeratinizing metaplasia*, is commonly found in the trigone of females during estrogen production and has been referred to as *pseudomembranous trigonitis*. It occurs in 36%–80% of apparently normal bladders and is most likely a normal variant that develops under hormonal influences. Women may have unrelated symptoms of cystitis, urethritis, and cystocele. In a biopsy study of 50 women with recurrent abacterial cystitis, squamous metaplasia of the trigone was present in 84%.

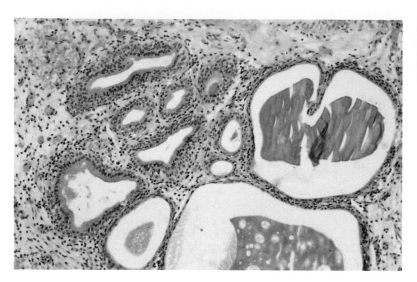

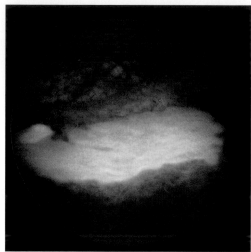

Figure 10.33 The whitish appearance of the mucosa of the trigone and proximal urethra is due to the presence of nonkeratinizing squamous metaplasia. This is a normal cystoscopic finding in women of reproductive age. (Courtesy of B. Bracken, MD, Cincinnati, Ohio)

Figure 10.32 Brunn's nests within the lamina propria dilate and fill with eosinophilic secretions to form cystitis cystica. The cysts are lined by flattened or stratified transitional epithelium. Cystitis cystica and cystitis glandularis (left) are frequently observed together. Cystitis glandularis has a luminal layer of non-mucus secreting columnar epithelium. Edema and chronic inflammation are variably associated.

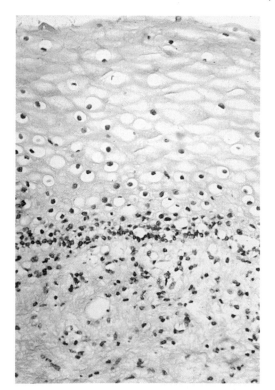

Figure 10.34 The metaplastic, nonkeratinizing squamous epithelium is composed of heavily glycogenated polygonal cells with ground-glass or vacuolated cytoplasm. Distinct intercellular bridges are absent. This appearance is similar to the hormonally responsive vaginal mucosa. (Reproduced with permission from Schumann and Weiss, 1981)

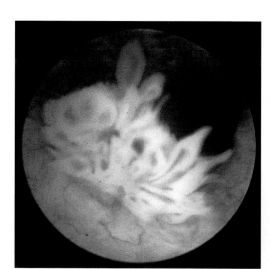

Figure 10.35 Cystoscopically, this condyloma acuminatum of the urethra has a papillary appearance indistinguishable endoscopically from a low-grade, superficial, transitional cell carcinoma. (Courtesy of B. Bracken, MD, Cincinnati Ohio)

Keratinizing squamous metaplasia is rarely confined to the trigone. It is usually the consequence of long-term irritation or chronic infection and may be associated with stones, diverticula, or schistosomiasis. Symptoms, including severe frequency, dysuria, and suprapubic pain, are generally related to associated inflammatory conditions or chronic vesical irritation. Pyuria and positive urine cultures may also be present. When extensive, keratinizing squamous metaplasia may decrease the bladder's capacity by interfering with contraction and dilatation. A cystogram may demonstrate a symmetric, small-capacity bladder. Keratinizing metaplasia, referred to as *leukoplakia*, occurs twice as frequently in the bladder as in the renal pelvis and ureter. Bladder involvement is four times more common in males. Renal colic with passage of desquamated epithelium resembling gritty flakes, soft stones, and white chalky membranes or tissue is pathognomonic of renal pelvic involvement. The latter may also produce a filling defect on intravenous pyelogram (IVP).

The majority of studies, particularly older ones, do not clearly separate these two types of squamous metaplasia with respect to frequency and association with bladder cancer. However, in view of the preceding discussion, it is not surprising that squamous metaplasia generally is reported to have a higher incidence in females at all ages and a predilection for the trigone (84% of cases). In a study by Widran and colleagues, 88% of patients with squamous metaplasia were women (16–93 years of age) and approximately 50% were younger than than 40. Although men with squamous metaplasia tend to be older, it is present in up to 20% of men after the fifth decade of life in comparison with 42%–100% of women at autopsy.

Review of the literature shows that carcinoma is present with squamous metaplasia in 10%–20% of cases at the time of diagnosis, but it may be adenocarcinoma, transitional cell carcinoma, or squamous cell carcinoma. In studies of squamous cell carcinomas, 16%–25% of patients had squamous metaplasia remote from or adjacent to the tumor. It has been observed, however, that tumors more frequently appear to arise from nonmetaplastic epithelium. In the study by Widran and colleagues, squamous metaplasia was associated with squamous cell carcinoma in less than 1% of women and in 15% of men, but no cases of squamous metaplasia progressed to cancer. Several additional studies have concluded that squamous metaplasia in females is not a precursor of cancer. Although it may have a greater malignant potential in males, documented progression in either sex is uncommon. In older studies based on relatively small numbers of patients, leukoplakia was reported to progress to cancer in up to 20% of cases.

MORPHOLOGY   Cystoscopically, pseudomembranous trigonitis appears as a usually well demarcated, often irregular white patch on the trigone (Fig. 10.33). Finely granular lesions may extend to the posterior lip of the bladder neck and upward to the ureteral orifices. There is frequently a rim of vascularity. Microscopically, this nonkeratinizing metaplasia resembles vaginal epithelium (Fig. 10.34). The stratified squamous epithelium is composed of polygonal cells with glycogenated cytoplasm that may have a vacuolated or ground-glass appearance. Because of its location in the trigone, it frequently is associated with Brunn's nests, cystitis cystica, and cystitis glandularis. Inflammatory infiltrates are not invariably present. This metaplastic lesion should be distinguished from condyloma acuminatum, which only rarely involves the bladder (Fig. 10.35) (see Chapter 18). Condylomata are flat or have a papillary configuration with a central stalk. They are frequently nonkeratinizing and have a hyperplastic squamous epithelium composed of cells with clear cytoplasm and slightly enlarged, hyperchromatic nuclei (koilocytes) (Fig. 10.36).

Grossly, keratinizing metaplasia (leukoplakia) appears gray-white, leathery, and parchmentlike or coral-like. Borders are sharply demarcated or may imperceptibly blend with the surrounding hyperemic mucosa (Fig. 10.37). The condition may be mistaken for encrusted alkaline cystitis, malakoplakia, or yeast infection. Microscopically, the well differentiated, mature, strati-

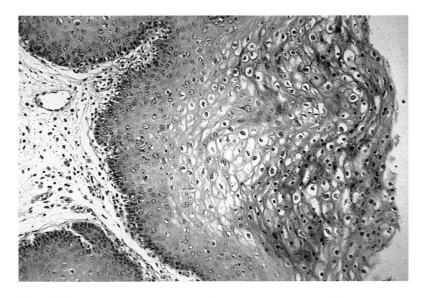

Figure 10.36 Koilocytes in the hyperplastic squamous epithelium are characteristic of condyloma. They have enlarged, irregular hyperchromatic nuclei with a surrounding halo of cleared cytoplasm. (Reproduced with permission from Schumann and Weiss, 1981)

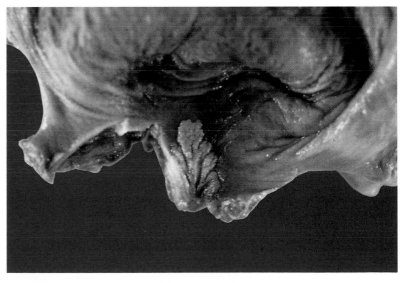

Figure 10.37 In this specimen, keratinizing squamous metaplasia has produced a sharply demarcated gray-white mucosal patch (leukoplakia) that resembles coral.

fied squamous epithelium has cells with eosinophilic cytoplasm, intercellular bridges, elongated rete, and variable surface keratinization (Fig. 10.38).

Intestinal Metaplasia

Columnar cell metaplasia may occur as a focal surface change (Fig. 10.39) or as a component of proliferative cystitis, that is, cystitis glandularis. Rarely, there may be extensive surface and glandular metaplasia characterized by the presence of columnar mucus-producing cells. These cases tend to occur with longstanding, marked chronic irritation or infection, as in association with exstrophy or pyocystis, or following bladder trauma. This form of widespread intestinal metaplasia should be distinguished from cystitis glandularis, as the literature suggests that intestinal metaplasia is a potentially premalignant lesion carrying a much greater risk for subsequent bladder carcinoma.

MORPHOLOGY In classic examples of intestinal metaplasia, the surface epithelium and glands limited to the lamina propria resemble colonic mucosa and are lined by a single layer of mucin-producing goblet cells with small, round, basally situated nuclei. Paneth cells may be identified at the base of the cryptlike glands, and argyrophil cells may also be present (Fig. 10.40). Mucin histochemistry with the periodate borohydride/KOH/PAS stain has shown the presence of O-acetylated sialomucin, which is also typ-

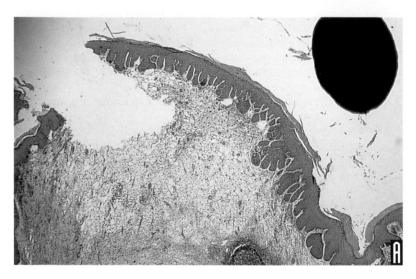

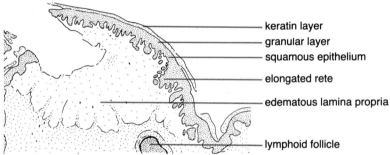

keratin layer
granular layer
squamous epithelium
elongated rete
edematous lamina propria
lymphoid follicle

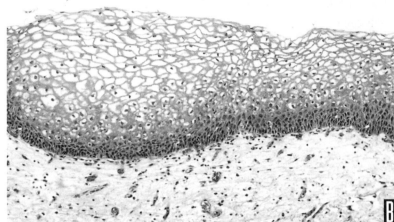

Figure 10.38 A, Mature, stratified squamous epithelium is present in keratinizing metaplasia, and a granular layer may exist beneath the keratin. Rete are typically elongated. Other findings of chronic bladder irritation are common, including the follicular cystitis shown in this photomicrograph. **B,** Focal absence of keratin and cytoplasmic clearing or vacuolization may resemble nonkeratinizing metaplasia or flat condyloma acuminatum. Deeper layers have eosinophilic cytoplasm and distinct intercellular bridges. This focus was adjacent to an invasive squamous cell carcinoma.

Figure 10.39 Columnar cell metaplasia of the surface epithelium is present in this bladder biopsy. The nonmucus-producing columnar epithelium is nonstratified, with basally oriented nuclei. Cytologic atypia is absent; however, an adjacent primary invasive adenocarcinoma was present in this bladder.

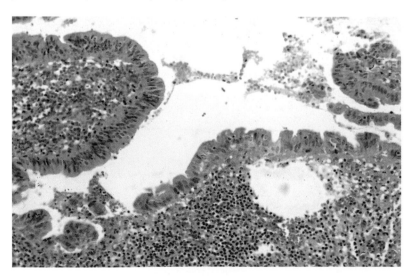

ically present in the epithelium of the terminal ileum and large intestine, as well as primary mucinous adenocarcinoma of the bladder. The lamina propria usually has marked edema and chronic, as well as acute, inflammation. Adjacent mucosa may demonstrate an earlier stage of metaplasia, with goblet cells on the surface or mucin-producing cells distributed throughout the thickness of the urothelium. The urine sediment typically shows an inflammatory background and contains large numbers of exfoliated cells. Colonic-type glandular fragments and individual cells distended with intracytoplasmic mucin should not be mistaken for mucinous or signet-ring cell adenocarcinoma.

Nephrogenic Adenoma

Nephrogenic adenoma is neither a neoplasm nor of renal origin but represents a peculiar form of immature urothelial metaplasia. The name is derived from its resemblance to primitive renal tubular structures. It has been reported most often in the bladder (82% of cases), but it may occur in the urethra (13%) and ureter (5%).

Most cases of nephrogenic adenoma have occurred in the setting of acute and/or chronic cystitis. Patients have ranged from 4–83 years of age (mean, 41 years), and two thirds have been males. A history of genitourinary operations or procedures—for example, multiple catheterizations—has been found in approximately 60% of patients. Other associated conditions have included calculi (14%), urinary tract trauma (9%), and renal transplantation (8%).

PATHOGENESIS   Although nephrogenic adenoma is generally considered metaplastic in origin, the possibility that it represents mesonephric or metanephric embryonic rests or choristomas of renal origin has been considered. Lectin histochemistry studies have shown that epithelia of nephrogenic adenoma and tubules in the mesonephric and metanephric kidney exhibit PNA receptor sites, which are not present in other proliferative and metaplastic urothelial lesions such as cystitis cystica, cystitis glandularis, and squamous metaplasia. Findings from ultrastructural studies have been inconclusive. Some suggest a urothelial derivation and others note a resemblance to epithelium of the thin limb of Henle's loop, collecting duct, or proximal convoluted tubule.

CLINICAL MANIFESTATIONS   Symptoms associated with nephrogenic adenoma include gross or microscopic hematuria, frequency, dysuria, nocturia, and other irritative manifestations. Lesions may remit following treatment of bladder infection, but in 30% of cases they have persisted or recurred with subsequent reinfection.

MORPHOLOGY   The majority of lesions are papillary (61%) or polypoid (15%), while the remainder are sessile, often raised, yellow nodules. The involved mucosa has also been described as granular, ulcerated, heaped-up and shaggy, cobblestone, and erythematous. Lesions are usually solitary, but they have been multiple (up to eight) in 18% of cases. Most are located in the trigone. While the

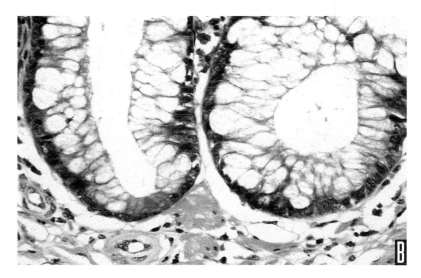

Figure 10.40 **A,** Intestinal metaplasia, particularly when associated with marked chronic inflammation, resembles colonic mucosa. **B,** Paneth cells with characteristic dense eosinophilic cytoplasm may be present at the base of the gland crypts. (**B:** Reproduced with permission from Schumann and Weiss, 1981)

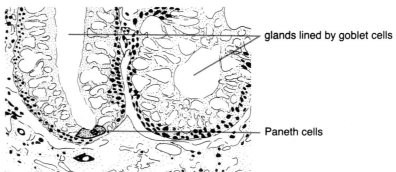

glands lined by goblet cells

Paneth cells

majority are small, they can range from microscopic to a size large enough to involve the entire bladder.

Microscopically, nephrogenic adenoma is composed of tubules, cysts, or papillae lined by a single layer of cells (Fig. 10.41). Foci may also demonstrate a diffuse pattern with solid tubules or tiny tubules simulating signet-ring cells. Cells are typically cuboidal or low columnar. They may be "hobnail" with intraluminal nuclear protrusions and have scanty, moderate or, rarely, abundant clear-to-eosinophilic cytoplasm. The tubules and cysts generally have empty lumina but may contain eosinophilic or basophilic fluid (Fig. 10.42), which is weakly positive with mucin stains. Tubules are surrounded by a PAS-positive basement membrane that may become thickened and hyalinized. The benign cytology, rarity of mitoses, presence of basement membrane, lack of reactive fibrous proliferation, and absence of muscle wall invasion help to distinguish nephrogenic adenoma from mesonephric adenocarcinoma (see Chapter 12). The lamina propria commonly has acute and chronic inflammation, and the mucosa may be ulcerated. Squamous metaplasia, intestinal (colonic) metaplasia, cystitis cystica, and cystitis glandularis may be associated findings.

MISCELLANEOUS PSEUDOTUMORS

INFLAMMATORY PSEUDOTUMORS

Inflammatory pseudotumors of the bladder (IPTB) are rare. Pseudosarcomatous stromal lesions of the genitourinary tract that develop at surgical sites are known as postoperative spindle cell nodules and more frequently occur in the prostate (see Chapter 13). Bladder lesions typically follow transurethral resection of a bladder tumor. However, proliferative spindle cell lesions of the bladder that resemble sarcomas can also occur without a recent history of instrumentation, trauma, or surgery. The terms *pseudosarcomatous fibromyxoid tumor* and *pseudosarcomatous myofibroblastic proliferation* have been used for these inflammatory pseudotumors. The stimulus for the reactive cellular proliferation, which resembles nodular fasciitis, is unknown.

CLINICAL MANIFESTATIONS IPTB can affect both children and adults. A female preponderance has been noted. Patients typically present with hematuria and a bladder mass, with or without dysuria.

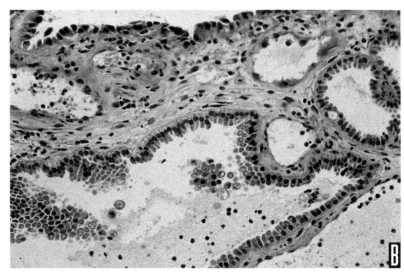

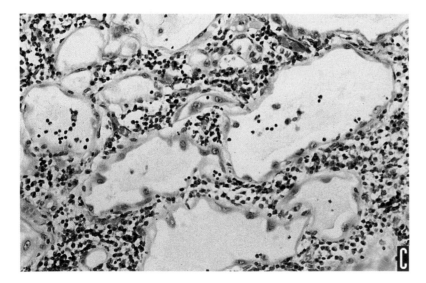

Figure 10.41 **A,** The thickened mucosal fold visible in this photomicrograph contains a nephrogenic adenoma within the expanded inflamed lamina propria. Beneath the intact urothelium are tightly packed tubules and microcysts with empty lumina, lined by a single layer of small cuboidal or flattened cells with scant, pale cytoplasm. **B,** In other foci, columnar cells with basal nuclei and more abundant eosinophilic cytoplasm are present. **C,** Nuclei may become enlarged and reactive with nucleolar prominence, but cytologic atypia is absent and mitoses are rare.

MORPHOLOGY Grossly, IPTB are firm or rubbery, nodular masses that are polypoid or pedunculated. They have ranged from 2–5 cm in greatest dimension. The cut surface is smooth, gray-white and gelatinous or mucoid (Fig. 10.43A). Surface ulcerations and hemorrhagic areas are common, but necrosis is absent. IPTB have no site predilection within the bladder. Although they may show only encroachment of superficial muscle bundles without destruction or replacement, most of the lesions reported in children have been locally aggressive, have shown infiltration of the muscularis propria of the bladder and, less commonly, extension into perivesical soft tissues.

Characteristic microscopic features include widely separated spindle cells set in a prominent myxoid stroma with little collagen, a chronic inflammatory infiltrate, and dispersed capillaries that are slit-

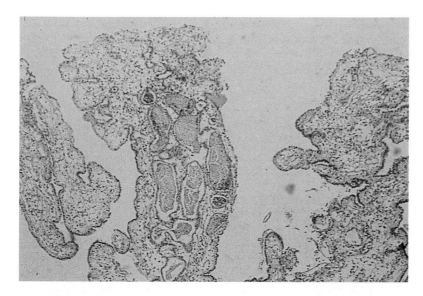

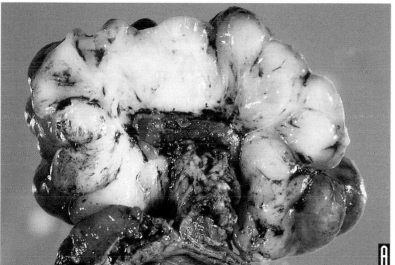

Figure 10.42 Nephrogenic adenomas may form delicate polypoid structures as well as papillae. Focally, tubules contain eosinophilic fluid. Cuboidal metaplasia is present on the surface of the papillae.

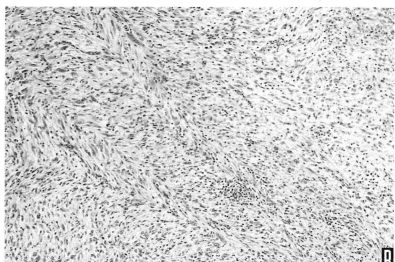

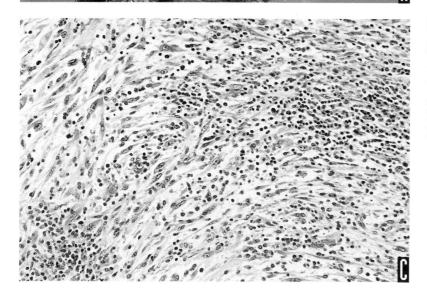

Figure 10.43 Inflammatory pseudotumor of the bladder. **A,** The tumor is pedunculated and has a nodular, gray-white gelatinous cut surface. Wide excision, which was performed after biopsy, showed no involvement of the muscularis propria. **B,** Microscopically, proliferating spindle cells form a vague fascicular pattern suggestive of a smooth muscle neoplasm. The stroma is myxoid and contains chronic inflammatory cells. **C,** The spindle cells have vesicular nuclei with prominent nucleoli and long, tapering eosinophilic cytoplasm. (Compare with Figs. 9.28, 12.56B, 12.58)

like or resemble granulation tissue (Fig. 10.43B–C). Inflammatory infiltrates, which consist of lymphocytes, plasma cells, neutrophils, mast cells, and eosinophils, are scattered throughout the lesion. Foci of densely cellular interlacing fascicles are common. The spindle cells have long, tapering eosinophilic cytoplasm with vesicular or slightly hyperchromatic nuclei that contain prominent nucleoli. Nuclear anaplasia and significant mitotic activity are lacking. Bizarre giant cells and cells that resemble "strap cells" or appear ganglionic may be observed. By electron microscopy, the spindle cells may have fibroblastic or myofibroblastic features. With immunohistochemistry, IPTB have been negative for epithelial membrane antigen, shown variable desmin expression, and have marked for vimentin, muscle specific actin and smooth muscle myosin. Focal immunoreactivity using a cytokeratin antibody cocktail (MAK6, AE1-AE3, and CAM 5.2) has been observed in several cases.

The major differential diagnosis is a low-grade leiomyosarcoma, particularly the myxoid variant (see Chapter 12). Lack of inflammatory cells and prominent blood vessels in deeper (i.e., nonulcerated) portions of the lesion, uniform cellularity, and an aggressive infiltrative margin with destruction of smooth muscle favor a diagnosis of leiomyosarcoma over IPTB. However, because of overlapping histologic, immunohistochemical, and ultrastructural features, distinction between them can be difficult. In addition, it is hazardous to make a definitive diagnosis on a limited biopsy specimen, particularly if superficial. When a confident distinction cannot be made, it is best to recommend wide excision or careful follow-up with cystoscopy and, if necessary, repeat biopsies.

ENDOMETRIOSIS

Urinary tract involvement by endometriosis may cause ureteral obstruction or result in a bladder wall mass (see Chapter 8). Rare cases of endometriosis have also been reported in males treated with estrogens for prostatic carcinoma who presented with hematuria secondary to an endometrioma of the posterior bladder wall. It is proposed that endometriosis in the male bladder results from hormonal stimulation of müllerian cell rests in the trigonal area, similar to endometriosis arising in the region of the prostatic utricle following prolonged estrogen therapy (see Chapter 13).

PRIMARY LOCALIZED AMYLOIDOSIS

Amyloidosis of the bladder may be part of the spectrum of primary (AL) or secondary (AA) systemic disease. Primary, localized amyloidosis of the genitourinary tract is rare and frequently a microscopic

finding, particularly in the seminal vesicles (1%–9% incidence at autopsy). However, at least 60% of reported urinary tract cases are localized to the bladder, and most cases of symptomatic amyloid disease of the bladder represent a solitary, localized, tumefactive process. There is no sex predilection, and lesions have occurred in patients 31–80 years of age (mean, 51 years).

PATHOGENESIS   Although the role of local bladder infection, allergy, or injury has been questioned, there are no consistent predisposing factors or disease, and the pathogenesis remains unclear. Amyloidosis is generally felt to result from aging and has been regarded as a senile type of amyloid. Most cases in the genitourinary tract have been shown to be of the light-chain (AL) type.

CLINICAL MANIFESTATIONS   Painless, gross hematuria is present in 85% of patients. Other associated urologic symptoms may include dysuria, nocturia, and frequency. Catastrophic hemorrhage may occur following cystoscopic biopsy.

The prognosis is more favorable than that for diffuse lesions resulting from systemic amyloidosis. Spontaneous regression of the localized tumefactive lesion has been commented upon, and transurethral resection, with or without fulguration, is generally curative, although local recurrences are possible. The diffuse lesions are more serious and may eventually require urinary diversion.

MORPHOLOGY   Bladder involvement may be localized or diffuse, and cystoscopic findings may be mistaken for single or multiple transitional cell carcinomas. Most localized amyloid occurs in the lateral walls and only rarely involves the trigone or anterior wall. Tumefactive lesions are typically broad-based and sessile, with thickening of the bladder wall that mimics an infiltrating neoplasm. The mucosal surface may be nodular, roughened, and ulcerated. Hemorrhagic ulcers and inflammatory excrescences may also be present.

Microscopically, globular masses of amyloid are present within the lamina propria and inner muscle layers (Fig. 10.44). The overlying epithelium may be polypoid. Deposits are also present in the walls of arteries and veins; however, a predominance of vascular deposits is more characteristic of systemic secondary amyloidosis. Amyloid has an affinity for Congo red dye and shows diagnostic apple-green birefringence under polarized light. It also shows metachromatic staining with crystal violet and thioflavin-T fluorescence. A foreign body giant cell reaction may be present at the margin of the amyloid deposits, but there is no plasma cell infiltrate.

Figure 10.44 Globular masses of amyloid in the connective tissue of the lamina propria are characteristic of primary localized amyloidosis. Vascular wall deposits are also present. The lamina propria is edematous and chronically inflamed. Amyloid is homogeneous, dense, and eosinophilic. Several foreign body giant cells are present.

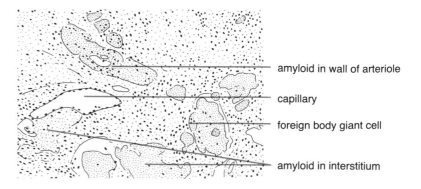

amyloid in wall of arteriole

capillary

foreign body giant cell

amyloid in interstitium

SECTION V

Neoplasms of the Urinary Tract

CHAPTER 11

Neoplasms of the Kidney, Renal Pelvis, and Ureter

NEOPLASMS OF THE KIDNEY

EPITHELIAL RENAL NEOPLASMS

CORTICAL ADENOMA

The cortical adenoma is the most common benign tumor of the kidney. Historically, any well differentiated tubular neoplasm less than 3 cm in diameter was considered an adenoma because of the rarity of metastases. However, reports have documented smaller tumors in adults and children that have metastasized and tumors larger than 10 cm in diameter that have not. Adenomas are most frequent in patients 40–80 years of age. The exact incidence is unknown since adenomas are asymptomatic and, therefore, often undetected. They are usually an incidental finding at autopsy (7% incidence in patients over 15 years of age) or in nephrectomies performed for another renal disease.

RELATIONSHIP TO RENAL CELL CARCINOMA There are many similarities between renal cell carcinoma (RCC) and adenoma: (1) both originate from proximal convoluted tubule epithelium; (2) they have no reliable distinguishing gross, histologic, histochemical, immunologic, or ultrastructural features; (3) adenomas arise more frequently in kidneys containing RCC; (4) both occur in the same age group (rarely in persons under 30 years old; more frequently with increasing age) and affect men two to four times more frequently than women; and

(5) both have a high incidence in tobacco users. When all renal tubular neoplasms are considered, a direct relationship is seen between tumor size and frequency of metastases. Bennington regards tubular neoplasms less than 3 cm in diameter that have not metastasized as latent cancers and proposes that *all* renal tubular neoplasms, regardless of size, should be regarded as carcinoma. Others believe that adenomas are the benign counterpart of RCCs and both are distinct entities, or that RCCs arise from adenomas.

Size is not a valid criterion for differentiating RCC from adenoma. Until more valid criteria are available, however, a diagnosis of adenoma should be made with caution and probably should be reserved for tubular neoplasms that are microscopically or grossly visible but not more than 1 cm in diameter. Larger neoplasms, particularly when encountered at surgery, should be regarded as RCCs with a potential for metastases and a prognosis that is statistically related to size.

MORPHOLOGY Grossly, adenomas are sharply demarcated, yellow or gray-white nodules that may protrude from the cortical surface (Fig. 11.1). Microscopically, they are unencapsulated and imperceptibly merge with surrounding parenchyma (Fig. 11.2). Growth patterns include papillae, occasionally within a cystic space (cystadenoma), small, uniform tubules, or solid nests (Fig. 11.3). Cells are small and uniform, have clear, vacuolated, or granular cytoplasm, and lack nuclear atypia. Features that suggest RCC, independent of size, include: (1) an expansile neoplasm that compresses the surrounding parenchyma, (2) capsular or venous invasion, (3) hemorrhage and necrosis, and (4) nuclear anaplasia (Fig. 11.4).

ONCOCYTOMA

Oncocytomas are rare, distinctive benign neoplasms of renal tubular origin that account for about 5% of all renal parenchymal neoplasms and are about 20 times less common than RCC. They have been reported to be multicentric in the same kidney in 5%–10% of cases and bilateral in about 3%; they occur rarely in polycystic kidneys. Oncocytomas show a predeliction for males (2.4:1); mean age at presentation is 64 years. Cytogenetic studies have shown karyotypic abnormalities that differ from RCC.

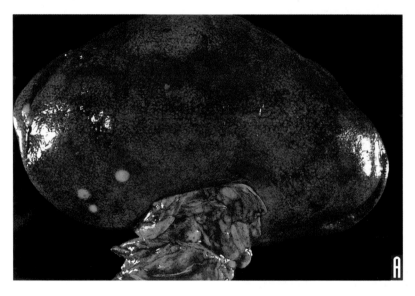

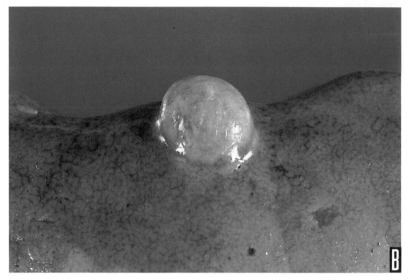

Figure 11.1 A, Cortical adenomas are a common incidental finding at autopsy and may be multiple. The three adenomas in this kidney are each less than 5 mm in diameter, slightly raised, sharply demarcated, gray-white, subcapsular nodules. **B,** This adenoma protrudes from the cortical surface. Although predominantly gray-white, there are multiple yellow areas, indicating that the adenoma is composed of both granular and clear cells.

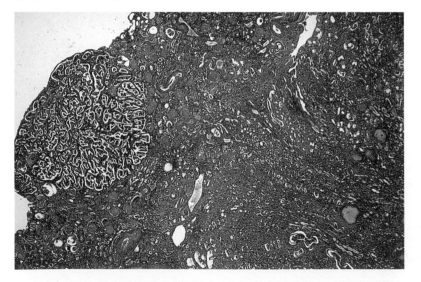

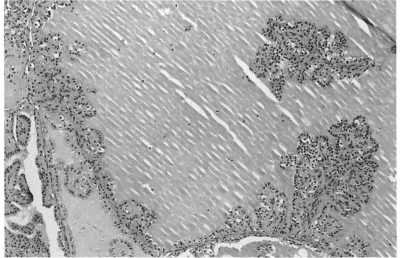

Figure 11.2 The unencapsulated tubular epithelial neoplasm in the subcapsular cortex (left) is an adenoma. It imperceptibly merges with the surrounding parenchyma, has a uniform papillary growth pattern, and lacks hemorrhage or necrosis.

Figure 11.3 In this view of a cortical adenoma associated with acquired renal cystic disease, papillae projecting into several microcysts are lined by a uniform layer of granular cuboidal cells. (This is the same case as Figure 11.8.)

CLINICAL MANIFESTATIONS Patients are typically asymptomatic, and the neoplasm is usually found incidentally at autopsy or during a radiologic workup of the urinary tract for other reasons. Gross hematuria and flank pain have occasionally been noted; however, the presence of a symptomatic renal mass should be regarded as suspicious for RCC. To date, no well documented case of oncocytoma has metastasized.

Although a characteristic angiographic "spoke-wheel" pattern with peripheral vessels radiating to the center is found in 50% of oncocytomas, RCCs may appear encapsulated and have a spoke-wheel pattern in up to 10% of cases. The arterial pattern in the oncocytoma is sharp, discrete, and very orderly, with no amorphous puddling or large arteriovenous lake formation (Fig. 11.5).

MORPHOLOGY Oncocytomas vary considerably in size and have ranged from 0.3–20 cm in diameter. Classically, they are well circumscribed and have a mahogany-brown cut surface (Fig. 11.6). A central stellate fibrotic scar is more common in larger tumors.

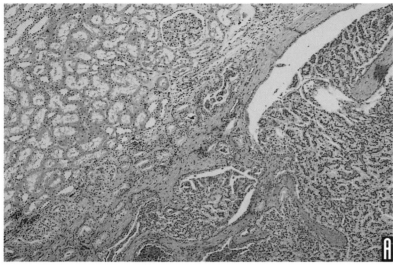

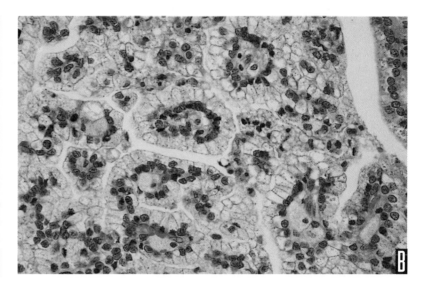

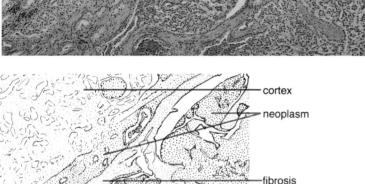

cortex

neoplasm

fibrosis

old hemorrhage

Figure 11.4 A, This 1.5-cm tubular epithelial neoplasm from a prospective renal transplant donor has microscopic features of RCC. At the interface with adjacent normal cortex, there is fibrosis, chronic inflammation, and old hemorrhage. **B,** Papillae are lined by columnar cells with abundant clear cytoplasm and basally oriented, slightly enlarged, hyperchromatic, irregular nuclei with nucleolar prominence.

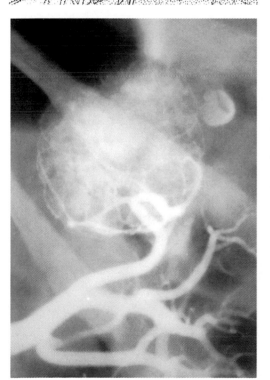

Figure 11.5 This angiogram, which demonstrates features common in, but not diagnostic of, an oncocytoma, shows a round, moderately vascular lesion. Although peripheral vessels radiate to the center, a "spoke-wheel" pattern is not apparent. (This is the same case as Figure 11.6.)

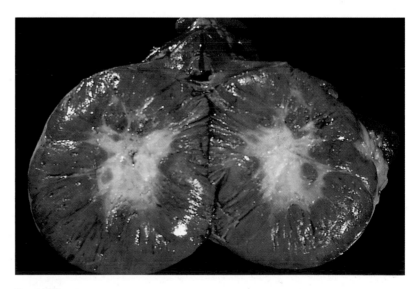

Figure 11.6 This large oncocytoma contains a central stellate scar and has a lobular appearance. (Reproduced with permission from Schumann and Weiss, 1981)

The radiating fibrous bands may give the cut surface a lobular appearance and the subcapsular surface a bosselated, almost cerebriform contour. Hemorrhage is uncommon, and cystic change is rare. The variegation typical of RCC, including yellow-tan foci, is not present, and there is no grossly evident necrosis or venous invasion.

Oncocytomas have a relatively homogeneous histologic and cytologic appearance. They are composed of uniform polygonal cells with a moderate amount of eosinophilic, granular cytoplasm. Diffuse organoid packeting of cells is prominent, especially centrally, in the relatively acellular, loose, edematous, fibrous scar (Fig. 11.7). There may be sheets of cells, with nests and cords separated by delicate fibrovascular septa. Less commonly, central lumina within cell packets focally form a tubular or alveolar pattern; lumina may dilate and form microcysts filled with acellular eosinophilic coagulum. Whether papillary foci may constitute a minor component is controversial. Microscopic capsular invasion with extension into perinephric fat is rare, and its prognostic significance remains unclear.

Oncocytomas may show low-grade nuclear atypia, although nuclei generally are uniform, round, and regular with fine chromatin, small nucleoli, and thick nuclear membranes; mitoses are absent. There may be a few multinucleated cells and cells with bizarre degenerative giant nuclei. The few oncocytomas that have been studied by flow cytometry have been composed of cells containing euploid DNA.

Oncocytomas are believed to arise from proximal convoluted tubules. However, an origin from the epithelium of distal convoluted tubules was suggested by the ultrastructural features observed in one study, including: (1) numerous, generally round-to-oval mitochondria with a paucity of other organelles; (2) extensive interdigitation and invagination of basal plasmalemma; (3) basement membrane protrusions into concavities of plasmalemma; and (4) sparse, blunt microvilli (no brush borders). Other studies have supported an origin from the thick ascending loop of Henle or collecting ducts, and the use of monoclonal antibodies specific for different nephron segments has yielded conflicting results regarding histogenesis.

It should be emphasized that RCCs may contain a variably prominent component of oncocytic cells, although these congeners of the oncocytoma lack the diffuse organoid packeting of cells and frequently demonstrate one or more of the following features: (1) necrosis, (2) clear cell foci, (3) ballooning distention of cytoplasm, (4) a predominant papillary pattern, (5) high-grade nuclear atypia with pleomorphism and macronucleoli, and (6) mitoses. In order to accurately diagnose RCCs that resemble oncocytoma, the tumor must be thoroughly sampled. A definitive diagnosis of oncocytoma should not be based on frozen section, needle biopsy, or fine-needle aspiration.

RENAL CELL CARCINOMA

RCC is relatively infrequent among malignant tumors in adults (not more than 3%). It is rare in children (1.5% of all tumors and 7% of all primary renal malignancies), in whom Wilms' tumor is 30 times more common. Its incidence, which averages 3.5 per 100,000 persons per year, increases exponentially with advancing age in both sexes. RCC accounts for about 85% of clinically manifest primary malignant renal tumors. It is two to three times more common in males and occurs primarily in patients over 40 years of age, with a peak incidence in the sixth to seventh decades of life. Bilateral RCCs, whether synchronous or metachronous, have been reported in up to 2% of cases.

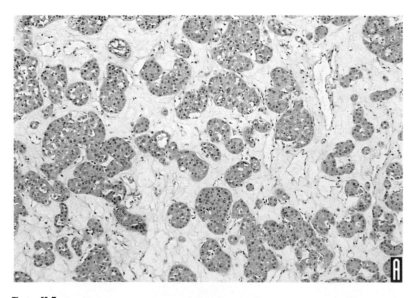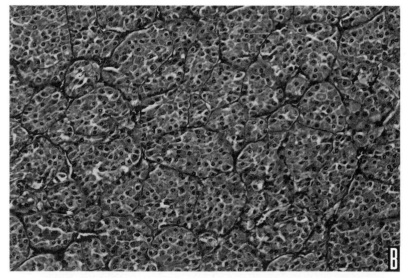

Figure 11.7 A, The central scar is composed of relatively acellular, loose, fibrous tissue. Organoid packeting of oncocytes is prominent. **B,** Peripherally, compact nests are separated by a delicate fibrovascular stroma. Oncocytomas are composed of a uniform population of tubular cells with abundant eosinophilic, granular cytoplasm and minimal nuclear atypia.

ETIOLOGY/PATHOGENESIS Most RCCs occur sporadically. In the rare cases having a familial distribution, a dominant pattern of inheritance is suggested. Rearrangement of the short arm of chromosome 3 has been described in both hereditary and sporadic forms of RCC. Patients with familial RCC are more likely to have multiple and/or bilateral tumors than solitary lesions and tend to develop tumors at an earlier age.

Patients with phacomatoses will more likely have multiple RCCs than solitary lesions. Von Hippel-Lindau disease and tuberous sclerosis (see Chapter 1) are two phacomatoses with a notably increased incidence of atypical renal cysts and RCC. Epithelial hyperplasia within the cysts appears to be linked to the development of RCC. This sequence of evolution is similar to RCC occurring with long-term hemodialysis, where 20% of patients with acquired renal cystic disease (see Chapter 3) develop renal tumors (up to 4% incidence of RCC) (Fig. 11.8). The association of polycystic kidney disease and RCC is also observed in autosomal dominant (adult) polycystic kidney disease (see Chapter 1), where there is a tenfold higher incidence of RCC (20% bilateral) (Fig. 11.9).

Although RCCs can be induced experimentally in laboratory animals by chemical, physical, and oncogenic viral agents, as well as by hormones such as estrogens, these do not appear to be etiologic factors in humans. There is a strong statistical association, however, with tobacco use, particularly cigars and pipes.

CLINICAL MANIFESTATIONS The classic triad of hematuria, pain, and a flank mass occurs in as few as 10% of patients with RCC and indicates advanced disease and a poor prognosis; about 50% of patients already have metastases. Painless gross or microscopic hematuria frequently indicates invasion of the collecting system and is usually a late event, occurring in more than 50% of patients at some stage.

Presenting signs and symptoms, which are frequently nonspecific and may be quite variable and nonurologic, include pyrexia, weight loss, fatigue, anorexia, nausea and vomiting, neuropathy, and myositis. Although fewer than 5% of patients present with symptoms from metastases, they are found in up to 33% of patients at diagnosis and may occur at unusual sites. Spontaneous regression of pulmonary metastases following nephrectomy has been reported.

Polycythemia, with or without leukocytosis and thrombocytopenia, exists in 2%–6% of patients and frequently is associated with elevated plasma erythropoietin levels. Other laboratory findings may include normochromic, normocytic anemia (25% of patients), an elevated sedimentation rate, and hypercalcemia, possibly related to tumor production of a parathormone-like substance. Reversible hepatic dysfunction with nontender hepatomegaly may be manifested by elevated serum levels of alkaline phosphatase, indirect bilirubin and alpha-2 globulin, and hypothrombinemia; liver biopsy shows nonspecific reactive hepatitis.

Urine cytology is of little value when diagnosing RCC, although it may be positive in late stages when the collecting system is invaded. Fine-needle aspiration cytology, which has been used to evaluate renal masses for more than three decades, is an accurate and simple diagnostic technique generally used with radiologic studies to establish the diagnosis of solid and cystic renal lesions. In the United States it has been used primarily for the identification and therapeutic evacuation of benign cysts (see Fig. 3.9); but in Scandinavia the technique is used routinely for the preoperative

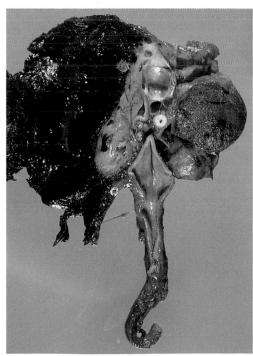
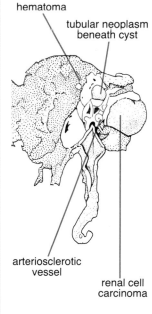

hematoma
tubular neoplasm beneath cyst
arteriosclerotic vessel
renal cell carcinoma

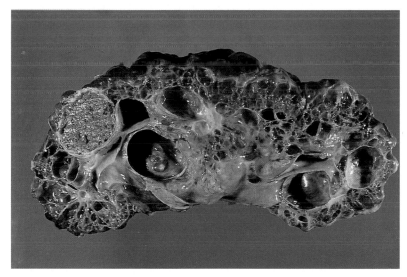

Figure 11.9 This kidney with typical findings of adult polycystic kidney disease contains a solitary RCC (left), which was an incidental finding in a patient who underwent bilateral nephrectomy prior to renal transplantation.

Figure 11.8 This kidney with acquired renal cystic disease contains a 2-cm RCC that has undergone hemorrhagic infarction. A small, tubular epithelial neoplasm bulges beneath a cyst wall, and parenchyma is compressed by a large perirenal hematoma. Chronic dialysis has caused marked arteriosclerosis.

diagnosis and grading of RCC (Figs. 11.10–11.13). RCC can be diagnosed in 72%–88% of cases without major complication or morbidity and without risk of needle (21 gauge or less) tract seeding. Clinical indications for performing fine-needle aspiration cytology of renal masses include: (1) confirmation of a diagnosis of RCC in nonoperative patients or prior to infarction therapy, (2) differentiation of RCC from retroperitoneal tumor or metastases, (3) staging of metastatic tumors (carcinomas or lymphomas), and (4) differentiation of an adrenal neoplasm from an upper-pole RCC.

The accuracy of radiologic diagnosis of renal masses approaches 95%. A solid RCC with angiography typically appears as a hypervascular mass and frequently has large vascular lakes, a disorganized vascular architecture, and arteriovenous shunts (Fig. 11.14). Evaluation of cystic masses should combine ultrasound, CT, and

Figure 11.10
Cytologic Grading of Renal Cell Carcinoma

	Tumor Grade		
Cytologic Characteristics	Well Differentiated	Moderately Differentiated	Poorly Differentiated
Cytoplasm	Usually foamy	Variable	Usually granular
Nuclear enlargement	Slight	Moderate	Marked
N/C ratio	Low	Variable	High
Nucleoli	+/- enlarged	Prominent, single	Prominent, irregular, +/- multiple
Pleomorphism	Absent	Slight	Prominent (including giant and spindle cells)
Cohesion	Strong	Moderate	Poor
Fragments	Sheets or groups (tubulopapillary)	Small groups	Few
Single cells	Few	Variable	Numerous

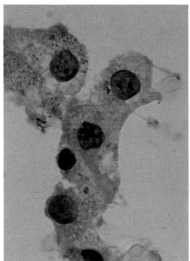
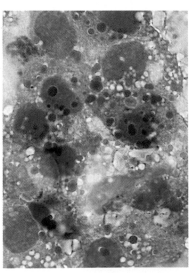
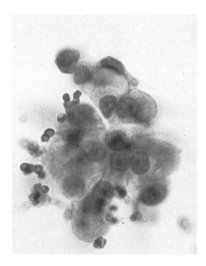
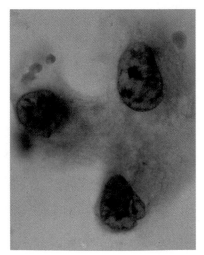
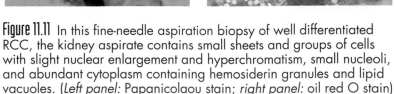

Figure 11.11 In this fine-needle aspiration biopsy of well differentiated RCC, the kidney aspirate contains small sheets and groups of cells with slight nuclear enlargement and hyperchromatism, small nucleoli, and abundant cytoplasm containing hemosiderin granules and lipid vacuoles. (*Left panel:* Papanicolaou stain; *right panel:* oil red O stain)

Figure 11.12 In these examples of fine-needle aspiration biopsies of moderately differentiated RCCs, cells show moderate nuclear enlargement and slight pleomorphism with chromatin clearing and single prominent nucleoli. Cytoplasm is vacuolated (left panel) or foamy (right panel) (Papanicolaou stain).

selective angiography. If radiologic findings are equivocal, fine-needle aspiration biopsy should be performed, particularly to distinguish a benign renal cyst from an "atypical" cyst suspicious for a cystic RCC. Radiologic indications for performing fine-needle aspiration cytology include: (1) an echo-free mass with irregular, poorly demarcated margins (ultrasound); (2) an avascular/hypovascular mass (angiography) (Fig. 11.15); (3) a "typical" cortical cyst with cloudy or hemorrhagic fluid; and (4) a suspected renal pelvic transitional cell carcinoma with negative urine cytologies.

MORPHOLOGY Although multiple tumors are present in the same kidney in up to 4.5% of patients, some may represent intraparenchymal metastases. More than 50% of tumors are larger than 6 cm in diameter at diagnosis.

RCCs typically appear as irregular, bosselated, cortical masses that protrude beneath the capsular surface and are sharply demarcated by a pseudocapsule composed of condensed connective tissue and compressed renal parenchyma. The cut surface is lobular and variegated (Fig. 11.16). Viable tumor glistens and is pale yellow to

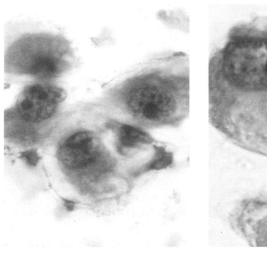
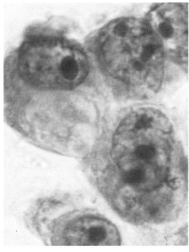

Figure 11.13 Fine-needle aspiration biopsies of poorly differentiated RCCs show cells that have prominent nuclear pleomorphism with chromatin clearing and single or multiple macronucleoli. Nucleus-to-cytoplasm ratios are high. In the left panel, perinuclear cytoplasm is distinctly granular (Papanicolaou stain).

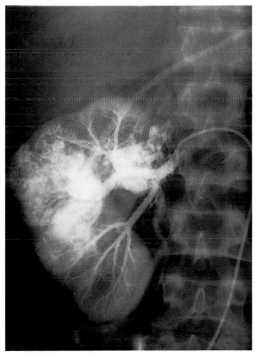
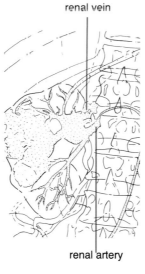

renal vein

renal artery

Figure 11.15 In this example of a papillary cystic RCC, the parenchymal phase of the selective renal arteriogram reveals a slightly irregular, almost completely avascular area (arrows). (This is the same case as Figure 11.26.) (Courtesy of H. Hawkins, MD, Cincinnati, Ohio)

Figure 11.14 An arteriogram of a solid RCC shows a hypervascular mass with a typical vascular pattern. Neovascularity in the course of the renal vein indicates tumor thrombus. (Courtesy of H. Hawkins, MD, Cincinnati, Ohio)

orange in lipid-rich areas and gray in lipid-poor tumors or sarcomatoid variants. Chromophobe RCCs are light brown or beige. Areas of necrosis are dull gray and opaque. Cystic degeneration and fibrosis with septa formation are common, as are areas of old and recent hemorrhage (Fig. 11.17). Extensive degeneration and necrosis occasionally produce a hemorrhagic mass with little identifiable neoplasm grossly or microscopically (Fig. 11.18). Cystic RCCs may occur with resorption of necrotic tumor or with a primary papillary cystadenocarcinoma (see Fig. 11.26); 3% of RCCs arise from a benign cyst.

RCCs demonstrate a variety of histologic patterns—tubular, papillary, alveolar, cords, nests and sheets, as well as sarcomatoid (Fig. 11.19). A rich capillary vascularity is typical. Collagenous stroma, which is generally inconspicuous, may be prominent and hyalin-

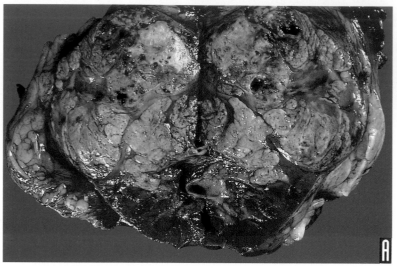

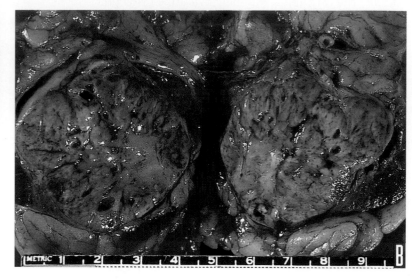

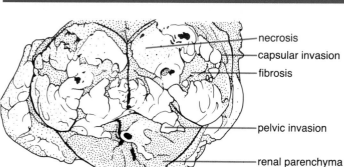

necrosis

capsular invasion

fibrosis

pelvic invasion

renal parenchyma

Figure 11.16 A, In this gross specimen, a large, lobulated, yellow-tan RCC replaces the upper and middle portions of the bivalved kidney. It has a variegated appearance secondary to hemorrhage, necrosis, and fibrosis. The renal capsule and pelvis are focally invaded. **B,** This RCC appears orange and has an eccentric stellate scar with small foci of cystic degeneration. It should not be mistaken for an oncocytoma. (**A:** Reproduced with permission from Schumann and Weiss, 1981)

Figure 11.17 The RCC in the lower pole of this kidney shows marked cystic degeneration with fibrosis and septa formation.

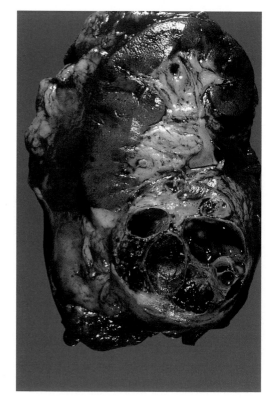

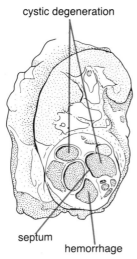

cystic degeneration

septum

hemorrhage

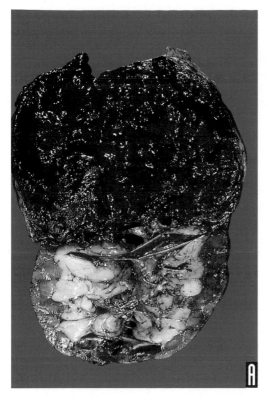

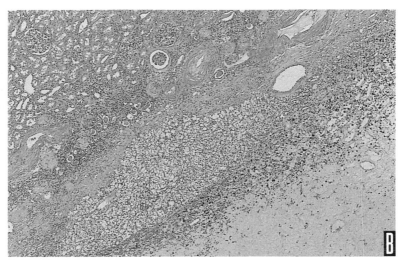

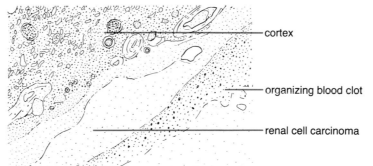

cortex

organizing blood clot

renal cell carcinoma

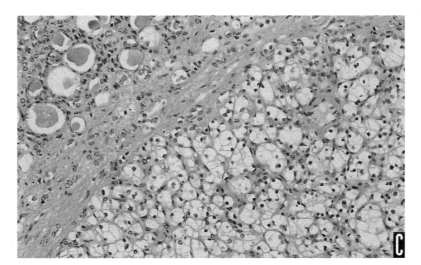

Figure 11.18 A, As in this gross specimen, RCC may present as a hemorrhagic cyst filled with blood clot. **B,** Microscopic examination of the interface with renal parenchyma demonstrates a focus of clear cell RCC, which should not be mistaken for lipid-laden histiocytes resulting from the hemorrhage. Thorough sampling of the peripheral fibrotic capsule is often required to document recognizable tumor. **C,** At higher magnification, the clear cells form discrete nests.

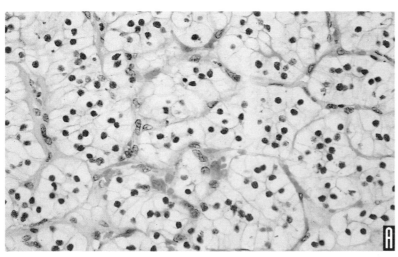

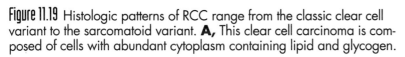

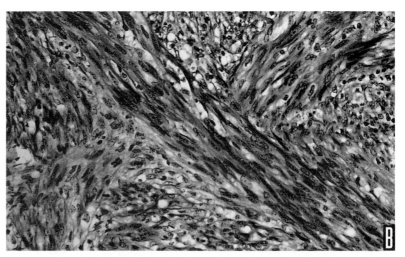

Figure 11.19 Histologic patterns of RCC range from the classic clear cell variant to the sarcomatoid variant. **A,** This clear cell carcinoma is composed of cells with abundant cytoplasm containing lipid and glycogen.

A rich capillary vascularity with scant intervening stroma separates the cell nests and is characteristic of RCC. **B,** Intersecting fascicles of anaplastic spindle cells are present in this sarcomatoid variant.

ized in areas of prior necrosis; myxoid areas are occasionally present. Foci of calcification may show osseous or cartilaginous metaplasia. Areas of hemorrhage and necrosis contain inflammatory cells, cholesterol clefts, and hemosiderin-laden macrophages. Clusters of foamy macrophages and laminated, calcified concretions (psammoma bodies) may be present, particularly in papillary tumors (Fig. 11.20). Amyloidosis is found in the tumor-bearing kidney or metastatic sites in 2%–3% of patients at autopsy.

RCCs may be of pure clear cell, granular cell, or mixed cell types, and foci of oncocyte-like cells may be present. Cells may be cuboidal, columnar, or ovoid to polygonal. Clear cells, which are large and frequently uniform, have abundant cytoplasm, distinct cell membranes, and relatively small nuclei. The clear cytoplasm is due to the abundance of neutral lipids (oil red O-positive), phospholipids (Sudan black-positive), and glycogen (periodic acid–Schiff [PAS]-positive). Ultrastructurally, these cells have little endoplasmic reticulum and Golgi and few mitochondria. Granular cells have

eosinophilic cytoplasm due to diminished lipid; increased organelles are found ultrastructurally, including numerous mitochondria, more highly developed Golgi, and endoplasmic reticulum with more frequent cytosomes and small amounts of particulate glycogen. Oncocytic cells, which have a coarsely granular eosinophilic cytoplasm, are packed with mitochondria.

The recently described chromophobe RCC consists of polygonal cells with sharply defined borders and voluminous lightly staining cytoplasm that appears finely reticular or flocculent (Fig. 11.21). In some tumors, variable numbers of cells show transitions to eosinophilic granular cytoplasm. Unlike clear cells, chromophobe cells contain little glycogen or lipid and show intensely positive staining for acid mucopolysaccharides (Hale's colloidal iron stain). Ultrastructurally, numerous microvesicles are present in both the typical chromophobe cells and the eosinophilic variants.

The following ultrastructural features of RCC resemble proximal convoluted tubule epithelium: (1) a brush border of tightly packed

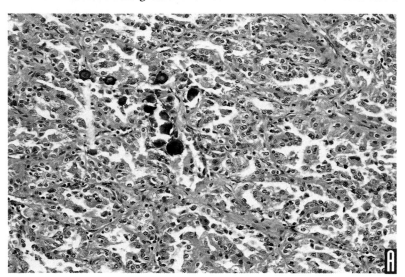

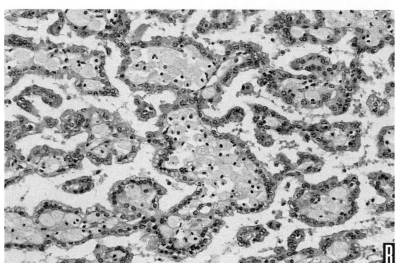

Figure 11.20 **A,** This granular cell RCC forms tubules and contains a focus of psammoma bodies, which are basophilic and have characteristic lamellations. **B,** Prominent foamy macrophages may be present in the stroma of papillary RCCs.

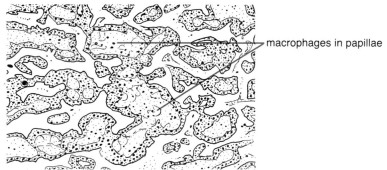

macrophages in papillae

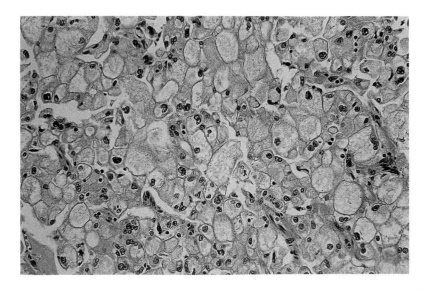

Figure 11.21 Chromophobe cells are polygonal and have abundant, finely reticular or flocculent appearing cytoplasm with distinct cell borders. (Courtesy of J. Eble, MD, Indianapolis, Indiana)

microvilli, (2) membrane-associated vesicles involved in pinocytosis, (3) membrane coating of extracellular material (glycocalyx), (4) infoldings of plasma membrane, and (5) abundant atypical, tortuous, or elongated mitochondria with bizarrely arranged cristae and amorphous dense bodies.

The reported expression of brush border antigen in 80% of cases further supports the hypothesis that RCC originates from proximal convoluted tubule epithelium in the vast majority of cases. RCCs also frequently coexpress cytokeratin and vimentin, but are negative for Tamm–Horsfall antigen.

Sarcomatoid variants constitute about 1.0%–1.5% of RCCs and are thought to derive from metaplastic transformation of the cells of the adenocarcinoma (Fig. 11.22). The sarcomatoid component may resemble rhabdomyosarcoma, fibrosarcoma, malignant fibrous histiocytoma, or liposarcoma, and some tumors have contained malignant bone and cartilage. Some of these mixed tumors may be derived from both epithelial and stromal elements and represent true carcinosarcomas. Thorough sampling of the tumor with careful light-microscopic examination of numerous sections should be performed before a diagnosis of primary renal sarcoma is made. Immunohistologic studies and electron microscopy may be needed to document an epithelial origin. Sarcomatoid RCCs must be distinguished from pleomorphic and spindle cell transitional cell carcinomas and Wilms' tumor, as well as from primary or metastatic sarcomas.

PROGNOSIS The prognosis for RCC is generally poor, with most deaths occurring in the first two years. The overall survival rate in both adults and children approaches 18%–27% ten years after nephrectomy. Prognosis has been correlated with both gross and microscopic features.

In general, the larger the tumor, the greater the likelihood of local extension, vascular invasion, and metastases. However, size alone does not indicate the degree of malignancy; about 2% of tumors larger than 10 cm in diameter have not metastasized at the time of diagnosis.

Gross features that predict prognosis are incorporated into a staging system:

Stage I   Tumor confined to kidney.
Stage II   Invasion of perinephric fat but confined to
           Gerota's fascia.
Stage IIIA Invasion of renal vein or vena cava.
Stage IIIB Metastases to regional lymph nodes.
Stage IIIC Both present.
Stage IVA Invasion of adjacent organs, other than adrenal.
Stage IVB Distant metastases.

Tumor stage at the time of diagnosis is the most important prognostic factor. Several studies, however, have shown that invasion of the renal vein (Fig. 11.23) does not significantly alter prognosis

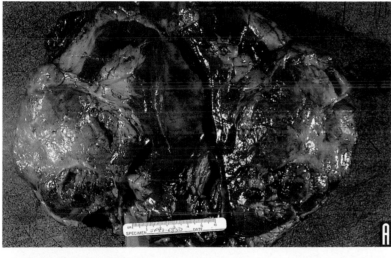

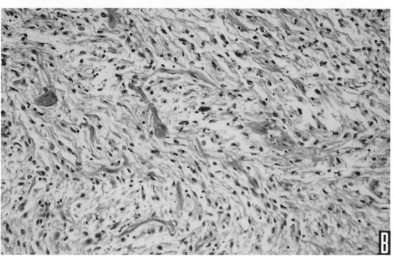

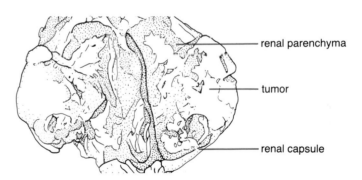

renal parenchyma

tumor

renal capsule

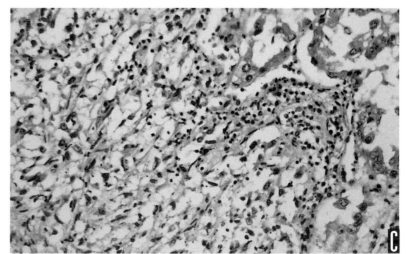

Figure 11.22 A, A sarcomatoid RCC, which invades the renal capsule in this gross specimen, appears gray-tan and has prominent degeneration and necrosis. **B,** An omental metastasis, which was initially biopsied, consists of anaplastic, vacuolated spindle cells supported by a delicate capillary stroma, suggesting the possibility of a liposarcoma. **C,** Thorough sampling of the renal mass documented merging of the liposarcomatous tumor with tubules lined by pleomorphic granular cells (right).

in patients who are otherwise stage I. RCC extends into the vena cava in 4%–10% of patients undergoing nephrectomy (Fig. 11.24). Pritchett and colleagues have shown that the level of vena caval tumor extension adversely affects five-year survival if there is atrial extension or if complete tumor resection is impossible.

Additional hematogenous routes of metastasis include retrograde flow to pelvic structures via the left spermatic or ovarian vein and spread via Batson's paravertebral venous plexus to the axial skeleton (Fig. 11.25). Metastases, present in up to 95% of patients at autopsy, most commonly involve the lungs (55%), lymph nodes, liver, and bone (33%), but may be found in virtually any organ.

Excluding sarcomatoid variants, which have a median survival of about six months, histologic patterns generally do not correlate with prognosis. Tumors that are more than 50% papillary, however, may have a better prognosis (Fig. 11.26).

Several studies have shown that pure clear cell tumors are less aggressive and have a lower metastatic rate than granular or mixed forms, and have a better prognosis for up to five years. Fuhrman

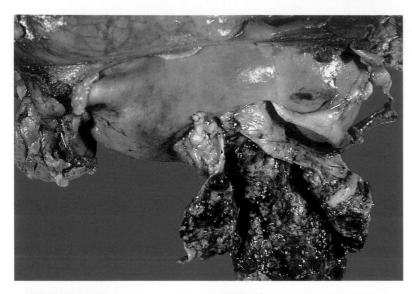

Figure 11.23 With massive venous invasion by RCC, the renal vein may become occluded by adherent tumor thrombus.

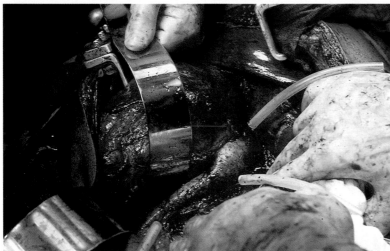

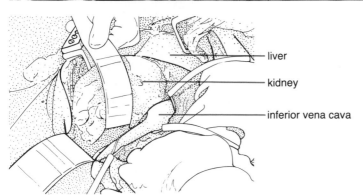

Figure 11.24 In this patient undergoing a radical nephrectomy, the inferior vena cava is distended by tumor thrombus. RCCs may extend proximally to the right atrium. (Coursey of J.E. Fowler, Jr., MD, Chicago, Illinois)

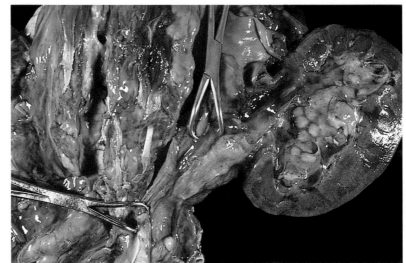

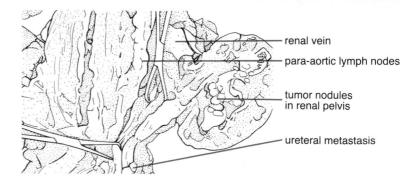

Figure 11.25 RCC (not shown) arising in the right kidney has metastasized to para-aortic lymph nodes. There are multiple, yellow-gray nodules in the renal pelvis. An obstructing metastatic nodule in the midureter has caused hydroureter and hydronephrosis. Retrograde lymphohematogenous spread also produced multiple submucosal and intramural nodules in the bladder.

and co-workers showed that both survival and metastatic potential can be predicted by a nuclear grading system (Fig. 11.27) that they developed:

Grade 1 Small (10 μ), round, uniform nuclei and inconspicuous or absent nucleoli (resemble normal tubular cells)

Grade 2 Slight nuclear enlargement (15 μ) and irregularities with small nucleoli

Grade 3 Moderate nuclear enlargement (20 μ) with obvious irregularities, pleomorphism, and prominent nucleoli

Grade 4 Similar to grade 3, with addition of bizarre, often multilobed nuclei and heavy chromatin clumps, or with sarcomatous features.

A relationship was also noted between cell type and nuclear grade: Clear cell tumors accounted for 93% of grade 1 tumors and only 5% of grade 3 and 4 tumors, while 57% of granular cell tumors were grade 3 or 4. In a study by Skinner and colleagues, nuclear grading had a definite, although limited, predictive value within stages I, III, and IV.

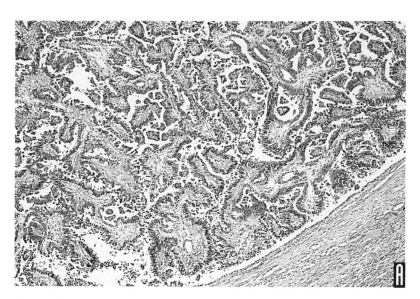

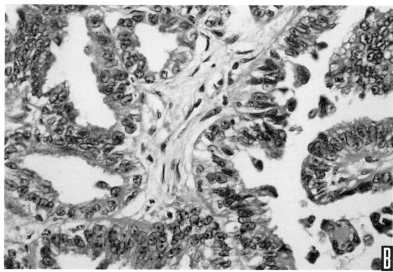

Figure 11.26 A, This intracystic RCC is predominantly papillary. B, Papillae and tubules in this tumor are lined by cuboidal-to-columnar cells with granular cytoplasm. (This is the same case as Figure 11.15.)

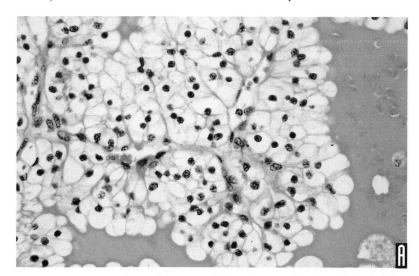

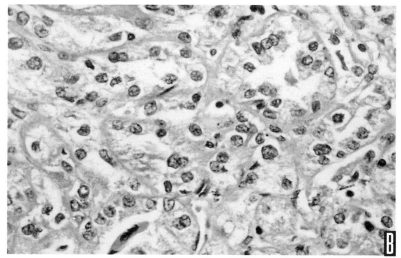

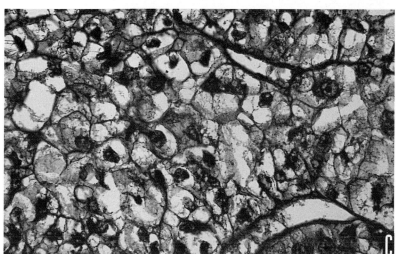

Figure 11.27 Histologic grading of RCC is based on nuclear characteristics. A, Grade 1; B, Grade 2; C, Grade 3. (A: Reproduced with permission from Schumann and Weiss, 1981)

DNA ploidy correlates with nuclear grade. In studies by Ljunberg and colleagues, aneuploid tumors showed more aggressive growth with spread outside the renal capsule, although metastatic potential and survival time were not predicted by the DNA content of the primary tumor. In comparison, the proportion of tumors with aneuploid DNA content was higher in the metastases; aneuploid metastases indicated a poor prognosis.

Collecting-Duct Carcinoma

The few well documented cases of this adenocarcinoma suggest that it represents less than 1% of RCCs. Unlike typical RCC, histologic, immunocytochemical, and ultrastructural features have supported origin from collecting ducts of Bellini. In the six patients reported by Fleming and Lewi, the mean age was 67 years, although patients have ranged from 13–83 years. Most patients have been male.

CLINICAL MANIFESTATIONS Patients with collecting-duct carcinoma may present with hematuria, an abdominal mass, or signs and symptoms of metastases. The majority of tumors are aggressive, with early dissemination leading to rapid death.

MORPHOLOGY These neoplasms have a characteristic medullary location with distortion of the pelvicalyceal system, infiltration into hilar tissue, and destuctive intrarenal spread that may not alter the outer contour of the kidney. They are typically firm, white or gray. Their borders are ill-defined, but may be distinctly papillary and friable. Massive hemorrage and necrosis are absent.

Microscopically, tumor infiltrating the renal parenchyma, as well as metastases, has a characteristic microcystic-papillary pattern associated with a prominent desmoplastic stromal reaction (Fig. 11.28). Dilated, branched, and anastomosing tubules are lined by a simple or multilayered, pleomorphic cuboidal or columnar epithelium that is mitotically active and forms papillae or pseudopapillae. Tubular, solid, and occasionally cribriform as well as spindle cell patterns may be observed. Focal, scant, intracellular mucin may be identified.

Microscopic invasion of intrarenal and hilar veins is common. Intratubular spread may be present, as may atypical hyperplasia and carcinoma in situ within collecting ducts of adjacent renal medulla. Growth within the renal pelvis may occur. Some tumors have formed a papillary adenocarcinoma composed of fibrovascular stalks and fronds lined by a single layer of uniform cuboidal cells with clear or faintly granular, eosinophilic cytoplasm. They show minimal nuclear pleomorphism and rare mitoses. Calcospherites (psammoma bodies) may be present. In one reported case, which was an unusual variant that appeared to arise from metaplastic glandular epithelium of the pelvis, both tumor and metaplastic epithelium had ultrastructural features typical of collecting duct epithelium. Adenocarcinomas of collecting duct origin mark for high-molecular weight cytokeratins as well as Ulex europaeus agglutinin (UEA-1), unlike convoluted tubular epithelium and RCCs.

Embryonal Renal Neoplasms
Congenital Mesoblastic Nephroma

Pure mesenchymal neoplasms in infants constitute 1%–10% of pediatric tumors and may be benign, indeterminate, or malignant. Congenital mesoblastic nephroma (CMN) is a benign tumor that typically presents in the perinatal period and is diagnosed in the early months of life. It rarely occurs in older children or young adults. CMN has been viewed as a stromal/leiomyomatous

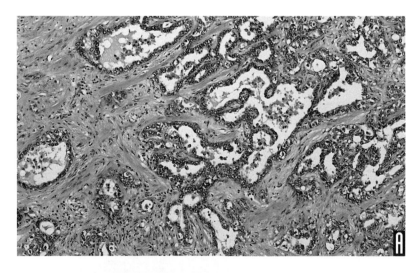

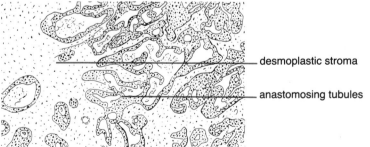

desmoplastic stroma

anastomosing tubules

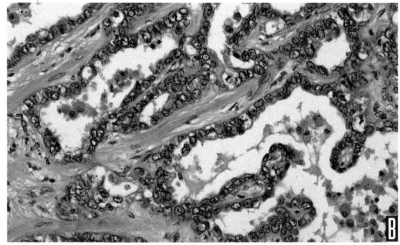

Figure 11.28 A, Collecting-duct carcinoma infiltrates as anastomosing tubules and causes a marked desmoplastic stromal reaction. **B,** High grade nuclear features and mitotic activity are present.

hamartoma, as well as a cytodifferentiated variant or even a precursor of Wilms' tumor. Ultrastructural and immunohistochemical studies have shown features consistent with myofibroblastic differentiation.

Nephrectomy is considered curative for CMN when performed during the neonatal period or up to three months of age. However, if the excision is incomplete and histologic features are atypical—particularly in a child three months of age or older—CMN may recur or metastasize.

MORPHOLOGY   CMNs are unilateral, solitary tumors that may range from less than 1 cm to 14 cm in diameter (Fig. 11.29A). Unlike leiomyomas in the adult kidney, CMN has a vague, unencapsulated junction with adjacent parenchyma and often extends beyond the renal capsule. The cut surface is uniform, gray-white to yellow-brown, tough, and finely trabeculated. Hemorrhage, cystic change with accumulation of clear fluid, and necrosis are rare.

Microscopically, CMN has a diffuse growth pattern and is interspersed with adjacent renal parenchyma without causing compression. It is composed of variably mature connective tissue cells arranged in interlacing bundles or whorls (Fig. 11.29B,C). The spindle-shaped fibromuscular cells have cigar-shaped vesicular nuclei with small basophilic nucleoli, no atypia, and variable mitotic activity (0–5 mitoses/10 hpf). There are thin-walled sinusoids and clusters of vascular structures. Myxoid regions, foci of extramedullary hematopoiesis, and skeletal muscle or cartilage may be present. Well differentiated tubular and glomeruloid structures may represent entrapped, dysplastic nephrons or a differentiated component of the tumor. Dysplastic elements and a prominent lymphoid infiltrate may exist at the margin.

An aggressive variant of mesoblastic nephroma, which appears to carry an increased risk for recurrence and metastases, has been reported as malignant mesenchymal nephroma, cellular variant of congenital mesoblastic nephroma, or atypical mesoblastic nephroma

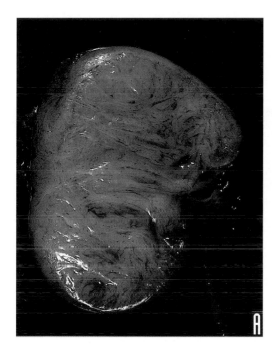

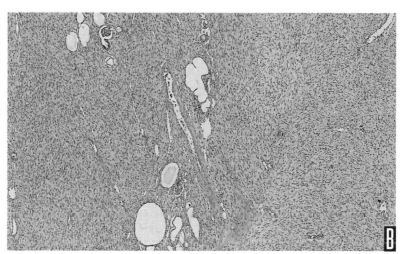

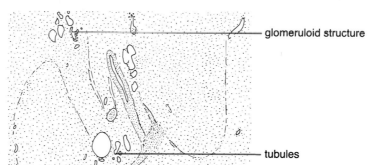

glomeruloid structure

tubules

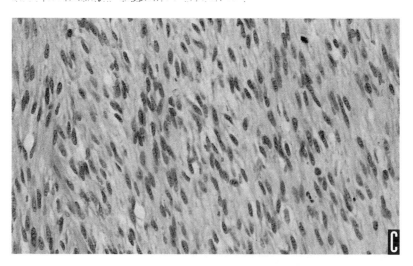

Figure 11.29 **A,** In this gross specimen, a yellow-tan, finely trabeculated CMN replaces most of the renal parenchyma. **B,** Microscopically, CMN is composed of spindle cells arranged in interlacing bundles or whorls. Glomeruloid structures and tubules are commonly interspersed. **C,** The fibromuscular spindle cells lack nuclear atypia, but may have occasional mitoses. (Courtesy of K. Bove, MD, Cincinnati, Ohio)

(Fig. 11.30). In comparison to the conventional mesoblastic nephromas described above, the atypical mesoblastic nephromas tend to be larger, bulging, white, fleshy tumors with frequent cystic change, hemorrhage, and necrosis. Microscopically, the uniform regular interlacing pattern is lost; cellularity and mitotic activity are increased (10–30 mitoses/10 hpf). Tumor cells, which are arranged in compact sheets, have scanty cytoplasm and oval to fusiform nuclei with clumped chromatin and nuclear irregularities. Clear cell sarcoma-like areas have been observed in a few neoplasms.

MULTILOCULAR CYST

Although multilocular cyst is presented elsewhere (see Chapter 2), it is probably related to cystic partially differentiated Wilms' tumor (see Fig. 2.11). Many authorities view it as a nephroblastoma with benign differentiation that may occur in association with Wilms' tumor, and have termed it cystic nephroma.

WILMS' TUMOR AND PRECURSOR LESIONS

Wilms' tumor (nephroblastoma) is a mixed renal tumor composed of metanephric blastema and its stromal and epithelial derivatives at variable stages of differentiation. Wilms' tumor characteristically affects young children, accounting for about 20% of all pediatric neoplasms; approximately 450 cases are diagnosed annually. The peak incidence is during the second year of life; 50% of cases are diagnosed before age three, and 75% before age five. Bilateral and familial nephroblastomas occur at a younger age than nephroblastomas in general. Children younger than one year of age have less than a 50% chance of bearing a classic Wilms' tumor. The fetal rhabdomyomatous nephroblastoma presents at an early age (mean, 20 months) and has a 33% incidence of bilaterality. Wilms' tumor shows no sex predilection, although cases associated with hemihypertrophy have a female preponderance.

Wilms' tumor in adults is rare; the oldest patient was 80 years of age. Many of the reported cases are probably RCCs with undifferentiated or sarcomatoid features. Two patients with bilateral tumors have been recorded.

The rare extrarenal Wilms' tumor is thought to arise from embryologic rests of renal tissue (pro-, meso-, or metanephros). Thorough histologic examination is required to exclude origin from within a teratoma.

PATHOGENESIS   Gestational factors suspected of playing a role in the pathogenesis of Wilms' tumor have not been statistically proven. Hereditary factors appear to be more relevant. In several

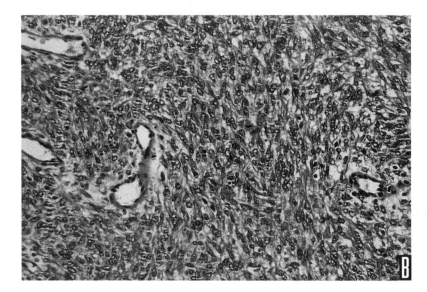

Figure 11.30 A, This atypical mesoblastic nephroma has a variegated cut surface due to marked hemorrhage as well as cystic degeneration with foci of necrosis. Viable tumor is fleshy and gray-white. **B,** Microscopically, sheets of closely packed cells with scanty cytoplasm are haphazardly arranged. The oval to fusiform nuclei are enlarged and hyperchromatic with clumped chromatin. Mitotic figures are present. (Courtesy of M. Wick, MD, St. Louis, Missouri)

Figure 11.31 The kidney on the left contains multiple gray-white, sharply demarcated Wilms' tumors. The mottling of the upper pole mass is due to focal hemorrhage and necrosis.

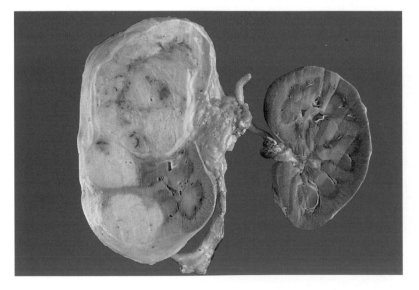

familial nephroblastomas, an autosomal-dominant mode of inheritance was suggested. Familial cases, however, are rare compared to the frequency of multifocal or bilateral tumors, and vertical transmission is almost nonexistent. Wilms' tumors are rarely seen in newborns, but in children less than 2 years old, precursor lesions consisting of hamartomatous remnants of aberrant metanephric differentiation are more common. Nephrogenic blastema is found in up to 1% of infants at autopsy, which is about 100 times the expected incidence of Wilms' tumor. They are rare as an incidental finding in older children or adults.

Clinicopathologic observations support Cohnheim's concept of the origin of cancer in embryonic rests, as well as the proposed two-mutation theory of oncogenesis proposed by Knudson and Strong, in which a prezygotic and a postzygotic gene mutation lead to the development of Wilms' tumor. There are two distinct groups of Wilms' tumors: (1) unilateral, nonfamilial tumors rarely associated with malformations; and (2) bilateral and/or familial tumors that may be associated with other malformations and occur at an earlier age. The first group represents the spontaneous, sporadic form arising from normal tissue after two or more postzygotic (somatic) mutational events. The second group represents the inherited form, in which persistent nephrogenic rests may be a manifestation of prezygotic mutation, with transformation to Wilms' tumor requiring only one additional error of replication. This theory of etiopathogenesis predicts that germ cell mutation should be associated with bilateral precursor lesions and postzygotic mutations with unilateral precursors. Chromosomal studies in Wilms' tumor have generally shown a normal karyotype. Deletion within the 11p13 band of chromosome 11 has been shown in tumor tissue of sporadic cases of Wilms' tumor without occurring in the normal somatic cells.

CLINICAL MANIFESTATIONS   Presenting symptoms depend on the tumor's size. An abdominal mass is present in more than 90% of cases, and abdominal pain is common. There may be fever, anorexia, nausea and vomiting, constipation, hypertension, and gross hematuria; venous obstruction leads to varicocele or leg edema. Erythropoietin levels without polycythemia may be elevated. About 25% of patients have metastatic disease at the time of diagnosis. Older children usually present with more advanced disease. Common sites of metastases include lung, liver, mediastinal nodes, adrenals, diaphragm, and retroperitoneum; bone metastases are rare (5% of cases). Metastases usually present within two years of diagnosis of the primary tumor. The risk period is calculated by the age at diagnosis plus nine months. Prognosis is more favorable if the tumor is diagnosed before two years of age.

ASSOCIATED CONDITIONS   The risk of Wilms' tumor developing in children with *sporadic aniridia* is about 33%. Associated abnormalities include microcephaly, developmental retardation, malformed ears, genitourinary anomalies, lumbosacral spina bifida with lipoma, and meningocele. *Hemihypertrophy* may involve a portion or an entire side of the body, or may be crossed. The hemihypertrophy–visceral neoplasia syndrome includes hepatoblastoma and adrenal carcinoma. The closely related Beckwith–Wiedemann syndrome of macroglossia, omphalocele, gigantism, adrenal cytomegaly, and visceromegaly is associated with Wilms' tumor. The syndrome of male pseudohermaphroditism, glomerulopathy, and nephrotic syndrome with Wilms' tumor (Drash syndrome) is rare. There are reports of Wilms' tumor associated with chromosomal disorders, for example, trisomy 18. Both Beckwith's syndrome and trisomy 18 are associated with metanephric blastemal remnants (nephroblastomatosis).

MORPHOLOGY   Wilms' tumor may be multifocal within a kidney (Fig. 11.31) or may appear as a diffuse subcapsular neoplastic cap; there is a 4%–6% incidence of bilaterality. Most nephroblastomas are large (median diameter, 12 cm), sharply demarcated tumors. A pseudocapsule is formed by compressed renal parenchyma, renal capsule, and perirenal tissue, but infiltrative margins may also be evident. The cut surface is soft, gray-tan, and bulging, with confluent lobules producing an encephaloid appearance (Fig. 11.32). Tumors with prominent stromal differentiation have a tougher texture, and focal hemorrhage or necrosis produces variegation. Variable cystic change may be present; tumors contain calcifications in up to 14% of cases. The cystic, partially differentiated

Figure 11.32 As in this typical specimen, Wilms' tumor is gray-tan and bulging, with a lobulated or encephaloid appearance. Slight variegation is due to recent and old hemorrhage. Compressed parenchyma forms a pseudocapsule. Renal vein invasion is present. (Reproduced with permission from Schumann and Weiss, 1981)

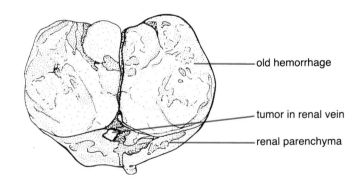

old hemorrhage

tumor in renal vein

renal parenchyma

nephroblastoma (Fig. 11.33) lacks solid, expansile masses and is totally multicystic, but may contain luminal papillonodules. The fetal rhabdomyomatous nephroblastoma is an expansile, sharply circumscribed tumor that tends to present as a polypoid intrapelvic growth (Fig. 11.34). The cut surface is tan-white with a prominent whorled fibromyomatous architecture.

Traditionally, Wilms' tumor has been viewed as a triphasic embryonal renal neoplasm with blastemal, stromal, and epithelial cell types, each of which may exhibit a variety of patterns or lines of differentiation (Fig. 11.35). *Blastema* is composed of closely packed, slightly ovoid cells with scanty cytoplasm. It is usually divided into circumscribed nodules or trabeculae by surrounding stroma. *Epithelial* differentiation may be minimal or prominent. Tubular formation within blastema may be central, eccentric, or marginal. Nephronic tubules and avascular glomeruloid structures are most common. The rare teratoid Wilms' tumor contains variable epithelial derivatives, including squamous, mucinous, ciliated, columnar, urothelial, argentaffin and argyrophil, neuroepithelial, neuroblast, neuroglia, and ganglion cells. The stroma is usually fibroblastic, with myxoid regions. Smooth muscle may be prominent; foci may contain undifferentiated spindle cells. A variety of mesenchymal derivatives are well recognized, including skeletal

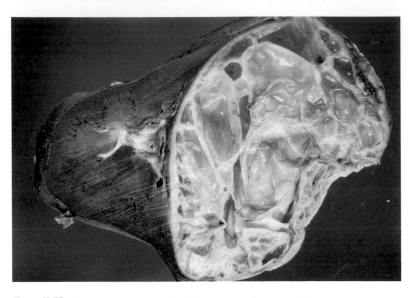

Figure 11.33 This cystic, partially differentiated nephroblastoma resembles a multilocular cyst.

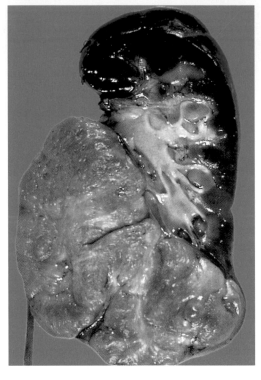

Figure 11.34 The fetal rhabdomyomatous nephroblastoma is an expansile, sharply circumscribed mass with a whorled, fibromyomatous appearance. (Reproduced with permission from Mahoney and Saffos, 1981. Courtesy of J. Mahoney, MD, Columbia, Missouri)

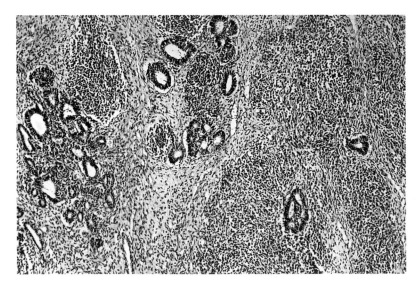

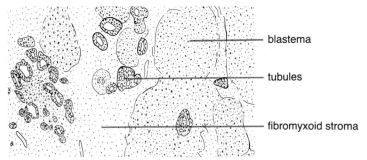

Figure 11.35 The classic triphasic Wilms' tumor contains circumscribed nodules of blastema showing variable epithelial differentiation and surrounded by fibromyxoid stroma. (Reproduced with permission from Schumann and Weiss, 1981)

muscle (frequent), well differentiated cartilage and fat cells, as well as blood and lymphatic vessels, osteoid and bone (uncommon), and lymphoid tissue (rare). Unlike teratomas, unequivocal heterotopic organogenesis is lacking. The uncommon cystic partially differentiated nephroblastoma contains blastemal cells and derivatives, and may have rhabdomyoblastic elements.

Examples of biphasic or monophasic Wilms' tumors that may be encountered include the monomorphous blastemal tumors and variants composed only of blastemal and fibromyxoid stromal elements (Fig. 11.36). The monomorphous epithelial variant consists of embryonic tubules that have lumens with a single layer of aligned cells and a distinct basement membrane (Fig. 11.37). Monomorphous epithelial tumors intermediate to Wilms' tumor and RCC contain epithelial cells with abundant granular or vesicular cytoplasm and are most common in adolescents and young adults. The rhabdomyomatous nephroblastoma contains prominent

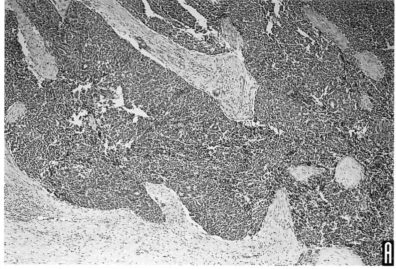

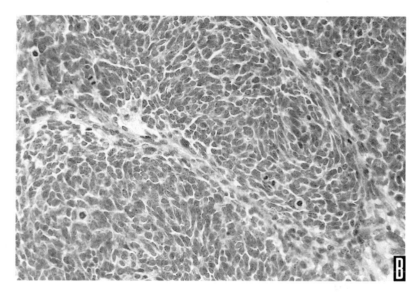

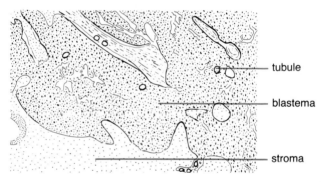

Figure 11.36 **A,** This Wilms' tumor is composed predominantly of blastema with intervening fibromyxoid stroma. Epithelial differentiation is minimal and consists of few nephronic tubules. **B,** Blastema is composed of small, closely packed cells with hyperchromatic, ovoid nuclei and scant cytoplasm. Mitotic figures, unless multipolar, are not a sign of anaplasia.

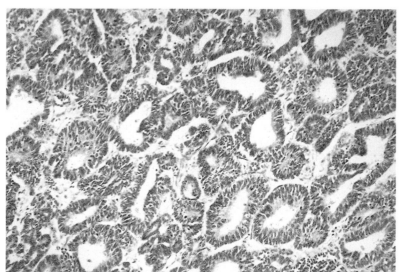

Figure 11.37 The monomorphous epithelial variant is considered a favorable histologic subtype of Wilms' tumor, and is composed of embryonic tubules.

(30%–95%), immature skeletal muscle haphazardly arranged in irregular bundles and fascicles (Fig. 11.38). Cells contain cross-striations and have paracentral oval nuclei with inconspicuous nucleoli and minimal atypia; mitoses average 1/10 hpf.

PRECURSOR LESIONS   At least one fifth of kidneys removed for Wilms' tumor have remnants of aberrant metanephric blastema, and the vast majority of bilateral tumors are associated with such hamartomas (Fig. 11.39A). These lesions include nodular renal blastema, metanephric hamartoma, and Wilms' tumorlet. Most of these lesions occur in the original nephrogenic zone—that is, in the subcapsular cortex or columns of Bertin; when multifocal or diffuse they compose the nephroblastomatosis complex. These precursor lesions generally lack the neoplastic undifferentiated stromal component characteristic of Wilms' tumor.

Nodular renal blastema is often multifocal and typically subcapsular in location or in the central portions of the columns of Bertin (Fig. 11.39B). The unencapsulated nodules, which are 100–300 μ in diameter, may have a thin, delicate, fibrous peripheral layer and fetal-type glomeruli at the edges. Blastemal cells look primitive, with scant cytoplasm and ovoid, hyperchromatic nuclei; there is little pleomorphism, and mitoses are rare. Rosettes or primitive tubules may be present within the nodules.

Metanephric hamartomas are also typically subcapsular and range from microscopic size to 2–3 cm in diameter. They may produce asymmetric lobules and deep interlobular clefts or may contain discrete nodules. Microscopically, they are composed of islands of blastemal cells and small, well developed tubules in a variable amount of dense, fibrous stroma (Fig. 11.40). The tubular epithelial cells are small and ovoid, and contain hyperchromatic nuclei with scant surrounding cytoplasm and no mitotic activity. They may form papillary fronds with psammoma bodies. In older patients, the stromal component is abundant and tubules are sparse.

Wilms' tumorlets are grossly visible, discrete nodules up to several centimeters in diameter. They are usually monomorphous and consist of proliferating embryonal renal blastema (see Fig. 11.40). They appear to develop in metanephric hamartomas and may show focally incomplete tubular differentiation. Intralobar tumorlets are usually polymorphous lesions with a prominent cystic component.

Nephroblastomatosis, as defined by Bove and McAdams, refers to a Wilms' tumor that develops in a setting of multifocal, discrete, superficial precursor lesions containing or derived from blastema. It is usually bilateral and causes nephromegaly. The subtypes are based on topographic distribution, but also show age differences at the time of clinical detection, including: (1) pancortical (infantile—the rarest type), (2) superficial diffuse (late infantile), and (3) multifocal (juvenile), which carries a substantial risk for developing Wilms' tumor.

Beckwith et al. have recently proposed a new classification and terminology for precursor lesions of Wilms' tumor based upon morphology and natural history. All precursor lesions are termed nephrogenic rests and are categorized as perilobar (PLNR) and intralobar (ILNR). Based upon gross and microscopic features, individual rests are subdivided into: a) nascent or dormant, b) maturing or sclerosing, c) hyperplastic, and d) neoplastic (adenomatous or nephroblastomatous). Nephroblastomatosis is classified as: a) PLNR only, b) ILNR only, c) combined PLNR and ILNR, and d) universal. This classification scheme had interesting clinical correlations which suggested pathogenetic heterogeneity for Wilms' tumors. Median age at diagnosis of Wilms' tumor was 36 months for PLNRs, 16 months for ILNRs, and 12 months if both types of rests were present. In addition, PLNRs were strongly associated with synchronous bilateral Wilms' tumors, and ILNRs with metachronous contralateral Wilms' tumors.

PROGNOSIS   One important prognostic factor for patients with Wilms' tumor is their clinicopathologic stage, which can be classified as:

Stage I   Limited to kidney and completely excised
Stage II   Extension beyond kidney, but completely excised

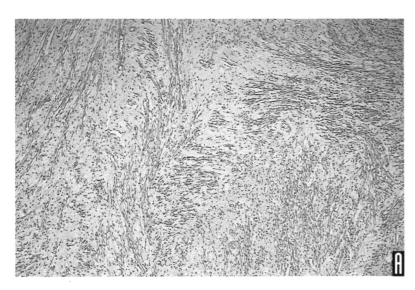
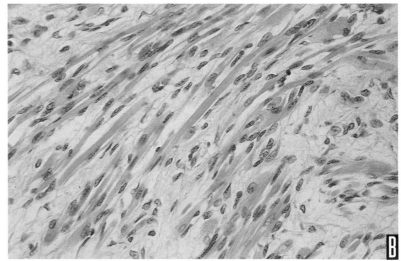

Figure 11.38 A, The rhabdomyomatous Wilms' tumor contains loose bundles and haphazard fascicles of skeletal muscle. **B,** The fetal-type skeletal muscle fibers have paracentral oval nuclei and eosinophilic cytoplasm with easily recognized cross-striations.

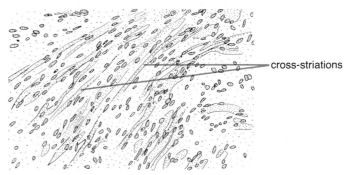

cross-striations

Stage III Extension beyond kidney; gross tumor remains in abdomen
Stage IV Hematogenous metastases.

Other prognostic variables are histologic subclassification that, like the clinicopathologic stage, is age-linked, and the presence of precursor lesions, which suggests the possibility of concurrent or subsequent bilateral tumors. Renal vein invasion and nodal metastases also influence prognosis.

The monomorphous epithelial variant has a better prognosis. The cystic partially differentiated nephroblastoma is associated with a benign outcome, and nephrectomy alone is probably curative, although occasional recurrences may develop. Unfavorable histologic subtypes are usually unilateral. The presence of undifferentiated "sarcomatous" stroma in a mixed Wilms' tumor does not imply an adverse prognosis. Cellular anaplasia within stromal (except skeletal muscle), epithelial, or blastemal cell lines, which defines anaplastic Wilms' tumor, is the major histopathologic correlate of tumor relapse and death due to tumor. Anaplasia is defined as marked nuclear enlargement to at least three times the diameter of adjacent nuclei of the same cell type, obvious hyperchromatism,

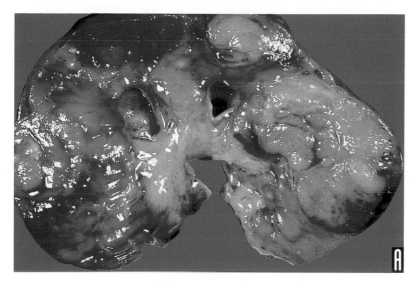

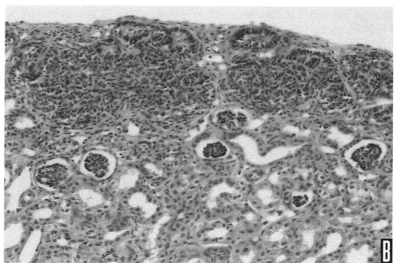

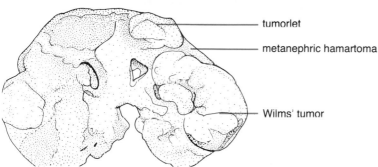

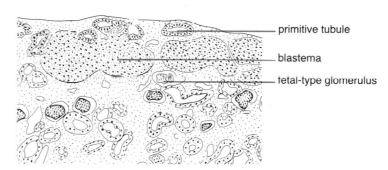

Figure 11.39 A, The Wilms' tumor in this kidney is associated with precursor lesions of the nephroblastomatosis complex. There are several tumorlets, one of which appears to arise in a metanephric hamartoma, and multiple ill-defined regions of cortical pallor.

B, Unencapsulated nodules of renal blastema are present in the subcapsular cortex. Blastemal nodules contain primitive tubules and are bordered by fetal-type glomeruli. (Courtesy of K. Bove, MD, Cincinnati, Ohio)

Figure 11.40 The subcapsular cortex adjacent to a Wilms' tumorlet contains a focus of nodular renal blastema and a metanephric hamartoma. The tumorlet is unencapsulated and consists of a monomorphous population of blastemal cells. (Courtesy of K. Bove, MD, Cincinnati, Ohio)

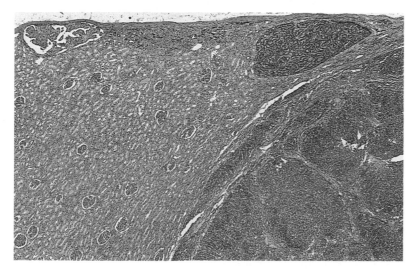

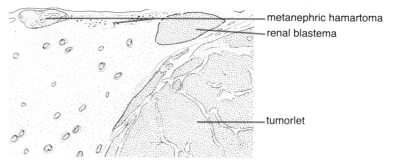

and multipolar mitotic figures (Fig. 11.41). Tumors that are predominantly blastemal or have anaplasia limited predominantly (> 60%) to the blastemal component may have an even higher relapse rate. Anaplasia may be extremely focal within the tumor; it can often be identified more easily in nodal or other metastatic sites, where it may be even more prognostically significant. Anaplasia is uncommon in tumors from patients less than two years old.

Clear Cell Sarcoma

Clear cell sarcoma of the kidney (CCSK), an uncommon and distinctive tumor that has never been documented in extrarenal sites, constitutes about 4% of all primary childhood renal tumors. It is characterized by a predilection for males (1.3–7.6:1) and a marked propensity to metastasize to bone. Age at presentation ranges from the neonatal period to about 15 years; most patients are less than

three years old. There have been no bilateral or multicentric tumors. Ultrastructurally, the tumor appears to arise from primitive mesenchymal cells, and it has been speculated that CCSK is the malignant counterpart of CMN.

CLINICAL MANIFESTATIONS CCSK has an aggressive clinical behavior and poor prognosis (39%–49% one-year actuarial survival). Patients may present with an abdominal mass or gross hematuria. Bone metastases occur in 42%–76% of cases, may be polyostotic, and almost always involve the skull.

MORPHOLOGY CCSK is a tan or gray-tan, bulging tumor with infiltrative margins (Fig. 11.42). It is typically firm, lobular, and whorled, but may have soft, fleshy areas separated by bands of necrosis; hemorrhage is uncommon. Cysts, which may be barely visible or large and multiloculated, usually occur at the tumor–kidney interface. CCSK may have a central or renal medullary origin.

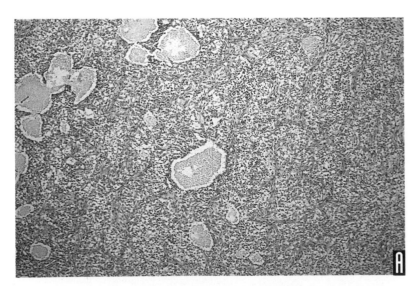

Figure 11.41 Blastema in this Wilms' tumor shows features of anaplasia. Enlarged, hyperchromatic nulcei and a multipolar mitosis (center) are present. (Courtesy of K. Bove, MD, Cincinnati, Ohio)

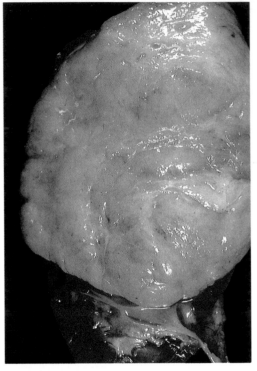

Figure 11.42 Clear cell sarcoma has a gray-tan, bulging cut surface that is lobulated and whorled. The tumor in this specimen has small foci of necrosis and barely visible cysts.

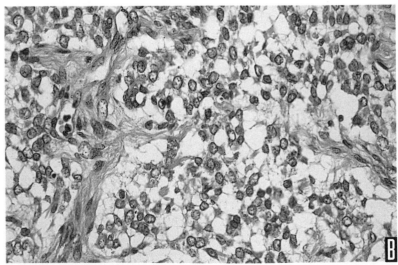

Figure 11.43 **A,** Microscopically, a prominent arborizing network of capillaries is evenly distributed throughout the clear cell sarcoma. Microcysts (upper left and center) may form in areas of stromal degeneration. **B,** The delicate fibrovascular stroma divides the tumor into nests and cords of cells. The polygonal tumor cells have clear to slightly granular cytoplasm and vesicular nuclei with indistinct nucleoli.

The classic and diagnostically distinctive histologic pattern of CCSK consists of a prominent, evenly distributed, arborizing network of delicate fibrovascular stroma with fine capillaries that divides the tumor cells into nests and cords (Fig. 11.43). Tumors are highly cellular and composed of haphazardly arranged polygonal cells with vesicular, round-to-oval nuclei, indistinct nucleoli, and clear to faintly eosinophilic (PAS-negative) cytoplasm.

Ultrastructurally, tumor cells differ from Wilms' blastema by the absence of basal lamina, epithelial differentiation, and transitional forms with stroma, and the presence of intermediate filaments, occasional primitive cell junctions, and extended cell processes. Glycogen and lipid are scant. The clear cell appearance is explained in part by the effect of formalin on perinuclear cytoplasmic filaments and the tendency of tumor cell extensions to infold the pale extracellular matrix.

Epithelial differentiation is classically absent; tubular structures represent entrapped, preexisting nephrons. Cysts may occur secondary to myxomatous degeneration (liquefaction) or arise from entrapped tubules.

Variant patterns include: (1) epithelioid–trabecular; tumor cells are parallel around vascular septa and may be columnar; cytoplasm is compact and more deeply stained; (2) fibrotic–hyalinized; the delicate fibrovascular stroma is replaced by broad bands of dense collagen, isolating individual cells and small clusters; (3) angiectatic (hemangiopericytoma-like), with dilated sinusoids; and (4) neurilemoma-like (15% of cases), with nuclear palisading (Fig. 11.44).

Malignant Rhabdoid Tumor

Malignant rhabdoid tumor of the kidney (MRTK) occurs in infants (median age, 13 months) and is one of the most lethal neoplasms of early life. It constitutes about 2% of malignant childhood renal tumors. There is no sex predilection. Although light-microscopic features suggest rhabdomyoblastic differentiation, it is speculated to be of neuroendocrine (APUD) origin. Morphologically similar primary neoplasms are encountered in soft tissues of infants, children, and adults, as well as in the central nervous system, liver, and thymus. MRTK has been associated with primary midline posterior fossa tumors resembling medulloblastoma or a primitive neuroectodermal neoplasm of indeterminate type.

CLINICAL MANIFESTATIONS Patients with MRTK have a high relapse rate shortly after diagnosis, regardless of the initial stage. Metastases rapidly appear, and survival time is short.

MORPHOLOGY Grossly, MRTK has infiltrating margins (Fig. 11.45). It is composed of sheets, cords, and nests of cells that may have an alveolar or trabecular arrangement (Fig. 11.46). Stroma may be condensed into broad, acellular, hyaline bands. Cells have eosinophilic, PAS-positive, granular cytoplasm and eccentric nuclei with frequently large, single, "owl-eye" nucleoli; cross-striations are absent. The hallmarks are large, hyaline, often globular, PAS-positive, diastase-resistant, cytoplasmic inclusions that show immunocytochemical vimentin positivity. Ultrastructurally, these

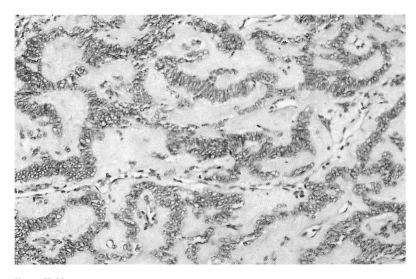

Figure 11.44 This epithelioid-trabecular variant of clear cell sarcoma shows hyalinization of the fibrovascular stroma. Tumor cells have indistinct cell borders and bland nuclei that appear almost empty.

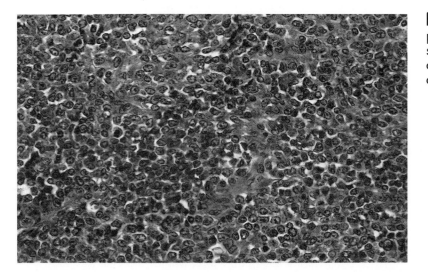

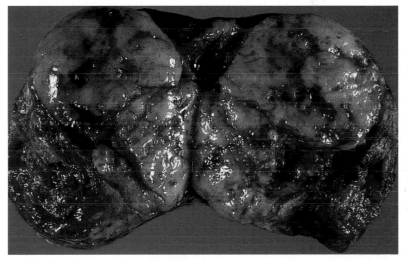

Figure 11.45 In this specimen of a malignant rhabdoid tumor with marked hemorrhage and necrosis, only a small remnant of upper-pole renal parenchyma is not infiltrated.

Figure 11.46 Microscopically, this malignant rhabdoid tumor is composed of sheets and ill-defined nests or cords of cells in areas where stroma is relatively inconspicuous. Tumor cells, which characteristically have an eccentric nucleus and a densely eosinophilic globular cytoplasmic inclusion, are reminiscent of rhabdomyoblasts.

inclusions correspond to parallel, intermediate filaments (6–9 nm in diameter) packed into perinuclear, nonmembrane-bound, concentric whorls (Fig. 11.47). The PAS-positive cytoplasmic granularity corresponds to larger filaments (10 nm in diameter) packed in elongated, gently curved bundles. Glycogen may also be abundant. Epithelial features include nexus-type cell junctions and tonofilament bundles; a basal lamina is absent.

The lack of immunoreactive myoglobin corroborates the ultrastructural findings, which fail to demonstrate skeletal muscle differentiation. The similarity of the filamentous cytoplasmic inclusion to those of some APUD tumors suggests a neural crest origin. Tumor cells coexpress vimentin and cytokeratin, but are negative for desmin, neurofilament, and S100 protein.

MESENCHYMAL RENAL NEOPLASMS

ANGIOMYOLIPOMA

Angiomyolipomas of the kidney are considered hamartomatous, but are composed of heterotopic tissue and are more precisely termed choristomas. They constitute less than 1% of surgically excised renal tumors. The female-to-male ratio is 2.6:1; mean age at presentation is 41 (range, 26–72 years). Angiomyolipomas are multiple in only 13%–30% of cases and bilateral in only 15%. The existence of a malignant form has been questioned; however, sarcomatous transformation with pulmonary metastases was recently documented.

Up to 50% of patients with angiomyolipomas have one or more features of the tuberous sclerosis complex, while about 80% of patients with complete or severe forms of tuberous sclerosis have angiomyolipomas. Multiple tumors, whether unilateral or bilateral, are more often associated with tuberous sclerosis. The tuberous sclerosis complex may vary in expression from a solitary renal tumor to the fully developed syndrome; renal cysts may also be present.

CLINICAL MANIFESTATIONS   The most common symptom is flank or abdominal pain due to intra- or perirenal hemorrhage or extrarenal extension. Pain may be sudden and severe or less intense and sporadic over several years. Hematuria and hypertension occasionally are the presenting symptoms. Bilateral multiple tumors may cause renal failure. Angiomyolipomas may also be an unsuspected radiologic finding.

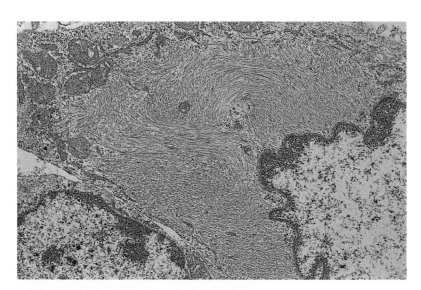

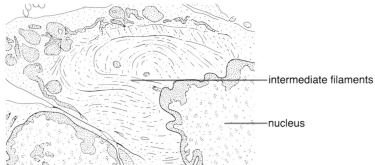

Figure 11.47 Ultrastructurally, the perinuclear cytoplasmic inclusions are nonmembrane-bound, concentric whorls of tightly packed intermediate filaments.

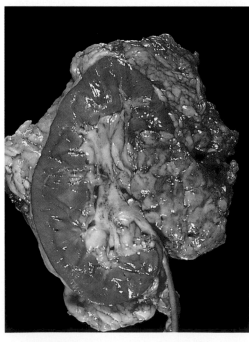
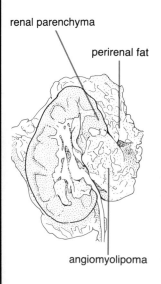

Figure 11.48 Angiomyolipomas containing large amounts of fat are lobulated yellow masses that merge with the perirenal adipose tissue. This tumor compresses the upper-pole renal parenchyma and has a circumscribed margin.

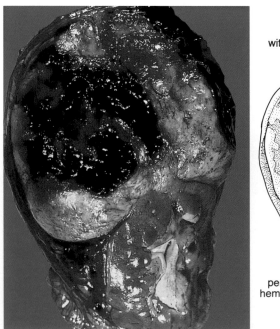
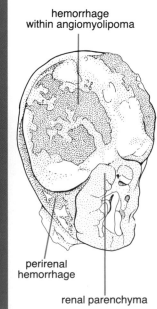

Figure 11.49 This large angiomyolipoma, which arises from the upper pole of the kidney, shows predominantly extrarenal growth. Acute massive hemorrhage within the tumor extends into the perirenal connective tissue.

Tuberous sclerosis is heredofamilial and believed to be due to a rare autosomal-dominant gene. Severely affected patients have the classic triad of mental retardation, epilepsy, and adenoma sebaceum; however, the tuberous sclerosis complex includes widely distributed hamartomatous lesions, such as retinal phakomas and visceral and cerebral angiomas.

MORPHOLOGY Angiomyolipomas may arise in the cortex or medulla and are frequently polar. They are round-to-oval, bulging masses with a smooth or bosselated surface, and can be up to 20 cm in diameter. Multiple satellite masses that are less than 1 cm in diameter may be present. The cut surface is yellow to gray, depending upon the proportion of fat and smooth muscle, and is lobulated (Fig. 11.48). Focal intrarenal or perirenal hemorrhage is common (Fig. 11.49); necrosis, cystic change, and calcification vary. Angiomyolipomas usually are circumscribed and show expansile growth, with replacement of parenchyma and compression of the collecting system. However, they may also be locally invasive, extending into the pelvis, or may have a predominant extrarenal growth pattern, penetrating through the renal capsule, infiltrating the retroperitoneal fat, and incorporating perirenal structures. Vascular invasion, however, is absent. Hamartomatous nodules within regional nodes should not be interpreted as metastases.

Microscopically, a variable mixture and organization of mature adipose tissue, blood vessels, and smooth muscle are seen; fat or smooth muscle may predominate (Fig. 11.50). The adult-type fat cells have a large, central lipid vacuole and an eccentric pyknotic nucleus. Smooth muscle cells contain longitudinal cytoplasmic myofibrils; nuclei are frequently hyperchromatic and moderately pleomorphic, and show frequent mitotic figures. Mono- and multi-nucleated giant cells may be present. The smooth muscle is usually arranged in sheets of interlacing fascicles, but may form perivascular collarettes, dissect between fat cells, demonstrate a hemangiopericytic pattern, or have an epithelioid appearance. Diastase resistant PAS-positive needle- and rodlike crystalloids may be observed, particularly in large epithelioid cells. The vascular component consists of tortuous, thick-walled muscular vessels that resemble arteries but lack a normal elastica and may be fibrotic (Fig. 11.51).

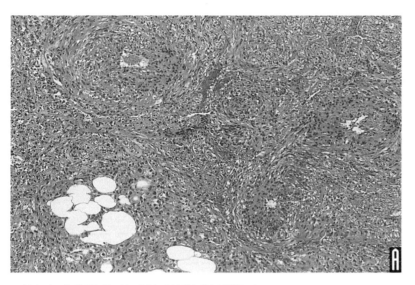

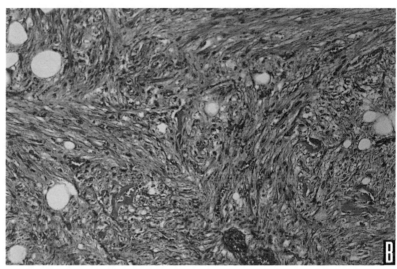

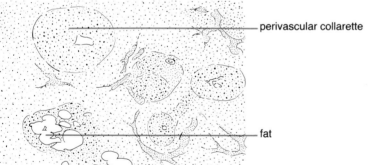

perivascular collarette

fat

Figure 11.50 **A,** Angiomyolipomas may contain only a scant amount of fat. A helpful diagnostic feature is the presence of vessels with perivascular collarettes of smooth muscle. **B,** Smooth muscle cells are arranged in sheets and interlacing fascicles and may show nuclear hyperchromatism, pleomorphism, and mitotic activity. (**A:** Courtesy of H. Levin, MD, Cleveland, Ohio)

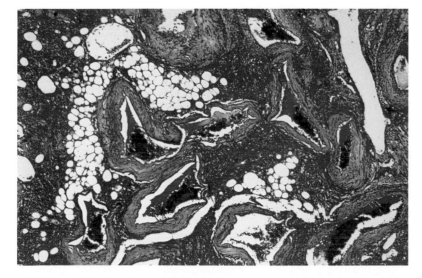

Figure 11.51 Microscopically, the large, tortuous, muscular vessels in angiomyolipomas lack a normal elastica typical of arteries and have fibrotic walls (trichrome stain).

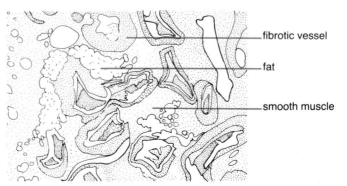

fibrotic vessel

fat

smooth muscle

The renal cysts in patients with tuberous sclerosis and angiomyolipoma(s) vary in diameter from several millimeters up to 8 cm and may be multiple. They may be lined by a distinctive hyperplastic epithelium (see Fig. 1.20) or flat, cuboidal, columnar, or urothelial cells (Fig. 11.52). A spindle cell stroma may surround the cysts.

RENOMEDULLARY INTERSTITIAL CELL TUMOR

Although previously termed *medullary fibroma*, these nonhamartomatous tumors are composed of renomedullary interstitial cells, which normally have an antihypertensive action. They are found in 26%–42% of autopsies and are multiple in about 50% of cases. Patients are typically over 50 years of age; there is no sex predilection.

MORPHOLOGY   Renomedullary interstitial cell tumors are white-to-pale-gray, round-to-oval, unencapsulated nodules with a diameter of 1–3 mm that compress surrounding parenchyma and have well defined margins (Fig. 11.53). Microscopically, they are composed of variable amounts of ovoid stromal cells with indistinct margins and vesicular nuclei embedded in a collagenous matrix that may be densely eosinophilic and hyalinized (Fig. 11.54). Entrapped tubules are common.

JUXTAGLOMERULAR CELL TUMOR

The juxtaglomerular cell tumor (JGCT) is derived from the specialized pericytes of the juxtaglomerular apparatus. It contains large amounts of extractable renin and is felt to be a specialized form of

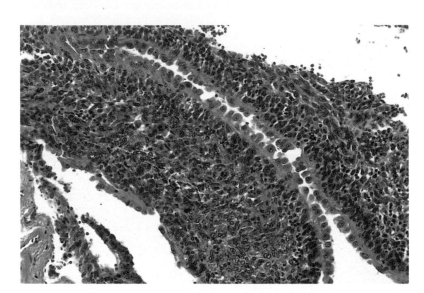

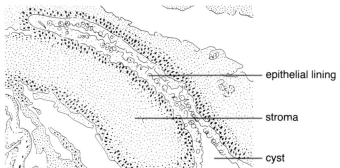

Figure 11.52 The presence of renal cysts and angiomyolipomas strongly suggests tuberous sclerosis. Cysts may be lined by columnar cells with eosinophilic cytoplasm and be surrounded by a spindle cell stroma. (This is the same case as Figure 11.50A.)

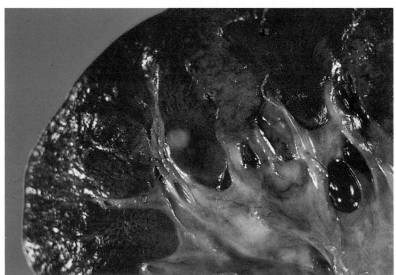

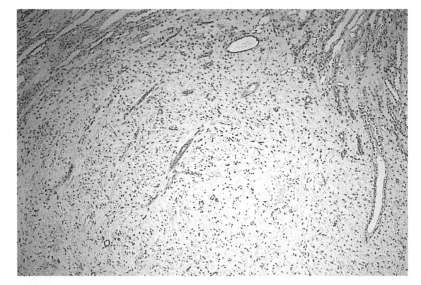

Figure 11.53 Grossly, the renomedullary interstitial cell tumor is typically a small, sharply circumscribed, gray-white nodule.

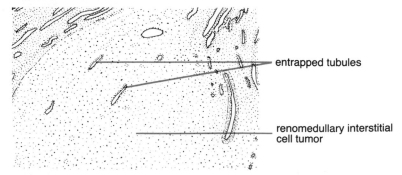

Figure 11.54 Microscopically, the renomedullary interstitial cell tumor is unencapsulated and commonly contains entrapped tubules. The tumor is composed of ovoid stromal cells embedded in collagen.

hemangiopericytoma that is biologically benign. This rare tumor shows no sex predilection and is primarily a lesion of the second decade, but has been reported in patients 2–58 years old.

CLINICAL MANIFESTATIONS   Patients present with severe hyperreninemic hypertension with secondary hyperaldosteronism and hypokalemia. Plasma renin levels may be increased two- to sevenfold. Headaches may be accompanied by polyuria or nocturia. Hypertension has preceded diagnosis by more than five years. Follow-up of patients after resection has shown no tumor recurrences or metastases.

MORPHOLOGY   JGCTs are small, gray-white-to-tan cortical neoplasms with pushing margins that may be less than 1 cm in diameter. They are typically solid but may have small, degenerative, fluid-filled cysts.

Microscopically, a thin rim of hyalinized collagen separates the tumor from compressed, atrophic parenchyma. Fibroblastic-like spindle cells and polyhedral cells form loosely cohesive trabecular cords set in a myxoid, delicately collagenous stroma. The stroma merges with areas containing nodular aggregates of small epithelioid cells with eosinophilic, slightly granular cytoplasm (Fig. 11.55). Individual cells and small cell clusters are surrounded by reticulin. A poorly formed swirling pattern may be present around the numerous venous and capillary channels. The stroma may be densely hyalinized focally.

Both spindle and polyhedral cells have smooth nuclear contours with evenly distributed chromatin and slight pleomorphism; mitoses are absent. Rare cells contain D-PAS-positive and Bowie-positive granules that have been identified as renin by immunofluorescence. Ultrastructurally, there are characteristic, small, membrane-bound, rhomboid-shaped (zinc-containing) granules, as well as numerous, larger, irregularly shaped cytoplasmic granules with an amorphous electron-dense matrix that represents the less diagnostic storage form of renin. Nonmyelinated axon terminals abut tumor cells, probably reflecting the normal sympathetic (adrenergic) innervation of juxtaglomerular cells.

MISCELLANEOUS BENIGN TUMORS

Benign mesenchymal tumors are about 100 times more common than sarcomas. They are found in 8%–11% of autopsies, are usually small and are clinically insignificant.

Cortical *fibromas* are rare; tumors composed of fat and smooth muscle are most common, particularly in women over 40 years of age. They average less than 5 mm in diameter and are rarely large and symptomatic. These choristomas may occur in pure form (*lipoma* and *leiomyoma*) or as a mixed cortical nodule *(myolipoma)* (Fig. 11.56).

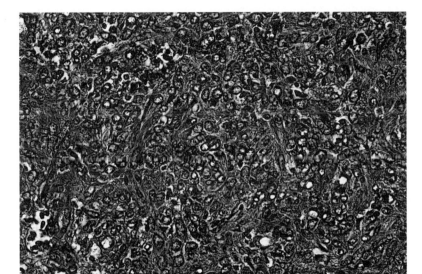

Figure 11.55 The juxtaglomerular cell tumor has a delicate collagenous stroma and a prominent venous or capillary vasculature. Cells are arranged in loosely cohesive trabecular cords. There are fibroblast-like spindle cells and focal nodular aggregates of small epithelioid cells with eosinophilic, slightly granular cytoplasm.

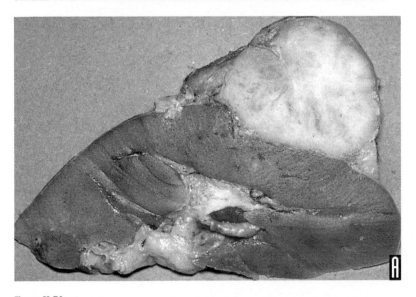

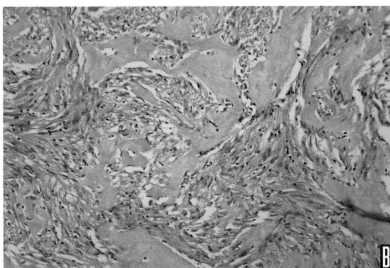

Figure 11.56 A, A large cortical nodule deforms the renal capsule in this gross specimen. It is sharply circumscribed and has a gray-white, whorled cut surface typical of a leiomyoma. **B,** Microscopically, the nodule is composed of benign smooth muscle cells and hyalinized collagen.

Leiomyomas are sharply circumscribed and do not contain entrapped tubules or glomeruloid structures. About 50% of myolipomas in patients without clinical evidence of tuberous sclerosis have a prominent angiomatous component and are histologically indistinguishable from angiomyolipomas occurring with tuberous sclerosis.

The relatively uncommon *hemangioma* is usually detected in the third to fourth decades of life. Hematuria is the presenting symptom in 95% of cases; colicky pain due to passage of blood clots is less common. Hemangiomas are typically located at the tips of the pyramids, are usually 3–4 mm in diameter, and may be multiple and bilateral. They are usually of the capillary type and consist of disorganized small vessels interspersed among compact clusters of endothelial cells with inconspicuous lumens. The cavernous type contains widely dilated channels.

Lymphangiomas, which are extremely rare, are usually found in infants and children. They are large, unencapsulated, multicystic lesions that may replace the majority of the kidney. The dilated vessels are lined by a single layer of endothelial cells.

Sarcomas

Sarcomas represent about 2%–3% of malignant renal neoplasms. They are generally encountered after the second decade of life and occur more frequently with advancing age. They are thought to arise from undifferentiated mesenchyme of the kidney or renal capsule. Leiomyosarcoma is most common, followed by liposar-

coma and hemangiopericytoma, and the rare rhabdomyosarcoma, osteogenic sarcoma, and malignant fibrous histiocytoma. Fibrosarcoma and angiosarcoma are virtually nonexistent. More than 50% of the renal sarcomas—including all liposarcomas—reported by Farrow and co-workers had a capsular location. These neoplasms must be differentiated from primary retroperitoneal sarcomas and sarcomatoid RCCs.

CLINICAL MANIFESTATIONS Because these invasive tumors are large, flank pain, mass, and hematuria are common. Nonspecific symptoms include fatigue, malaise, and weight loss. Hypoglycemia is sometimes associated with hemangiopericytoma. Osteogenic sarcomas and occasional leiomyosarcomas show radiologic calcifications.

MORPHOLOGY *Leiomyosarcomas* are eccentric, firm, bosselated, bulging masses that elevate or invade the renal capsule (Fig. 11.57). The cut surface is light gray to tan, whorled, and lobulated; hemorrhage, cystic change, fibrosis, and calcification may be present. Well differentiated tumors are composed of plump spindle cells with oblong, blunted nuclei and variable amounts of cytoplasm with longitudinal myofibrils (trichrome stain). Poorly differentiated tumors contain large, round, or irregular cells with large, single, or multiple hyperchromatic nuclei. The degree of differentiation and nuclear anaplasia is not a reliable prognostic indicator; mitotic rate is the best histologic criterion of malignancy, and extrarenal invasion carries a poor prognosis.

Figure 11.57 A, The leiomyosarcoma, unlike its benign counterpart, is typically large, infiltrates renal parenchyma and capsule, and has foci of hemorrhage and necrosis. **B,** Microscopically, it may have pushing borders that compress renal parenchyma (upper left). Spindle cells are arranged in interlacing fascicles. **C,** Increased cellularity, nuclear anaplasia, and, particularly, mitotic rate are histologic features of malignancy.

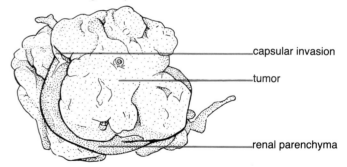

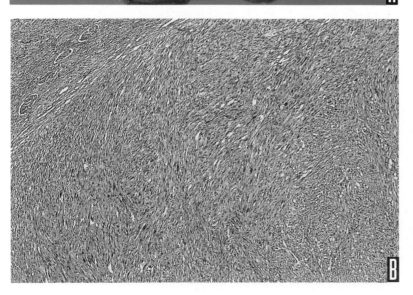

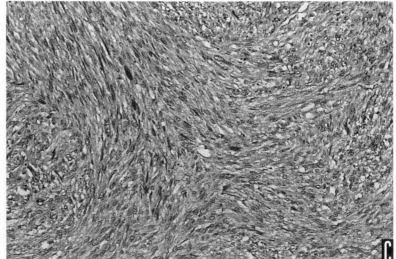

Liposarcomas are typically large, bulky neoplasms that may appear well circumscribed but often extend into perirenal fat. The cut surface may be uniformly lobulated and yellow, mucoid and slimy, or variegated with bright yellow, gray-white, or pink-red areas and foci of cystic change, hemorrhage, and necrosis. Histologic subtypes, including the myxoid liposarcoma, resemble those encountered in soft tissue.

Hemangiopericytomas are typically firm, multinodular, well circumscribed tumors that compress renal parenchyma, but they may be grossly invasive. The cut surface is pale gray-pink, red-brown, or yellow. Microscopically, endothelial-lined vascular channels are separated by solid aggregates of round-to-fusiform cells with pale cytoplasm, indistinct cell borders, and round-to-oval vesicular nuclei. As with hemangiopericytomas located elsewhere, malignant potential is difficult to predict from the histologic appearance; more aggressive tumors commonly have a higher mitotic index.

The storiform–pleomorphic type of *malignant fibrous histiocytoma* is an aggressive neoplasm composed of spindle cells in a collagenous stroma intermixed with variable numbers of plump histiocytes and scattered bizarre giant cells.

The *pleomorphic rhabdomyosarcoma* is a pink-gray, multinodular tumor containing strap cells with eosinophilic, fibrillary cytoplasm and cross-striations in a background of anaplastic spindle cells and giant cells.

Renal osteogenic sarcoma is yellow-white and well circumscribed; small anaplastic spindle cells form variably calcified osteoid.

PRIMARY HEMATOPOIETIC TUMORS

Renal Lymphoma
Primary extranodal lymphomas occur in the genitourinary tract much less commonly than secondary involvement. They are more common in the kidney than in the bladder, but account for less than 1% of primary extranodal lymphomas.

CLINICAL MANIFESTATIONS Secondary renal lymphoma frequently is clinically silent, but kidney involvement may be the earliest manifestation of systemic disease, with presentation as a focal renal tumor mimicking a primary renal neoplasm. Presenting symptoms include flank or abdominal pain and mass, weight loss, painless hematuria, and, rarely, renal failure. At the time of diagnosis, "primary" renal lymphoma is often widespread.

MORPHOLOGY Renal lymphoma is a firm, homogeneous, gray tumor that may occur as single or multiple, well circumscribed, parenchymal nodules, as a diffusely infiltrating neoplasm, or as an invasive, predominantly hilar mass (Fig. 11.58).

Plasmacytoma
Extramedullary plasmacytomas account for 3% of all plasma cell tumors; about 78% arise in the upper respiratory tract. Solitary plasmacytomas, whether in bone or soft tissues, show evidence of dissemination in 90% of cases up to 20 years after presentation. Primary plasmacytomas of the kidney are extremely rare, and reported cases have frequently been associated with antecedent, solitary plasmacytoma elsewhere.

CLINICAL MANIFESTATIONS Patients may present with a palpable abdominal mass, gross hematuria, or Bence Jones proteinuria. Radiologic evaluation may show small amounts of mottled calcifications within a tumor that has neovascularity and a moderate tumor blush on angiogram.

MORPHOLOGY Firm, light-tan nodules or a pink-gray, homogeneous, infiltrating mass may be present, occasionally with renal capsular extension and renal vein involvement. Microscopically, the tumor is composed almost exclusively of clusters and sheets of plasma cells in a scant, delicate connective tissue stroma.

NEOPLASMS OF THE RENAL PELVIS AND URETER

MESENCHYMAL NEOPLASMS

Benign mesenchymal neoplasms, such as leiomyoma, neurilemoma, lipoma (see Fig. 8.22), and angioma, rarely arise in the renal pelvis or ureteral wall. Their malignant counterparts are virtually nonexistent, although leiomyosarcomas have been rarely reported.

FIBROEPITHELIAL POLYP

Fibroepithelial polyps most often occur in the ureters of young adult men. They may be multiple, and rarely occur in the renal pelvis; no bilateral lesions have been reported. Etiologic factors are unknown.

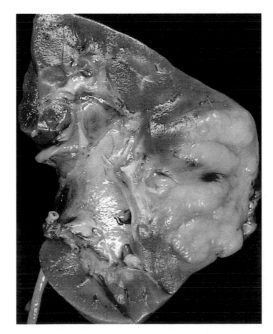

Figure 11.58 Lymphoma in this kidney presented as a primary renal neoplasm. The mass consists of multiple, confluent, gray-white parenchymal nodules. (Courtesy of J.T. Wolfe III, MD, Charlotte, North Carolina)

Intermittent flank pain is the most common symptom; dysuria and hematuria are less frequent. A long, narrow, radiolucent filling defect is seen on IVP.

The majority of fibroepithelial polyps occur in the upper-third of the ureter (Fig. 11.59). They are typically solitary and form an elongated (up to 5 cm), slender, lobulated projection, but may be polypoid with multiple branching projections. They are solid and firm, and have a smooth, intact mucosal surface. Microscopically, normal or hyperplastic urothelium covers loose, vascular, edematous, fibrous stroma that may be inflamed.

UROTHELIAL NEOPLASMS

Urothelial tumors of the renal pelvis account for 7%–8% of all malignant renal tumors. Primary malignant renal parenchymal tumors occur four to five times more frequently than malignant tumors of the pelvis and ureter combined, which include transitional cell carcinomas (TCCs) (approximately 90%), squamous cell carcinomas (approximately 10%), adenocarcinomas (1%), and undifferentiated carcinomas (1%). Carcinoma of the renal pelvis is $2\frac{1}{2}$ times more frequent than ureteral carcinoma. The majority (66%–75%) of ureteral tumors occur in the distal one third.

These carcinomas occur almost exclusively in adults and increase in frequency with age, having a peak incidence in the sixth to seventh decades of life. There is a male preponderance for both pelvic (3:1) and ureteral (2:1) tumors.

TCCs are frequently multicentric and may be synchronous (30%–40%) or metachronous. Bilateral tumors are present in 3%–10% of cases; 11% present with a concurrent bladder tumor. There is a 20%–64% incidence of tumors in the ureteral remnant after incomplete ureterectomy, related to the presence of frequent epithelial abnormalities (hyperplasia, dysplasia, carcinoma in situ) peripheral to the original tumor and reflecting a field change. Subsequent bladder tumor incidence is 20%–50%, almost always within three years after a renal pelvic tumor.

Carcinomas of the bladder are 50–70 times more common than pelviureteral tumors. In patients with bladder cancer, ureteral carcinoma in situ occurs in 8.5% and invasive cancer in 8.5%; the coincidence is higher in patients with multifocal and high-grade vesical TCCs.

PATHOGENESIS   Metaplastic and neoplastic changes are often associated with inflammation and/or calculi in the renal pelvis or ureter. Chemical carcinogens, which are an occupational hazard in certain industries (e.g., dye-stuff, rubber, and plastic), include beta-naphthylamines and benzidene, but these are more frequently associated with bladder cancer. Coffee and tobacco have also been implicated. Consumption of large amounts of phenacetin predisposes to carcinoma of the pelvis at a rate at least 40 times that expected in the normal population. There is an increased incidence of TCC in patients with Balkan nephropathy, which shows no sex predilection, may be bilateral (10%), and is commonly associated with chronic renal failure (approximately 40% of patients).

CLINICAL MANIFESTATIONS   Gross, painless hematuria is the most common presenting symptom; cystoscopy reveals bloody efflux from the ureteral orifice or protruding fronds in 30% of distal ureteral tumors. Patients may also have flank pain, urinary frequency, pyuria and dysuria, an abdominal mass, fever, and weight loss. There may be a history of chronic urinary tract infection or calculi.

Urinary cytology is a valuable adjunct and detects about 60% of TCCs of the renal pelvis and 70% of TCCs of the ureter (approximately 70% grade III and 30%–45% grade II). Retrograde ureteral catheterization increases yield, and brush biopsy decreases the false-negative rate to about 15%. Grade I lesions are generally undetectable. In equivocal cases, fine-needle aspiration biopsy of the kidney should be performed (Fig. 11.60).

Because of the multicentricity of TCCs, complete nephroureterectomy with removal of a cuff of bladder is the procedure of choice.

MORPHOLOGY   Papillary TCCs are frequently bulky, soft, pink-tan, sessile, or pedunculated tumors that have an arborescent, occasionally lobular, translucent and glistening surface formed by a

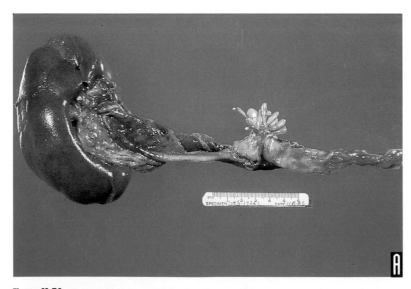

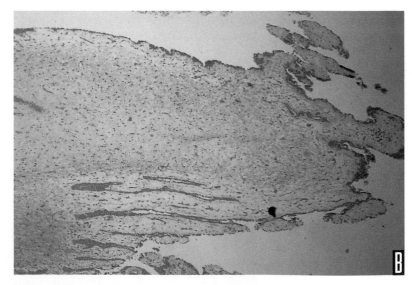

Figure 11.59 **A,** The fibroepithelial polyp in this specimen has a characteristic location in the upper one third of the ureter. It forms a polypoid intraluminal mass with multiple fingerlike projections.

B, Microscopically, the polyp has a loose, edematous-appearing fibrous stroma. (Courtesy of J. Crissman, MD, Detroit, Michigan)

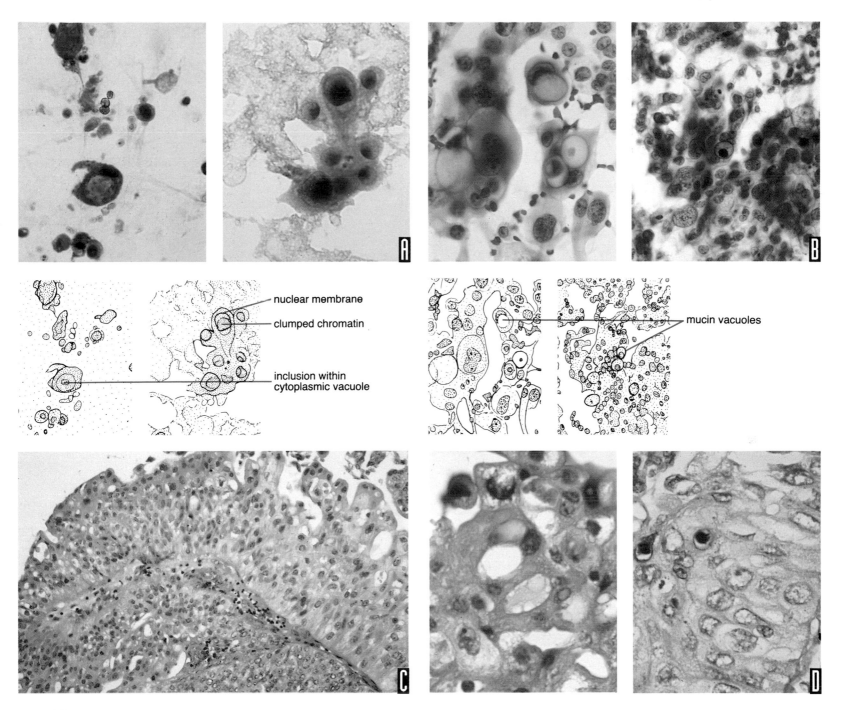

Figure 11.60 **A,** Routine cytologic evaluation in this case of suspected renal pelvic neoplasm is suspicious for TCC. The left panel (ureteral urine), shows single, degenerated urothelial cells with pyknotic nuclei, including one with its nucleus displaced by a cytoplasmic vacuole containing an inclusion. In the right panel (ureteral brush), a small, papillary urothelial fragment contains cells with enlarged, hyperchromatic, slightly irregular nuclei showing central chromatin clumping with loss of detail (Papanicolaou stain). **B,** Fine-needle aspi-

ration biopsy yielded papillary epithelial fragments and single cells with enlarged, hyperchromatic, pleomorphic nuclei having prominent nucleoli. Occasional cells have intracytoplasmic mucin vacuoles that displace nuclei. The findings are consistent with a grade II–III papillary TCC (*Left panel:* Papanicolaou stain; *right panel:* PAS stain with diastase). **C,** Histologically, the pelvic neoplasm in the nephrectomy is a grade II papillary TCC. **D,** Vacuolated cells within the papillae contain mucin (*Right panel:* PAS stain with diastase).

myriad of delicate filiform projections (Fig. 11.61). Nonobstructing tumors may fill the renal pelvis, whereas obstructing tumors of the ureteropelvic junction or in the ureter may be small (Fig. 11.62).

Squamous cell and undifferentiated carcinomas are typically solid, large, flat, slightly raised or rounded tumors that are frequently ulcerated and invasive (Fig. 11.63). Adenocarcinomas are heaped-up, nodular, mucoid tumors that may form hemorrhagic papillary fronds. Calculi and changes of chronic pyelonephritis are often present with squamous cell carcinoma and adenocarcinoma.

Pathologic diagnosis should include the cell type(s), pattern of growth, grade, and extent of invasion (Fig. 11.64), as well as evaluation of urothelial abnormalities remote from the tumor(s).

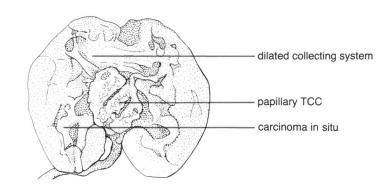

Figure 11.61 In this specimen, a papillary TCC (grade II–III) forms a polypoid mass that obstructs the ureteropelvic junction. Filiform projections are present on the surface. The lower-pole calyces (left side) have a granular mucosa that proved histologically to be carcinoma in situ.

— dilated collecting system

— papillary TCC

— carcinoma in situ

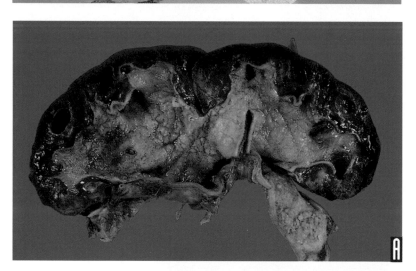

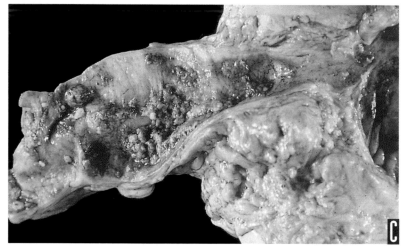

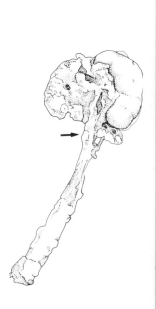

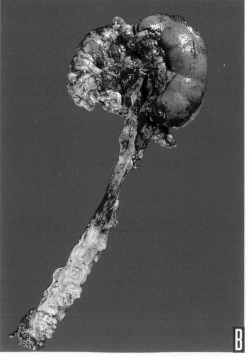

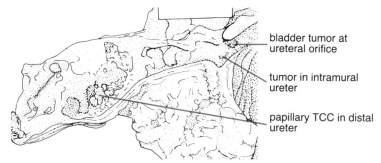

bladder tumor at ureteral orifice

tumor in intramural ureter

papillary TCC in distal ureter

Figure 11.62 A, The mucosa of the dilated collecting system and ureter is diffusely dull, thickened, granular to nodular, and microscopically had extensive carcinoma in situ. Small, ill-defined papillary tumors are present in the proximal ureter. Hydronephrosis and hydroureter were due to lower urinary tract obstruction. **B,** In this nephroureterectomy specimen, the distal segment of ureter contains multiple small, papillary TCCs that obstruct the lumen. The dilated proximal ureter also contains a papillary TCC (arrow). **C,** This autopsy specimen illustrates why nephroureterectomy with removal of a cuff of bladder is the recommended surgical procedure for TCC of the upper urinary tract. Papillary TCCs are present in the distal prevesical segment of the ureter, the intramural portion of the ureter, and in the bladder mucosa adjacent to the ureteral orifice.

Histologic features and grading of urothelial neoplasms are discussed elsewhere (see Chapter 12).

PROGNOSIS Although frequently correlated with grade, tumor stage is the best guide in predicting the tumor's biologic behavior and assessing prognosis. A system for staging urothelial tumors of the upper urinary tract is as follows:

Stage O Noninvasive
Stage A Invasion of lamina propria
Stage B Invasion of pelvic or ureteral muscle
Stage C Invasion through muscle layer into peripelvic or periureteral adipose tissue or renal parenchyma
Stage D Regional or distant metastases.

A staging system for ureteral tumors is presented below:

Stage I Noninvasive papillary TCC or carcinoma in situ
Stage II Invasion of lamina propria
Stage III Invasion of muscularis or extension beyond muscularis in the intrarenal portions of the renal pelvis if confined to the kidney
Stage IV Invasion through muscularis with involvement of adjacent structures and/or metastases.

The overall five-year survival for renal pelvic TCC after nephroureterectomy is about 50% (stage A, 100%; stage B, 65%; stage C, 34%; stage D, 0%). For ureteral tumors, five-year survival is 62% for stage I, 25% for stage II, 33% for stage III, and 0% for stage IV.

Multifocal or diffuse carcinoma in situ is an unfavorable prognostic sign and predicts the development of metachronous bladder carcinomas.

SECONDARY NEOPLASMS OF THE UPPER URINARY TRACT

Secondary neoplasms of the kidney and ureter may result from direct extension of retroperitoneal sarcomas and lymphomas. Ureteral involvement commonly results in hydronephrosis (see Chapter 8). This section deals with metastatic neoplasms of the kidney.

SARCOMA

Metastatic sarcomas may occur as isolated, limited metastases or may represent massive terminal dissemination.

METASTATIC CARCINOMA

Renal metastases are found at autopsy in approximately 5%–8% of patients with carcinoma and are bilateral in 70%–80% of cases. Virtually any carcinoma may metastasize to the kidney; however, the most common primary sources are the breast and the lung (about 25%) (Fig. 11.65), intestine (about 11%), and opposite kidney (about 8%). Up to 28% of RCCs metastasize to the opposite kidney. Fine-needle aspiration biopsy is useful for documenting metastases. Special stains are frequently helpful in differentiating metastatic adenocarcinoma (D-PAS-positive) from RCC (oil red O-positive) (Fig. 11.66).

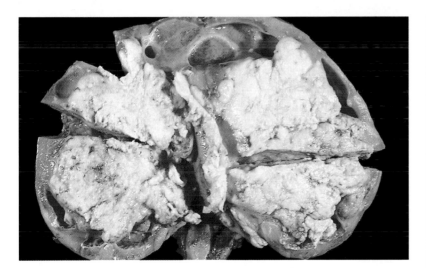

Figure 11.63 The dilated pelvicalyceal system of this hydronephrotic kidney is filled with a squamous cell carcinoma.

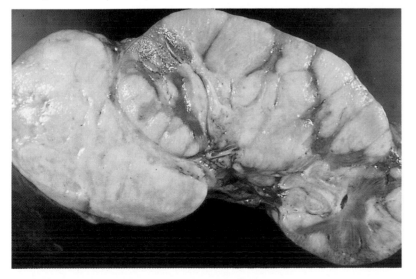

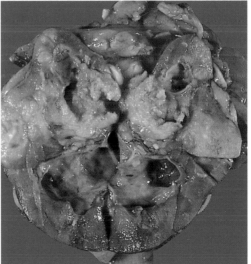

Figure 11.64 This papillary TCC arising in the upper pole of the kidney shows obvious gross invasion of the renal parenchyma. Cases with parenchymal invasion may be mistaken radiologically for RCC.

Figure 11.65 Carcinoma of the lung commonly metastasizes to the kidney. As shown in this specimen, metastases are also frequent in the adrenal gland (left), which is completely replaced by tumor.

Leukemia and Multiple Myeloma

Leukemic infiltration of the kidney occurs in 24%–63% of cases and may cause renal enlargement of up to two to three times normal size. Pale gray-pink or gray-white infiltrates are usually limited to the outer cortex and produce geographic mottling (Fig. 11.67). Microscopically, the interstitial infiltrates are diffuse or irregularly confluent, unlike lymphomatous infiltrates, which are typically discrete and nodular. Renal involvement by multiple myeloma may produce diffuse or nodular lesions.

Lymphoma

Only the lung is more frequently affected by secondary deposits of lymphoma than the kidney, and among metastases to the kidney, only lung and breast are more common. Lymphomatous infiltrates occur at autopsy in about 33% of patients dying of malignant lymphoma (46%–63% non-Hodgkin's and 13% Hodgkin's lymphoma), and are bilateral in 75% of cases. About 90% of secondary renal lymphomas result from hematogenous dissemination, and not more than 10% from direct invasion by retroperitoneal tumor.

In most cases, renal involvement is associated with retroperitoneal lymphoma, and the extent of the renal lesions parallels the retroperitoneal disease.

CLINICAL MANIFESTATIONS Most cases are discovered during routine evaluation for generalized disease. Antemortem diagnosis is made in only about 5% of cases of non-Hodgkin's lymphoma. Clinical manifestations are infrequent and often nonspecific. Renal involvement may produce urinary tract symptoms (dysuria, hematuria), abdominal pain, or a mass. The kidneys can be massively infiltrated by lymphoma and still have relatively normal function; only 0.5%–2% of deaths from lymphoma are attributable to uremia secondary to renal involvement. Fine-needle aspiration biopsy can be used to stage lymphomas and document renal involvement (Fig. 11.68).

MORPHOLOGY Grossly, multiple discrete nodules are more common than a circumscribed, solitary parenchymal nodule or diffuse infiltrate (Fig. 11.69). Initially, tumor proliferation is interstitial, with preservation of normal renal structures; with continued growth and parenchymal destruction, infiltrates become expansile and eventually confluent (Fig. 11.70).

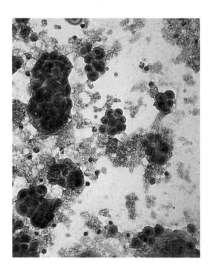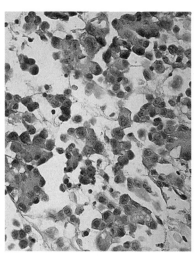

Figure 11.66 Fine-needle aspiration biopsy of the kidney from a patient with pulmonary and renal masses contains papillary and glandular epithelial fragments. The presence of intracytoplasmic mucin (right panel, center) excludes RCC and is consistent with metastatic adenocarcinoma (*Left panel:* Papanicolaou stain; *right panel:* mucicarmine stain).

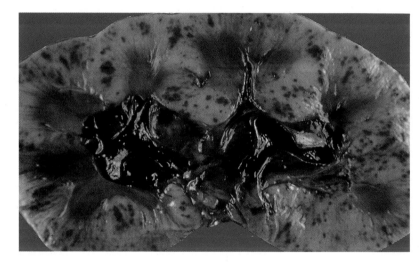

Figure 11.67 Leukemic infiltrates are diffusely present throughout the cortex of this kidney. Parenchymal and pelvic mucosal hemorrhages are secondary to severe thrombocytopenia.

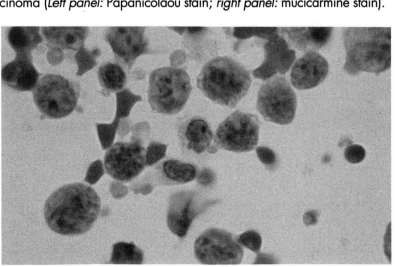

Figure 11.68 Fine-needle aspiration biopsy from a patient with known lymphoma contains a relatively monomorphous population of large lymphocytes with prominent nucleoli and scant cytoplasm. Unlike epithelial malignancies, the cells occur singly rather than in cohesive fragments (Papanicolaou stain).

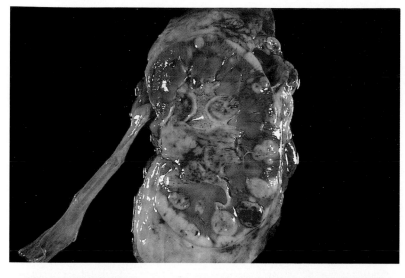

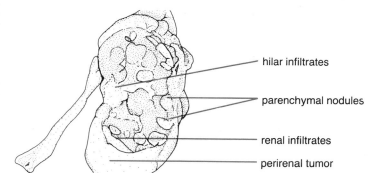

Figure 11.69 This kidney contains multiple, discrete nodules and confluent infiltrates of lymphoma; perirenal and hilar infiltrates are also present. This patient died from extensive retroperitoneal lymphoma.

hilar infiltrates

parenchymal nodules

renal infiltrates

perirenal tumor

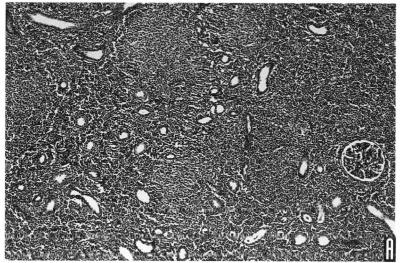

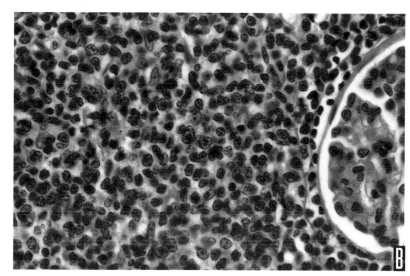

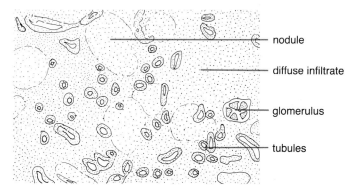

nodule

diffuse infiltrate

glomerulus

tubules

Figure 11.70 **A,** The presence of nodular and diffuse lymphocytic infiltrates in the renal cortex is consistent with involvement by a B-cell lymphoma. **B,** At higher magnification, the infiltrate is composed of a mixture of large and small lymphocytes with scattered, small, cleaved cells typical of a follicular center cell lymphoma. (**A,B:** Reproduced with permission from Schumann and Weiss, 1981)

CHAPTER 12

Bladder Neoplasms

BENIGN EPITHELIAL NEOPLASMS

TRANSITIONAL CELL PAPILLOMA

Transitional cell papillomas constitute not more than 2%–3% of all primary bladder tumors. The much higher incidence (up to 30%) reported in some series, the associated rates of recurrence (31%–60%), and progression to carcinoma (10%–52%) reflect the lack of consistent diagnostic criteria. Some authors continue to regard grade 1 papillary transitional cell carcinoma (TCC) as a papilloma. However, papilloma, as defined by the World Health Organization panel, has a better prognosis with very few recurrences and is probably a benign lesion biologically as well as histologically.

MORPHOLOGY Papillomas are usually single. Rarely, diffuse papillomatosis the mucosa is extensively replaced by delicate papillary processes and has a velvety appearance.

Microscopically, urothelium that is not more than six cell layers thick covers thin, delicate, fibrovascular papillary excrescences (Fig. 12.1). The urothelium is indistinguishable from normal bladder mucosa and shows normal maturation, with individual cells oriented parallel to each other and perpendicular to the basement membrane. Nuclear abnormalities such as enlargement and hyperchromatism are absent. Mitotic figures are rare and, if present, basally located.

INVERTED PAPILLOMA

Inverted papillomas, which constitute less than 1% of all urinary tract tumors, occur most often in the sixth decade of life and are six to seven times more common in men than in women. Although they have a predilection for the trigone, they are also common in the bladder neck and posterior urethra, and have been reported in the renal pelvis and ureter. Inverted papillomas are almost always single, nonrecurrent, and self-limiting. Although a potential for malignant transformation has been reported, inverted papillomas are generally regarded as benign and show no relationship to carcinogen exposure. They are thought to develop by proliferation of basal cells of the surface urothelium analogous to hyperplastic Brunn's nests or from cystitis cystica and cystitis glandularis (i.e., so-called Brunnian adenoma).

Gross, painless hematuria is the most frequent symptom. Bladder outlet obstruction is also common.

MORPHOLOGY Inverted papillomas may be up to 7.5 cm in diameter, but the majority are less than 3 cm. They are pedunculated, polypoid or sessile, firm, and have a smooth, glistening, gray-white surface.

Microscopically, inverted papillomas have a characteristic endophytic growth pattern and are confined to the lamina propria. In the classic trabecular type, invaginated, anastomosing cords and sheets of urothelial cells are attached to the uninterrupted, normal, atrophic, or slightly hyperplastic mucosal surface (Fig. 12.2). The urothelial cells, which are arranged compactly, lack the fibrovascular cores typical of exophytic papillary TCCs. Cords are surrounded by connective tissue of the lamina propria. There is peripheral palisading of cells with an outer layer of cuboidal cells and a surrounding basement membrane. Microcysts lined by flattened cells and containing eosinophilic (periodic acid–Schiff [PAS]-positive, mucicarmine-positive, alcian blue-positive) material are common. Foci of nonkeratinizing squamous metaplasia may be present. There may be a few mildly atypical nuclei, but nucleolar prominence and mitotic figures are absent. A symmetric unit membrane, which is not a specific morphologic marker for malignancy, has been demonstrated ultrastructurally in luminal cells.

The glandular type of inverted papilloma resembles polypoid cystitis cystica and cystitis glandularis. It is characterized by multiple round-to-oval, solid nests of proliferating urothelial cells with microcystic pseudoglandular structures and true glands lined by mucin-secreting columnar cells surrounded by several layers of urothelial cells. Intestinal metaplasia with goblet cells may be present.

VILLOUS ADENOMA

Benign glandular neoplasms of the bladder are exceedingly rare. In spite of the remarkable metaplastic potential of urothelium, only a few examples of villous adenoma have been reported, each in association with cystitis glandularis. The prognosis and behavior of these adenomatous papillary neoplasms are unclear; malignant transformation has not been observed.

MALIGNANT EPITHELIAL NEOPLASMS

Although carcinomas are classified by cell type into transitional cell (urothelial), squamous cell, glandular, and small cell undifferentiated types, mixed carcinomas are common. Spindle cell or giant cell carcinomas must be differentiated from sarcomas and carcinosarcomas.

Regardless of cell type, clinicopathologic stage (Fig. 12.3) is the most important parameter for planning treatment and determining prognosis of patients with bladder cancer. It has been shown that clinical staging, when compared with pathologic staging, is inaccurate in about 30%–50% of cases, primarily because of the inability to adequately assess depth of invasion and regional lymph node involvement.

TRANSITIONAL CELL CARCINOMA

TCC, which accounts for about 90% of bladder carcinomas, is classified by growth pattern into the following types: (1) papillary

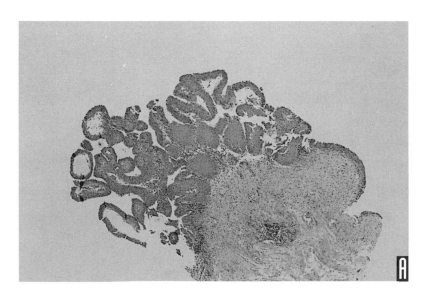

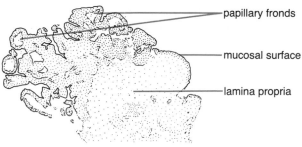

papillary fronds

mucosal surface

lamina propria

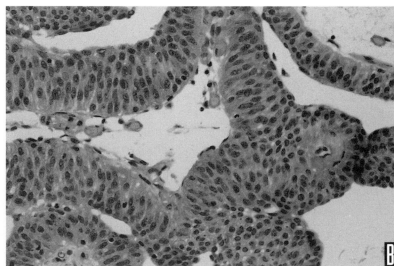

Figure 12.1 A, In this microscopic view of transitional cell papilloma, branching papillary fronds supported by fibrovascular connective tissue protrude from the mucosal surface. **B,** Urothelium lining the papillae is not thickened and shows orderly maturation with relatively preserved polarity. The slight nuclear enlargement and irregularities are atypical features, suggesting that this lesion is a grade I papillary TCC.

(approximately 70%); (2) papillary and infiltrating (approximately 20%); (3) sessile, nodular, and infiltrating (approximately 10%); and (4) nonpapillary, noninvasive, i.e., carcinoma in situ (CIS).

TCC of the bladder is rare before the age of 40 or 50 years. Its incidence increases with age; peak death rate is between 65 and 75 years. In general, males have a two- to fivefold greater incidence than females. CIS affects males ten times more frequently than females; most patients are in the sixth to seventh decade of life. In populations at high risk, TCCs occur at a younger age (30–40 years), and the incidence is increased 10- to 50-fold.

Urothelial tumors are very rare in patients less than 20 years of age, but can occur in children as young as two years old. They are usually unifocal, papillary TCCs (grade I) and, with rare exceptions, are not invasive or recurrent.

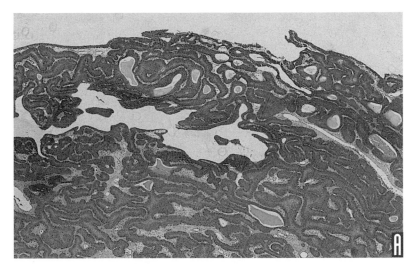

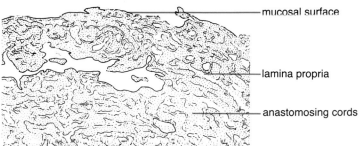

mucosal surface

lamina propria

anastomosing cords

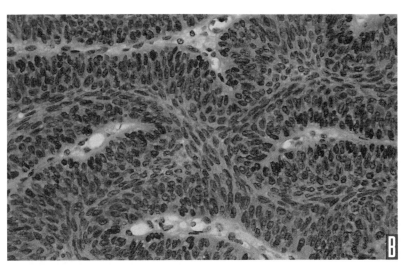

Figure 12.2 **A,** Inverted papillomas, which have an endophytic growth pattern, are composed of anastomosing cords of urothelial cells within the lamina propria. The overlying mucosal surface is smooth and generally uninterrupted. Trabeculae lack a central fibrovascular core. They are either solid or contain microcysts filled with mucinous material. **B,** The compactly arranged cords are surrounded by connective tissue. Urothelial cells, which may be spindle or squamoid, lack significant cytologic atypia.

Figure 12.3
Comparison of Jewett-Strong-Marshall (JSM) and American Joint Commitee (AJC) Classifications of Bladder Cancer

Extent of Tumor	JSM		AJC
Superficial	0	Epithelial	TIS, Ta (papillary carcinoma confined to mucosa)
	A	Lamina propria	T_1
	B_1	Superficial muscle (≤ one half depth)	T_2
Deep	B_2	Deep muscle	T_{3a}
	C	Perivesical fat	T_{3b}
Metastatic	D_1	Adjacent organs	T_{4a}
			T_{4b} (fixation to pelvic or abdominal wall)
		Regional lymph nodes	N^+
	D_2	Postregional lymph nodes or distant metastases	
			M^+ (metastatic lesions other than lymph nodes)

Modified from Prout, 1979.

PATHOGENESIS Epidemiologic studies have shown that bladder cancer results mainly from exposure to chemicals in the environment. Aromatic amines are well documented carcinogens; the most dangerous compounds include benzidine, 2-naphthylamine, and para-aminodiphenyl. Cancer results from long exposure (2–20 years) and has a latent period of 5–30 years. High-risk occupations include dye (aniline), rubber, and leather industries.

The incidence of bladder cancer is two- to threefold higher in smokers. It is estimated that cigarette smoking may account for as much as 30%–50% of bladder cancer in men.

Dietary factors such as tryptophan are thought to induce bladder cancer by acting as promoters. Artificial sweeteners (cyclamate and saccharin) act as promoters in experimental animals.

An increased risk of developing bladder cancer is associated with a variety of urinary tract diseases, including bladder lithiasis, chronic infection, and diverticula. Bladder cancers associated with schistosomal infection are predominantly squamous cell; malformations such as a patent urachus and exstrophy are predominantly associated with adenocarcinomas.

Iatrogenic causes of bladder cancer include phenacetin, cyclophosphamide, and radiation.

There appear to be two distinct pathways in the pathogenesis of bladder neoplasia. Papillary tumors are commonly produced in experimental animals exposed to carcinogens; invasion is rare. Epithelial hyperplasia, with concomitant or subsequent dysplasia, precedes and accompanies the formation of papillary tumors that carry supporting fibrovascular connective tissue. Experimentally induced invasive carcinomas are predominantly of squamous type and develop from atypical squamous metaplasia. Nonpapillary tumors (i.e., CIS) are the major source of invasive and metastasizing carcinomas in humans. Both experimental and clinical observations suggest that CIS develops from urothelial dysplasia.

CLINICAL MANIFESTATIONS In general, clinical signs of bladder cancer are dominated by macroscopic hematuria. Cystitis that causes hematuria, particularly when no organisms are present, requires follow-up to exclude a TCC. Other symptoms include bladder pain or irritation with dysuria and frequency. Locoregional invasion may cause nonspecific symptoms related to compression of nerves, ureters, and veins. Complete urinary retention is uncommon.

At least 80% of patients with CIS of the bladder present with irritative bladder symptoms suggestive of cystitis (frequency, dysuria, urgency, and suprapubic discomfort) but without evidence of infection. A history of transurethral resection of the prostate for these symptoms is common. In comparison with other forms of bladder cancer, hematuria is less common (approximately 20% of patients). The mean duration of symptoms prior to definitive diagnosis is generally less than two years. The intensity of symptoms reflects the extent of mucosal disease. A positive urinary cytologic diagnosis without associated symptoms is found in not more than 10% of patients. CIS is only rarely diagnosed as an incidental finding at cystoscopy.

CIS is commonly a multifocal or panurothelial lesion. The base of the bladder and trigone, including the ureteral orifices, are the most common locations. Ureteral CIS is found at cystectomy in 6%–60% of cases and is most common in the juxtavesical segments, but has a low rate of progression (approximately 3%). There is, however, an increased risk of upper urinary tract tumors with multifocal CIS and distal ureteral involvement; new tumors develop at an average of 61 months. Involvement of prostatic ducts and the urethra, which occurs in 18%–45% of cases, may cause pseudoprostatitis and penile voiding symptoms, respectively.

CIS is the initial presenting form of urothelial malignancy in approximately 1% of cases; unexpected microinvasion may be

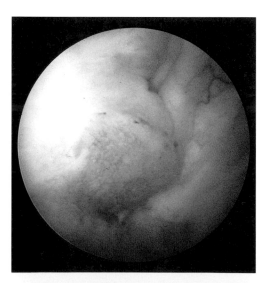

Figure 12.4 In this cystoscopic view, the discrete, localized, velvety area represents CIS. There is mucosal erythema lateral to a ureteral orifice with adjacent, more normal-appearing bladder mucosa. (Courtesy of B. Bracken, MD, Cincinnati, Ohio)

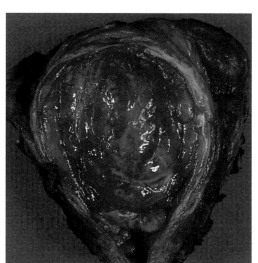

Figure 12.5 This cystectomy was performed for diffuse CIS. The mucosa is granular and erythematous, with hemorrhagic areas marking sites of extensive denudation. There are multiple, poorly defined areas with a cobblestone appearance.

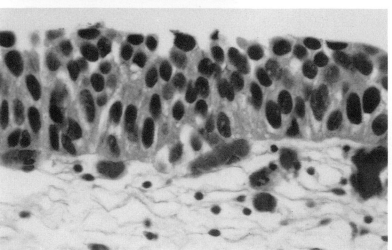

Figure 12.6 In this microscopic view of the small-cell type of CIS, there is no evidence of maturation, and polarity is lost. Nuclei are hyperchromatic, have inconspicuous nucleoli, and show frequent molding because of the high N/C ratios. (Reproduced with permission from Schumann and Weiss, 1981)

found in up to one third of cystectomy specimens. Recurrences of CIS commonly follow transurethral resection of a localized lesion: 30% occur in the first three months, 60% by six months, and 85% by one year. About 50% of patients with primary CIS develop invasive carcinoma in four to six years, and 80% do so within ten years. More often, CIS accompanies synchronous or metachronous papillary tumors or frankly invasive nonpapillary TCC.

Approximately 70% of all bladder cancers are localized to the bladder at the time of diagnosis, and less than 10% show clinical evidence of distant metastases. Five-year survival rates for patients with invasive bladder cancer following cystectomy plus adjuvant radiation therapy are 35%–52%; distant metastases occur in 30%–50% of patients, usually within 12–18 months. The most common metastatic sites, in addition to regional lymph nodes, are lungs, liver, and bone.

CARCINOMA IN SITU AND UROTHELIAL DYSPLASIA

MORPHOLOGY   CIS is best appreciated through the cystoscope (Fig. 12.4). Lesions have a granular, cobblestone, or velvety erythematous appearance and are slightly raised; marked denudation may produce hemorrhagic areas (Fig. 12.5). CIS rarely has a well

defined perimeter because of the frequent association of hyperplasia or dysplasia at the border. Comedolike yellow elevations correspond to involvement of Brunn's nests. Only rarely is no lesion identified cystoscopically. Hematoporphyrin derivative can localize dysplastic and neoplastic mucosal lesions, which show red fluorescence when irradiated with blue-violet light.

Microscopically, CIS is defined as a lesion in which the entire thickness of urothelium shows grade III dysplasia. Cells have a high nuclear-to-cytoplasmic (N/C) ratio, which causes cellular crowding and nuclear molding. Loss of sequential maturation and polarity produces a haphazard, disorderly appearance. The classic type of CIS, which is less common, is composed of small cells with hyperchromatic nuclei and inconspicuous nucleoli (Fig. 12.6). The more frequent large cell type contains cells with variable hyperchromatism. Nuclei are large and irregular, with coarse chromatin and prominent nucleoli; mitoses are frequent (Fig. 12.7). Urothelium with CIS lacks cohesiveness, and denuding cystitis is frequently seen in biopsy specimens. A single discontinuous layer of malignant urothelial cells may adhere to the basement membrane, or CIS may be seen in Brunn's nests beneath the denuded mucosa (Fig. 12.8). Cytologic examination of bladder biopsy supernatants is a useful diagnostic adjunct (Fig. 12.9). Two histologic patterns of intra-

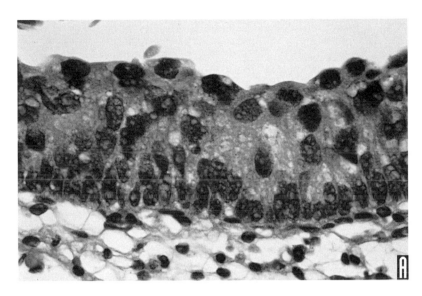

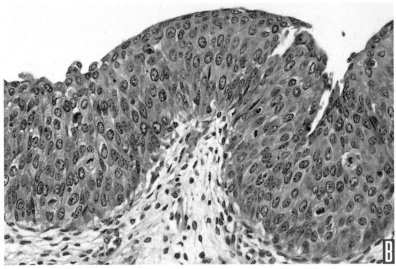

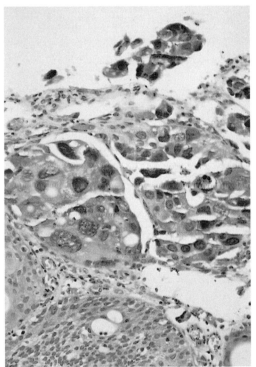

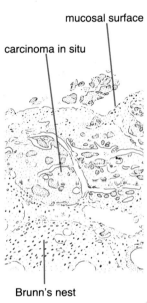

mucosal surface

carcinoma in situ

Brunn's nest

Figure 12.8 Beneath the denuded mucosal surface is a focus of CIS replacing Brunn's nest.

Figure 12.7 A, At the same magnification as Fig. 12.6, the entire thickness of urothelium with the large-cell type of CIS is occupied by cells with large, hyperchromatic, irregular nuclei. **B,** In this example of CIS, nuclei are large and have prominent nucleoli but are less hyperchromatic and more uniform in appearance; mitoses are frequent. Because anaplasia is less striking in this variant, it might be diagnosed as grade II CIS by some pathologists.

epithelial spread of CIS should be recognized. Malignant cells may grow along the basement membrane in a lepidic fashion and lift up the existing benign urothelium (Fig. 12.10). With pagetoid spread, malignant cells are dispersed within the urothelium as single cells or small cell groups (Fig. 12.11).

Urine cytology, which is critical to diagnosing CIS, is positive in 85%–100% of cases. Because there is marked exfoliation, the urine sediment is typically very cellular and contains individual cells as well as small syncytial fragments in a clean background (Figs. 12.12, 12.13).

Urothelial dysplasia includes a range of abnormalities from normal to CIS and is graded mild, moderate, or severe (Fig. 12.14). Histologically, basal and intermediate cells become polygonal, with loss of cytoplasmic clearing and the normal perpendicular orientation; mitotic activity is increased. Nuclei are crowded secondary to enlargement, show notching with one or two sharp angulations, indentations or creases, and may contain prominent nucleoli. Chromatin has increased granularity but is evenly distributed.

Grading of dysplasia is based on a comparison with the degree of pleomorphism observed in papillary TCCs. Mild dysplasia

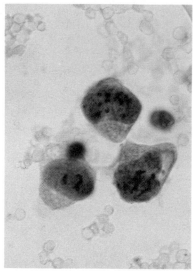

Figure 12.9 The bladder biopsy supernatant in a case of CIS with denuding cystitis contains a small urothelial fragment (left panel) and single cells (right panel) with high N/C ratios, marked nuclear irregularities, and prominent nucleoli (Papanicolaou stain).

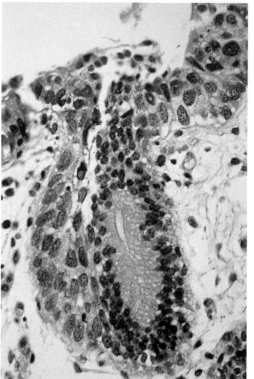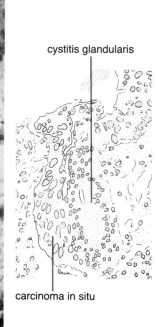

cystitis glandularis

carcinoma in situ

Figure 12.10 CIS is extending in a lepidic fashion into a focus of cystitis glandularis. The malignant cells are located between the basement membrane and metaplastic columnar cells. This undermining pattern of intraepithelial spread may also occur in the surface urothelium.

Figure 12.11 With pagetoid spread of CIS, the large malignant cells are irregularly distributed within the urothelium and do not occupy the full thickness.

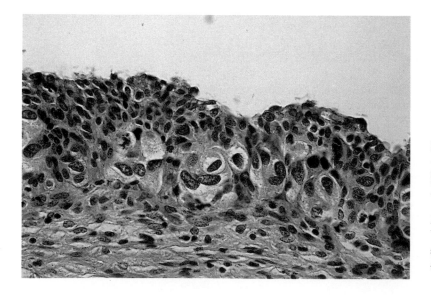

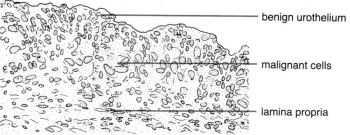

benign urothelium

malignant cells

lamina propria

shows the features of grade I, moderate dysplasia of grade II, and severe dysplasia of grade III. From a conceptual and clinical standpoint, mild-to-moderate (low-grade) dysplasia may have malignant potential. Severe (high-grade) dysplasia should be considered neoplastic. It differs from CIS by the preservation of cellular cohesion, and absence of full thickness changes with preservation of superficial cells (Fig. 12.15). In practice, the distinction between severe dysplasia and CIS may be arbitrary. Because the clinical (and biologic) implications are identical, this is not an important differentiation.

Uniformity in classifying mucosal dysplasia and CIS is lacking. Some flat, noninvasive counterparts of grade II papillary TCC are diagnosed as grade II CIS (see Fig. 12.7B). In addition, some experts object to the term *dysplasia*, preferring to regard these mucosal changes as grades (I–III) of CIS or intraepithelial neoplasia to reflect the concept of a progressive continuum of neoplastic change.

At present, the biology, course, and prognosis of urothelial dysplasia are unclear. The histologic diagnosis should be viewed as identifying a patient at risk for developing a new or recurrent neoplasm. Invasive TCC may arise not only from severe dysplasia but

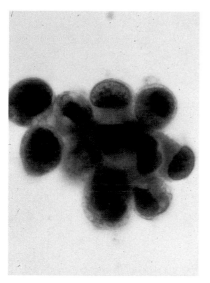 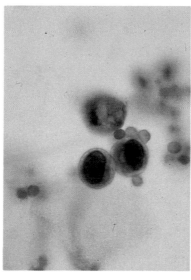

Figure 12.12 The small urothelial fragment (left panel) and individual cells (right panel) in this urine sediment exfoliated from a small cell type of CIS. The small, relatively uniform cells have enlarged, markedly hyperchromatic nuclei that lack distinct nucleoli (Papanicolaou stain). (This is the same case as Figure 12.9.)

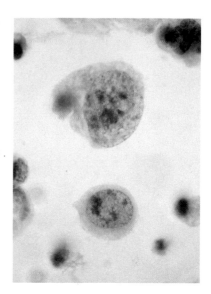

Figure 12.13 *Left:* This urine sediment from a patient with large cell CIS contains a syncytial urothelial fragment with large pleomorphic nuclei. Chromatin is coarsely granular, and macronucleoli are seen. *Right:* Single, malignant cells with similar features are present in a clean background. CIS developed following long term cyclophosphamide therapy (*Both panels:* Papanicolaou stain). (Courtesy of G. Farrow, MD, Rochester, Minnesota)

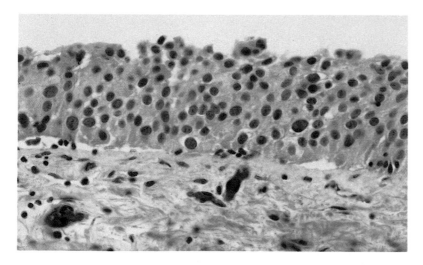

Figure 12.14 In this example of low grade (moderate) urothelial dysplasia, there is loss of cytoplasmic clearing, altered cell polarity, and irregular crowding of nuclei, which are enlarged, hyperchromatic, and focally notched.

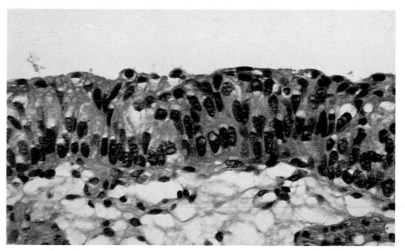

Figure 12.15 Although polarity is not totally lost and there is maturation to superficial cells, the degree of pleomorphism present in this severely dysplastic urothelium approaches CIS. It should be considered neoplastic, and carries a high risk for invasion.

occasionally from flat urothelium that appears to show low-grade dysplasia (Fig. 12.16). The demonstration of ABO(H) blood-group isoantigen deletion may help to identify "low-grade CIS." With DNA Feulgen cytophotometry, dysplasias are characterized by a predominance of tetraploid DNA values, and CIS (grade III) by a high percentage of aneuploid cells. Pleomorphic microvilli revealed by scanning electron microscopy of bladder biopsies and urinary cytologic specimens is not a specific marker of preneoplastic hyperplasia or malignancy and is observed with reversible lesions.

Denudation is not a feature of dysplasia. Dysplastic cells do not exfoliate into the urine in great numbers. They can be identified by their increased nuclear size, nuclear notching, granular chromatin, and tendency to occur in small, loose clusters (Fig. 12.17). The cytodiagnosis of urothelial dysplasia requires follow-up with cytology, endoscopy, and selected site mucosal biopsies to provide a definitive diagnosis and rule out a more serious lesion.

PAPILLARY TRANSITIONAL CELL CARCINOMA

MORPHOLOGY Cystoscopically, papillary TCCs resemble red sea anemones, with branching excrescences attached to a central connective tissue stalk (Fig. 12.18). Secondary and tertiary stalks often

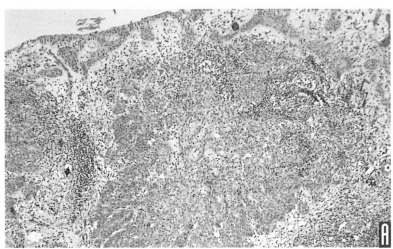

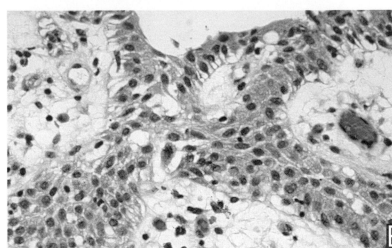

Figure 12.16 A, In this microscopic view, an invasive tumor within the lamina propria arises from flat urothelium. It forms confluent nests and has pushing margins. **B,** The overlying flat urothelium shows moderate nuclear enlargement and mild hyperchromatism more consistent with low-grade dysplasia than with CIS.

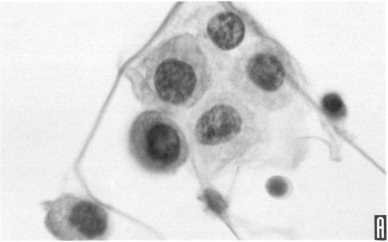

Figure 12.17 A, Mildly dysplastic urothelial cells form a loose cluster and have enlarged, centrally placed nuclei with granular chromatin and irregular borders. **B,** An isolated severely dysplastic urothelial cell, such as this one, is a cytologic finding worrisome for a high grade

TCC, including CIS. The enlarged nucleus has a discrete notch, chromatin clumping and clearing, and an irregularly shaped macronucleolus (**A,B:** Papanicolaou stain). (**A:** Reproduced with permission from Schumann and Weiss, 1981)

show complex branching. Tumors with long, fingerlike single branches are usually low-grade. High-grade papillary tumors, which often have poorly formed fronds, appear as solid, invasive neoplasms in about 90% of cases and are commonly associated with CIS. Single or multiple tumors may be present (Figs. 12.19, 12.20).

Papillary TCCs are lined by thickened urothelium (more than seven cell layers) and are graded I–III according to the degree of nuclear pleomorphism and alteration in cellular maturation. Grade I tumors, which constitute up to 30% of TCCs, show orderly maturation with preserved superficial cells. There is slight-to-moderate

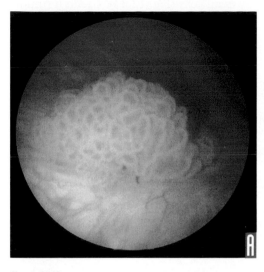
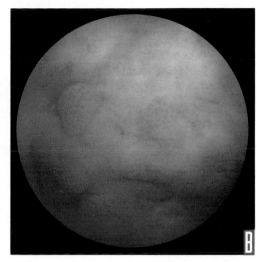
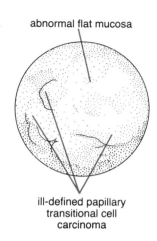

abnormal flat mucosa

ill-defined papillary transitional cell carcinoma

Figure 12.18 Cystoscopic findings frequently predict the histologic grade of papillary TCCs and are useful in assessing adjacent urothelium. **A,** Discrete grade II papillary TCC (Ta or T₁) is surrounded by normal mucosa. **B,** Multiple grade II papillary TCCs (Ta or T₁) are ill-defined due to surrounding mucosal abnormalities. This lack of definition between the malignant and benign mucosa makes definitive transurethral resection uncertain. (**A,B:** Courtesy of B. Bracken, MD, Cincinnati, Ohio)

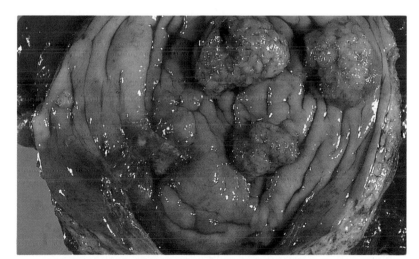

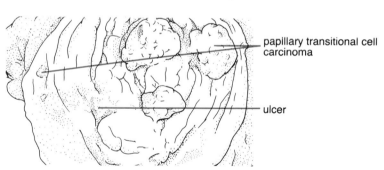

Figure 12.19 This cystectomy specimen contains three large and two small papillary TCCs. Transurethral resection of an additional papillary tumor, which documented muscle invasion, has left an ulcerated area in the right posterolateral wall.

papillary transitional cell carcinoma

ulcer

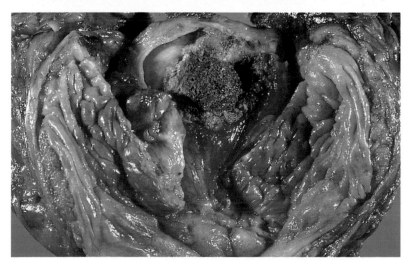

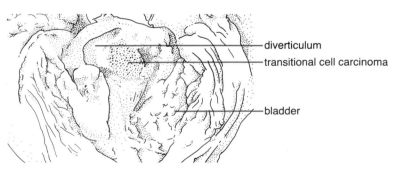

Figure 12.20 In this specimen, a large diverticulum in the posterior bladder wall contains a necrotic high-grade TCC. Cystectomy was performed following preoperative radiation therapy.

diverticulum

transitional cell carcinoma

bladder

nuclear enlargement, slight hyperchromatism, and slight pleomorphism (Fig. 12.21). A normal (diploid) DNA content, absence of marker chromosomes, and preservation of surface blood-group antigens characterize these well differentiated papillary tumors, which are rarely invasive but carry the risk for developing recurrent (5%–20% higher grade), invasive TCCs.

Grade I–II tumors may contain elongate or squamoid cells (Fig. 12.22).

Grade II papillary TCCs show a variable loss of superficial cells with altered maturation, disturbed polarity, and loss of cytoplasmic clearing (Fig. 12.23). Moderate-to-marked nuclear enlargement with nuclear crowding, moderate hyperchromatism, and variable pleomorphism are present; mitoses are common. Variants may have a rosettelike or pseudoglandular arrangement or may contain columnar, spindle, clear, or small cells (Fig. 12.24). Grade II tumors are heterogeneous with respect to aneuploidy (approximately 33%

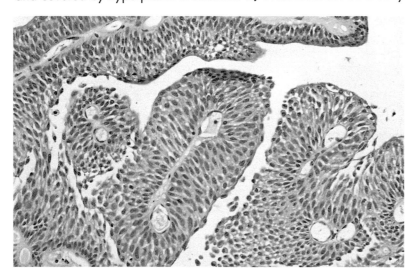

Figure 12.21 A, In this grade I papillary TCC, papillae are well formed and covered by hyperplastic urothelium. **B,** Urothelium shows orderly

maturation to superficial cells. The slightly hyperchromatic nuclei are crowded together secondary to mild-to-moderate enlargement.

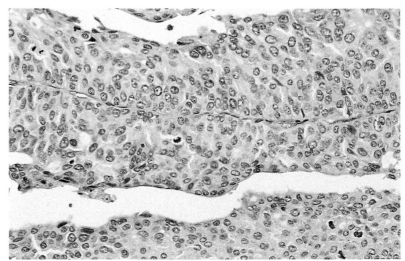

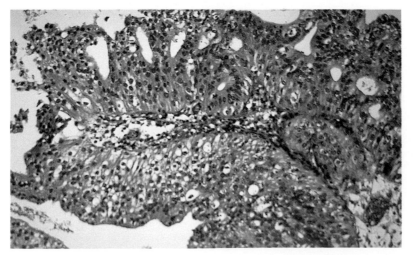

Figure 12.22 In this papillary TCC, grade I–II cells are elongate, which gives the urothelium a squamoid appearance.

Figure 12.23 This grade II papillary TCC shows altered nuclear polarity with increased pleomorphism and mitotic activity. Nuclei are moderately enlarged and appear vesicular.

Figure 12.24 This grade II papillary TCC contains pseudoglandular spaces surrounded by flattened urothelial cells, as well as lumina lined by columnar cells.

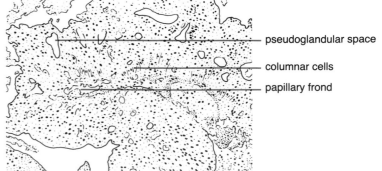

pseudoglandular space

columnar cells

papillary frond

of cases), blood-group antigen expression, and morphologic chromosomal abnormalities. Invasion by these carcinomas is common (approximately 50% of cases), and they are frequently associated with hyperplasia, dysplasia, or CIS in the adjacent urothelium.

Grade III papillary TCCs constitute 19%–34% of TCCs. Evidence of maturation and polarity is lost, and there is marked exfoliation of cells (Fig. 12.25). Nuclear enlargement, hyperchromatism (coarse and irregular), and pleomorphism are marked; mitoses are prominent, and single or multiple macronucleoli are common. These tumors typically lack surface blood-group antigens (up to 94% of cases), are aneuploid, and contain marker chromosomes. High-grade papillary tumors are typically invasive; differentiation

from nonkeratinizing squamous cell carcinoma may be difficult. Severe dysplasia or CIS can usually be identified in the adjacent urothelium.

Mixed urothelial carcinomas, which account for less than 10% of all bladder cancers, do not differ prognostically from pure TCCs. These tumors contain a component of squamous and/or glandular differentiation, which may occur in up to 50% of grade III TCCs (papillary or sessile) (Figs. 12.26, 12.27).

Overall, the accuracy of urine cytology in the diagnosis of TCC has ranged from 25%–100% (mean, approximately 70%). Results, however, should be correlated with cystoscopic findings and are influenced by histologic grade; about 20%–60% of grade I and

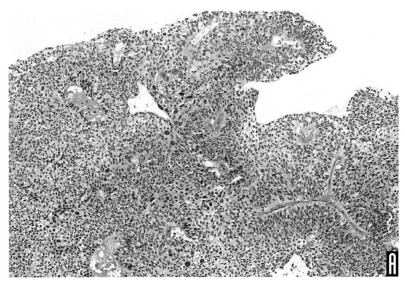

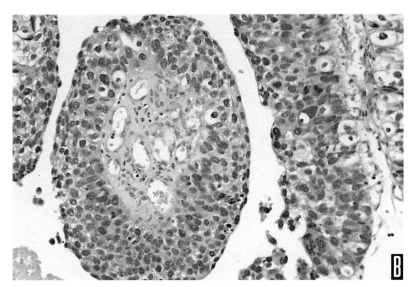

Figure 12.25 A, Grade III papillary TCCs frequently appear solid because papillae are poorly formed. **B,** There is marked nuclear enlargement, hyperchromatism, and pleomorphism with macronucleoli. The urothelium, which shows loss of polarity, may not be hyperplastic because of cell exfoliation.

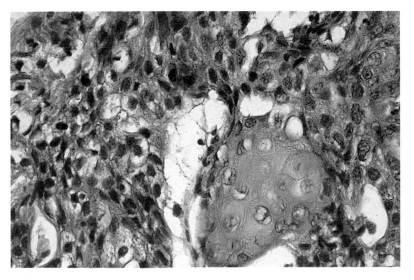

Figure 12.26 High-grade TCCs with focal squamous differentiation (center) should not be misdiagnosed as SCC.

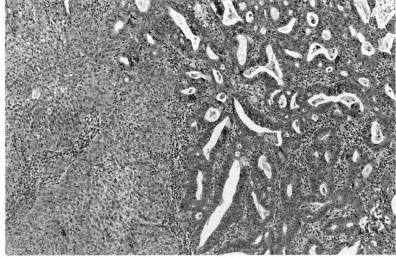

Figure 12.27 This mixed urothelial carcinoma contains an invasive high-grade TCC and adenocarcinoma (right).

75%–100% of grade II–III papillary TCCs are detected cytologically (Figs. 12.28–12.30). Specificity is 95%–99% and sensitivity is 66%–85%; cytohistologic correlation is possible in about 75%–90% of cases. False-negative cytologic studies reflect the difficulty in detecting grade I papillary TCCs. In bladder washings, a positive or suspicious diagnosis in the presence of a grade I papillary tumor may reflect sampling of neoplastic urothelium at other sites. False-positives (1%–12%) must be distinguished from unconfirmed positives. The cytologic diagnosis of a TCC may precede cystoscopic diagnosis by up to five years.

PROGNOSIS   TCC represents a polychronotopical malignant diathesis (i.e., multiple with respect to time and place) (Fig. 12.31). Among patients with superficial tumors, 40%–70% have true recurrences or new occurrences (10%–20% higher grade), most often within one to two years following the primary diagnosis; progression to a higher stage occurs in about 30%.

In addition to establishing the diagnosis, the pathologist is responsible for predicting the biologic potential of TCC. Tumor characteristics that are considered risk factors for recurrence and have predictive value with respect to progression (i.e., invasion and metastases) must be evaluated for complete classification. Diagnoses should include the configuration (sessile versus papillary), grade, and pathologic stage, particularly the presence of muscular, lymphatic, or vascular invasion. Associated mucosal abnormalities (hyperplasia, dysplasia, CIS) should be noted. Selected-site, cold-cup biopsies from the posterior midline, dome, lateral to the ureteral orifices, and approximately 2 cm from the evident lesion have been recommended. Size (larger than 3–4 cm), multiplicity (more than three tumors), and rate of recurrences (more than one per year) adversely affect prognosis and can be evaluated clinically.

Additional biologic predictors of poor prognosis include: (1) deletion of ABO(H) blood-group antigens (predictive value, about 70%) and alterations in Thomsen–Friedenreich (T) antigen, which is normally cryptic (Figs. 12.32, 12.33); (2) presence of marker chromosomes (e.g., ring or A-1 chromosomes); and (3) demonstration of aneuploidy by flow cytometry or DNA cytophotometry. These special procedures may be best applied to assessing dysplasia and the heterogeneous group of grade II papillary TCCs.

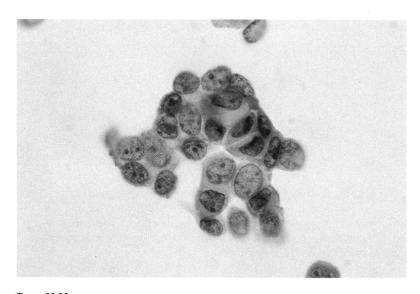

Figure 12.28 This urothelial fragment from a grade I papillary TCC shows nuclear crowding and molding secondary to increased N:C ratios. The enlarged nuclei have membrane indentations and finely granular chromatin with slight clumping and clearing (Papanicolaou stain).

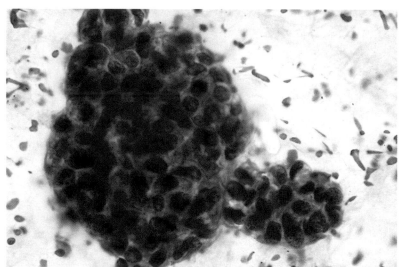

Figure 12.29 In this grade II papillary TCC, a papillary fragment (left) with altered cellular maturation contains enlarged, hyperchromatic nuclei that are tightly packed and occasionally molded (Papanicolaou stain).

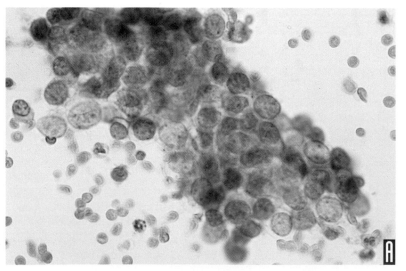

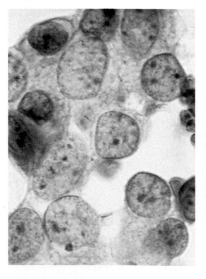
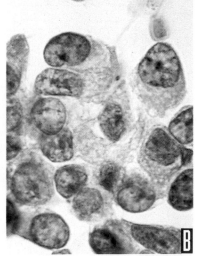

Figure 12.30 A, This large sheet of malignant urothelial cells from a grade III TCC shows prominent nuclear molding. **B,** Urothelial fragments have a syncytial arrangement. Nuclei are markedly enlarged, hyperchromatic, and pleomorphic, with coarsely granular, irregularly clumped chromatin and small or large nucleoli (**A,B:** Papanicolaou stain). (Reproduced with permission from Schumann and Weiss, 1981)

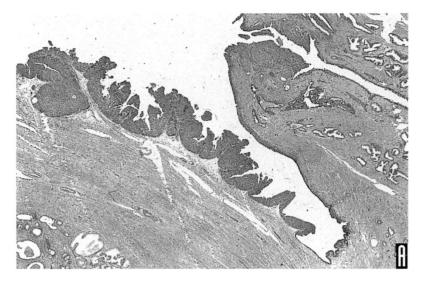

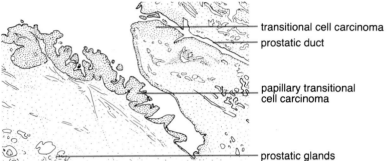

transitional cell carcinoma
prostatic duct

papillary transitional
cell carcinoma

prostatic glands

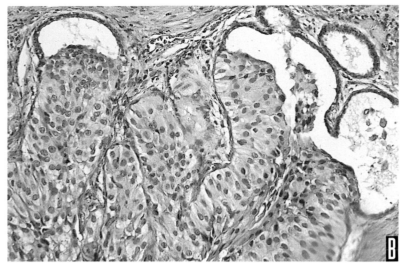

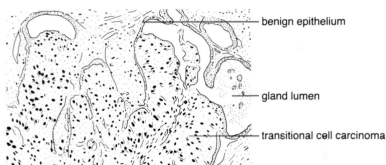

benign epithelium

gland lumen

transitional cell carcinoma

Figure 12.31 **A,** Cystoprostatectomy performed for TCC of the bladder yielded this specimen, which shows a noninvasive papillary tumor in the prostatic urethra near the verumontanum. TCC is present at the opening of a prostatic duct. **B,** Extension along ducts into the prostate gland may be mistaken for a primary TCC in a needle biopsy or transurethral resection of the prostate.

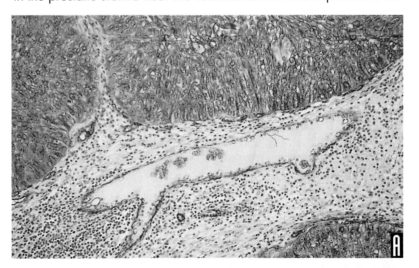

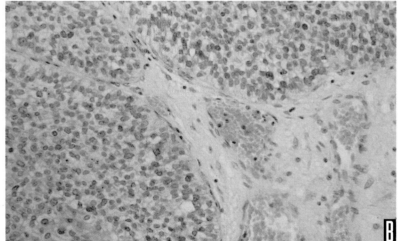

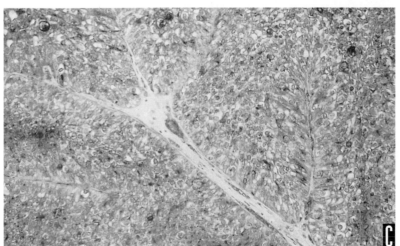

Figure 12.32 **A,** This noninvasive grade II papillary TCC shows staining for blood-group antigen A. Neoplastic cells, the endothelium, and RBCs are positive. **B,** The tumor shows a negative reaction for spontaneous expression of T-antigen. **C,** A positive reaction for "cryptic" T-antigen followed treatment with neuraminidase. Tumor cells, as well as endothelial cells and RBCs, react with the biotinylated arachis (**A:** ABC immunoperoxidase method; **B,C:** biotinylated PNA-Vectastain-hematoxylin). (Courtesy C. Limas, MD, Minneapolis, Minnesota)

Squamous Cell Carcinoma

Squamous cell carcinoma (SCC) of the bladder occurs infrequently in the Western hemisphere, representing only 5%–7% of bladder carcinomas. In areas such as Egypt, Africa, and the Middle East, where schistosomiasis (*Schistosoma haematobium*) is prevalent, SCC is the most common form of bladder cancer (55%–70%). SCC

should be distinguished from high-grade TCC with focal squamous differentiation. In contrast with TCC, there is an almost equal sex distribution.

PATHOGENESIS Squamous metaplasia (see Chapter 10) is often identified at the periphery of the infiltrating carcinoma or at sites remote from the tumor (16%–25%). However, SCC frequently

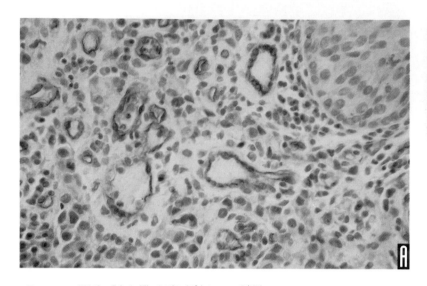

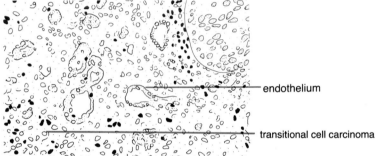

endothelium

transitional cell carcinoma

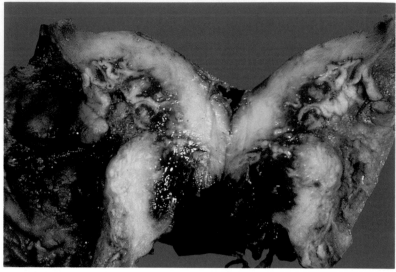

Figure 12.34 SCC partially fills a bladder diverticulum and infiltrates perivesical fat in this gross specimen. The adjacent bladder mucosa shows keratinizing squamous metaplasia.

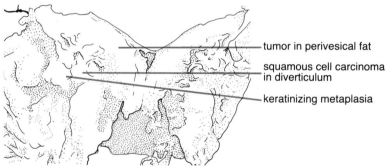

tumor in perivesical fat

squamous cell carcinoma in diverticulum

keratinizing metaplasia

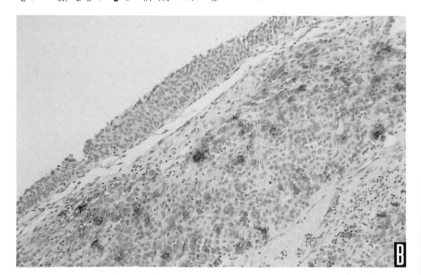

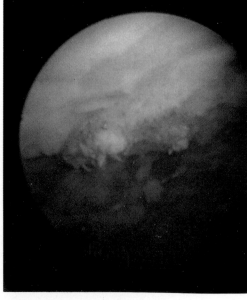

Figure 12.35 SCC in the dome of the bladder has a keratinized surface. The background shows defined, patchy erythematous areas with partial keratinization. (Courtesy of B. Bracken, MD, Cincinnati, Ohio)

Figure 12.33 A, This invasive grade III TCC lacks blood-group antigen A. The neoplastic cells are negative, while the vascular endothelium is strongly positive (ABC immunoperoxidase method). **B,** T-antigen expression is spontaneous. Invasive tumor cells show a positive reaction, while the overlying mucosa is negative (biotinylated PNA-Vectastain-hematoxylin). (Courtesy of C. Limas, MD, Minneapolis, Minnesota)

appears to arise from nonmetaplastic epithelium. Leukoplakia has been documented as a precursor lesion in up to 20% of cases.

CLINICAL MANIFESTATIONS SCCs characteristically develop without a prior history of vesical malignancy and present as a solitary invasive tumor. They are often the cell type seen in bladder diverticula (Fig. 12.34) or in paraplegics with chronic indwelling catheters. Patients commonly have a history of urethral stricture, calculous disease, or chronic urinary tract infection. They often present with obstructive symptoms and an abnormal intravenous pyelogram (IVP), irritative bladder symptoms, or signs of advanced disease (weight loss, back or pelvic pain). SCCs are rapidly growing,

aggressive tumors that tend to present at an advanced stage. Overall five-year survival ranges from 10%–48%.

MORPHOLOGY While SCCs are usually ulcerating and infiltrating neoplasms, they may be exophytic or fungating (Figs. 12.35, 12.36). Because these tumors may be bulky and frequently have a necrotic infected surface or are covered by keratin debris, it is often difficult to obtain an adequate biopsy, particularly for documentation of muscle invasion (Fig. 12.37). A biopsy specimen should be obtained from the junction of tumor and normal tissue.

Well differentiated (grade I) SCCs show orderly maturation and minimal pleomorphism (Fig. 12.38). Sheets of squamous cells have

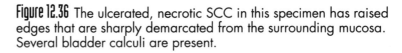

Figure 12.36 The ulcerated, necrotic SCC in this specimen has raised edges that are sharply demarcated from the surrounding mucosa. Several bladder calculi are present.

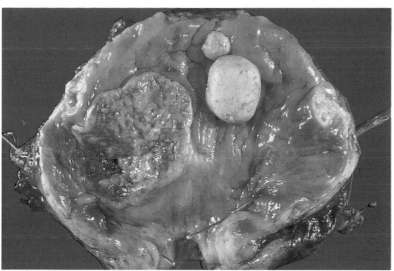

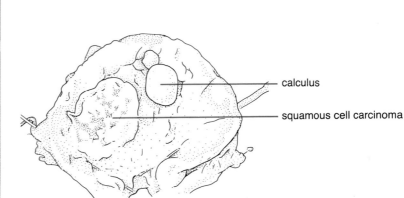

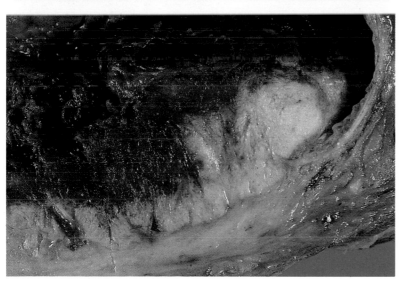

Figure 12.37 It is difficult to obtain adequate biopsies from an exophytic SCC such as this one. The surface is covered with necrotic keratin debris and the bulk of the tumor is intravesical. The bladder wall deep to the SCC is infiltrated by gray-white tumor.

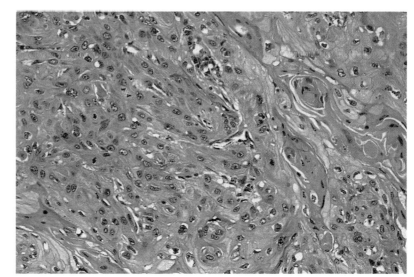

Figure 12.38 In this well differentiated SCC, sheets of polygonal keratinizing cells with intercellular bridges produce extracellular keratin and form pearls.

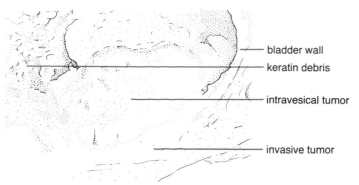

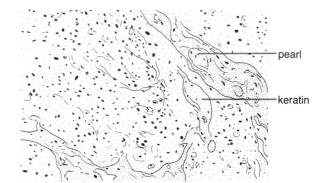

a peripheral basal layer, a broad zone of large, polygonal intermediate cells with prominent intercellular bridges, frequent individual cell keratinization with concentric aggregation (keratin pearls), and abundant extracellular keratin production. Moderately differentiated (grade II–III) SCCs are solid tumors that infiltrate in broad sheets and show disordered maturation with an increased proportion of basal-type cells, mild-to-moderate pleomorphism, and dyskeratosis (Fig. 12.39). Extracellular keratin and pearls are less evident. Occasional tumors are composed of large, clear cells. In poorly differentiated (grade IV) SCCs, there is minimal maturation and infrequent keratinization. These tumors contain a high proportion of undifferentiated cells with marked nuclear pleomorphism and numerous mitotic figures, scattered dyskeratotic cells, and occasional pearls. The small cell anaplastic variant resembles an oat cell carcinoma. Although high-grade tumors are more often advanced, grade provides little prognostic information.

ADENOCARCINOMA

Adenocarcinomas, which constitute about 2% of all primary malignant epithelial tumors, reflect the metaplastic potential of urothelium that persists into adult life. They are the most common malignant tumor (about 80%) arising in the exstrophic bladder and occur more frequently in areas where schistosomiasis is endemic. In general, adenocarcinomas are most common during the sixth to seventh decades of life and occur two times more frequently in males than in females. Those of urachal origin occur more often in younger patients than do other forms of bladder cancer. Adenocarcinomas must be distinguished from high-grade TCCs with a glandular component. In comparison with TCCs, which characteristically are multifocal and have a high recurrence rate, adenocarcinomas are typically solitary and show a predilection for the trigone. The majority of bladder adenocarcinomas are metastatic. The possibility of metastases from adjacent or distant sites, including colon and breast, should be ruled out.

CLINICAL MANIFESTATIONS Gross hematuria and dysuria are common symptoms of adenocarcinoma. Patients may also present with irritative voiding symptoms, urinary retention, or flank pain; ureteral obstruction is particularly common with signet-ring cell carcinomas. Nonurachal adenocarcinomas have a clinical course similar to that of invasive TCC, and prognosis depends on stage (overall five-year survival is less than 25%). The pattern (lung, liver, and bone) and frequency of metastases are similar to those of TCC. Since adenocarcinomas occurring with exstrophy are usually diagnosed early, they metastasize less frequently. Urachal adenocarcinomas have a poor prognosis and tend to involve the entire urachus as well as extend into the space of Retzius. The signet-ring cell variant is characterized by a rapidly progressive and fatal course (mean, 7½ months), with extension into adjacent organs and seeding of the peritoneal cavity.

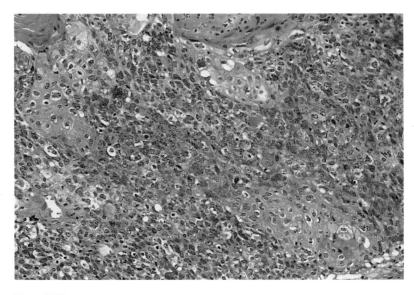

Figure 12.39 This moderately differentiated SCC has numerous basal-type cells growing in sheets, which show focal disorderly maturation to keratinizing squamous cells, with moderate nuclear pleomorphism.

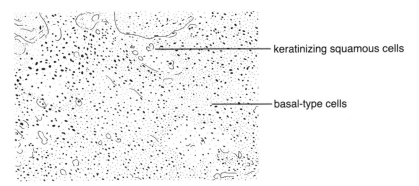

keratinizing squamous cells

basal-type cells

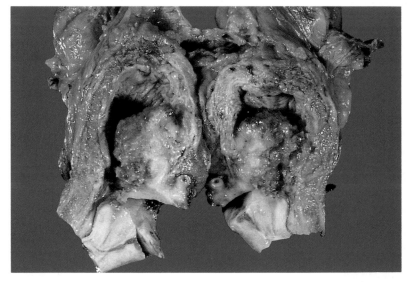

Figure 12.40 The invasive papillary adenocarcinoma arising from the posterior wall of this bisected bladder has a characteristic mucinous surface.

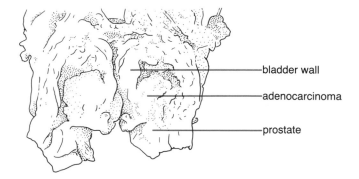

bladder wall

adenocarcinoma

prostate

MORPHOLOGY Adenocarcinomas characteristically appear as mucus-covered, papillary, or nodular sessile masses (Figs. 12.40, 12.41). The signet-ring cell variant is diffusely infiltrative and produces marked thickening and stiffening of the bladder wall similar to linitis plastica of the stomach; the mucosa appears edematous, hypertrophied, and focally hemorrhagic. Predominantly intramural tumors located in the dome or anterior wall and covered by normal or ulcerated urothelium should be considered urachal carcinomas clinically; pathologically, they are usually glandular, but may be TCCs or mixed carcinomas since the urachus is normally lined by urothelium (Fig. 12.42).

Histologic variants most commonly resemble enteric adenocarcinomas and are frequently mucus producing. Papillary and glandular tumors are composed of columnar cells with variable mucin

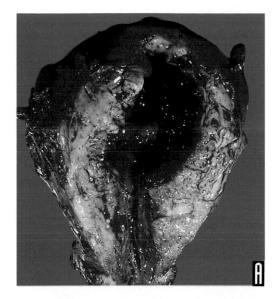

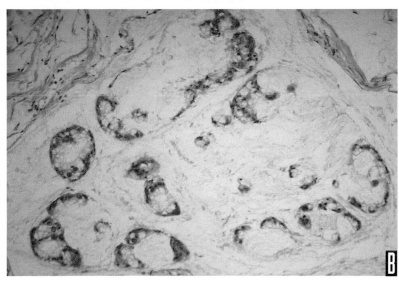

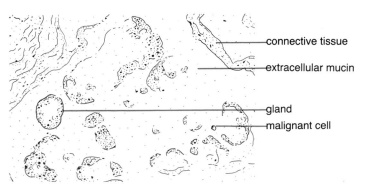

Figure 12.41 A, In this specimen, the bladder wall is diffusely thickened by an infiltrating colloid carcinoma and has a glistening, gelatinous, or mucoid appearance. The mucosa is hemorrhagic and lacks a discrete mass. **B,** Colloid carcinomas contain glands and individual cells floating in pools of extracellular mucin. Columnar cells with intracytoplasmic mucin resemble intestinal goblet cells.

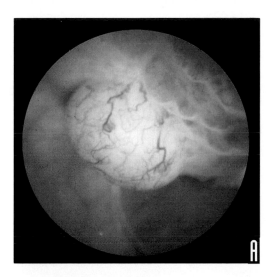

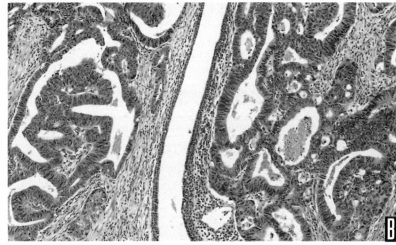

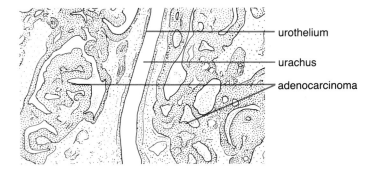

Figure 12.42 A, The intact, normal mucosa in the bladder dome is stretched by a tumor that appears to be invading the bladder from an intramural or extravesical source. These cystoscopic findings are characteristic of a urachal adenocarcinoma. **B,** This urachal adenocarcinoma arose in the wall of the bladder dome. The microscopically patent urachus is lined by a thin layer of urothelium. Papillae and glands are lined by stratified columnar epithelium. (**A:** Courtesy of B. Bracken, MD, Cincinnati, Ohio)

production (Fig. 12.43). Colloid carcinomas contain clusters of cuboidal or columnar cells within lakes of mucin (see Fig. 12.41B). Infiltrating signet-ring cell carcinomas are often associated with extensive fibrosis (Fig. 12.44). The presence of CIS, which may contain signet-ring cells, helps to distinguish this variant from metastatic gastric or breast (lobular) carcinoma. Mesonephric adenocarcinomas, which are most often trigonal, are composed of clear cells (mucin-negative) and may have glands, trabeculae, or papillae lined by hobnail cells (Fig. 12.45).

SMALL CELL UNDIFFERENTIATED CARCINOMA

Small cell undifferentiated carcinomas (SCUCs) are rare bladder neoplasms that have a predilection for elderly men. They may occur in pure form or as the major component of a mixed carcinoma. Although neuroendocrine cells have been documented in normal and metaplastic bladder mucosa, and primary carcinoid tumor has been reported, it is more likely that SCUC is derived from a multipotential mucosal stem cell capable of divergent differentiation.

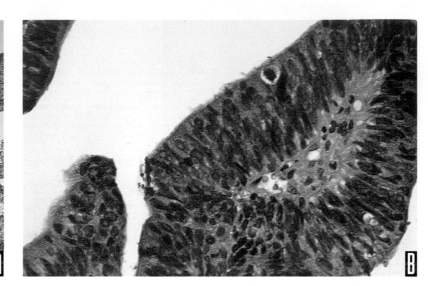

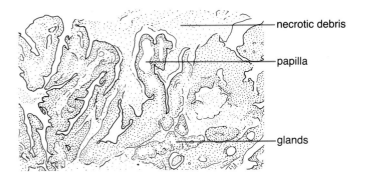

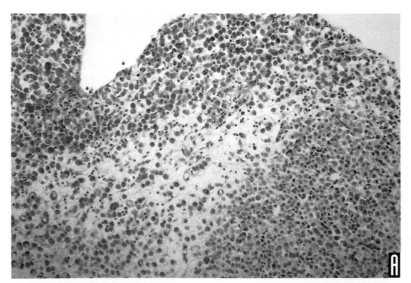

Figure 12.43 **A,** Adenocarcinomas of the bladder, which are commonly papillary and glandular, resemble intestinal neoplasms. The luminal surface of this tumor is covered with necrotic cellular debris and mucin. **B,** Like the urachal adenocarcinoma shown in Figure 12.42, adenocarcinomas of the bladder contain stratified columnar epithelium. Intracytoplasmic mucin may be absent.

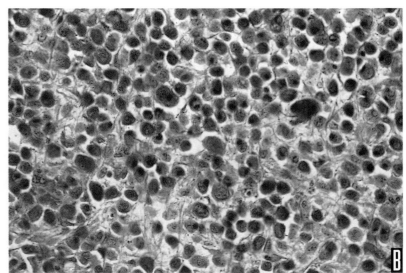

Figure 12.44 **A,** The lamina propria contains a dense, cellular infiltrate of neoplastic cells. Overlying urothelium is denuded. **B,** Numerous cells contain mucin vacuoles. Those with displaced nuclei have

a signet-ring cell appearance (PAS stain with diastase). The presence of CIS confirmed a bladder origin for this signet-ring cell carcinoma.

CLINICAL MANIFESTATIONS   Clinical presentation is similar to that of other forms of bladder cancer; the majority of patients have gross hematuria. Ectopic adrenocorticotropic hormone (ACTH) production, hypercalcemia, and hypophosphatemia have been reported. SCUC is an aggressive neoplasm with an extremely poor prognosis (median survival, five months); metastases occur early and are widespread.

MORPHOLOGY   Most tumors form large, ulcerated, polypoid intraluminal masses (Fig. 12.46). Microscopically, intermediate and oat cell variants occur. The lymphocytelike, polygonal, or fusiform cells have scant cytoplasm and hyperchromatic nuclei with a "salt-and-pepper" appearance and inconspicuous nucleoli. A high mitotic rate and tumor necrosis are characteristic; vascular invasion is common.

SCUCs frequently express one or more epithelial markers (cytokeratin, epithelial membrane antigen, or human milk fat–globule protein) and neuroendocrine markers (neuronspecific enolase, chromogranin, Leu 7, or serotonin). By electron microscopy, neurosecretory (150–250 nm) granules are usually present, and tumor cells may have dendritelike processes, form intercellular lumina, or contain cytoplasmic tonofilaments.

SCUCs are frequently associated with other forms of in situ or invasive carcinoma, including a minor (up to 10%) component of adenocarcinoma, transitional cell, squamous cell, or spindle cell carcinoma, or carcinoid tumor.

Spindle Cell Carcinoma

The patient with this rare variant of invasive transitional cell or squamous cell carcinoma usually presents at an advanced stage and has a poor prognosis. Histologically, spindle cell carcinoma is composed of interlacing sheets of anaplastic spindle cells with variable amounts of cytoplasm that merge imperceptibly with

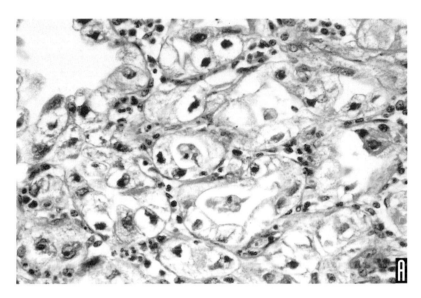

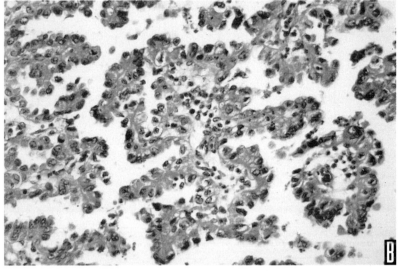

Figure 12.45 A, In this microscopic view of mesonephric adenocarcinoma, glands are lined by cells with abundant, clear cytoplasm. Nuclear pleomorphism is one feature that distinguishes this lesion from its apparently benign counterpart, the nephrogenic adenoma. **B,** Papillae lined by cells with apical nuclei (hobnail cells) are characteristic. Nuclei are enlarged and hyperchromatic.

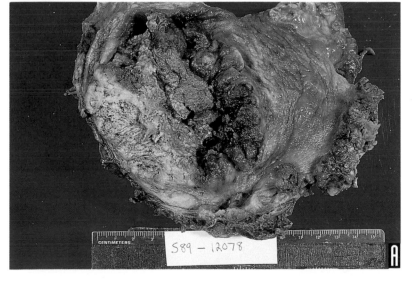

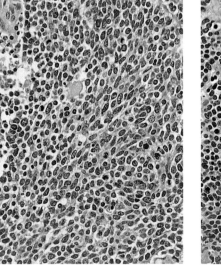

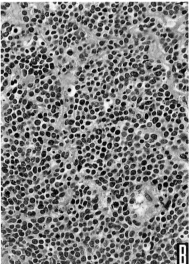

Figure 12.46 A, The large necrotic intraluminal mass in this cystectomy specimen is a small cell undifferentiated carcinoma. **B,** Microscopically, it contains both intermediate and oat cell variants. The fusiform (left panel) and lymphocyte-like (right panel) cells have scant cytoplasm and small hyperchromatic nuclei with inconspicuous nucleoli. Numerous mitotic figures and individual cell necrosis are present. (Courtesy of S. McClure, MD, Akron, Ohio).

the relatively well demarcated epithelial component (Fig. 12.47). Tumor giant cells may be numerous (Fig. 12.48). When the invasive carcinoma is not sampled, these tumors may be mistaken for a primary sarcoma such as leiomyosarcoma. The immunohistochemical demonstration of cytokeratin is helpful in confirming epithelial differentiation. Unlike carcinosarcomas, there is no malignant mesodermal component.

Spindle cell carcinomas should be distinguished from urothelial carcinomas with a pseudosarcomatous stroma, in which widely spaced, evenly distributed spindle-shaped stromal cells with abundant eosinophilic to amphophilic cytoplasm have bizarre, hyperchromatic nuclei (Fig. 12.49). These atypical cells, which may be multinucleated, have a degenerative appearance and lack mitotic figures.

MALIGNANT MESODERMAL MIXED TUMORS

Malignant mesodermal mixed tumors are rare, highly malignant bladder tumors composed of carcinomatous and differentiated sarcomatous elements (carcinosarcoma). They occur three times more commonly in men than in women; most patients are elderly (mean, 62 years). Carcinosarcomas should be distinguished from spindle cell carcinoma, primary osteosarcoma, and the rare sarcoma coexistent with a separate TCC, although all have an equally poor prognosis. Additionally, these tumors must be distinguished from carcinomas with benign osteocartilaginous stromal metaplasia.

Patients typically present with hematuria of recent onset. Although metastases occur, deaths are frequently due to local spread and resultant complications.

Figure 12.47 Spindle cell carcinomas show imperceptible merging between infiltrating nests of carcinoma and anaplastic spindle cells. The malignant spindle cells, which have lost their epithelial features, form interlacing sheets and resemble an undifferentiated sarcoma.

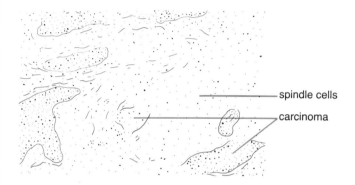

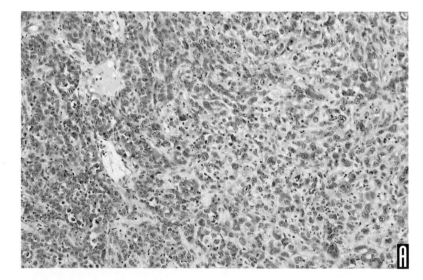

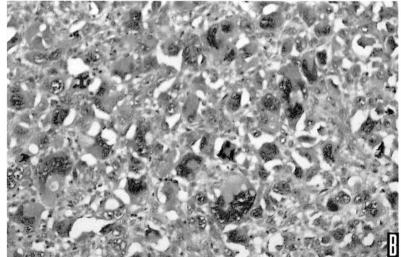

Figure 12.48 A, This spindle cell carcinoma contains sheets of undifferentiated carcinoma (left) that gradually transform into a pleomorphic malignant neoplasm (right). **B,** In this focus, there are bizarre, pleomorphic, mononucleate, and multinucleate giant cells.

MORPHOLOGY Carcinosarcomas are bulky, infiltrating neoplasms that frequently form a large polypoid or fungating intravesical mass. They are less commonly papillary, pedunculated, or sessile. Microscopically, the malignant epithelial and mesenchymal elements are distinct and, although intimately admixed, rarely show transition. TCC is the most frequent epithelial component, but SCC (about 20%) and adenocarcinoma (about 33%) are also common. In 25%–50% of tumors, the malignant mesenchymal element consists of bone, cartilage, or skeletal muscle (Fig. 12.50). Leiomyosarcoma or fibrosarcoma may also be present. Occasional tumors contain a component of undifferentiated carcinoma or sarcoma. Metastases may be pure carcinoma, pure sarcoma, or mixed.

BENIGN MESENCHYMAL NEOPLASMS

Benign mesenchymal tumors are uncommon. Hemangiomas, lipomas, granular cell tumors, and adenomatoid tumors are occasion-ally observed. Neurofibromas may occur in patients with von Recklinghausen's disease (Fig. 12.51).

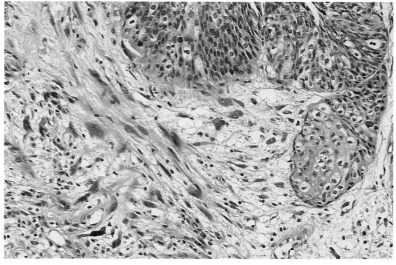

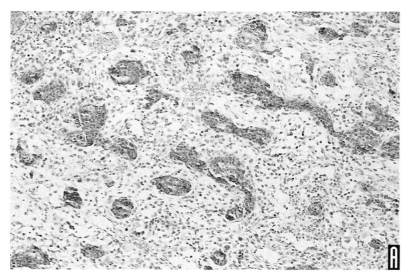

Figure 12.49 Atypical spindle cells in the lamina propria have eosinophilic cytoplasm and variably enlarged, hyperchromatic nuclei. This pseudosarcomatous stroma was associated with a grade II TCC (upper right) that showed multifocal superficial invasion. (Courtesy of R. Young, MD, Boston, Massachusetts)

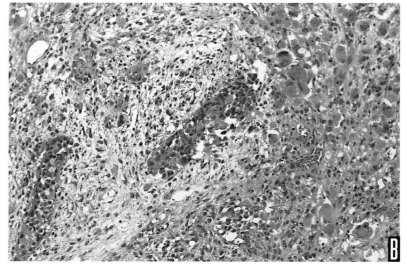

Figure 12.50 A, Malignant mesodermal mixed tumors contain a carcinoma and a sarcoma, which may be focally undifferentiated. **B,** Rhabdomyoblastic differentiation is common. The carcinomatous component is admixed but remains distinct from the sarcoma.

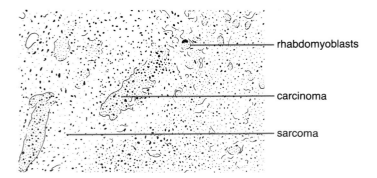

LEIOMYOMA

Leiomyomas constitute approximately 35% of benign mesenchymal neoplasms and show no sex predilection. Intramural or extravesical tumors are usually an incidental finding and are, in general, asymptomatic unless the patient's urinary tract function is affected. Endovesical tumors may cause gross hematuria and irritative or obstructive symptoms.

Leiomyomas are sharply circumscribed, firm masses that may be calcified or show cystic change. Endovesical tumors are sessile or pedunculated. Microscopically, sheets of smooth muscle cells are arranged in parallel bundles and interlacing fascicles (Fig. 12.52). Nuclear atypia and mitoses are absent.

MALIGNANT MESENCHYMAL NEOPLASMS

EMBRYONAL RHABDOMYOSARCOMA

Rhabdomyosarcomas account for 10%–15% of solid malignant tumors in children; 15%–27% of these tumors arise in the genitourinary tract. Embryonal rhabdomyosarcoma of the bladder, however, is a rare tumor. It predominates in the first few years of life, accounting for the initial peak incidence of bladder cancer, and shows a male preponderance. These very aggressive neoplasms occasionally occur in older children but are rare in adults.

Patients may present with complete urinary retention or hematuria and dysuria. Radiologic evaluation frequently shows a multilobed intravesical mass.

MORPHOLOGY Embryonal rhabdomyosarcomas of the bladder exhibit a predilection for the prostatic urethra. With botryoid sarcomas, the bladder becomes partially or completely filled with translucent, grapelike masses that are broad-based and multicentric (Fig. 12.53). Microscopically, the polyps have a loose, edematous stroma covered by intact urothelium (Fig. 12.54). A cellular zone beneath the mucosa makes up the cambium layer. The tumor is composed predominantly of primitive (undifferentiated) small spindle cells with hyperchromatic nuclei. Poorly differentiated skeletal muscle cells have prominent eosinophilic cytoplasm. Rounded and elongate rhabdomyoblasts (strap cells), however, are relatively sparse, and cross-striations may be difficult to identify.

ADULT-TYPE RHABDOMYOSARCOMA

Adult-type rhabdomyosarcomas predominate in patients over the age of 40 but occasionally occur in children. These bulky, infiltrating sarcomas are composed of large, anaplastic muscle cells showing varying degrees of differentiation. Cross-striations may be iden-

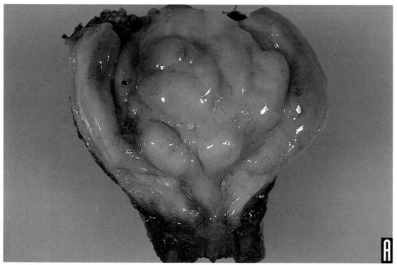

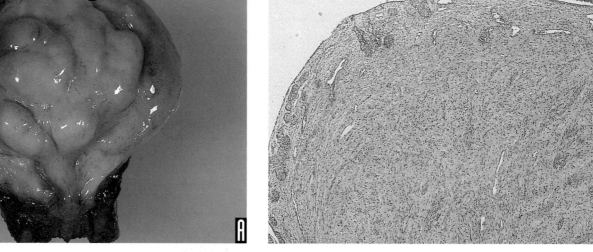

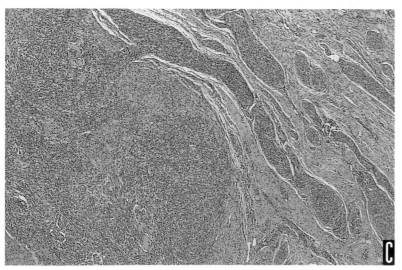

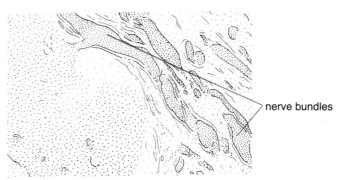

nerve bundles

Figure 12.51 A, In this specimen, a plexiform neurofibroma of the bladder has produced multiple, nodular, submucosal masses. **B,** Microscopically, the firm submucosal masses are composed of proliferating cells dispersed within a loose collagenous matrix. Neurites are focally present (right). **C,** Tortuous, hypercellular nerve bundles within the bladder wall are surrounded by neurofibromatous tissue. An unencapsulated, densely cellular area (left) contains disorganized bundles and whorls of spindle cells.

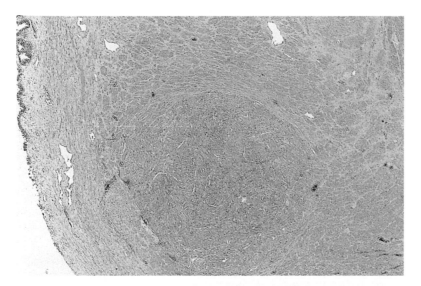

Figure 12.52 This small intramural leiomyoma appears sharply circumscribed. It is composed of spindle cells arranged in interlacing fascicles and merges with the smooth muscle bundles of the bladder wall.

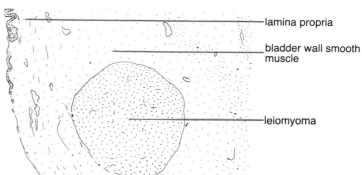

lamina propria

bladder wall smooth muscle

leiomyoma

Figure 12.53 As seen in this specimen, the botryoid type of embryonal rhabdomyosarcoma produces broad-based, translucent, polypoid masses.

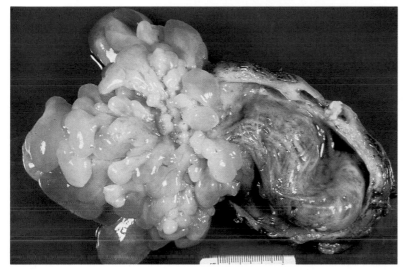

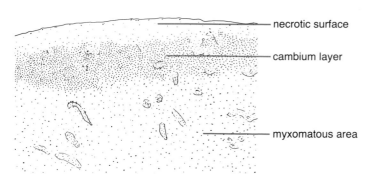

necrotic surface

cambium layer

myxomatous area

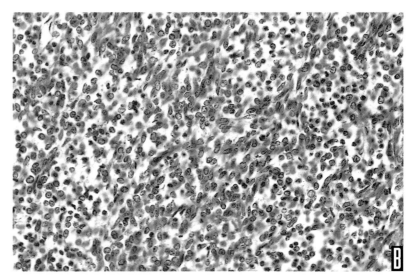

Figure 12.54 A, The grapelike masses occurring in botryoid sarcomas are hypocellular and appear myxomatous. A cambium layer, which consists of a submucosal zone of markedly increased cellularity, is characteristic. **B,** This variant of embryonal rhabdomyosarcoma contains primitive, round-to-oval mesenchymal cells.

tified in rhabdomyoblasts, which are large, eosinophilic cells with an eccentric nucleus and large nucleolus (Fig. 12.55).

Leiomyosarcoma

Leiomyosarcoma is an uncommon neoplasm of the bladder. It occurs with approximately the same frequency as rhabdomyosar-

coma during the second decade of life, but is more common in older patients; most patients are over 40 years of age. Prognosis depends upon grade; low-grade tumors tend to recur locally rather than metastasize.

MORPHOLOGY Low-grade tumors form intramural nodules covered by intact mucosa (Fig. 12.56A). High-grade neoplasms are

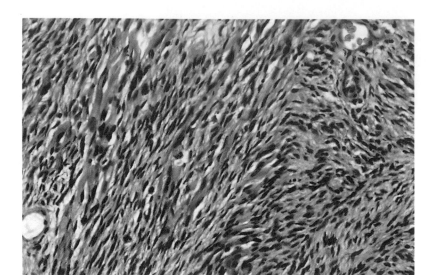

Figure 12.55 The spindle-cell variant of rhabdomyosarcoma is composed of bundles of elongate rhabdomyoblasts that have tapered eosinophilic cytoplasm and cross-striations.

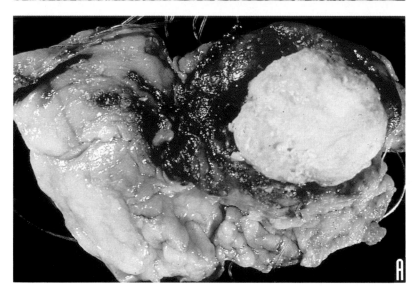

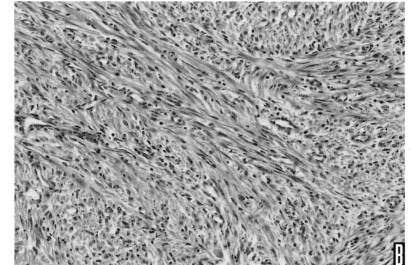

Figure 12.56 A, The discrete, gray-white mass protruding into the bladder lumen is a low-grade leiomyosarcoma. **B,** Microscopically, cellularity is slightly increased and an interlacing fascicular pattern, char-

acteristic of a smooth muscle neoplasm, is maintained. There is only mild nuclear enlargement and hyperchromatism. (Courtesy of R. Young, MD, Boston, Massachusetts)

Figure 12.57 This leiomyosarcoma shows obvious atypia. Enlarged, hyperchromatic, pleomorphic nuclei, as well as mitotic figures, are present.

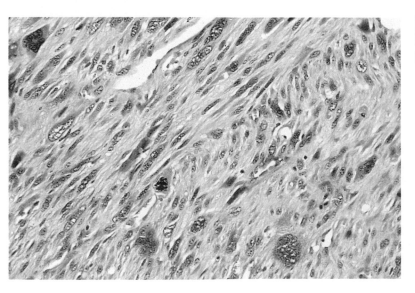

bulky and infiltrative; mucosal ulcerations are common. Myxoid leiomyosarcomas appear gelatinous.

Microscopically, leiomyosarcomas, like their benign counterpart, are composed of spindle cells arranged in parallel bundles and interlacing fascicles. Histologic grade is determined by the degree of cellularity, nuclear atypicality, and mitotic activity; necrosis is variable (Figs. 12.56B, 12.57).

Cytologic atypia may be slight or absent in the myxoid variant (Fig. 12.58). Although the absence of a prominent vascular stroma and diffuse inflammatory infiltrate is helpful in distinguishing this variant from a myxoid inflammatory pseudotumor (see Fig. 10.43), a demonstration of infiltrative and destructive margins is required for a definitive diagnosis of malignancy.

MISCELLANEOUS NEOPLASMS

PARAGANGLIOMA

Paragangliomas, which constitute about 0.06% of all bladder tumors, occur in children and adults (mean age, 41 years) and show no sex predilection. They are thought to arise from persistent small nests of paraganglionic tissue that have migrated to the bladder with sympathetic ganglia.

CLINICAL MANIFESTATIONS The classical clinical triad consists of paroxysmal hypertension; gross, intermittent, terminal, painless hematuria; as well as micturitional attacks of headache, shortness of breath, sweating, and pallor. Urinary secretory products include catecholamines or their metabolites (vanillylmandelic acid, metanephrine, or normetanephrine). Malignant, metastasizing tumors that secrete dopa or dopamine have been reported.

MORPHOLOGY Paragangliomas have ranged from 3 mm to 5.5 cm in diameter. Although most commonly located in the trigone in or near the ureteral orifices, they may occur in the dome and lateral walls. They are typically intramural and may produce a bulging, intraluminal, cauliflowerlike mass and mucosal ulcerations (Fig. 12.59). When placed in dichromate fixatives (e.g., Zenker's) or 10% potassium iodide, the tumor changes from gray-white to dark brown.

Microscopically, the majority of tumors are poorly circumscribed. Thin, richly vascular septa surround nests and cords of large polyhedral cells (Zellballen) that have eosinophilic, granular cytoplasm and

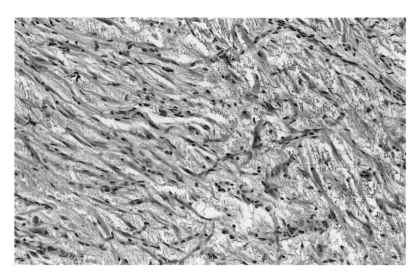

Figure 12.58 This myxoid leiomyosarcoma lacks an interlacing fascicular pattern. The neoplastic smooth muscle cells, which have tapered, eosinophilic cytoplasm, are separated by the myxoid stroma and appear haphazardly arranged. Scattered cells have enlarged nuclei, but hyperchromatism is minimal and nucleoli are not prominent. Small, nonbranching, thin-walled vessels are present. (Courtesy of R. Young, MD, Boston, Massachusetts)

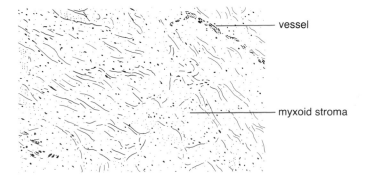

vessel

myxoid stroma

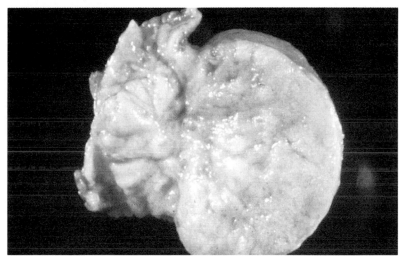

Figure 12.59 The paraganglioma in this specimen bulges beneath the mucosal surface of the bladder (right). The cut surface is lobulated and gray-white.

central ovoid nuclei (Fig. 12.60). Cellular and nuclear enlargement may be present, as well as neuroblastlike cells or ganglionlike cells. Cytoplasmic neurosecretory granules are present ultrastructurally.

CHORIOCARCINOMA

Choriocarcinoma of the bladder, which is extremely rare, has occurred predominantly in men. Similar extragonadal, nongestational, β-HCG–positive tumors occur in the stomach and lung. These neoplasms are thought to arise from a somatic cell that has undergone retrodifferentiation or transformation into a cell type functionally and morphologically similar to trophoblasts. Origin in a patient with an antecedent high-grade TCC has been reported.

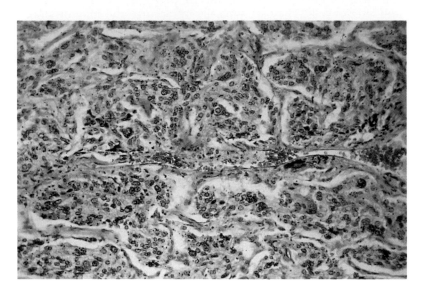

LYMPHOMA

In comparison with secondary bladder involvement, which occurs in about 10% of cases of systemic lymphoma, primary lymphoma of the bladder is rare. While it may occur at any age, most patients are 40–60 years old; females are affected more frequently than males. Origin from submucosal lymphoid follicles is suspected.

Primary bladder lymphoma presents as solid, rounded, predominantly submucosal masses covered by intact urothelium. They may form polypoid excrescences and lead to mucosal ulcerations. Most cases are non-Hodgkin's lymphomas.

Figure 12.60 Paragangliomas demonstrate a Zellballen pattern, with nests and cords of large polyhedral cells surrounded by thin, richly vascular septa. Scattered cells have enlarged nuclei.

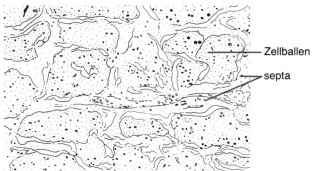

SECTION VI

Lesions of the Prostate and Seminal Vesicles

CHAPTER 13

Nonneoplastic Lesions of the Prostate and Seminal Vesicles

VARIANTS OF PROSTATITIS

Acute and chronic forms of prostatitis are extremely common but poorly understood inflammations that are caused by infectious and, occasionally, noninfectious agents. Several uncommon variants of prostatitis are often confused, both clinically and pathologically, with carcinoma.

ACUTE BACTERIAL PROSTATITIS

Acute, suppurative inflammation of the prostate is invariably due to bacterial infection. It most commonly affects sexually active individuals and is rare before the onset of puberty.

PATHOGENESIS Retrograde spread of organisms from the urethra appears to be the usual route of infection. Less often, bacterial prostatitis may result from urinary dissemination of an acute pyelonephritis or cystitis. Lymphatic or hematogenous seeding from extraneous foci may also occur. Not surprisingly, the distribution of responsible pathogens is similar to that of urinary tract infections. Prior to the development of antibiotic agents, *Neisseria gonorrhoeae* was the most common cause of acute prostatitis. Currently, other gram-negative organisms predominate, particularly strains of *Escherichia coli*. Species of *Klebsiella, Enterobacter, Pseudomonas, Proteus, Serratia,* and gram-positive organisms may also produce acute prostatitis.

CLINICAL MANIFESTATIONS Patients with acute prostatitis usually have a combination of systemic and localized symptoms. Fever, chills, malaise, myalgia, and arthralgia are accompanied by lower back pain, urinary urgency and frequency, dysuria, painful defecation, and perineal tenderness. Purulent urethral discharge, particularly on awakening, is common, but hematuria is unusual.

The correct diagnosis can be suspected after review of the symptoms. On rectal examination, the prostate is enlarged, boggy to palpation, and extremely tender. Prostatic massage, which generally produces a purulent urethral discharge, should be gentle due to the associated extreme pain and potential risk of bacteremia.

The diagnosis requires verification of an intraprostatic infection and identification of the offending organism. This is best achieved by quantitative, differential cultures of urine and prostatic secretions. Specimens obtained include: (1) the first 10 mL of voided urine, (2) midstream urine, (3) any prostatic secretions expressed by gentle massage, and (4) urine passed after prostatic massage. Patients with urethritis have their highest bacterial counts in the first specimen; patients with cystitis have their highest bacterial counts in the second specimen; patients with acute prostatitis have their highest counts in massaged secretions or postmassage voided urine. When the midstream specimen indicates an acute cystitis, it is difficult to exclude a coexisting prostatitis. Under these conditions, the urine should be sterilized by administering nitrofurantoin, penicillin G, or ampicillin for several days, followed by a repeat of the localization cultures.

Treatment of acute prostatitis requires prolonged (at least 30 days) antibiotic therapy with an agent to which the organism is known to be sensitive and which will reach the prostate in bactericidal concentrations. Trimethoprimsulfamethoxazole is currently the standard agent for gram-negative infections.

MORPHOLOGY Biopsy specimens are seldom obtained from patients with acute prostatitis. Instead, clinical features and bacterial cultures suffice for the diagnosis in virtually all individuals. Occasionally, acute prostatitis is present in prostatic tissue removed for nodular hyperplasia or other reasons. Except in rare hematogenously or lymphogenously disseminated infections, the inflammation begins in the prostatic ducts and acini. Aggregates of neutrophils accumulate in the ducts and glands, along with secretions and cell debris. Acute prostatitis may remain localized to only a portion of the gland or may result in diffuse disease. Eventually, the ducts and acini are destroyed and the infection spreads to involve the surrounding parenchyma (Fig. 13.1). Further necrosis and liquefaction may lead to the development of an abscess.

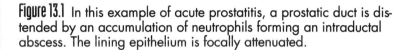

Figure 13.1 In this example of acute prostatitis, a prostatic duct is distended by an accumulation of neutrophils forming an intraductal abscess. The lining epithelium is focally attenuated.

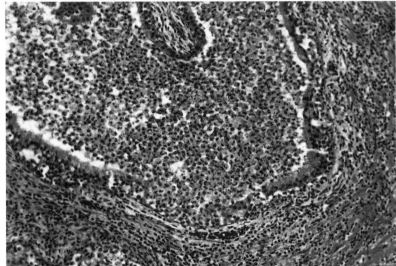

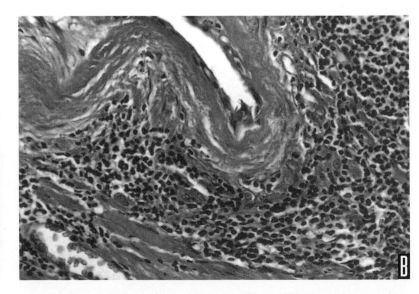

Figure 13.2 A, The numerous prostatic calculi seen in this prostatectomy specimen from a patient with chronic prostatitis are surrounded by zones of chronic inflammation. **B,** Long-standing inflammation may produce periductal fibrosis and distortion of the lumen.

Chronic Bacterial Prostatitis

PATHOGENESIS Factors promoting the development of chronic bacterial prostatitis are only partially understood. As with infections at other locations, any process impeding the flow of urine or prostatic secretions may lead to secondary infection. Normal prostatic secretions have antibacterial properties due to the presence of a zinc-containing polypeptide known as prostatic antibacterial factor. Men with chronic bacterial prostatitis have decreased levels of zinc in their prostatic fluid, but it is uncertain whether this promotes infection or is one of its consequences. Once a chronic infection is established, bacteria may be protected from both endogenous antibodies and exogenous antimicrobial agents by becoming incorporated in prostatic calculi.

CLINICAL MANIFESTATIONS The relationship between acute and chronic prostatitis is unclear. While an association is sometimes suggested, the two conditions may be unrelated, because acute prostatitis does not predispose to chronic disease and the onset of chronic prostatitis is not typically heralded by an acute infection. It is clear that patients with chronic prostatitis experience acute exacerbations.

As with acute disease, chronic bacterial prostatitis is usually associated with *E. coli* infection, but other coliform and gram-positive organisms have been implicated in some cases. Patients may be completely asymptomatic, but most have mild, often vague symptoms including lower back pain, dysuria, perineal pain or discomfort, and low-grade fever. A rectal examination may be completely normal. Quantitative cultures of urine and postmassage secretions, as described for acute prostatitis, are typically necessary to document bacterial prostatitis. Culture of an ejaculate may substitute for massage-induced secretions. Characteristically, patients with recurrent exacerbations culture the same organism throughout their clinical course.

Because medical management of chronic prostatitis often requires long-term, suppressive antibiotic therapy, it is important to verify a bacterial pathogenesis. Many otherwise excellent antibiotics are of little value in treating chronic prostatitis because they do not penetrate the prostatic parenchyma at bactericidal levels in the absence of acute inflammation. Trimethoprim is the antibiotic of choice because it easily infiltrates the prostatic tissues and is effective against most pathogens. Trimethoprim is almost always used in association with sulfamethoxazole, although it is unclear if the latter makes a measurable contribution. Rifampin, which also effectively penetrates the prostatic tissues, may be a valuable adjuvant to trimethoprim in problematic cases, although it should not be used alone because of its tendency to stimulate the development of resistant strains.

Chronic prostatitis is difficult to cure. Antimicrobial therapy most likely results only in long-term suppression of the infection. Surgical management is usually avoided. Transurethral resection of the prostate is not effective unless all of the infected tissue is removed. Prostatectomy carries a generally unacceptable risk of postsurgical impotence and urinary incontinence. The procedure, however, may be employed as a last resort in cases not controlled by other means.

MORPHOLOGY Biopsy is not generally helpful in diagnosing chronic bacterial prostatitis. Foci of chronic inflammation are often present in prostatic tissue, particularly in association with prostatic calculi (Fig. 13.2), nodular hyperplasia, or adenocarcinoma. These should not be interpreted as evidence of chronic bacterial infection. Conversely, lack of inflammation in a biopsy specimen does not exclude infection. The invariably focal nature of chronic prostatitis accounts for such sampling errors.

Tuberculous and Mycotic Infection

CLINICAL MANIFESTATIONS Tuberculous infection of the prostate or seminal vesicles, which is extremely uncommon, usually accompanies more obvious infection elsewhere in the genitourinary tract. Most patients have no prostatic symptoms. Infection is documented by culture or microscopic examination of seminal fluid or tissue. Atypical mycobacterial infections, most commonly seen in immunocompromised individuals, may also involve the prostate and seminal vesicles.

Isolated fungal infection of the prostate is extremely uncommon. Most patients with mycotic prostatitis have generalized disease. Blastomycosis, cryptococcosis, histoplasmosis, candidiasis, and coccidioidomycosis have been documented to involve the prostate under these circumstances. Coccidioidomycosis has also been shown to cause isolated prostatic disease after dissemination from a pulmonary focus.

MORPHOLOGY Tuberculous infection of the prostate or seminal vesicles produces caseating granulomas that may be visible grossly as zones of liquefied, "cheeselike" necrosis. (Fig. 13.3). Microscopically, it is characterized by an infiltrate of epithelioid, often multin-

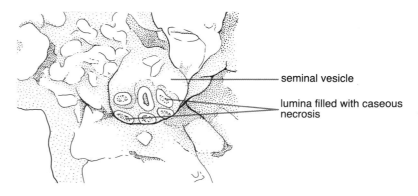

Figure 13.3 In this specimen of tuberculosis of the seminal vesicle, the vesicle has been transected. The lumina are filled with caseating necrotic material typical of a tuberculous granuloma.

seminal vesicle

lumina filled with caseous necrosis

ucleated, histiocytes (Fig. 13.4). Because a variety of infectious and noninfectious processes may produce identical images, definitive diagnosis requires culture or identification of acid-fast organisms. Most mycotic infections of the prostate also produce a granulomatous inflammatory response (Fig. 13.5). Silver methenamine stains highlight fungal forms (Fig. 13.6).

Some fungi, such as *Coccidioides immitis*, have a highly characteristic microscopic appearance. *Cryptococcus neoformans* is noted for its mucicarmine positivity in tissue sections. Other fungi may require culture for specific identification.

Malakoplakia of the Prostate

Malakoplakia, which has been described in a wide variety of extraurinary sites, is an uncommon process with a predilection for the urinary tract. The bladder is the most frequent location; prostatic involvement is rare. This rare prostatic lesion warrants mention because its clinical presentation may be confused with carcinoma.

PATHOGENESIS Malakoplakia represents a chronic bacterial infection, usually with *E. coli* or other coliforms, in which bacteria are phagocytosed by histiocytes but are incompletely digested. A defect in host lysosomal response has been postulated as a possible cause, but the exact mechanism is unclear.

CLINICAL MANIFESTATIONS Patients are typically middle-aged or elderly men with nonspecific symptoms referable to the prostate. Rectal examination typically demonstrates an enlarged, firm, and frequently nodular gland highly suspicious for carcinoma.

MORPHOLOGY Microscopically, a dense, inflammatory infiltrate replaces the prostatic glands and stroma. The predominant cell is a large, epithelioid, typically mononuclear histiocyte with abundant eosinophilic-to-vacuolated cytoplasm. Within the cytoplasm of scattered histiocytes are eosinophilic inclusions known as Michaelis–Gutmann bodies, which are targetlike intracellular structures representing mineralized remnants of bacterial cell walls. They can easily be visualized with a periodic acid-Schiff (PAS) stain (Fig. 13.7).

Nonspecific Granulomatous Prostatitis

After exclusion of prostatic granulomas of known pathogenesis, there remains a controversial group of lesions referred to as nonspecific granulomatous prostatitis.

PATHOGENESIS As the terminology implies, the cause or causes of nonspecific prostatitis are unknown. Spillage of prostatic fluid due to rupture of ducts and acini has been proposed as one mechanism for the development of granulomatous inflammation.

CLINICAL MANIFESTATIONS Granulomatous prostatitis, which is unusual before the age of 50 years, typically occurs in the seventh decade of life. The clinical history frequently suggests a lower urinary tract infection, with fever, urgency, burning on urination, and symptoms of minimal-to-moderate prostatic obstruction. Cystoscopy may demonstrate an associated cystitis. Transrectal palpation of the prostate leads to the clinical suspicion or strong consideration of carcinoma in a high percent-

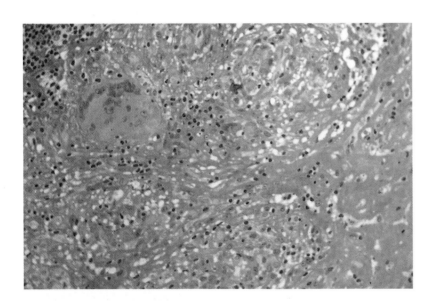

Figure 13.4 The multinucleated giant cells and necrosis (right) in this photomicrograph are typical of tuberculous prostatic infection. Culture or microscopic identification of organisms is necessary to confirm the diagnosis.

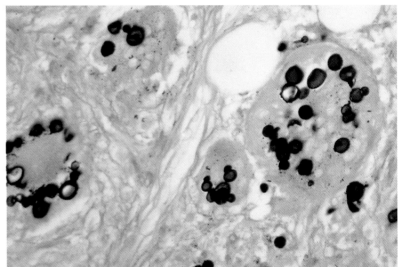

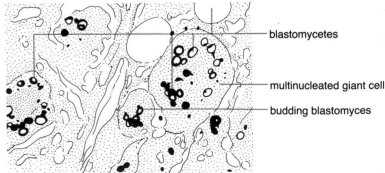

blastomycetes

multinucleated giant cell

budding blastomyces

Figure 13.5 Multiple, large, brown-staining yeast forms of blastomycosis are present in this photomicrograph. Budding yeast have a characteristic broad base (silver methenamine stain).

age of patients; findings suggestive of carcinoma include fixation of the gland, diffuse firmness, and nodularity.

MORPHOLOGY Grossly, the zones of prostatic involvement are nodular, firm, and tan to yellow, an appearance highly suggestive of prostatic carcinoma. Microscopically, this process is characterized by a nodular granulomatous infiltrate replacing the prostatic acini and stroma. Ruptured ducts and acini with leakage of secretions into the surrounding stroma are common. Multinucleated histiocytes are invariably present (Fig. 13.8).

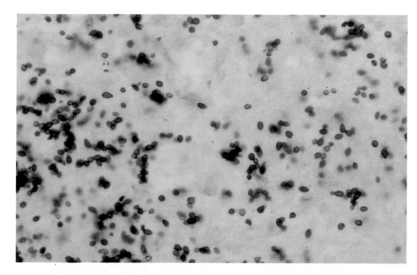

Figure 13.6 Numerous organisms approximately the size of erythrocytes can be seen in this example of histoplasmosis of the prostate. They are much smaller than those found in blastomycosis. Buds tend to be narrow-based. Culture is desirable to confirm the diagnosis.

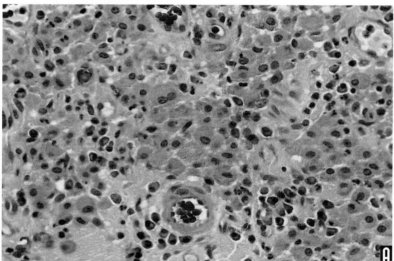

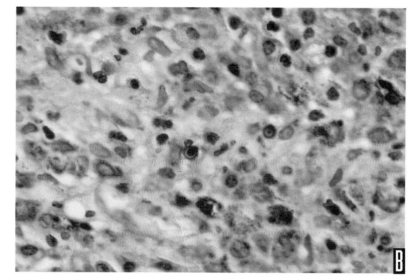

Figure 13.7 A, Sheets of histiocytes with abundant eosinophilic cytoplasm characterize prostatic malakoplakia. Michaelis–Gutmann bodies within the cytoplasm of these cells are difficult to see in this H&E-stained section. **B,** Targetlike Michaelis–Gutmann bodies here stain strongly with PAS stain. Ultrastructurally, these are aggregates of incompletely digested microorganisms.

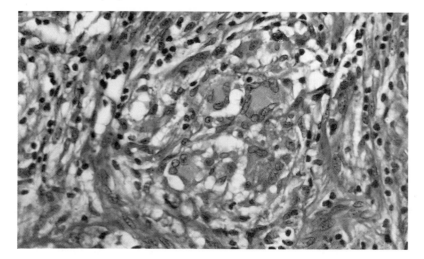

Figure 13.8 In nonspecific granulomatous prostatitis, a chronic inflammatory cell infiltrate with granulomatous aggregates of multinucleated histiocytes does not indicate infection. This reaction may represent a response to ruptured ducts, with leakage of secretions into the stroma.

In some instances, large numbers of histiocytes have foamy or xanthomatous cytoplasm due to the phagocytosis of lipid. The term xanthogranulomatous prostatitis has been applied to such cases, but they are simply a variant of nonspecific prostatitis (Fig. 13.9). Large granulomas may have centers undergoing liquefactive necrosis, but caseous necrosis such as that seen in tuberculous infections is absent. The stroma surrounding the granulomas may be fibrotic or demonstrate muscular hyperplasia. About 10% of cases contain prominent eosinophils.

Because the granulomatous inflammation may partially obscure an accompanying carcinoma, histologic sections must be carefully examined to exclude this possibility. The diagnosis of nonspecific granulomatous prostatitis is one of exclusion, and stains for microorganisms must also be performed.

Postsurgical Necrobiotic Prostatic Granuloma

This variant of prostatitis is a microscopically distinctive lesion that, when present, is always seen in prostatic tissue obtained following a biopsy or transurethral resection. The interval between the initial surgery and removal of the granuloma-containing specimen has varied from over four years to only a few days.

PATHOGENESIS Postsurgical prostatic granulomas appear to represent a reproducible response to the trauma of previous surgery. The association with prior transurethral resections has sug-

gested that this may be a response to cautery-induced damage. However, several cases of postsurgical granuloma have occurred following needle biopsy without cautery. Similar changes have also been described in the bladder wall following surgery, suggesting that injured prostatic glands and/or stroma are not required for these changes to develop.

CLINICAL MANIFESTATIONS It is highly unlikely that the granulomas produce any symptoms in addition to those that prompt the initial and subsequent procedures. Virtually all patients have had nodular hyperplasia or prostatic adenocarcinoma as their underlying lesions, and complaints were ascribed to these primary processes. There is no evidence that postsurgical granulomas are of any clinical importance, except for their potential confusion with other granulomatous processes, such as tuberculosis or allergic prostatitis.

MORPHOLOGY Postsurgical granulomas are usually too small to be grossly visible, but their microscopic appearance is highly characteristic. A central, circular to irregularly shaped zone of fibrinoid necrosis is surrounded by a rim of palisading epithelioid histiocytes, with a resulting image indistinguishable from a rheumatoid nodule (Fig. 13.10). The zone of necrosis typically measures less than 2 mm in greatest dimension, but in occasional lesions a sinuous tract of necrosis may extend throughout the specimen. Inflammation in the surrounding stroma, consisting of lymphocytes

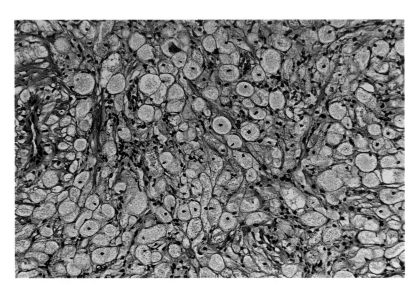

Figure 13.9 The xanthogranulomatous prostatitis in this photomicrograph is a variant of nonspecific prostatitis characterized by numerous lipid-laden histiocytes.

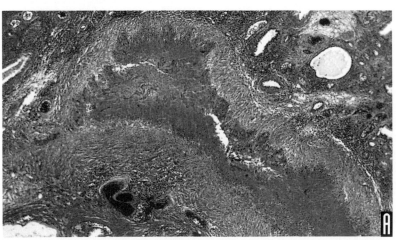

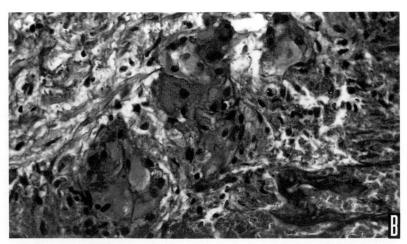

Figure 13.10 A, At low power, a sharply demarcated zone of necrosis is situated within the prostatic stroma in this illustration of postsurgical necrobiotic granuloma. **B,** At high power, the histiocytic cells surrounding the zone of necrosis (below right), can be seen in detail.

and plasma cells, is generally minimal. Scattered eosinophils may be present and can be numerous in some cases, particularly in those with a short interval between initial and subsequent biopsy. Multinucleated histiocytes may also be present in the intervening stroma. The usually multiple granulomas average four to five per specimen.

Nodular Prostatic Hyperplasia (Benign Prostatic Hypertrophy)

The normal prostate gland slowly enlarges from birth until puberty, when it undergoes a much more rapid increase in size. This enlargement may continue into the third decade of life before it stabilizes. Beginning at about 45 years of age, the prostate typically begins to follow one of two divergent courses. It may very slowly atrophy, a process that can continue for the remainder of the patient's life. More frequently, the prostate begins to develop progressive changes of nodular hyperplasia. The age at which this change begins as well as the rate at which it progresses are highly variable. Only a minority of patients become clinically symptomatic. The frequency of both symptomatic and asymptomatic prostatic enlargement increases with age. Randall reported evidence of partially obstructive nodular hyperplasia in 20% of males in the sixth decade of life, 30% in the seventh decade, and 40% in the eighth decade. The frequency of asymptomatic hyperplasia follows a parallel course, but the condition is much more common. Up to 95% of males in their eighth decade have evidence of nodular hyperplasia at autopsy.

PATHOGENESIS   Any theory that explains the development of nodular hyperplasia must account for several well known facts. It is an age-related process that is extremely uncommon before the age of 40 years. It does not occur in males who have had bilateral orchiectomy prior to the onset of puberty, and regression of disease is common following orchiectomy. The androgen dihydrotestosterone is present at high levels in the prostatic tissues. Finally, nodular hyperplasia can be induced in animals by androgen administration. A hormonal mechanism, therefore, is certainly involved.

However, a unifying theory detailing the initiating events and the roles of circulating- versus tissue-androgen levels, end-organ sensitivity, and pituitary feedback has not been developed.

CLINICAL MANIFESTATIONS   Prostatic enlargement without associated secondary changes is asymptomatic. Patients with nodular hyperplasia typically present with signs and symptoms of urinary obstruction or, less commonly, infection.

As the prostate enlarges, it distorts the prostatic urethra. When nodular hyperplasia predominantly involves the lateral lobes, it compresses the urethra to a ribbonlike structure. Median lobe involvement may be confined below the bladder, in which case the bladder is elevated with angulation of the urethra. If the enlarged median lobe protrudes into the bladder, it forms a pedunculated mass that may obstruct the urethral orifice by functioning as a ball valve. Obstruction may be acute, with associated bladder dilatation, or chronic, with secondary hypertrophy of the bladder musculature. The increased intravesicular pressure that occurs with hypertrophy of the detrusor muscle may lead to the formation of bladder diverticula, failure of the ureteral valves, urinary reflux, hydronephrosis, and renal insufficiency.

If the urethral obstruction is partial and chronic, as is usually the case, patients present with gradually increasing symptoms, including urinary frequency, nocturia, a sensation of incomplete voiding, decrease in the diameter and force of the urinary stream, difficulty in initiating or terminating urination, and posturination dribbling. Acute urinary retention may occur in previously asymptomatic individuals, but it is more commonly superimposed on chronic incomplete obstruction.

MORPHOLOGY   Nodular hyperplasia consists of a benign proliferation of prostatic epithelium, fibrous tissue, and smooth muscle. The relative amounts of each of these elements can vary tremendously, producing distinctly different gross and microscopic images. Nodular hyperplasia typically involves the periurethral prostatic tissue composing the so-called lateral and median lobes (Fig. 13.11). As the nodules expand, they compress a rim of muscle and fibrous tissue, producing a pseudocapsule that separates them from the surrounding prostate.

If the fibromuscular components predominate, the prostate may be diffusely enlarged or may contain firm, solid nodules. If the

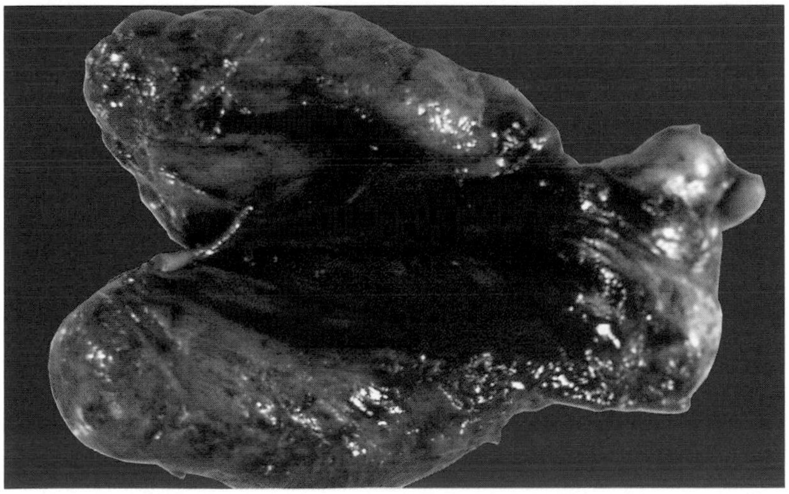

Figure 13.11   In this prostatectomy specimen, hyperplasia of the lateral and median lobes produces a distinctly three-lobed mass.

hyperplasia is predominantly glandular, the glands are often visible grossly as spongy or multicystic nodules (Fig. 13.12).

Microscopically, a fibromuscular component is invariably present either in association with epithelial hyperplasia or as pure mesenchymal nodules devoid of epithelial elements (Fig. 13.13). The epithelial component of nodular hyperplasia consists of aggregates of glands, that vary in size, with larger glands predominating. In some glands the epithelium may have a flattened, even atrophic, appearance (Fig. 13.14). Most commonly, however, there is epithelial hyperplasia in the form of papillary glandular infoldings, which may bridge glandular spaces in some sections, leading to confusion with cribriform carcinoma (Fig. 13.15). This pattern may be particularly prominent when the cells are composed of abundant clear cytoplasm. The term florid benign papillary/cribriform hyperplasia has been applied to this process (Fig. 13.16).

Microscopic distinction of nodular hyperplasia from carcinoma is usually not difficult if cytologic features are carefully evaluated. The epithelium of nodular hyperplasia is two cells in thickness. The outer, or basal, cell layer is often conspicuous, but it may be flattened and focally difficult to visualize. It is composed of small cells with uniform nuclei and little cytoplasm. The inner layer consists of cells with a columnar shape as well as prominent eosinophilic-to-clear cytoplasm. Most important, cell nuclei are uniform, and nucleoli are small or absent. Mitotic figures, which are extremely rare, never have an atypical configuration. The junction between the glands and stroma is sharply defined, without the blurred margin seen at the edges of carcinomatous glands.

It should be remembered that carcinoma may arise in, or at least be closely associated with, foci of epithelial hyperplasia. For this reason, histologic sections must be carefully studied to avoid overlooking such areas. Less commonly, the epithelium of nodular hyperplasia may show atypical cytologic or architectural features that fall short of overt carcinoma. These changes, which are discussed in more detail below, often signal the presence of carcinoma elsewhere in the prostate. Nonneoplastic secondary processes may also be present in nodular hyperplasia. Changes such as infarction, squamous metaplasia, basal cell hyperplasia, and chronic inflammation are discussed elsewhere in this chapter.

ATYPICAL EPITHELIAL HYPERPLASIA/DYSPLASIA

Careful observers of prostatic morphology have invariably encountered "borderline" proliferations possessing some, but not all, of the features of adenocarcinoma. A variety of terms has been applied to these lesions, whose exact relationship to carcinoma remains unclear. They may represent early neoplasms or may be atypical hyperplasias that lack the critical aberrations required for true carcinomas. For our purposes, we include them among the nonneoplastic proliferations, acknowledging the arbitrary nature of this classification. No convincing demonstration has shown that these atypical hyperplasias actually give rise to invasive adenocarcinomas; considering the limitations of sampling and study, this is not surprising. Since they are found much more frequently in prostatic tissue containing

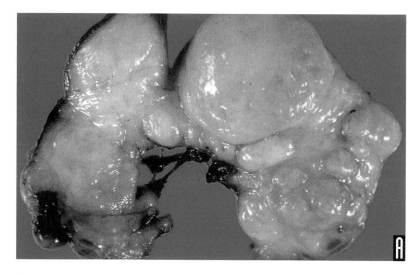

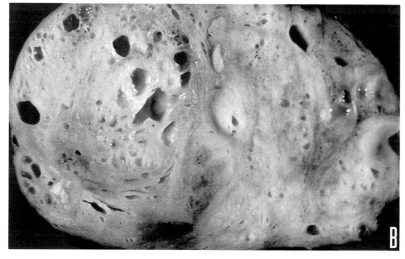

Figure 13.12 A, This prostatic cut section shows the multinodular nature of the hyperplasia. Cystic spaces are not grossly visible in this specimen. **B,** In contrast to **A,** the hyperplastic nodules in this prostate are distinctly cystic. The zone of red discoloration at the bottom represents a small infarct. India ink has been applied to the external surface of the specimen to demarcate the resection margin.

Figure 13.13 This characteristic fibromuscular variant of nodular hyperplasia consists of a mixture of glandular and fibromuscular elements. In some nodules, the latter components proliferate to the exclusion of epithelium.

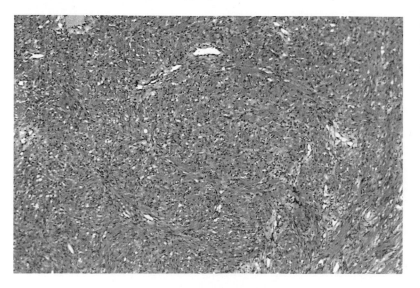

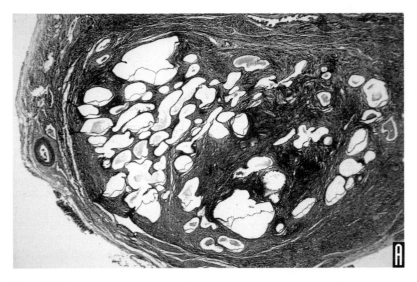

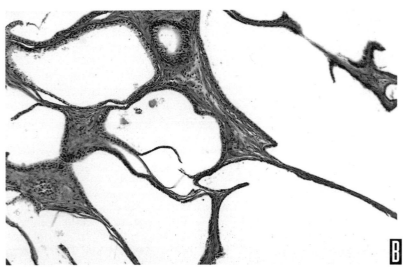

Figure 13.14 A, The cystic, glandular form of nodular hyperplasia seen here exhibits sharply circumscribed borders containing cystically dilated glands. The simple, nonpapillary configuration and large size of the glands exclude carcinoma, even at this low magnification. **B,** At higher magnification, the cysts are lined by a flattened layer of epithelium.

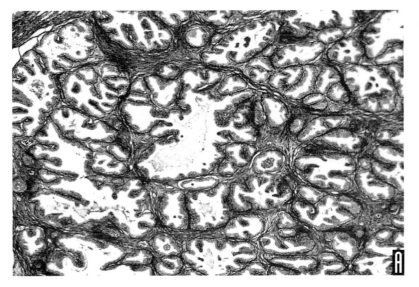

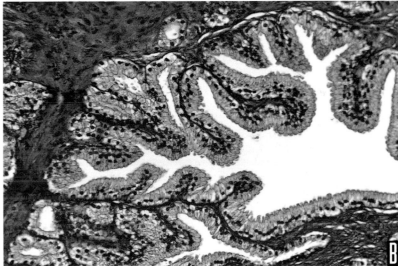

Figure 13.15 A, This example of nodular hyperplasia with papillary epithelial hyperplasia represents the more common pattern, in which there is a papillary proliferation of epithelial cells lining enlarged glands. The occasional cribriform structures that may be formed should not be confused with carcinoma. **B,** The epithelial cells in this medium-power photomicrograph have a tall, columnar configuration with uniform, basally located nuclei. Delicate fibrovascular stalks form the center of the papillae.

Figure 13.16 The florid papillary/cribriform variant of epithelial hyperplasia illustrated here may be confused with adenocarcinoma. The epithelial cells frequently have clear cytoplasm. Distinction of this process from adenocarcinoma rests on the cytologic blandness of the epithelial cells.

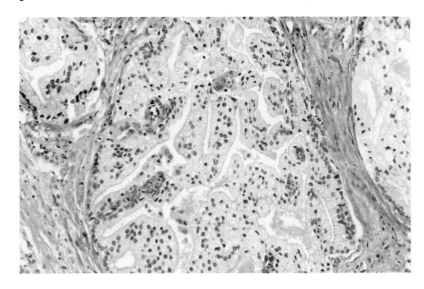

clear-cut adenocarcinoma than in similar specimens of benign prostate, they may be viewed, at the very least, as a marker of neoplasia. Their presence should stimulate a thorough search of all available material for an associated carcinoma.

Most of the initial work in the United States relating to these atypical proliferations was done by McNeal and colleagues, who have recognized two very different histologic patterns that seem to be associated with prostatic adenocarcinoma. One is predominantly a cytologic aberration; the other represents an architectural atypia with little or no cytologic derangement (see below).

INTRADUCTAL DYSPLASIA

CLINICAL MANIFESTATIONS Intraductal dysplasia is detected microscopically as an incidental finding in prostatic tissue removed for other reasons, particularly nodular hyperplasia and adenocarcinoma. Foci of dysplasia were found by McNeal and Bostwick in 82% of prostates containing carcinoma and only 43% of benign prostates. The frequency of dysplasia in benign glands rose slightly with age but not as rapidly as the frequency of carcinoma. The dominant grade of dysplasia also correlates with the presence or absence of carcinoma. Grade I dysplasia predominated with virtually equal frequency in benign and carcinomatous prostates; however, grades II and III dysplasia were dominant in only 8% of benign prostates as opposed to 44% of prostates containing carcinoma.

MORPHOLOGY Intraductal dysplasia is fundamentally a cytologic abnormality occurring within prostatic ducts and acini, having an otherwise normal configuration. Grade I dysplasia is characterized by cellular crowding and multilayering, accompanied by an increase in and variability of nuclear size (Fig. 13.17). Nuclear chromatin is normal; nucleoli are small and infrequent. Grade II dysplasia is similar to grade I, except that nuclear chromatin is increased and small nucleoli are slightly more common (Fig. 13.18). Grade III dysplasia is distinguished by the presence of numerous, large, typically eosinophilic nucleoli identical to those seen in invasive prostatic adenocarcinoma (Fig. 13.19). Solid papillations without central cores are common. Cells within these papillae may show

marked nuclear crowding, with pyknosis of the central nuclei. There may also be occasional intraluminal bridges resembling those seen in cribriform carcinoma.

ATYPICAL ADENOMATOUS HYPERPLASIA

CLINICAL MANIFESTATIONS As with intraductal dysplasia, this is an asymptomatic process detected incidentally in prostatic tissue removed for other reasons. The clinical features of this condition have not been as well documented as those of intraductal dysplasia, due in part to considerable variation in the criteria that distinguish atypical hyperplasia from well differentiated adenocarcinoma. A perusal of published illustrations will identify histologically similar lesions labeled as hyperplasia, atypical hyperplasia, adenosis, and well differentiated adenocarcinoma. We follow the criteria outlined by Gleason and reviewed below to distinguish these closely related lesions. As will be discussed in Chapter 14, the biologic behavior of these processes also follows a continuum, such that well differentiated adenocarcinoma (Gleason score 2) is seldom, if ever, associated with metastases. Thus, the controversy surrounding nomenclature is not associated with clinically important biologic differences.

MORPHOLOGY Microscopically, atypical hyperplasia consists of an abnormal proliferation of small, relatively uniform glands that show little or no cytologic atypia (Fig. 13.20). The Veterans Administration Cooperative Urologic Research Group has suggested the following criteria: (1) abnormally compact cluster of glands with an expansile, rather than infiltrative, growth pattern; (2) uniformity in size of glands; (3) relatively small, simple glands with rounded lumina; and (4) glands that may be focally lined by a single layer of epithelial cells. These features are shared by well differentiated adenocarcinoma, with the important exception that the latter has at least a few epithelial cells with prominent nucleoli larger than 1 μ in diameter. (For comparison, a red blood cell is approximately 5 μ in diameter in a standard formalin-fixed, paraffin-embedded section.) Thus, the presence of prominent nucleoli distinguishes atypical adenomatous hyperplasia from adenocarcinoma.

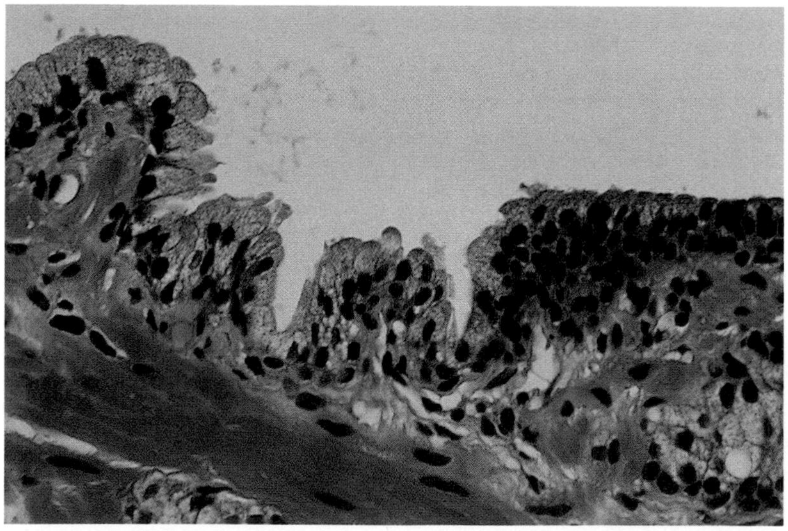

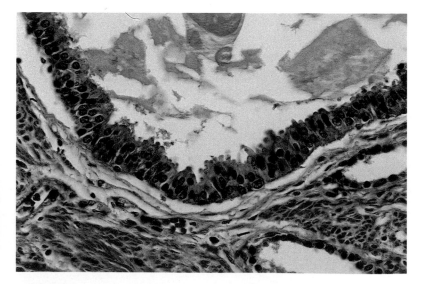

Figure 13.17 In this example of mild intraductal dysplasia, the normal epithelial cells at the left contrast with the cells at the right, which exhibit cellular crowding, multilayering, and an increase in nuclear size. Changes of this mild degree may not be important, as they are seen with equal frequency in both benign and malignant prostatic specimens.

Figure 13.18 As seen in this photomicrograph, moderate intraductal dysplasia exhibits more cellular crowding, disorganization, and variation in nuclear size than does the milder form seen in Figure 13.17.

Metaplastic and Pseudoneoplastic Lesions
Basal Cell Prostatic Hyperplasia

CLINICAL MANIFESTATIONS This benign, nonneoplastic process is known by a variety of terms, including basal cell adenoma, "fetalization" of the prostate, and embryonal hyperplasia. It is an asymptomatic, incidental finding in prostatic tissue removed for nodular hyperplasia. Apparently unrelated foci of adenocarcinoma have also been described in association with this change. Patients, who are typically over 60 years of age, present with obstructive symptoms related to their accompanying nodular hyperplasia. Basal cell hyperplasia has no intrinsic clinical importance, but lack of familiarity with it may lead to confusion with true neoplasms such as adenocarcinoma, adenoid cystic tumor, transitional cell carcinoma, or small cell undifferentiated carcinoma.

MORPHOLOGY Basal cell hyperplasia is an acinar lesion that is always closely associated with more conventional glandular hyperplasia. Areas of transition between the two are common. The basal cells usually form sharply circumscribed nests in the prostatic stroma, often with palisading of the peripheral cell layer (Fig. 13.21).

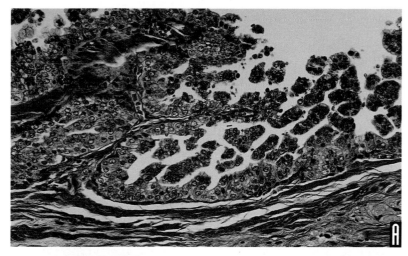

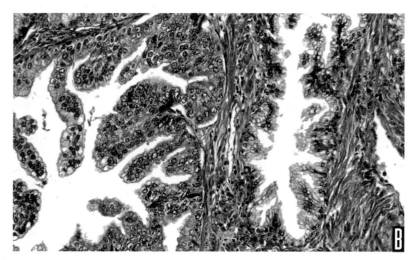

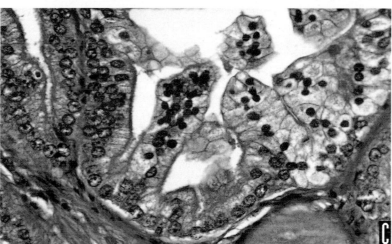

Figure 13.19 A, The cytologic features of severe intraductal dysplasia are not apparent at this magnification, but a papillary architecture is obvious. **B,** The severely dysplastic gland on the left contrasts with the cytologically normal gland on the right. **C,** The sharp junction of dysplastic and cytologically normal epithelial cells is illustrated in this high-power photomicrograph. The dysplastic cells have enlarged nuclei with occasional prominent nucleoli. (Compare nuclear size in this illustration with the examples in Figures 13.17 and 13.18 taken at the same magnification.)

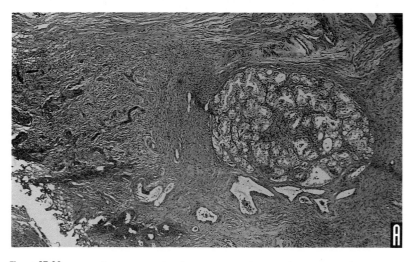

Figure 13.20 A, In the atypical adenomatous hyperplasia seen here, small, irregular, closely packed glands form a circumscribed nodule. **B,** At higher power, the epithelial cells in atypical adenomatous hyperplasia lack the prominent nucleoli of adenocarcinoma. A two- cell layer is present focally. Distinction of atypical adenomatous hyperplasia from well differentiated adenocarcinoma may be problematic and somewhat arbitrary.

Central lumina containing eosinophilic secretory material may be present in some cell nests. Aggregates of basaloid cells may also be seen "budding" from the periphery of typical hyperplastic glands. Cytologically, these are small cells with uniform nuclei and scant amounts of cytoplasm. Nucleoli may be prominent, but mitoses are rare or absent, and an infiltrative growth pattern is never seen. Confusion with carcinoma is avoided by noting the complete lack of nuclear pleomorphism (see Fig. 13.22B). The proliferating basal cells do not stain for prostatic-specific antigen or prostatic acid phosphatase.

Sclerosing Adenosis of the Prostate Gland

PATHOGENESIS This microscopically distinctive and worrisome lesion may be viewed as a variant of atypical adenomatous hyperplasia, although it is usually considered as a separate entity. Encountered in about 2% of prostatic specimens, its pathogenesis is unknown. It is unclear whether sclerosing adenosis should be considered a benign neoplasm or a reactive proliferation. As yet, there has been no evidence that sclerosing adenosis is a marker for carcinoma.

CLINICAL MANIFESTATIONS To date, cases of sclerosing adenosis have been incidental findings in patients undergoing transurethral resections for urinary obstruction due to prostatic enlargement. Accordingly, patients are generally older, with a mean age of approximately 70 years.

MORPHOLOGY Nodules of sclerosing adenosis have measured up to 1 cm in diameter in resection specimens. Most often, however, they are encountered as microscopic foci in curettings. At low-power, these are worrisome cellular proliferations with irregularly shaped glands "infiltrating" a spindle cell stroma (Fig. 13.22). At higher magnification, many of the glands are surrounded by a well-formed basement membrane (Fig. 13.23); others have a recognizable two-cell layer. Gland lumina may be empty, contain eosinophilic secretions, or, occasionally, contain intraluminal crystalloids. Although intraluminal crystalloids show a strong association with prostatic adenocarcinoma, they can be encountered in other benign lesions such as atypical adenomatous hyperplasia. Cell cytoplasm may be eosinophilic or vacuolated. The epithelial cells may show mild to moderate cytologic atypia, and occasional examples may contain cells with enlarged nucleoli.

The spindled stromal cells are cytologically uniform, resemble fibroblasts (Fig. 13.23A), and are separated by a collagenous to somewhat myxoid matrix. A clear-cut smooth muscle stromal component, analogous to the normal prostatic stroma, is absent. Immunohistochemical stains for cytokeratin and muscle specific actin will highlight the outer cell layer of the glands, which appears to have myoepithelial features. Scattered spindled stromal cells will also label for these antigens. These staining features are valuable in distinguishing sclerosing adenosis from adenocarcinoma. The latter neoplasm lacks a cytokeratin- or actin-positive basal cell layer.

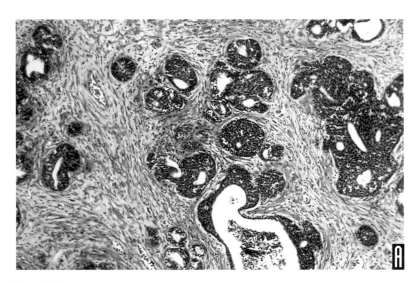

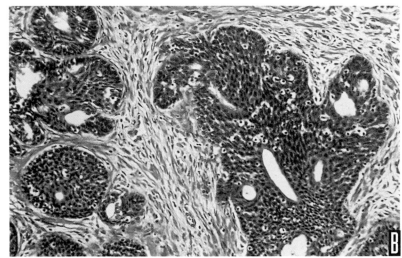

Figure 13.21 A, In basal cell hyperplasia, cuffs of basal cells surround central lumina of prostatic acini. **B,** Viewed at high power, the basal cells have uniform nuclei that lack the cytologic features of adenocarcinoma.

Figure 13.22 Sclerosing adenosis of the prostate gland has an alarming low-power appearance, with small, irregularly shaped glands in a cellular, spindle-cell stroma.

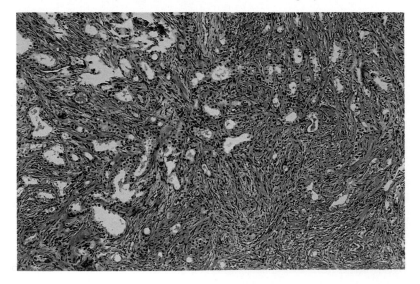

Squamous Metaplasia and Prostatic Infarct

CLINICAL MANIFESTATIONS As with many entities discussed in this section, squamous metaplasia of the prostate is an asymptomatic, incidental finding that may be misdiagnosed as a more ominous process. Commonly occurring in association with a prostatic infarct, it may also be seen as an apparently isolated lesion following estrogen administration, or may be associated with chronic infection.

Focal prostatic infarction is found in up to 25% of patients with nodular hyperplasia. Edema and inflammation developing in response to an infarction may lead to acute urinary retention or hematuria. Elevated serum acid phosphatase is present in about one third of patients.

MORPHOLOGY Squamous metaplasia is usually too small to be detected grossly, although, in retrospect, small squamous pearls may be present as tiny white flecks. Microscopically, squamous metaplasia consists of bland, keratinizing or glycogenated squamous epithelium that replaces the normal ductal or acinar lining cells. As the squamous component proliferates, it may obliterate the preexisting ductal or acinar lumina, resulting in nests of mature squamous cells (Fig. 13.24).

Prostatic infarcts, if large and well developed, may be visible grossly as circumscribed, soft, discolored nodules (see Fig. 13.12B). Microscopically, they are irregular, sharply defined zones of coagulative necrosis. Both glandular and stromal components are affected. Hemorrhage may exist in the infarcted area, and there may be an infiltrate of polymorphonuclear leukocytes. Squamous metaplasia arising in an infarct begins in the marginal tissue at the edge of the necrosis. Both acini and ducts are involved. As the infarct heals, fibroblasts proliferate in the stroma, and squamous, as well as glandular, epithelial cells repopulate the necrotic acini.

Postsurgical Pseudosarcomatous Nodules

In 1984 Proppe, Scully, and Rosai reported eight examples of an unusual spindle cell proliferation in the genitourinary region. All of the patients had undergone prior surgery in the area of the spindle cell tumor from five weeks to three months previously.

PATHOGENESIS The exact nature of these spindle cell nodules remains unclear. They are apparently reactive stromal proliferations stimulated in some fashion by prior surgery. A close relationship to other pseudosarcomatous stromal reactions such as nodular and proliferative fasciitis is suggested on the basis of morphologic similarities.

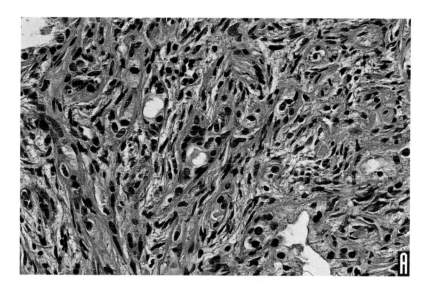

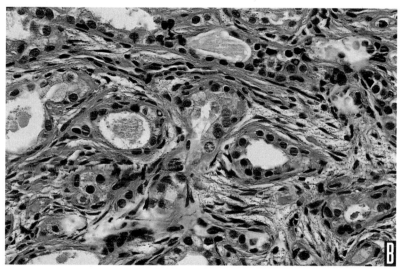

Figure 13.23 A, At higher magnification, the glands of sclerosing adenosis are distorted by the surrounding stroma. A well formed basement membrane surrounds the glands, and there is no cytologic atypia. **B,** The glands of sclerosing adenosis exhibit mild variation in nuclear size. Well formed basement membranes and an outer cell layer are visible around several glands.

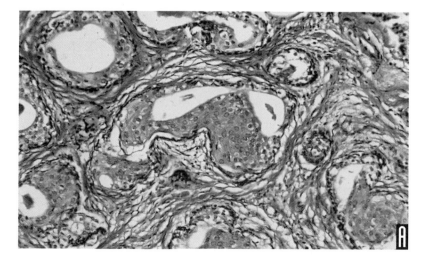

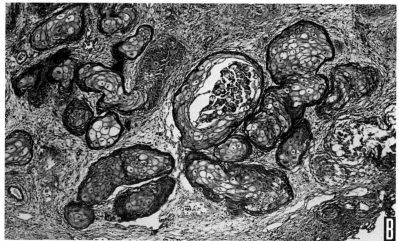

Figure 13.24 A, The prostatic acini in this illustration contain nests of metaplastic squamous cells without an associated infarct. **B,** After prolonged estrogen therapy, squamous metaplasia with clear, glycogenated cytoplasm is common.

CLINICAL MANIFESTATIONS Four of the lesions developed in women and involved the vagina. The remaining four occurred in men: three developed in the prostatic urethra, one in the bladder. The male patients had required prior transurethral resection for nodular prostatic hyperplasia or transitional cell carcinoma of the bladder.

Two of the male patients complained of hematuria. A third patient developed symptoms of urinary obstruction. The fourth patient's lesion was detected in a routine follow-up biopsy. The first three lesions were visualized at cystoscopy and described as unusual looking masses or heaped-up tumor. In most instances, incomplete resections (as judged for malignant lesions) were performed, yet all of the patients remained disease free 9-60 months later.

MORPHOLOGY The lesions had a highly characteristic and uniform microscopic appearance. Intersecting fascicles of plump spindle cells interdigitated with delicate capillaries. Stromal collagen or hyalinization was inconspicuous or focal. A storiform growth pattern was absent. Surface ulceration, together with an inflammatory infiltrate, was invariably observed. Extravasated erythrocytes formed rows and clusters between the spindle cell component in a pattern reminiscent of Kaposi's sarcoma (Fig. 13.25).

Spindle cells had prominent eosinophilic-to-amphophilic cytoplasm. Slightly enlarged nuclei were relatively uniform, with delicate chromatin and small nucleoli. Mitotic figures were numerous, but obviously atypical forms were not seen. Ultrastructural studies identified the proliferating spindle cells as fibroblasts.

This newly documented pseudosarcomatous postsurgical reaction is described in detail because of its alarming microscopic appearance and potential for confusion with a true sarcoma. The history

of prior surgery, the generally small size of the lesion, and, most important, the lack of objective nuclear anaplasia or atypical mitoses aid in this distinction.

Pseudoinfiltration of Skeletal Muscle and Nerve

MORPHOLOGY These two histologic variants found in otherwise normal prostatic tissue may easily be mistaken for carcinoma. Approximately 17% of prostate glands have skeletal muscle fibers within the prostatic parenchyma that may be closely associated with glandular epithelium (Fig. 13.26). The presence of glands that seem to infiltrate skeletal muscle in a biopsy specimen may lead to the erroneous conclusion that a carcinoma has infiltrated the prostatic capsule and extended into the surrounding musculature. Attention to the microscopic features of the glands and awareness of this normal anatomic variation prevent confusion.

Perineural invasion is a common, diagnostically useful finding in prostatic adenocarcinoma. It is also a frequent feature of carcinomas occurring at other locations. Perineural, or even intraneural, invasion is not, however, fully diagnostic of carcinoma. Benign epithelial proliferations may occasionally demonstrate perineural or intraneural growth. Several recent studies have convincingly documented benign prostatic glands in the perineural space, and Cramer illustrated benign glands within a nerve. Interestingly, he postulated that this may represent nerve growth around preexisting glands, rather than the converse. Whatever the mechanism, benign epithelium, prostatic or otherwise, is occasionally found in close association with peripheral nerves (Fig. 13.27). This should not lead to an a priori diagnosis of carcinoma. The latter interpretation rests solely on the morphologic features of the epithelium in question.

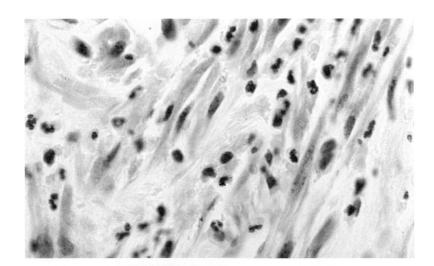

Figure 13.25 This postsurgical pseudosarcomatous nodule is an unusual proliferation whose cellularity and mitotic rate may lead to confusion with sarcoma. Cellular pleomorphism is minimal, however, and atypical mitotic figures are not seen. The inflammatory infiltrate is common. Extravasated red blood cells between widely separated, proliferating spindle cells are characteristic of this process.

Figure 13.26 Skeletal muscle fibers may be present within the prostatic capsule. Benign glands "invading" these muscle bundles must not be misinterpreted as adenocarcinoma infiltrating extraprostatic muscle.

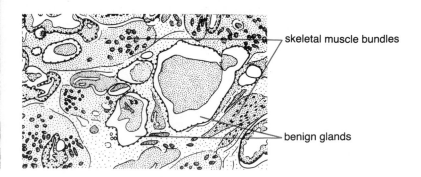

skeletal muscle bundles

benign glands

Seminal Vesicle Atypia

MORPHOLOGY Needle biopsies and cytologic aspirations of the prostate frequently traverse one of the seminal vesicles, yielding tissue fragments or exfoliated epithelial cells from the latter structures. This would be of no consequence except for the fact that the seminal vesicles in about 75% of adult males contain cells that could be confused with prostatic carcinoma by the unwary pathologist or cytologist. Fortunately, these cells are well documented, although their pathogenesis is poorly understood. Similar changes occur in the epididymis (see Chapter 17).

Epithelial cells with enlarged, hyperchromatic nuclei appear in the seminal vesicle at about the time of puberty, increasing in numbers with age. Initially, there is a moderate gain in nuclear size, with a coarse clumping of nuclear chromatin. As the amount of nuclear material increases, it forms a homogeneous, densely staining mass that fills an even larger nuclear volume. Some nuclei reach gigantic proportions, with diameters ten or more times greater than normal. Mitoses are uniformly absent.

Distinction from prostatic carcinoma in needle biopsy and fine-needle aspiration cytology specimens is based on cytologic features. The seminal vesicle cells have uniform, often "inkblot," enlarged nuclei. Nucleoli and mitoses are absent. Cells with large nuclei also have increased cytoplasm so that the nuclear-to-cytoplasmic ratio remains relatively normal. Finally, the seminal vesicle epithelium typically contains prominent lipofuscin pigment (Fig. 13.28). When larger specimens are available, the characteristic architecture of the seminal vesicle is a further distinguishing feature.

Prostatic Atrophy

Atrophy of prostatic glands and stroma, like nodular hyperplasia, is an age-related process. Unlike nodular hyperplasia, however, it is of no clinical importance except for its potential confusion with adenocarcinoma.

Atrophic changes may predominate in prostatic specimens, but often they occur in concert with areas of hyperplasia. The end result of combined stromal and glandular atrophy is a zone of tightly packed, small glands, an image reminiscent of adenocarcinoma (Fig. 13.29). The atrophic epithelial cells are low, cuboidal, or flattened; the underlying basal cell layer may be difficult to discern. Distinction from adenocarcinoma is most easily made based on cytologic features. The nuclei in prostatic atrophy are small and hyperchromatic, without nucleoli.

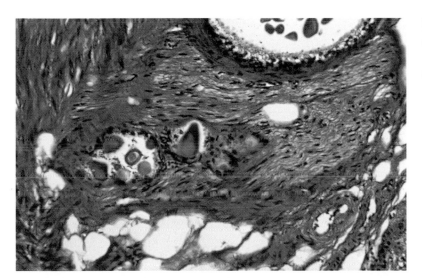

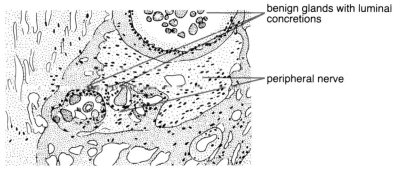

Figure 13.27 Perineural and intraneural invasion are common features of adenocarcinoma, but this phenomenon is rarely associated with benign glands. The lack of nuclear features of malignancy in such glands allows distinction. (Courtesy of S.F. Cramer, MD, Rochester, New York)

benign glands with luminal concretions

peripheral nerve

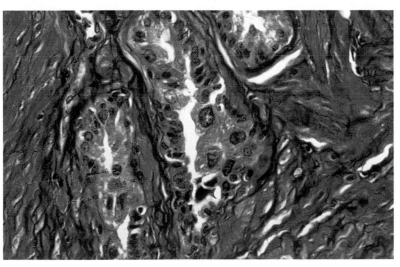

Figure 13.28 When the seminal vesicle is penetrated during needle biopsy of the prostate, the atypical cells may be confused with prostatic carcinoma. Although the nuclei are large, they lack nucleoli and often resemble inkblots. The presence of yellow-brown lipofuscin pigment in the cytoplasm is typical of seminal vesicle epithelium.

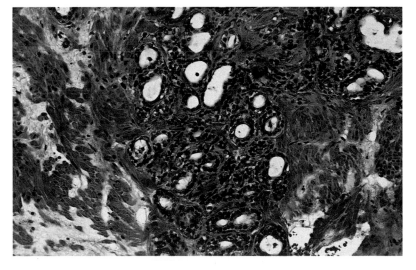

Figure 13.29 In prostatic glandular atrophy, small, tightly packed, atrophic glands are composed of cuboidal cells with uniform, small nuclei. Nucleoli are not present.

CHAPTER 14

Neoplastic Lesions of the Prostate and Seminal Vesicles

EPITHELIAL POLYPS OF THE PROSTATIC URETHRA

A histologically diverse group of polypoid epithelial proliferations may arise in the prostatic urethra. They are impossible to distinguish endoscopically, but important clinical distinctions mandate their separation.

PATHOGENESIS The origin of these polyps is speculative. Although prostatic or adenomatoid polyps may not be neoplasms in the narrow sense of the term, controversy regarding this point warrants their inclusion in this chapter, as does their occasional association with carcinoma.

Theories that account for the presence of prostatic-type epithelium in the prostatic urethra include ectopic urethral prostate, prolapse of prostatic epithelium into the urethra, and prostatic metaplasia of transitional epithelium. The origin of adenomatoid polyps is also unclear. An early theory suggested that they were a hamartoma of mesometanephric tissue; ultrastructural studies have both supported and refuted this point. A resemblance to adenomatoid tumors of the mesothelial type (see Chapter 17) has not been demonstrated. Negative immunocytochemical studies for prostatic markers also make prostatic origin unlikely. The most plausible possibility is an unusual metaplasia of transitional epithelium, probably secondary to longstanding irritation.

CLINICAL MANIFESTATIONS Prostatic polyps occur in a broad age range, with a median age at presentation of 50 years. The most common presenting complaint is gross hematuria. Symptoms of dysuria, urinary tract infection, or hemospermia may occasionally be present.

While patients with prostatic-type polyps do not typically have histories of antecedent urinary tract abnormalities or prior surgery, patients with adenomatoid-type polyps have often had previous surgery, longstanding partial obstruction, or repeated infections.

Cystoscopically, prostatic and adenomatoid polyps produce papillary or frondlike masses. The posterior portion of the prostatic urethra is almost invariably involved, but other regions may also be affected. Both prostatic and adenomatoid polyps occasionally occur in the bladder's trigone region.

Transurethral resection is the treatment of choice for epithelial polyps of the prostatic urethra. Polyps with prostatic-type epithelium almost never recur. Recurrence of adenomatoid-type polyps is much more common, but it may be managed by repeat excision.

MORPHOLOGY

PROSTATIC-TYPE POLYPS Grossly, these are small lesions, usually less than 1 cm in size after removal. Intact lesions may have a papillary appearance. Microscopically, there is typically a mixed papillary-acinar configuration with widely varying amounts of each component. The epithelium lining the papillae and acini is identical to that of the normal prostate. Beneath a surface layer of columnar cells with clear-to-pale eosinophilic cytoplasm, discrete cell borders, and basal nuclei lies a basal layer of flattened cells. Mitotic figures are not seen, and an inflammatory cell component is usually absent. Prostatic-type polyps stain strongly positive with immunocytochemical markers for prostatic epithelium, such as prostatic-specific antigen (Fig. 14.1).

ADENOMATOID POLYPS These polyps are composed of complex papillary and tubular epithelium overlying an edematous, often chronically inflamed stroma. The epithelium consists of a single layer of predominantly cuboidal cells with granular, eosinophilic cytoplasm (Fig. 14.2). Many cells contain intracytoplasmic vacuoles. Some cells may have a "hobnail" shape with enlarged nuclei and a basal cytoplasmic constriction. Immunocytochemical stains for prostatic acid phosphatase as well as prostatic-specific antigen are negative. Adenomatoid polyps must be distinguished from rare clear cell papillary adenocarcinomas that arise in the bladder or urethra. The latter are far more common in females than in males, occur in older individuals, and grow focally as sheets of clear cells with pleomorphism and mitotic activity.

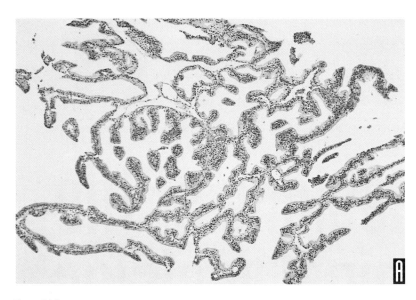
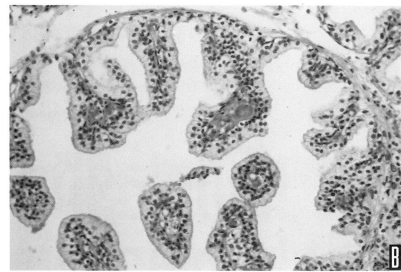

Figure 14.1 **A,** This prostatic-type urethral polyp illustrates the typical delicate papillary and glandular architecture. **B,** Seen at higher magnification, the epithelial cells are identical to those of the normal prostate.

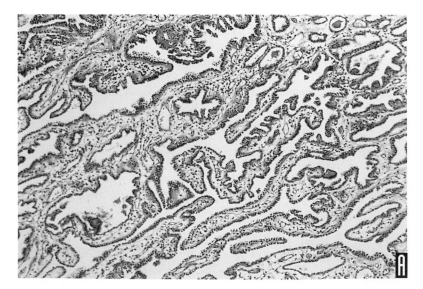
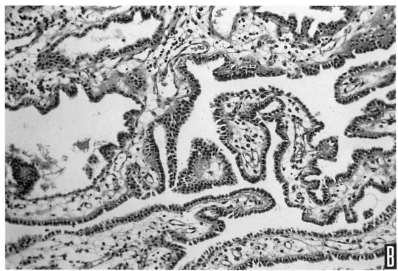

Figure 14.2 **A,** This adenomatoid urethral polyp exhibits a complex glandular and papillary pattern similar to that of prostatic-type polyps. **B,** At higher magnification, the lining epithelial cells are cuboidal and lack the prominent cytoplasm of prostatic-type epithelial cells.

"ENDOMETRIOID" ADENOCARCINOMA OF THE PROSTATIC URETHRA AND DUCTS

Melicow and Pachter were the first to recognize an unusual adenocarcinoma arising in the region of the prostatic utricle that strongly resembled endometrial adenocarcinoma. Several years later, Melicow and Tannenbaum reported a series of six such cases. Many larger series have been published subsequently.

PATHOGENESIS The prostatic utricle is widely believed to represent, at least in part, a vestigial müllerian structure. The location and appearance of these neoplasms initially suggested that the tumors were of müllerian origin and represented true endometrial-type adenocarcinomas.

   Subsequent studies of clinical behavior, morphologic features, and antigen expression have effectively excluded the above hypothesis. "Endometrioid" adenocarcinoma of the prostate has been shown to respond, in some instances, to androgen depletion and estrogen administration, the reverse of what would be expected for a müllerian-derived neoplasm. These tumors are frequently closely associated with more typical patterns of prostatic ductal and acinar adenocarcinoma. Every immunocytochemical study has documented the presence of prostatic acid phosphatase and prostatic-specific antigen in the tumor cells, markers which are always absent from uterine endometrial tumors. It thus seems certain that "endometrioid" prostatic adenocarcinoma is a misnomer applied to a variant of prostatic ductal adenocarcinoma that superficially resembles uterine endometrial adenocarcinoma.

CLINICAL MANIFESTATIONS Patients with "endometrioid" prostatic adenocarcinoma tend to be older males, typically no younger than their seventh decade. Obstruction and hematuria are the most common presenting complaints. Cystoscopy invariably demonstrates a papillary, exophytic mass protruding from the prostatic ducts in the region of the utricle (verumontanum). Rectal examination often documents an enlarged prostate due to nodular hyperplasia or an associated conventional adenocarcinoma.

   Therapy varies, depending in large part on the presence or absence of other forms of carcinoma. Transurethral resection has been successful in the treatment of purely exophytic tumors. Although initially believed to be an indolent neoplasm, "endometrioid" prostatic adenocarcinoma has been shown, in larger series, to have a biologic behavior approximating that of conventional prostatic adenocarcinoma.

MORPHOLOGY As noted above, these tumors have a microscopic appearance strikingly similar to that of uterine adenocarcinoma. A papillary and cribriform arrangement of complex glands is typical. The neoplastic cells have a stratified columnar appearance with prominent eosinophilic cytoplasm. Nuclear pleomorphism is usually moderate or marked; mitotic figures are abundant. Cytoplasmic mucin is absent or sparse. Prostatic-specific antigen and prostatic acid phosphatase are immunocytochemically demonstrable (Fig. 14.3).

TYPICAL (ACINAR) PROSTATIC ADENOCARCINOMA

Prostatic adenocarcinoma is by far the predominant malignancy of the male genitourinary system. Although it is the second most common cancer in males and the most frequent carcinoma in nonsmoking males, it remains poorly understood; very little is known about its causative factors. The dramatic increase of both latent and clinically detectable carcinoma with advancing age is well recognized. Age-matched incidence rates demonstrate considerable geographic and racial variation, some of which must be ascribed to extraneous biasing factors. Nonetheless, some reported regional and racial fluctuations appear to accurately reflect differences in cancer incidence. Prostatic adenocarcinoma is much less common in Asians, as compared with whites and blacks. Considerable regional variation in incidence also exists among individual races.

PATHOGENESIS Whether individuals migrating from low- to high-incidence regions tend to acquire prostatic carcinoma at the higher rate has not been conclusively determined. Some studies have suggested a slightly increased cancer rate after migration, which implies that an environmental factor may be involved. Cadmium has been implicated as a carcinogen, but other environmental carcinogens have not been identified.

   Androgens play a permissive role in the evolution and maintenance of prostatic carcinoma, but they are probably not carcinogenic per se. Eunuchs do not develop these tumors, and the partial tumor regressions that often follow orchiectomy are well known.

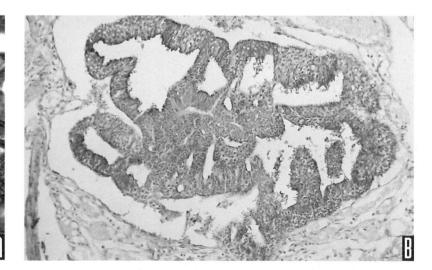

Figure 14.3 A, In "endometrioid" adenocarcinoma, the tumor, which arises in the prostatic ducts or urethra, is light-microscopically indistinguishable from adenocarcinoma of the endometrium. **B,** Prominent staining for prostatic-specific antigen supports the concept that these tumors arise from prostatic epithelium, in spite of their dramatic resemblance to müllerian-derived uterine tumors (anti-prostatic-specific antigen, hematoxylin).

There is no demonstrable relationship between circulating serum levels of sex steroid hormones and the development of prostatic carcinoma.

CLINICAL MANIFESTATIONS Prostatic carcinoma has two biologically distinctive forms. Latent (stage A) carcinoma is not clinically detectable, appearing as an incidental finding in prostatic tissue removed for other reasons. Except for rare high-grade tumors discovered fortuitously and tumors extensively involving the gland (stage A2), small foci of latent carcinoma are associated with little increased mortality and often require no specific treatment. It has been postulated that these tumors, although morphologically identical to clinical carcinomas, lack critical promoting factors for growth, invasion, and metastasis. Clinically detectable prostatic carcinomas, in contrast, typically present as advanced lesions, often with extraprostatic extension or metastases.

Prostatic carcinoma, unless associated with other conditions such as nodular hyperplasia or prostatitis, does not typically produce symptoms until it reaches an advanced state. Extraprostatic extension as well as metastases are frequent at the time of diagnosis and, if documented, rule out the only potentially curative procedure, radical prostatectomy. Metastases typically involve regional and para-aortic lymph nodes and bone (Fig. 14.4). In bone, they characteristically evoke an intense osteoblastic reaction manifested radiographically as increased bone density. Because prostatic carcinomas often arise in the posterior portion of the gland, just beneath the capsule, obstructive symptoms are not an early manifestation, whereas transcapsular extension is common.

The typically posterior location of prostatic carcinoma and its firm-to-rock-hard consistency do allow for detection by digital rectal examination. Not all indurated, firm prostates contain carcinoma, since a variety of inflammatory processes may produce an identical consistency. Firm prostatic nodules represent carcinoma in at least 50% of cases, however, and require pathologic study. Digital rectal examination is also valuable in detecting extraglandular spread, typically manifested as a blurring of the prostatic mar-gins. This technique is not highly sensitive, however, and misses small foci of capsular penetration. Other, more advanced techniques to clinically detect capsular invasion, such as computed tomography (CT), transrectal ultrasonography, and magnetic resonance imaging (MRI), have met with limited success.

All patients with clinical evidence of prostatic carcinoma require microscopic confirmation, which may be achieved in various ways. Needle biopsy by a transrectal or perineal approach is typically used for small, rectally palpable lesions. Transrectal fine-needle aspiration cytology has been shown to be a quick, sensitive, and specific means of diagnosis (Fig. 14.5). Because many passes may be made through the gland without injury by fine-needle aspiration, sampling error may be less than with a large-bore needle biopsy. Patients with bulky carcinomas producing obstruction may have their diagnosis confirmed by material removed for palliation by transurethral resection.

STAGING Although several different clinical staging systems have been applied to prostatic carcinomas, the most popular approach (below) employs four major categories with several important subdivisions. The definitions of the subdivisions vary slightly in different reports.

Stage   A   Tumors in this group are not clinically detectable or suspected.
        A1 Tumor is well differentiated, and it is present in three or fewer microscopic foci or involves less than 5% of the resected tissue.
        A2 Tumor is poorly differentiated, regardless of the amount of involvement. Alternately, if well differentiated, it involves greater than 5% of the resected prostatic tissue or is present in four or more microscopic foci.
Stage   B   Tumors in this group are evident on digital rectal examination but are clinically confined to the prostate.
        B1N This is the classic "Jewett nodule," a palpable, well circumscribed mass less than 1.5 cm in diameter.

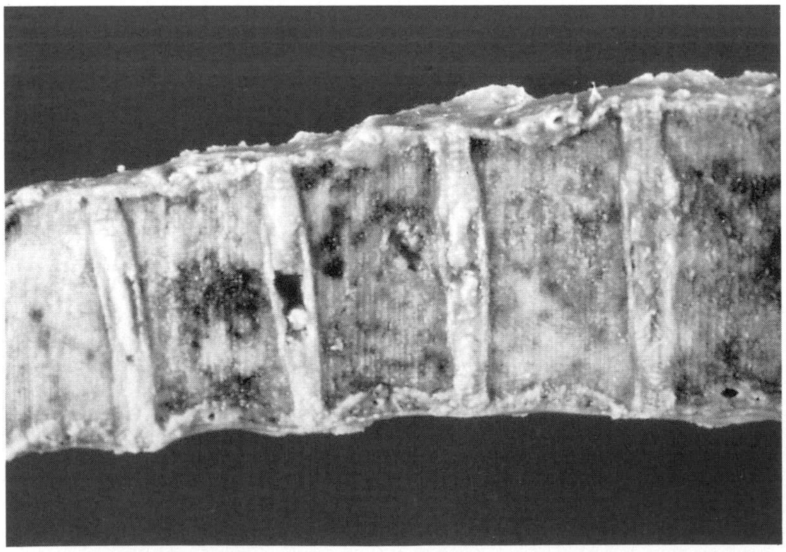

Figure 14.4 Prostatic adenocarcinoma typically metastasizes to bone—in this case to vertebrae—where it evokes an intense osteoblastic reaction. The dense white areas correspond to tumor deposits with associated new bone formation.

B1 The lesion is slightly larger, usually less than 2 cm in diameter. It may be more poorly demarcated than a B1N tumor but does not involve the entire lobe.

B2 The tumor is more diffuse and poorly demarcated, involving all of one lobe or both lobes of the prostate on palpation.

Stage C The tumor is clinically evident on rectal examination, extending beyond the confines of the prostate gland into the surrounding soft tissues or seminal vesicles. There is no clinical evidence of metastatic disease.

Stage D Metastatic disease is clinically detectable.

D1 Metastases are confined to pelvic lymph nodes below the aortic bifurcation.

D2 Metastases involve lymph nodes above the aortic bifurcation, bone, or other viscera.

MORPHOLOGY Prostatic adenocarcinomas, which are difficult to recognize grossly in a prostatectomy specimen, may be virtually impossible to detect in transurethral resection chips or needle biopsies. Distinctly yellow areas are suspicious and should be thoroughly

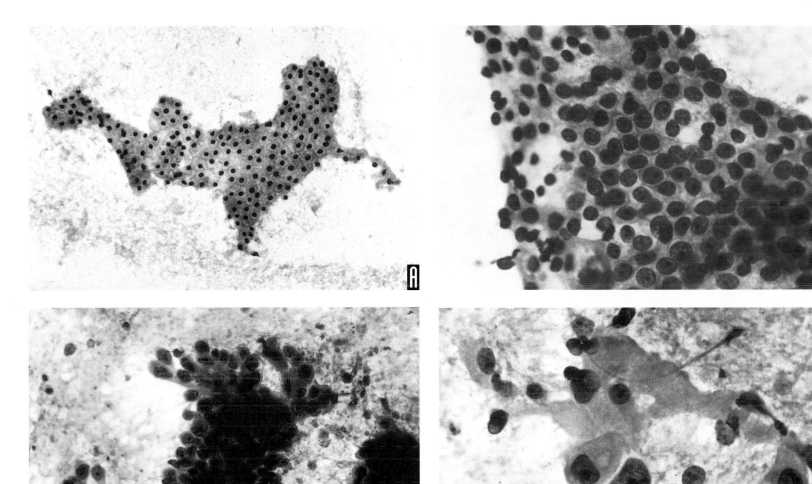

Figure 14.5 **A,** Sheets of glandular cells obtained by fine-needle aspiration of the prostate illustrate the uniform, small nuclei and lack of nucleoli characteristic of benign prostatic cytology specimens. **B,** Well differentiated prostatic adenocarcinoma consists of sheets of cells with larger nuclei and obvious nucleoli. **C,** Irregular clumps of cells with enlarged nuclei and prominent nucleoli characterize moderately differentiated prostatic adenocarcinoma in cytologic preparations. (Compare the nuclear size with that in **A,** at the same magnification.) **D,** Poorly differentiated adenocarcinoma has pleomorphic nuclei with prominent nucleoli, making the distinction from benign obvious (**A-D:** Papanicolaou stain).

sampled, although many carcinomas have the same tan-gray color as the normal prostatic stroma (Fig. 14.6). Cystic areas usually represent zones of hyperplasia. Many prostatic carcinomas arise in, or at least involve, the posterior portion of the gland. However, most of them are multifocal lesions with components in the median and lateral lobes. Some tumors clearly spare the posterior prostatic tissue.

As with most neoplasms, the microscopic criteria for prostatic malignancy are easy to list, but their application may be more problematic. Carcinomas producing clinical signs and symptoms (stage B and above) typically constitute a large portion of the biopsy material and display sufficient architectural and cytologic pleomorphism as to be easily distinguished from normal or hyperplastic glands.

Microscopically, most prostatic adenocarcinomas are distinctly glandular lesions. The glands are characteristically lined by a single layer of cells, in contrast to the two-cell layer seen in normal and hyperplastic glands (see Fig. 13.16). A typically infiltrative growth pattern and a blurring of the glandular margin is best shown by focusing up and down through the lesion. Glands may grow back-

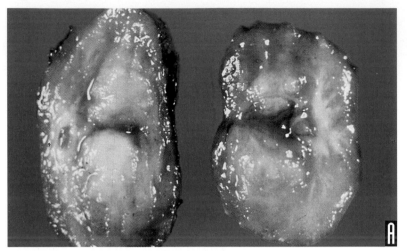

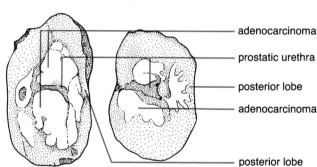

adenocarcinoma

prostatic urethra

posterior lobe

adenocarcinoma

posterior lobe

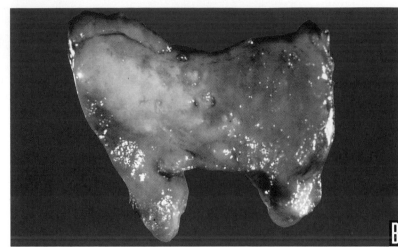

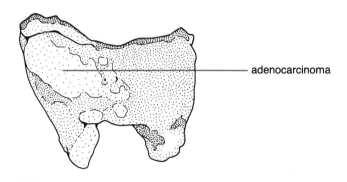

adenocarcinoma

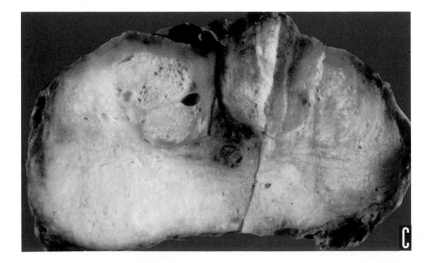

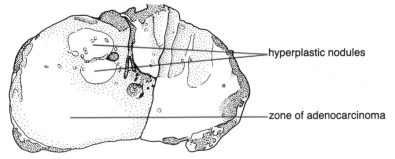

hyperplastic nodules

zone of adenocarcinoma

Figure 14.6 A, Although many prostatic carcinomas arise in the posterior portion of the gland, this is not invariably the case. Here a yellow zone of coloration in the periurethral region corresponds to adenocarcinoma involving both lateral lobes. **B,** This adenocarcinoma is also yellow and fills one lateral lobe. **C,** The adenocarcinoma in this example is more typically located in the posterior portion of the gland. Cystic areas represent zones of nodular hyperplasia unrelated to the carcinoma.

to-back, with no intervening stroma. Perineural invasion is strong, but not inviolate, evidence in favor of carcinoma (Fig. 14.7). Cytologically, the neoplastic cells have enlarged, uniform to mildly pleomorphic nuclei and, usually, prominent eosinophilic nucleoli. The microscopic appearance varies with the grade of the lesion, as discussed below. In addition to evaluating tumor grade, pathologic examination should evaluate capsular (Fig. 14.8) and seminal vesicle involvement.

Between 10% and 23% of acinar-forming prostatic adenocarcinomas contain intraluminal crystallike structures referred to as crystalloids. These are easily recognized in routine hematoxylin and eosin-stained sections and are often associated with amorphous,

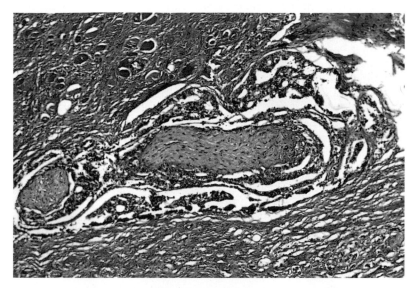

Figure 14.7 In this photomicrograph, a small nerve is surrounded by nests of adenocarcinoma. Such perineural infiltration is a strong, but not inviolate, feature of carcinoma.

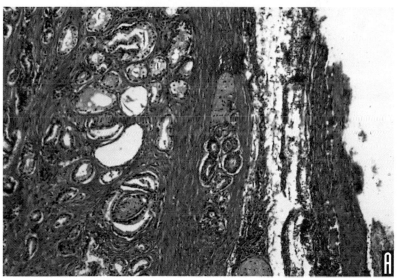

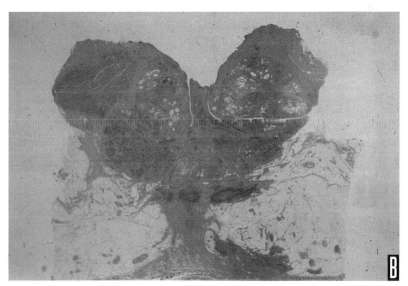

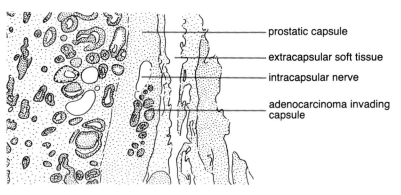

prostatic capsule
extracapsular soft tissue
intracapsular nerve
adenocarcinoma invading capsule

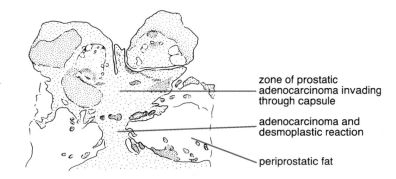

zone of prostatic adenocarcinoma invading through capsule
adenocarcinoma and desmoplastic reaction
periprostatic fat

Figure 14.8 A, In the example of prostatic adenocarcinoma shown here, glands of adenocarcinoma have extended into the capsule but have not penetrated to the pericapsular fat. **B,** The adenocarcinoma has extended through the prostatic capsule and into the surrounding fat, evoking a desmoplastic reaction. It is easy to appreciate how the latter change may be palpable transrectally.

intraglandular eosinophilic secretions. The crystalloids, which are also eosinophilic, may assume a variety of shapes, including rods, needles, rhombi, prisms, hexagons, and plates (Fig. 14.9). Ultrastructurally, crystalloids generally lack the periodicity of true crystals, and their exact composition remains unknown. Nonetheless, prostatic crystalloids may occasionally be diagnostically pertinent because of their strong association with adenocarcinoma. Although they are occasionally seen in atypical or benign glands adjacent to an adenocarcinoma, they are rarely present in normal or hyperplastic glands devoid of carcinoma.

DETECTION OF CLINICALLY LATENT CARCINOMA   The most time-consuming diagnostic problem in prostatic pathology is the exclusion of latent carcinoma in prostatic tissue removed for the treatment of nodular hyperplasia. A twofold problem arises. First, the carcinoma must be present in the examined tissue, leading to the question of how thoroughly prostatic specimens should be sectioned; second, the tumor must be recognized microscopically. It

can be argued that this second step represents a less important pitfall, since carcinomas underdiagnosed microscopically are invariably very well differentiated, focal tumors unlikely to progress. Occasionally, however, incomplete sampling of prostatic tissue may fail to detect a high-grade, clinically unsuspected tumor present in a resection specimen but not examined microscopically.

The question of how thoroughly prostatic transurethral resection specimens should be sampled to avoid missing potentially aggressive but clinically unsuspected carcinoma has been the subject of several studies. Although the methods employed and conclusions obtained vary somewhat, the consensus is the same. It is neither technically feasible nor necessary in terms of patient prognosis to completely section transurethral resection specimens. In one study, all stage A2 carcinomas were detected by embedding and sectioning 6 g of randomly selected prostatic chips. Histologic examination of 12 g of tissue detected all stage A2 tumors and 90% of incidental carcinomas, including all carcinomas deemed to have potential clinical significance.

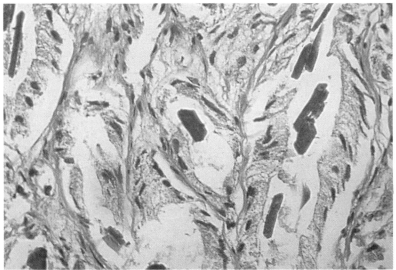

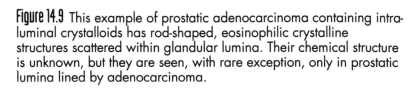

Figure 14.9 This example of prostatic adenocarcinoma containing intraluminal crystalloids has rod-shaped, eosinophilic crystalline structures scattered within glandular lumina. Their chemical structure is unknown, but they are seen, with rare exception, only in prostatic lumina lined by adenocarcinoma.

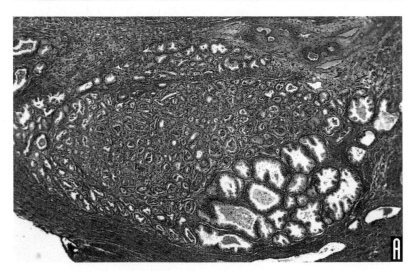

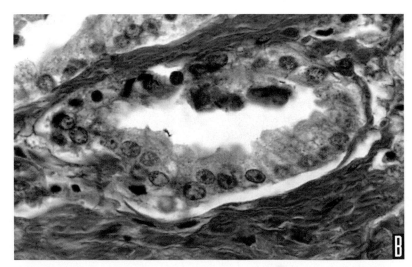

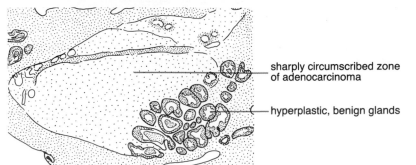

sharply circumscribed zone of adenocarcinoma

hyperplastic, benign glands

Figure 14.10 A, This prostatic adenocarcinoma, classified as Gleason grade 1, forms a sharply circumscribed aggregate of small, uniform glands. At this magnification, distinction from atypical adenomatous hyperplasia is not possible. The larger surrounding glands are hyperplastic. **B,**The presence of large nucleoli in the glandular cells has been used to distinguish low-grade carcinoma from atypical adenomatous hyperplasia. This is an admittedly arbitrary distinction that, fortunately, has little if any biologic importance. Intraluminal crystalloids are also present.

GRADING A dozen or more systems for the pathologic grading of prostatic adenocarcinoma have been proposed. At least six have been shown to correlate with clinical course. Some of these systems are based solely on the tumor's growth pattern; some, solely on the cytology of the cells; others, on a combination of histologic and cytologic features.

The best documented and most widely applied approach to grading prostatic carcinomas was developed by Gleason, based on material accumulated by the Veterans Administration Cooperative Urologic Research Group (VACURG). This approach provides prognostic information in addition to that supplied by the clinical stage. It relies, with minor exceptions, only on the architectural pattern of the tumor and has a high level of reproducibility. Gleason's system derives a score for each carcinoma based on the sum of the grades assigned to the most prominent and secondary architectural patterns. If the tumor consists solely of one grade, that number is doubled to determine the score. Careful statistical analysis also revealed that the sum of the grades assigned to the most prominent and secondary growth patterns is more predictive of outcome than the grade of either the most prominent or the worst growth pattern.

GLEASON GRADE 1 The tumor forms separate, round-to-oval glands of uniform size. The glands are closely packed, but the mass of glands has a sharply defined margin at its interface with the surrounding prostate (Fig. 14.10). The microscopic distinction between grade 1 carcinoma and atypical adenomatous hyperplasia (see Chapter 13) is problematic. The presence of large nucleoli is generally accepted as the distinguishing feature in carcinoma. In Gleason's study, this pattern was present in about 3.5% of carcinomas.

GLEASON GRADE 2 The tumor forms individual glands of similar size and shape but with somewhat more variation than in grade 1. There is more stroma separating individual glands, and the glandular aggregates are not as well circumscribed (Fig. 14.11). This pattern was present in 24% of the cases in Gleason's study.

GLEASON GRADE 3 Two distinctly different histologic images are included in this grade. The most common variant is a continuation of the previous patterns. Single, separate glands of irregular size and shape are usually more widely dispersed in the stroma. The glands may be larger, smaller, or similar in size to those in grades 1 and 2. Typically, they are highly variable in size and have angulated shapes (Fig. 14.12). Occasionally, the glands are closely packed but not fused, as in grade 4. The tumor outline is irregular, without a well defined boundary.

The second pattern in grade 3 has a papillary/cribriform architecture. Typically, large, ductlike structures with circular, sharply circumscribed edges contain cribriform, back-to-back glands and, less

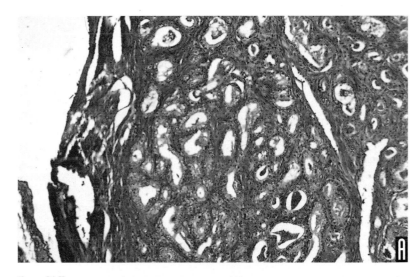

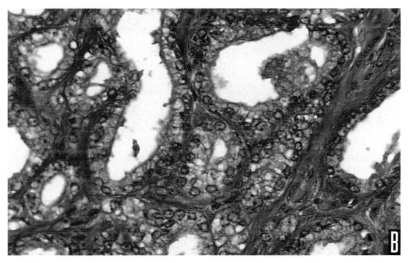

Figure 14.11 **A,** In this prostatic adenocarcinoma, greater variation in glandular size, more stroma between the glands, and a more infiltrative margin distinguish Gleason grade 2 carcinoma from the much less common grade 1 pattern. **B,** Carcinomatous glands are composed of a single layer of cells. The nuclei are enlarged and have prominent nucleoli.

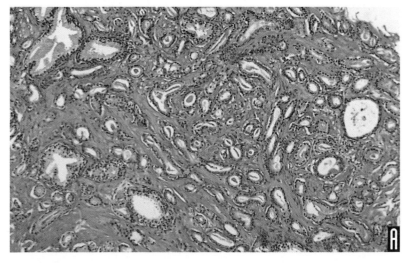

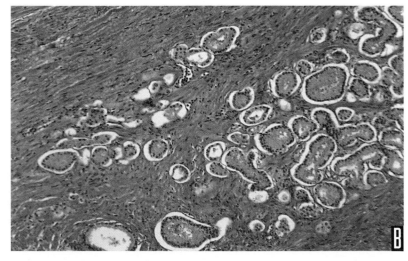

Figure 14.12 **A,** The Gleason grade 3 carcinoma shown here represents an extension of the changes seen in the grade 2 pattern. The glands are even more irregular in size and shape. The tumor is distinctly infiltrative, without any of the circumscription characterizing grade 1 and 2 lesions. **B,** The diffuse infiltration of single, irregular glands is evident in this photomicrograph. Small foci such as this are common in needle-biopsy specimens.

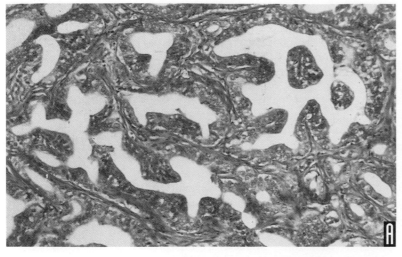

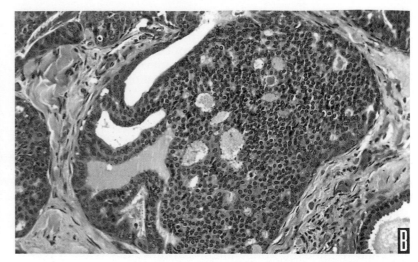

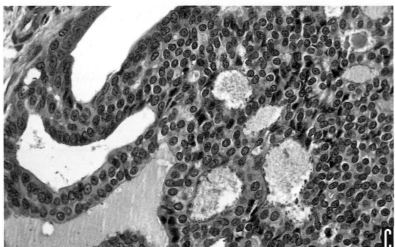

Figure 14.13 A, This prostatic adenocarcinoma exhibits a papillary/cribriform pattern. Large, carcinomatous glands with papillary infoldings are assigned a grade of 3. Distinction from florid papillary/cribriform hyperplasia is based on cytologic features. **B,** In this example, the grade 3 carcinoma cells form closely packed, cribriform aggregates within a ductlike structure. **C,** On higher-power view, the cytologic features of the malignant cells are apparent. Nuclei are enlarged, and occasional nucleoli are present.

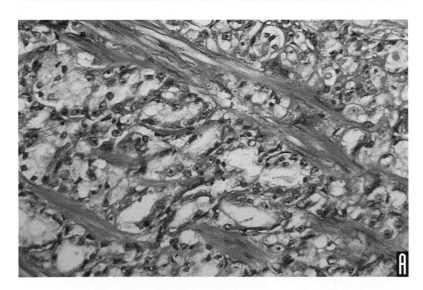

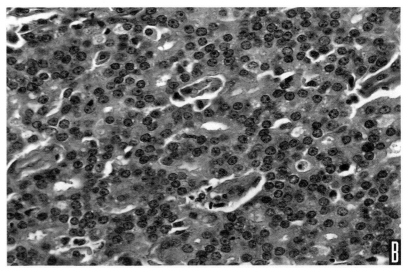

Figure 14.14 A, The most common grade 4 variant of prostatic adenocarcinoma is the fused-gland pattern seen here. Back-to-back glands without intervening stroma infiltrate the prostate. **B,** This photomicrograph shows another example of the fused-gland pattern in which the carcinoma grows as an infiltrating sheet of cells containing scattered lumina.

frequently, papillary infoldings (Fig. 14.13). In many instances, both grade 3 patterns are present in one case. Grade 3 is the most common form of prostatic carcinoma, present in 88% of the VAC-URG cases.

GLEASON GRADE 4 Two variants are included under grade 4. The characteristic feature is a "fused-gland" pattern in which large, irregular masses of neoplastic glands coalesce and branch (Fig. 14.14). In contrast to the sharply circumscribed, ductlike pattern seen as a variant of grade 3, these fused aggregates of tumor irregularly infiltrate the prostatic stroma. The second variant of grade 4 is the one conces-

sion to cytologic appearance encompassed in this system. Prostatic adenocarcinomas composed of cells with prominent clear cytoplasm, strongly resembling a clear cell renal carcinoma, are designated as grade 4 (Fig. 14.15). A grade 4 pattern was present in 12% of the VACURG cases.

GLEASON GRADE 5 Encompassing several growth patterns, this grade usually consists of diffusely infiltrating tumor cells with only abortive attempts at gland formation or occasional signet-ring cells to identify the tumor as an adenocarcinoma (Fig. 14.16). A second, less common pattern of grade 5 is composed of sharply circum-

Figure 14.15 This Gleason grade 4 prostatic adenocarcinoma exhibits a less common "hypernephroid pattern," which consists of sheets of cells with clear cytoplasm, closely resembling renal cell carcinoma.

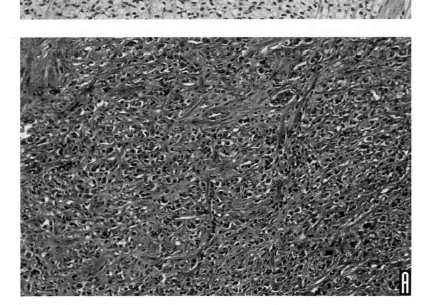

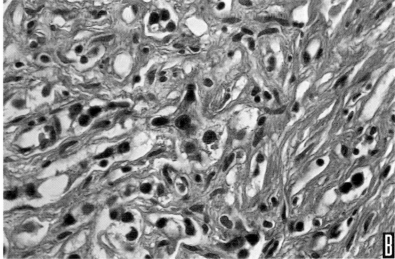

Figure 14.16 A, When prostatic adenocarcinomas such as the example here no longer form glands but infiltrate the stroma as single cells, they are considered grade 5, highly aggressive neoplasms. **B,** Highly pleomorphic cells infiltrate the stroma singly and in small strands. There is no gland formation.

scribed cords and nests of epithelial cells with only occasional, tiny glandular lumina (Fig. 14.17). This pattern is often associated with central necrosis in the cell nests, creating an image similar to that of mammary comedocarcinoma (Fig. 14.18). Grade 5 was present in 23% of the VACURG cases.

IMMUNOCYTOCHEMICAL MARKERS FOR PROSTATIC CARCINOMA Cell-specific markers for prostatic epithelium developed soon after the widespread application of immunoperoxidase staining to routinely processed, paraffin-embedded tissue sections. Both prostatic-specific acid phosphatase and prostatic-specific antigen (Fig. 14.19) have repeatedly proved to be sensitive markers for benign and malignant prostatic cells. Antibodies to these antigens may be of considerable value when applied to biopsy or aspiration cytology specimens containing metastases from clinically undetected prostatic primary tumors (Fig. 14.20).

Even poorly differentiated neoplasms, those most likely to cause diagnostic difficulty, are often positive with these techniques. It must be remembered, however, that these procedures are not 100% sensitive. Occasional poorly differentiated prostatic carcinomas are completely negative or only focally positive. Thus, negative staining does not exclude prostatic origin.

Prostatic-specific acid phosphatase and prostatic-specific antigen have also demonstrated marked specificity for prostatic epithelium. In several large series, normal and neoplastic tissues of nonprostatic origin have been negative with these markers. There have, however, been rare examples of renal cell carcinoma, islet cell carcinoma, carcinoma of the breast, and gastrointestinal carcinoid tumor that have reacted with these markers, particularly prostatic-specific acid phosphatase. As with any immunocytochemical marker, interpretation must not be based solely on staining positivity but must include morphologic and clinical considerations. It is likely, particularly in poorly differentiated neoplasms, that random gene activations occasionally lead to the inappropriate expression of prostatic markers by nonprostatic neoplasms.

PROGNOSIS The prognosis for prostatic adenocarcinoma depends on interrelated factors, including the stage and grade of the tumor, its amenability to complete surgical resection, the patient's age and serum acid phosphatase, as well as prostate specific antigen levels. Well differentiated stage A1 tumors are now generally accepted as indolent lesions. In contrast, patients with stage A2 disease typically have more poorly differentiated tumors and a high incidence (30%–40%) of regional lymph node metastases; the

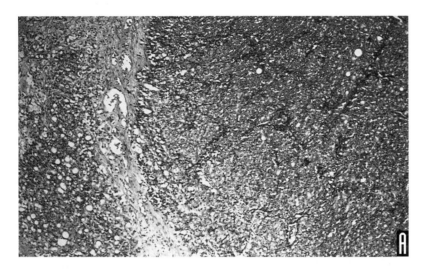
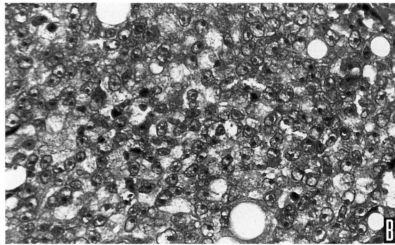

Figure 14.17 A, The expansile pattern of grade 5 prostatic carcinoma consists of large, circumscribed cell masses with little or no evidence of gland formation. **B,** Higher magnification demonstrates that the expansile masses are composed of sheets of pleomorphic cells without glandular differentiation.

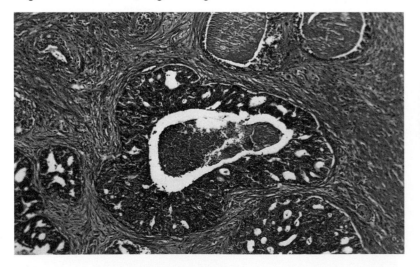
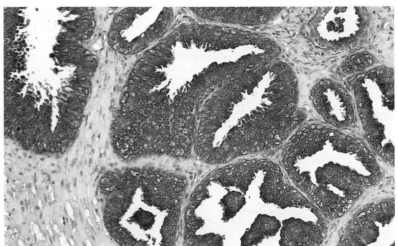

Figure 14.18 This grade 5 prostatic adenocarcinoma exhibits a comedocarcinoma pattern. Circumscribed nests of carcinoma are similar to those seen at low power in the cribriform variant of grade 3 carcinoma. The presence of a central area of necrosis distinguishes this pattern from grade 3.

Figure 14.19 Antiprostatic-specific antigen also produces strong positive (brown) staining in columnar cells of normal prostatic acini. As with prostatic acid phosphatase, basal cells do not stain (antiprostatic-specific antigen, hematoxylin).

presence of such metastases converts the patient to stage C disease. Stage B1 tumors, particularly the classic stage B1N nodules, have a lower frequency of metastatic disease than do stage A2 lesions. Survival drops dramatically as the tumor stage progresses to stage B2. Many patients in the latter group have clinically occult extraglandular extension in their resection specimens, rendering their tumors pathologic stage C carcinomas. Once patients become inoperable for cure with stage C and D disease, carcinoma-related mortality is inevitable. Duration of survival varies tremendously for inoperable patients depending on the efficacy of palliative measures, including hormonal manipulation and radiation therapy for symptomatic metastases.

Unusual Variants of Prostatic Carcinoma

Mucinous Adenocarcinoma

This term has been applied to prostatic adenocarcinomas in which at least 25% of the tumor tissue consists of lakes of extracellular mucin. Such tumors are rare, accounting for only six of approximately 1600 prostatic carcinomas studied at Memorial Hospital in New York. It is unclear whether mucinous prostatic adenocarcinomas exhibit clinical behavior that differs from their conventional counterparts. Epstein and Lieberman's study suggests that these tumors are less responsive to hormonal manipulation in the form of orchiectomy or estrogen therapy.

MORPHOLOGY Normal and hyperplastic prostatic acini produce mucosubstances, but these do not typically stain with the standard, somewhat insensitive mucicarmine stain. It is not widely recognized that 63%–90% of prostatic adenocarcinomas are positive with this technique (Fig. 14.21). In fact, mucicarmine positivity may be of diagnostic benefit when confronted with occasional problematic lesions. Other differential staining techniques, such as the alcian blue-PAS stain, can also document acid mucin production in tumor cells.

Because of their infrequency, prostatic tumors with large aggregates of extracellular mucin may be confused with metastases. However, immunocytochemical stains for prostatic-specific antigen and prostatic acid phosphatase are typically positive. The unusual architecture of mucinous adenocarcinoma with epithelial

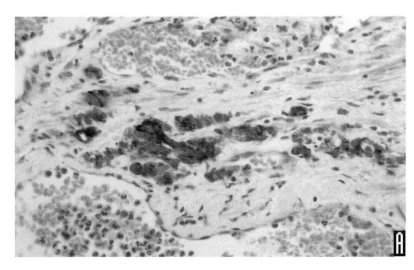

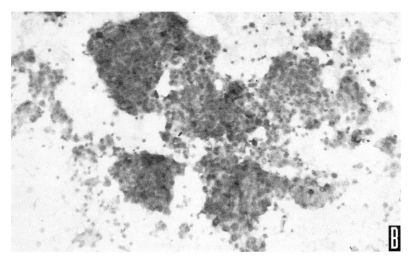

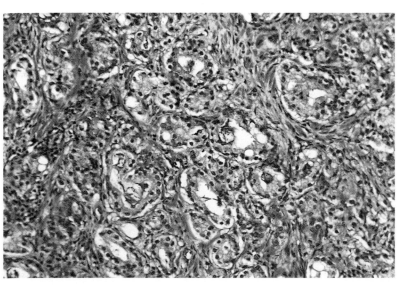

Figure 14.20 **A,** The true test of a tissue-specific marker is its ability to stain poorly differentiated metastases from clinically undetected primary tumors. In this figure, antiprostatic-specific antigen stains a biopsy specimen containing metastatic high-grade adenocarcinoma, strongly supporting a prostatic origin. **B,** Antibodies directed against prostatic-specific antigen and prostatic acid phosphatase may also be applied to needle aspiration cytology specimens. Positive staining for the latter in this pulmonary metastasis supports a prostatic origin (**A:** antiprostatic-specific antigen, hematoxylin; **B:** antiprostatic acid phosphatase, hematoxylin).

Figure 14.21 Even histologically, typical prostatic adenocarcinomas such as the one in this photomicrograph often stain positively (red) with the mucicarmine technique, in contrast to normal or hyperplastic prostatic tissue. This stain may thus be valuable as a diagnostic adjunct (mucicarmine).

islands separated by mucinous pools does not readily allow grading by the Gleason system (Fig. 14.22). Most of these tumors have associated areas of more conventional carcinoma that may be graded with this technique.

ADENOID BASAL CELL TUMOR

Tumors that are morphologically similar to adenoid cystic carcinoma of the salivary glands rarely arise in the prostate. Although these prostatic neoplasms have also been labeled adenoid cystic carcinomas, their biologic behavior is less clear-cut. There are no well documented examples of prostatic adenoid cystic carcinomas that exhibited metastases. Reed has suggested that even though these lesions are morphologically similar to a well recognized form of salivary gland carcinoma, they appear to be benign in the prostate. He has suggested the term adenoid basal cell tumor.

MORPHOLOGY These adenoid neoplasms are frequently associated with zones of basal cell hyperplasia as described in Chapter 13 (see Fig. 13.21). The adenoid component is an expansile or infil-

trating mass composed of islands of cells with scant, basophilic cytoplasm. Cells at the periphery of the islands may form palisades. Characteristically, the islands have a cribriform appearance with multiple lumenlike structures containing mucoid material or, less commonly, eosinophilic hyalinized masses (Fig. 14.23).

"CARCINOID TUMOR"

Ultrastructural, immunocytochemical, and routine silver staining techniques have demonstrated that the normal prostate contains numerous endocrine-paracrine cells. Over fifteen years ago, Azzopardi and Evans documented that such cells could exist in otherwise conventional-appearing prostatic adenocarcinomas. More recently, prostatic neoplasms have been reported with the light-microscopic features of a carcinoid tumor; neuroendocrine cells have also been demonstrated with special techniques. Such tumors are often associated with zones of typical prostatic adenocarcinoma. The carcinoid component stains with prostatic-specific antigen and prostatic acid phosphatase. These observations suggest that "carcinoid tumor" of the prostate represents an adenocarcinoma exhibit-

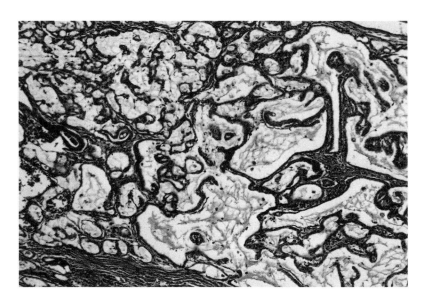

Figure 14.22 Some prostatic adenocarcinomas produce abundant extracellular mucin, which forms large pools in the stroma. Such carcinomas are not readily amenable to Gleason grading, and may be confused with metastases from gastrointestinal primary tumors.

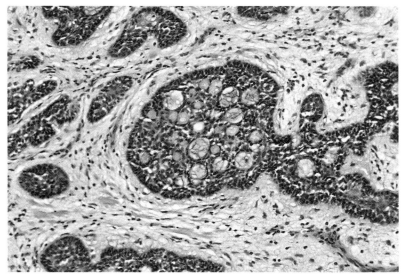

Figure 14.23 This typical adenoid basal cell tumor of the prostate is characterized by cribriform arrays of basaloid cells. The lumina in the cribriform areas are filled with mucinous material or hyalinized eosinophilic globules.

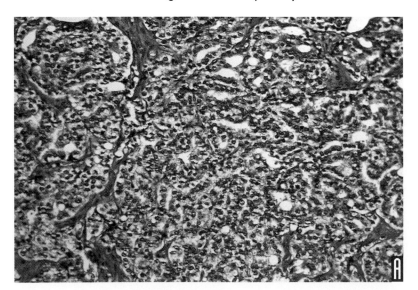

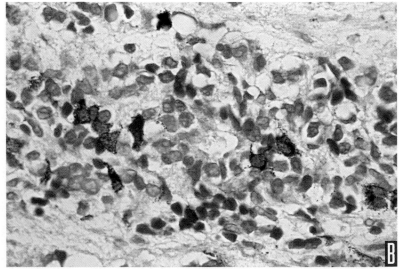

Figure 14.24 A, In prostatic carcinoidlike tumor, nests of cells with uniform nuclei and a glandular-trabecular growth pattern resemble gastrointestinal carcinoid tumors. **B,** Argyrophil stain demonstrates

numerous positive (brown) cells in a prostatic carcinoidlike tumor (Churukian-Schenk stain).

ing partial neuroendocrine differentiation, rather than a distinctive tumor derived from neural crest cells. The biologic significance of the carcinoidlike component remains unclear.

MORPHOLOGY Light-microscopically, the carcinoidlike areas may be indistinguishable from carcinoid tumors occurring elsewhere in the body. Typically, there are nests and sheets of monotonous, polygonal cells. Nuclei are uniformly round, and the cells have amphophilic-to-eosinophilic, granular cytoplasm. Areas of gland formation are inconspicuous or absent. Argyrophil stains such as the Grimelius or Churukian-Schenk stain are focally positive (Fig. 14.24); however, as discussed above, immunocytochemical stains for prostatic-specific antigen and prostatic acid phosphatase are also reactive. Electron microscopy may demonstrate dense core granules consistent with neurosecretory-type granules.

SMALL CELL CARCINOMA

Small cell carcinomas, histologically identical to oat cell carcinomas of the bronchial tree, are rare prostatic neoplasms that often develop during the clinical progression and "dedifferentiation" of typical adenocarcinomas. Their emergence signals the patient's rapid demise. The biologic behavior of prostatic small cell carcinoma thus appears to be analogous to that of small cell or oat cell carcinomas occurring at other locations. Ectopic adrenocorticotropic hormone (ACTH) production has been documented for one prostatic tumor of this type. Another was associated with the development of Cushing's syndrome.

MORPHOLOGY The light-microscopic appearance of these lesions is similar to that of conventional oat cell carcinoma of the lung. Small cells with inconspicuous cytoplasm and hyperchromatic nuclei form sheets and diffusely infiltrate the prostatic stroma (Fig. 14.25). Nuclei may exhibit "molding" when closely apposed to neighboring cells. The mitotic rate is extremely high, and there are broad zones of necrosis. Occasional rosettelike structures consisting of annular arrays of cells surrounding a central nonvascular space or fibrillary mass are present. Prostatic small cell carcinomas frequently merge with zones of typical prostatic adenocarcinoma.

Immunocytochemical stains for prostatic-specific markers may be absent in the small cell component but are present in any associated conventional adenocarcinoma. This loss of expression of cell-specific antigens reflects the poorly differentiated, anaplastic nature of the

small cell component. Argyrophil stains may be negative or focally reactive. Ultrastructural studies usually document dense core granules consistent with at least focal neuroendocrine differentiation. This does not imply origin from neuroendocrine precursor cells and probably represents divergent differentiation of neoplastic acinar epithelium.

TRANSITIONAL CELL CARCINOMA OF THE PROSTATE

Transitional cell carcinomas may involve the prostate by three distinctive routes: (1) they may arise de novo in the distal prostatic ducts; (2) primary transitional cell neoplasms of the bladder may invade the prostate by direct extension; or (3) transitional cell carcinomas may begin in the prostatic urethra, extending along the prostatic ducts, into the underlying gland. This distinction is not always possible, as many patients with apparently discontinuous prostatic disease also have multifocal involvement of the bladder and urethra. The second and third forms of prostatic transitional cell carcinoma are discussed in Chapter 12.

CLINICAL MANIFESTATIONS Patients with transitional cell carcinoma of the prostatic ducts typically present with obstructive symptoms and hematuria. The age range is similar to that of prostatic adenocarcinoma. Serum acid phosphatase levels are normal unless there is an accompanying adenocarcinoma. If osseous metastases develop, they are predominantly osteolytic, in contrast to the osteoblastic metastases of prostatic adenocarcinoma. Transitional cell prostatic carcinomas tend to be cytologically high-grade, rapidly growing tumors that are unresponsive to hormonal manipulation.

If the tumor is confined to the prostatic ducts without evidence of stromal invasion, conservative therapy such as transurethral resection is indicated. Stromal invasion is associated with lymphatic spread and a poor prognosis. There are only occasional five-year survivors. The average survival is approximately 23 months. In one series by Johnson and co-workers, all six patients with primary prostatic disease had invasive lesions. In contrast, 9 of 14 patients with associated transitional cell carcinoma of the bladder had only intraductal prostatic involvement.

MORPHOLOGY Transitional cell carcinoma of the prostate is a high-grade, nonpapillary neoplasm with microscopic features identical to those of more common transitional cell carcinomas of

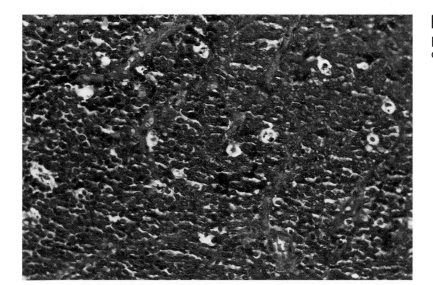

Figure 14.25 Carcinomas light-microscopically indistinguishable from pulmonary oat cell carcinoma occasionally arise in the prostate, usually in association with areas of more conventional adenocarcinoma.

the bladder (Fig. 14.26). The intraductal component consists of ducts replaced by nests of pleomorphic cells, often with central necrosis. Zones of squamous metaplasia may be present. Multiple microscopic sections may be necessary to document stromal invasion, which also resembles invasive carcinoma of the bladder with nests and single pleomorphic cells infiltrating the surrounding stroma.

Distinction of high-grade prostatic transitional cell carcinoma from prostatic adenocarcinoma has important clinical implications, as the former tumors do not respond to hormonal manipulation. In problematic cases, immunohistochemistry may be of discriminatory value. Transitional cell carcinomas will not label for prostatic mark-

ers such as prostatic specific antigen (Fig. 14.27). Unlike prostatic adenocarcinomas, many transitional cell carcinomas will display at least focal positivity for carcinoembryonic antigen (Fig. 14.28).

RARE PROSTATIC NEOPLASMS

ADENOSQUAMOUS AND SQUAMOUS CELL CARCINOMA

Malignant squamous cells may sometimes arise in the prostate, alone or in combination with adenocarcinoma (Fig. 14.29). The appearance of such cells should not be confused with the more

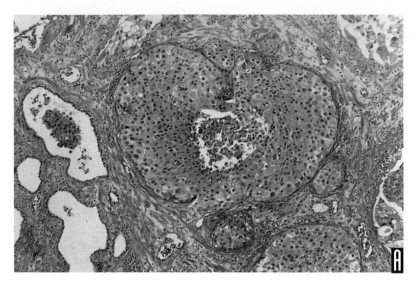

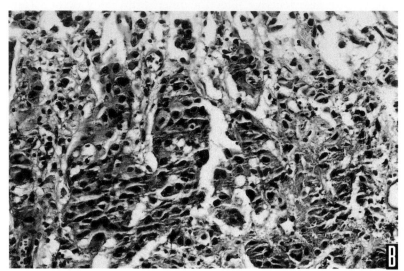

Figure 14.26 A, Transitional cell carcinomas may arise in the prostatic ducts or extend into the ducts from an initial focus in the prostatic urethra. These tumors are cytologically identical to analogous lesions of

the bladder and urethra. **B,** Invasive transitional cell carcinomas are characteristically composed of highly pleomorphic cells without any evidence of squamous or glandular differentiation.

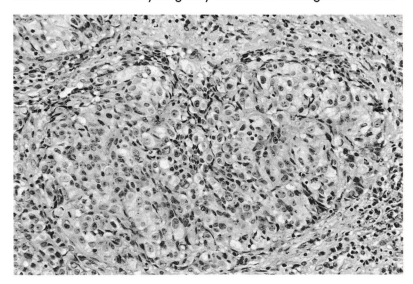

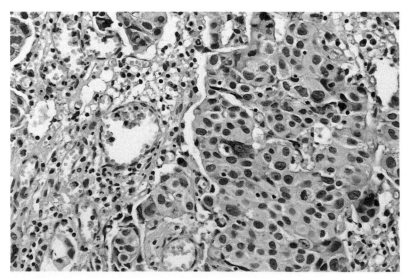

Figure 14.27 This prostatic transitional cell carcinoma is negative for prostatic specific antigen.

Figure 14.28 Rare cells in this prostatic transitional cell carcinoma exhibit staining for carcinoembryonic antigen

common benign squamous metaplasia that follows infarction or estrogen therapy. Squamous metaplasia secondary to estrogen therapy may involve benign glands (see Fig. 13.24) or it may affect areas of carcinoma. The distinction of squamous cell carcinoma from squamous metaplasia, with or without associated adenocarcinoma, is based on the presence of cellular pleomorphism and mitotic activity in the former. It is unclear whether prostatic squamous cell carcinoma arises from squamous metaplasia or glandular epithelium. A ductal origin is unconfirmed. Squamous cell carcinoma in combination with adenocarcinoma (adenosquamous carcinoma) appears to be more frequent than pure squamous carcinoma. At least two studies have documented the presence of prostatic acid phosphatase in the squamous cells, a finding that could potentially be of value for rare metastatic lesions from an undocumented primary tumor. There are too few cases to assess biologic behavior or the possible effects of hormonal manipulation.

Fibroadenoma and Cystosarcoma Phyllodes

Rarely, the prostate may give rise to mixed epithelial and mesenchymal proliferations analogous to those seen in the breast. The most common proliferations arise focally in nodular hyperplasia and resemble mammary fibroadenoma. These nodules are composed of prostatic acini and ducts with epithelial cells that stain positively for prostatic markers. Unlike typical nodular hyperplasia, the closely associated fibromuscular component distorts the glandular elements, producing irregular, angulated, branching lumina. The stroma is cytologically uniform and has a cellularity no greater than that of normal or hyperplastic prostate (Fig. 14.30). It is unlikely that such nodules represent true neoplasms; their clinical course is invariably benign.

There are other, less common stromal/epithelial proliferations in which the epithelial component remains benign, but the mesenchymal component is hypercellular or overtly malignant in appearance. Such tumors are analogous to mammary cystosarcoma phyllodes. These lesions may follow a recurrent, locally aggressive course, often with increasing cellularity, pleomorphism of the stromal component, and gradual loss of the epithelial elements.

Carcinosarcoma

Prostatic neoplasms composed of a mixture of malignant epithelial and stromal elements are extremely uncommon. Most purported examples of carcinosarcoma represent carcinomas with a pleomorphic, mesenchymal-like component. Such "pseudosarcomatous" carcinomas, which can occur throughout the body, are particularly common in the kidney (see Chapter 11).

Sarcoma

Malignant stromal tumors of the prostate account for only about 0.1% of prostatic neoplasms. Rhabdomyosarcomas, leiomyosarcomas, fibrosarcomas, and malignant fibrous histiocytomas have been

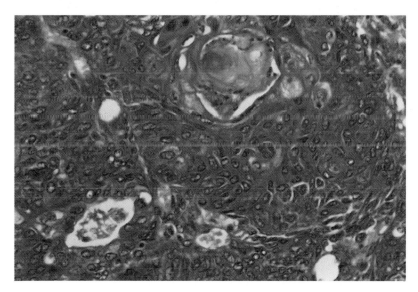

Figure 14.29 Prostatic carcinomas exhibiting squamous differentiation are extremely uncommon.

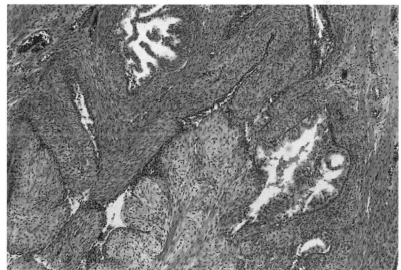

Figure 14.30 In prostatic fibroadenoma, mixed epithelial and mesenchymal proliferations occasionally closely resemble fibroadenoma of the breast. Glandular lumina in this example are distorted by proliferating mesenchymal nodules. The stroma in this case is benign, but rarely it may have a more cellular or overtly sarcomatous appearance. The latter lesions are analogous to mammary cystosarcoma phyllodes.

reported. Prostatic rhabdomyosarcoma tends to occur in children and young adults (Fig. 14.31), whereas other prostatic sarcomas typically develop later in life. Myogenic (smooth or skeletal muscle) differentiation may be documented immunocytochemically with antibodies directed against actin or desmin (Fig. 14.32). Sarcomas exhibiting skeletal muscle differentiation also react with myosin, myoglobin, or antirhabdomyoblast antibodies.

LYMPHOMA

Primary extranodal lymphomas may rarely arise in the prostate, or the prostate may be the site of recurrence for lymphomas originating elsewhere. A variety of subtypes of non-Hodgkin's lymphoma may be seen. In one series of seven primary prostatic lymphomas and six secondary lymphomas involving the prostate, survival averaged 14 months, with no difference in survival between primary and secondary disease.

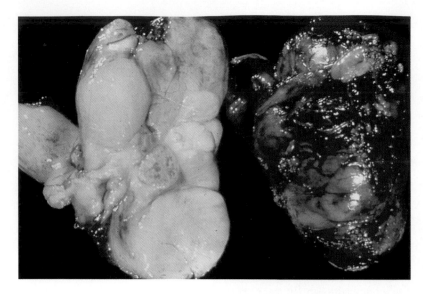

Figure 14.31 In this specimen of prostatic rhabdomyosarcoma, the prostate is enlarged by multiple nodules of white-tan tumor.

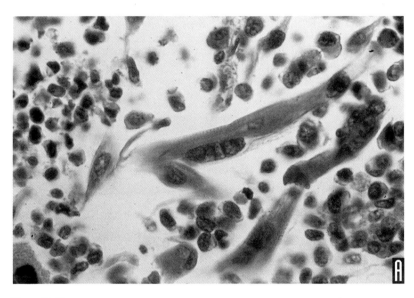

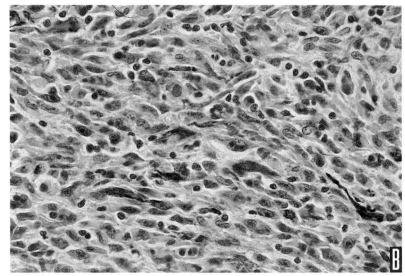

Figure 14.32 A, Microscopically, prostatic rhabdomyosarcomas are usually of the embryonal type and are composed predominantly of small cells with little evidence of differentiation. Rare "strap" cells may be found in some tumors with more obvious skeletal-muscle features. **B,** In problematic cases, staining for muscle markers such as desmin or muscle-specific actin may be helpful.

SECTION VII

Lesions of the Testis and Associated Structures

CHAPTER 15

Nonneoplastic Lesions of the Testis

TESTICULAR ABSENCE FROM THE SCROTUM

One or both testes are absent from the scrotum at birth in about 4% of term and 30% of premature male infants. Among the latter group, the testes usually descend to their proper position by three months of age. Sudmann reported that 85% of males with undescended testes had apparently normal, cryptorchid gonads, 12% had retractile or "pseudocryptorchid" testes, and 3% did not have testes. Testicular absence from the scrotum may also be seen in dysgenetic testis, hypogonadotropic hypogonadism, a variety of "intersex states," ectopic testis, as well as rudimentary testis.

CRYPTORCHIDISM

CLINICAL MANIFESTATIONS Cryptorchidism refers to the arrest of a testis in its descent along the normal pathway and its subsequent failure to reside in the scrotum. Cryptorchid testes have a predilection for the right side of the body. About 80% are arrested in the inguinal region; 20% are located intra-abdominally. Bilateral cryptorchidism is seen in about 25% of patients. An inguinal hernia is a common accompanying feature.

MORPHOLOGY Between two years of age and puberty, progressive interstitial and tubular fibrosis leads to irreversible damage, which continues to develop into adulthood (Fig. 15.1). Whether cryptorchid testes are intrinsically abnormal has been the subject of considerable debate. Nistal and colleagues studied biopsy specimens from 203 undescended testes, concluding that although 26% were normal or had mild changes ascribable to increased temperature, the remainder showed a variety of abnormalities that probably reflected varying degrees of gonadal dysgenesis.

ASSOCIATED ANOMALIES AND COMPLICATIONS Detecting cryptorchidism early in life is essential. The association with subsequent testicular neoplasia, particularly germ cell tumors, mandates removal of undescended testes detected after the onset of puberty. Some surgeons advocate removal of all cryptorchid testes discovered after six years of age because of frequent abnormalities in spermatogenesis and occasional germ cell tumors. Germ cell neoplasia occurs from 10 to 50 times more often in undescended testes as compared with normal testes. Intra-abdominal testes carry a higher risk than inguinal testes. There is also a slightly increased risk of neoplasia in the contralateral, normally descended gonad.

RETRACTILE, ECTOPIC, AND UNFORMED TESTES

CLINICAL MANIFESTATIONS Whereas cryptorchid testes are arrested at some point along the normal pathway of descent, the *retractile* or pseudocryptorchid testis is a gonad that retains sufficient mobility to ascend out of the scrotum, returning to its normal position. *Ectopic testes* are those that have become positioned in a deviant location. Approximately 5% of extrascrotal testes are ectopic. They are commonly located in the superficial inguinal region or lateral to the inguinal ring. In transverse ectopias, both of the testes descend through the same, usually left, inguinal ring.

As noted above, 3% of apparently undescended testes are due to the congenital absence of one (monorchism) or both (anorchism) gonads.

MORPHOLOGY Retractile and ectopic testes do not have distinguishing morphologic features. If a retractile testis spends most of its time in the inguinal canal, it may undergo changes similar to those seen in cryptorchidism. Extrascrotal ectopic testes also undergo fibrotic changes with time.

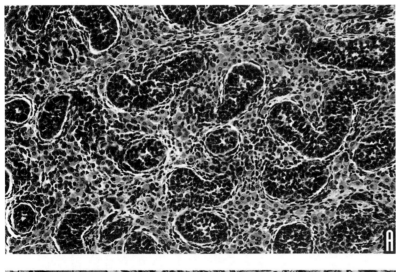
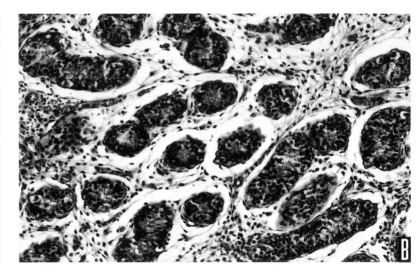
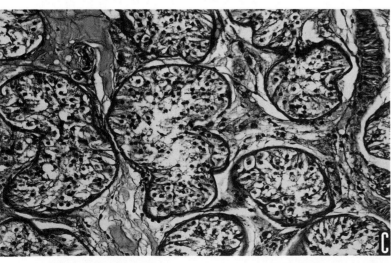
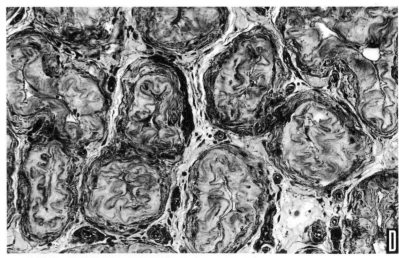

Figure 15.1 A, An undescended fetal testis consists of small, densely cellular tubules with unapparent lumina. The surrounding stroma contains prominent Leydig cells. **B,** In this undescended prepubertal testis from a six-year-old, well formed tubular lumina have not yet developed. There is no evidence of germ cell proliferation. The surrounding stroma lacks prominent Leydig cells. **C,** Microscopic examination of this cryptorchid testis, removed shortly after the onset of puberty, shows enlarged tubules and well developed lumina. Spermatogonia are present, but there is no evidence of spermatogenesis. Peritubular fibrosis is beginning to develop. **D,** In this histologic section of a cryptorchid testis, removed from a 25-year-old man, the seminiferous tubules have become completely sclerotic.

In patients with monorchism or anorchism, a small nodule of tissue is frequently found in the inguinal canal. When biopsied, it consists of a segment of normal or atrophic vas deferens, with or without an associated epididymis. Leydig cells may be present in a highly vascularized fibrous stroma, but seminiferous tubules are absent. It has been postulated that a functional fetal testis was present but regressed.

TESTICULAR TORSION

Although the majority of patients with testicular torsion are prepubertal, sporadic cases may occur at any age. At the time of torsion, some individuals may be engaged in strenuous physical activity, but many are inactive or even asleep. Testicular torsion requires rapid surgical intervention to preserve gonadal function. Generally, surgical manipulation within 6–10 hours is required to prevent necrosis. Only about 20% of testes can be salvaged when more than 12 hours have elapsed from the onset of symptoms.

PATHOGENESIS Testicular torsion is usually due to a developmental hypermobility caused by an elongated or redundant mesorchium, the so-called bell-clapper deformity. This defect, which may be familial, is commonly bilateral. Because of the frequent bilaterality, an orchiopexy-type surgical fixation should be performed on the contralateral testis. Other predisposing conditions include an abnormally loose attachment of the epididymis and, perhaps, a low-set, spiral insertion of the cremaster muscle.

CLINICAL MANIFESTATIONS Torsion is almost invariably accompanied by the acute onset of testicular or, in rare cases, referred pain, together with nausea. The overlying scrotal skin shows edema and inflammation, which increases in severity with the duration of symptoms. Prominent scrotal inflammation usually indicates longstanding torsion with little chance of testicular salvage.

DIAGNOSTIC STUDIES A number of radiologic as well as ultrasonographic techniques have been developed to aid in preoperative diagnosis and to assess viability at the time of surgery. Doppler ultrasonography is a rapid, noninvasive technique that relies on a shift in the frequency of sound waves as they are reflected by moving blood cells. The absence or marked restriction in blood flow caused by torsion is easily detected with this technique, the opposite testis serving as a control. Acute epididymitis, a condition often clinically confused with torsion, produces markedly increased blood flow. Doppler studies may occasionally be false-negative in patients with longstanding torsion, because increased scrotal blood flow sometimes develops secondary to prolonged torsion, masking the underlying testis.

Testicular perfusion has also been studied using short-lived radioisotopes and scrotal scanning. This procedure has successfully diagnosed patients with longstanding symptoms and delineated an infarcted testicular appendage from involvement of the testis itself. The use of fluorescein dye at the time of surgery can assess testicular viability. After the testis is manually detorsioned, a small bolus of sodium fluorescein is given intravenously; after 5–10 minutes, the testis is examined under ultraviolet light. Bright green fluorescence indicates that blood flow has been reestablished. If the testis remains dark and engorged, an orchiectomy is performed.

MORPHOLOGY The gross and microscopic findings in testicular torsion are those of hemorrhagic infarction caused by the obstruction of venous blood flow for some varying period of time before the restriction of arterial flow. Sudden obstruction of both arterial and venous blood flow is quite rare in testicular torsion, producing a coagulative necrosis without hemorrhage. Grossly, the testis is usually enlarged, dark red or brown, and may have extravasated blood visible beneath the tunica. The tunica's normally glistening surface may be dulled by the presence of a fibrinous exudate. The cut surface is dark red to black (Fig. 15.2).

The first microscopic change in hemorrhagic infarction is the distention of the interstitial space by extravasated erythrocytes. At this

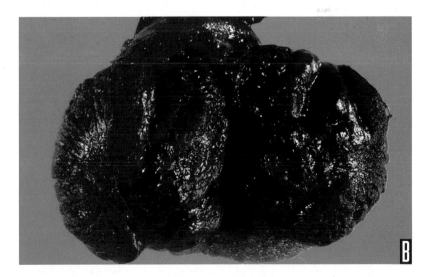

Figure 15.2 **A,** In this gross specimen of torsion of a prepubertal testis, obstruction of venous drainage has created a hemorrhagic infarct. The extravasated blood has altered with time, assuming a black coloration. **B,** In this case of recent torsion of an adult testis, venous obstruction has produced marked congestion and early hemorrhagic infarction.

stage, the seminiferous tubules appear normal, but they are widely separated by the stromal expansion. As the process continues, the tubular cells undergo necrosis, which is manifested microscopically by an absence of staining when hematoxylin is applied. Ultimately, the tubules collapse within the organizing hemorrhage (Fig. 15.3).

INTERSEXUALITY

Intersexuality refers to the presence of conflicting phenotypic sexual features. The reader is referred to the suggested readings for a more complete discussion of the endocrinologic, genetic, and phenotypic features of the entities included in this section. Wheeler and Rudy have subclassified the intersex states into five categories (reviewed below) on the basis of their gonadal histology.

True Hermaphrodism

True hermaphrodites are usually 46XX or mosaics and phenotypically male. By definition, they possess gonads containing both testicular and ovarian elements. About 2% of affected patients develop gonadal tumors, usually of the germ cell type, with the majority

being seminomas. Ovarian-type epithelial tumors and sex cord stromal tumors occur less often.

Considerable variation in gonadal morphology is possible. Most common, however, is an ovotestis with a contralateral ovary (Fig. 15.4). By definition, the testicular component of the ovotestis must contain seminiferous tubules, and the ovarian portion must have developing follicles. A uterus is also typically present.

Male Pseudohermaphrodism

CLINICAL MANIFESTATIONS   Male pseudohermaphrodites have ambiguous or overtly feminine external genitalia in association with gonads showing only testicular differentiation. Almost all are karyotypically 46XY. At least five subtypes of male pseudohermaphrodism have been described. The most common are the male adrenogenital syndromes and the testicular feminization syndrome.

Male adrenogenital syndromes are due to enzymatic defects in testosterone synthesis. Five metabolic variants have been reported, each due to a distinct abnormality in testosterone production. The *testicular feminization syndrome* is a sex-linked abnormality in androgen receptors that renders the patient's cells completely unresponsive to testosterone stimulation. The phenotypic results include

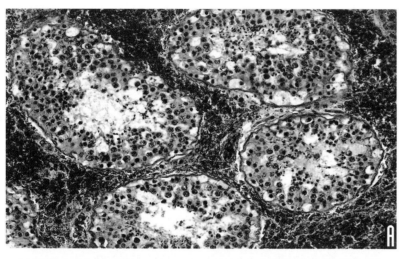

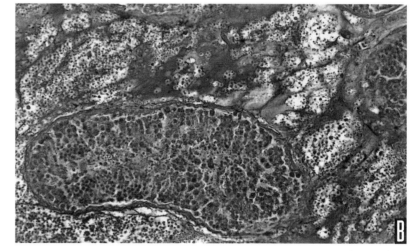

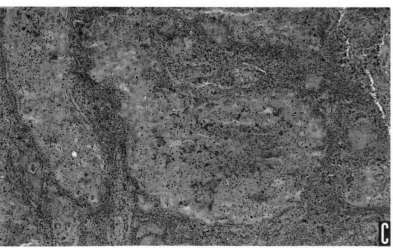

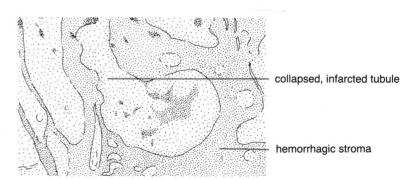

collapsed, infarcted tubule

hemorrhagic stroma

Figure 15.3 **A,** The initial microscopic manifestation of testicular torsion consists of erythrocyte extravasation into the peritubular parenchyma. At this stage, the intratubular constituents appear normal. **B,** As the vascular compromise progresses, the tubular cells undergo coagula-

tive necrosis. Their outline remains unchanged, but nuclear staining with hematoxylin has been lost. **C,** Eventually, testicular torsion leads to collapse of the tubules, seen here as irregular eosinophilic areas.

unequivocally female external genitalia and body habitus in a 46XY individual with levels of circulating testosterone equal to or greater than those in a normal adult male.

MORPHOLOGY In the adrenogenital syndrome, the testes vary in microscopic appearance but are typically immature, resembling normal prepubertal testes, except for the occasional presence of hyperplastic, or even neoplastic, often bilateral stromal cell nodules with microscopic and functional similarities to adrenal cortical cells (Fig. 15.5). The term "testicular tumor of the adrenogenital syndrome" has been applied to these nodules, most of which will regress following corticosteroid administration. Nonregressing nodules may represent true benign neoplasms. Metastases have not occurred.

In the testicular feminization syndrome, the vagina ends blindly. The uterus, fallopian tubes, and ovaries are absent. The testes are

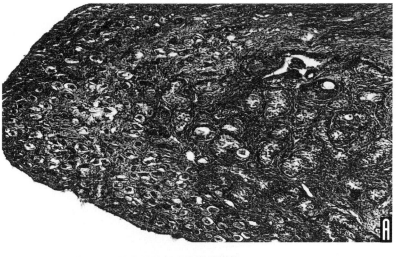

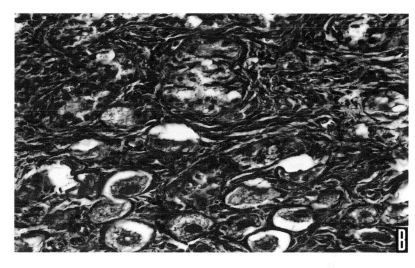

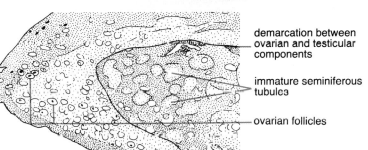

demarcation between ovarian and testicular components

immature seminiferous tubules

ovarian follicles

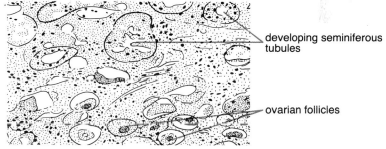

developing seminiferous tubules

ovarian follicles

Figure 15.4 **A,** In this ovotestis from a true hermaphrodite, ovarian follicles form a C-shaped configuration surrounding a zone of immature seminiferous tubules. **B,** At the junction of ovarian and testicular elements in an ovotestis, ovarian follicles abut developing seminiferous tubules.

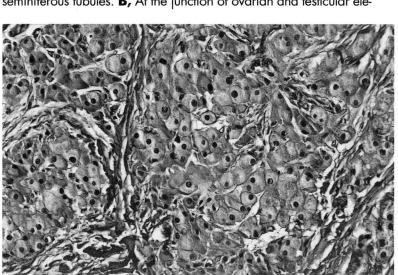

Figure 15.5 The "testicular tumor of the adrenogenital syndrome" consists of nodules of cells with prominent, eosinophilic cytoplasm, resembling adrenal cortical cells. Unlike Leydig cells, Reinke crystals are absent.

located in the inguinal canal or the abdomen (Fig. 15.6). Bilateral inguinal hernias in a phenotypically female infant should suggest the possibility of this condition.

Microscopically, the testes in testicular feminization resemble normal prepubertal testes, if removed in early childhood. Postpubertally, the Leydig cells become hyperplastic and tumorlike nodules of Sertoli cells may be seen (Fig. 15.7). There is an approximately 22% incidence of gonadal neoplasia, principally seminoma, in testes not removed before 30 years of age.

FEMALE PSEUDOHERMAPHRODISM

Female pseudohermaphrodites are karyotypically 46XX individuals with varying degrees of genital ambiguity in whom the ovaries are microscopically normal but unstimulated. Most cases are due to a form of adrenogenital syndrome in which abnormal cortisol production leads to elevated levels of adrenocorticotropic hormone (ACTH). This in turn leads to overproduction of virilizing adrenal steroids, which also suppress the pituitary production of gonado-

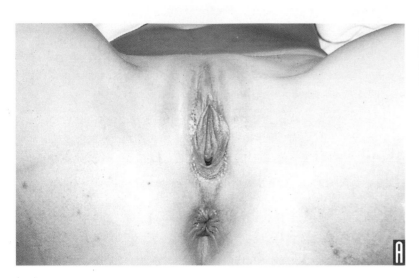

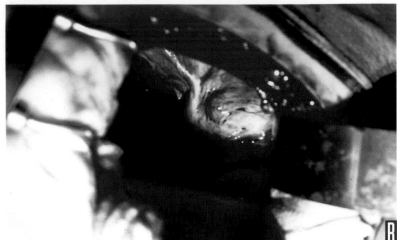

Figure 15.6 A, In testicular feminization syndrome, the external genitalia and body habitus are those of a normal female. **B,** Surgical exploration of the patient revealed bilateral abdominal testes and a blind-ending vagina without uterine, tubal, or ovarian structures. (Courtesy of J.E. Fowler, Jr., MD, Chicago, Illinois)

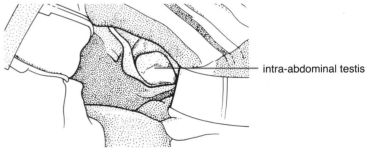

intra-abdominal testis

Figure 15.7 Nonneoplastic proliferations of hyperplastic Sertoli cells may be seen in cryptorchid testes, regardless of pathogenesis, but they are especially common in testicular feminization.

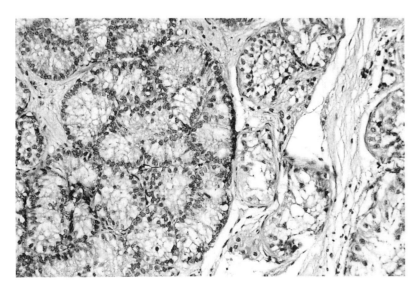

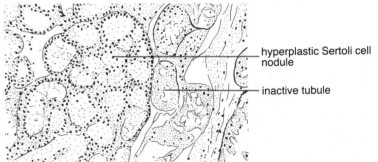

hyperplastic Sertoli cell nodule

inactive tubule

tropins. A second, smaller group of cases involves patients whose mothers received exogenous androgens during pregnancy or had androgen-secreting cortical neoplasms.

GONADAL DYSGENESIS

The term *gonadal dysgenesis* generally refers to the presence of bilateral streak gonads. The most common form of gonadal dysgenesis is Turner's syndrome (45XO or mosaicism), but patients may also be karyotypically normal males or females. Patients with Turner's syndrome or XX karyotype are phenotypic females. XY individuals with gonadal dysgenesis may be phenotypically male or female.

The streak gonads in these patients consist of little more than elongated condensations of fibrous stroma resembling ovarian stroma (Fig. 15.8). Scattered germ cells may be seen, but they disappear during the first several years of life. Up to 33% of XY individuals with gonadal dysgenesis develop mixed gonadoblastomas and seminomas.

MIXED GONADAL DYSGENESIS

Mixed gonadal dysgenesis is defined as the presence of an abnormal testis on one side and a rudimentary or streak gonad contralaterally. Patients usually have ambiguous, asymmetric genitalia, persistent müllerian duct structures, and a Y chromosome (usually as part of a mosaic karyotype).

Microscopically, the streak gonad is identical to that seen in "pure" or bilateral gonadal dysgenesis. Gonadoblastoma occurs in about one third of patients; 30% of these develop a seminomalike germ cell tumor.

INFERTILITY

Factors accounting for infertility are at least partially male-derived in 50% of couples who seek medical attention for this problem. Adequate evaluation usually necessitates a semen analysis for sperm count, morphology, and motility; endocrinologic evaluation, including luteinizing hormone (LH), follicle-stimulating hormone (FSH), and testosterone levels; and, in many cases, testicular biopsy. Proper study of a testicular biopsy specimen for infertility requires careful examination of the seminiferous-tubule architecture, thickness of the basement membrane, nature of the interstitial (Leydig) cells, and status of the germ cell epithelium. The possible morphologic findings characteristic for infertility are: (1) normal histology, (2) testicular immaturity, (3) sloughing of germ cell epithelium, (4) hypospermatogenesis, (5) maturation arrest, (6) Sertoli cells only (germ cell aplasia), and (7) peritubular fibrosis and hyalinization. Although these categories are useful guidelines, many testicular biopsies do not fit neatly into a single subgroup, and mixed patterns are common. The clinical causes (when known) as well as morphologic features of each category are discussed separately.

NORMAL HISTOLOGY

CLINICAL MANIFESTATIONS The most common cause of azoospermic infertility in a man with a histologically normal testicular biopsy is duct obstruction. This condition, which may be congenital or acquired, accounts for about 12%–14% of male infertility cases. Congenital obstruction usually occurs in the distal portion of the epididymis or proximal portion of the vas deferens and may be amenable to surgical reconstruction. Cystic fibrosis in males is associated with severe atresia or absence of the excretory ducts, but such patients have testicular changes as well. Occlusion may also result from infections, particularly tuberculosis or gonorrhea involving the epididymis.

Obstruction is not the only cause of infertility associated with normal testicular histology, but it almost always produces azoospermia. Infertile men with normal or only slightly decreased sperm counts and morphologically normal testes may have unrepresentative biopsies, toxic or metabolic abnormalities without microscopic counterparts, or immotile sperm.

MORPHOLOGY The seminiferous tubules from normal, postpubertal testes contain a complex mixture of Sertoli cells and germ cells in various levels of maturation. The process of spermatogenesis involves several mitotic divisions and a single meiotic (reduc-

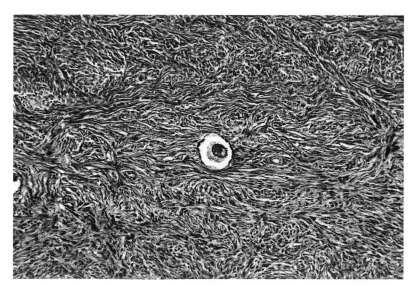

Figure 15.8 This microscopic view of a streak gonad came from a patient with Turner's syndrome who lacked well formed ovaries. The tissue, which was removed from the region of the ovarian ligament, consists of ovarianlike fibroblastic stroma and rare follicles.

tion) division (Fig. 15.9). Meiotic division in males can only take place in an environment that is several degrees lower than physiologic temperature, such as in the scrotum. The apparently absolute nature of this requirement has overridden evolutionary attempts to locate such genetically valuable structures in a less vulnerable location. Ovarian meiotic divisions occur during embryologic development and do not require lower temperature.

Normal spermatogenesis proceeds as "waves of maturation" throughout the seminiferous tubules. In any tubular section, most of the germ cells are at the same level of development. Sertoli cells are recognized by their peripheral location, columnar shape, and oval nuclei with uniform chromatin oriented radially around the tubules. The most undifferentiated germ cells, termed *spermatogonia*, tend to be located peripherally, just beneath the tubular basement membrane. Spermatogonia undergo a mitotic division, providing one cell for maturation and one new spermatogonium to perpetuate the stem cell line. The cell destined to mature gradually moves toward the lumen, enlarges, becoming a *primary spermatocyte*. Each primary spermatocyte undergoes a meiotic divi-

sion to form two smaller *secondary spermatocytes*. Almost immediately, the secondary spermatocytes undergo a final mitotic division to form four haploid *spermatids*. The spermatids undergo maturation with compaction of the nuclear chromatin to form mature *spermatozoa*. During the final stages of development, the spermatids are buried in the cytoplasm of Sertoli cells, from which they receive nutrients. Spermatozoa are typically immotile until mixed with prostatic secretions.

Infertile males with normal light-microscopic biopsies and sperm counts should undergo motility studies, including ultrastructural examination. In the immotile cilia syndrome, there is an absence of ciliary dynein arms that is often accompanied by other ultrastructural abnormalities.

Testicular Immaturity

Testicular immaturity accounts for only about 1% of patients seeking medical attention for symptomatic infertility. Because patients with immature testes suffer from prepubertal gonadotropin insuffi-

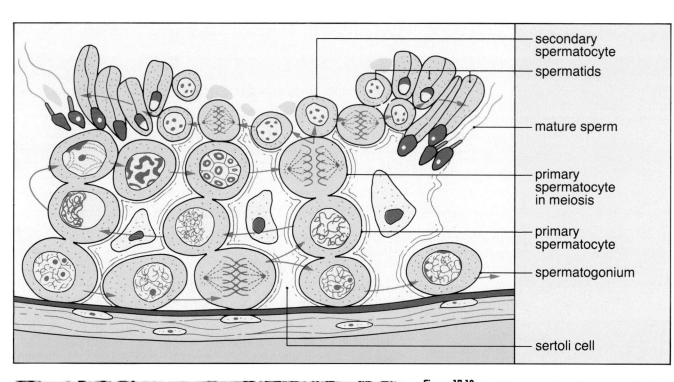

secondary spermatocyte

spermatids

mature sperm

primary spermatocyte in meiosis

primary spermatocyte

spermatogonium

sertoli cell

Figure 15.9 This schematic traces the developmental stages of mature spermatozoa. Because maturation moves in "waves" through the tubules, germ cells are at approximately the same stage of development in a real tubular cross-section.

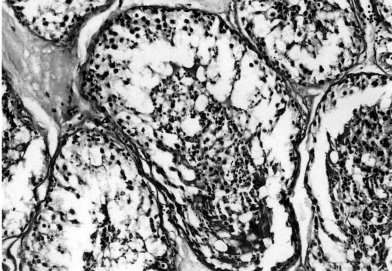

Figure 15.10 In this example of germ cell sloughing, the central portion of the seminiferous tubules filled with aggregates of germ cells at varying stages of development.

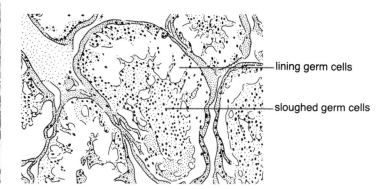

lining germ cells

sloughed germ cells

ciency and sexual immaturity, they are unlikely to complain of infertility. Treatment with exogenous gonadotropins results in sexual maturation, but most patients remain infertile. Another cause of immature testes is prepubertal androgen excess, from either an exogenous source or an androgen-producing neoplasm. The high level of circulating androgens inhibits pituitary gonadotropin secretion. Biopsy specimens from these adult males are histologically identical to normal prepubertal testes (see Fig. 15.1).

Sloughing of Germ Cells

Intraluminal aggregates of immature germ cells are a common finding in males with low sperm counts. The causes of tubular sloughing, as well as its natural course, are unclear. It is often found in patients with varicoceles and following vasectomy or mumps orchitis.

The lumina of the seminiferous tubules are partially or completely obstructed by disorganized, free-floating, cellular masses of immature germ cells (Fig. 15.10). The surrounding tubular lining may appear hypocellular. A diagnosis of sloughing should be made only if more than half of the tubules are affected. Leydig cells appear normal, but there may be mild peritubular fibrosis.

Hypospermatogenesis

CLINICAL MANIFESTATIONS   Underproduction of spermatozoa is one of the most common morphologic findings in oligospermic males, accounting for 30%–51% of testicular biopsies for infertility. A variety of causes have been reported, including malnutrition, chronic illness, chronic exposure to environmental heat, febrile illness, toxins, Down's syndrome, hypothyroidism, Cushing's syndrome, and exogenous corticosteroids. Unfortunately, many cases are idiopathic.

MORPHOLOGY   The seminiferous tubules are of normal or slightly reduced diameter. Cells in all stages of spermatogenesis are decreased such that the germ cell elements remain in approximately normal proportions and mature sperm are present. These features allow distinction from maturation arrest. Because of the loss of germ cells, the tubular lining is thinned and the lumen is correspondingly enlarged (Fig. 15.11). Hypospermatogenesis may be qualitatively graded as mild, moderate, or severe. The correlation with sperm count is imperfect, however, probably because of limited sampling. Severe cases of hypospermatogenesis may be difficult to distinguish from germ cell aplasia (see Sertoli cell-only syndrome, below). Indeed, many cases of germ cell anaplasia may represent an end stage of hypospermatogenesis.

The morphologic findings, with one exception, do not suggest a causative agent. In the fertile eunuch syndrome, the testes typically show hypospermatogenesis and, in addition, marked diminution or absence of Leydig cells.

Maturation Arrest

CLINICAL MANIFESTATIONS   Maturation arrest is one of the most common variants of male infertility, accounting for roughly 40% of cases in one series. Patients are typically azoospermic or severely oligospermic. Reported causes include uremia, Down's syndrome, XYY karyotype, cystic fibrosis, adrenogenital syndrome, febrile illness, exposure to environmental heat, glucocor-

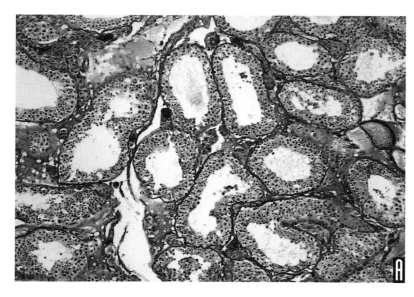

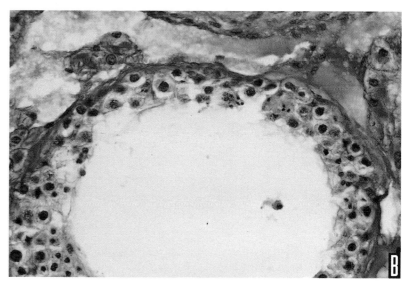

Figure 15.11 A, At low magnification, the intratubular lining in a patient with hypospermatogenesis appears thinned, and the lumen is correspondingly enlarged. **B,** A high-power view demonstrates that although the overall germ cell activity is markedly diminished, developing spermatids are still present, a feature distinguishing this lesion from maturation arrest.

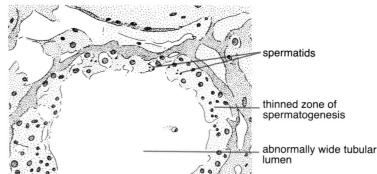

spermatids

thinned zone of spermatogenesis

abnormally wide tubular lumen

ticoid excess, and mumps orchitis. Many of these conditions are also causes of hypospermatogenesis. The morphologic features of maturation arrest do not allow prediction of the underlying pathogenesis.

MORPHOLOGY The microscopic hallmark of maturation arrest is an abrupt cessation in germ cell maturation at a specific point in development (Fig. 15.12), usually at the diploid primary spermatocyte stage prior to the important meiotic division. It may also occur at the secondary spermatocyte or spermatid stage. Although the level of arrest varies from patient to patient, it remains constant throughout the tubules of a given testis. No defects are noted in the Sertoli cells, Leydig cells, or basement membrane of the seminiferous tubules.

GERM CELL APLASIA [SERTOLI CELL–ONLY SYNDROME]

CLINICAL MANIFESTATIONS Some 10%–20% of infertile males have germ cell aplasia, as evidenced by testicular biopsies essentially devoid of germ cell epithelium. Azoospermia and elevated serum-FSH levels are accompanying clinical findings. Sexual development is normal. Germ cell aplasia was originally regarded as a congenital defect in germ cell migration. Although some cases may be congenital, others are acquired as the end stage of a variety of processes producing hypospermatogenesis. Conditions associated with germ cell aplasia include chemotherapy, XYY karyotype, Down's syndrome, uremia, varicocele, radiation, adrenogenital syndrome, and mumps orchitis.

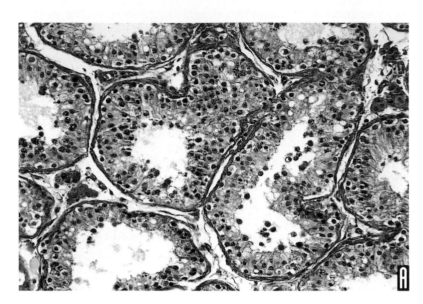

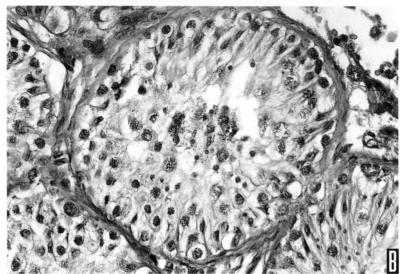

Figure 15.12 Examples of maturation arrest. **A,** The thickness of the germ cell epithelium in this low-power view is approximately normal. No spermatids are seen, but such tubules are common in normal testes because of the wavelike maturation of spermatozoa. When all of the tubules assume this pattern, the patient has maturation arrest. **B,** Many of the germ cells have similar nuclear characteristics and appear to be arrested at the primary spermatocyte stage.

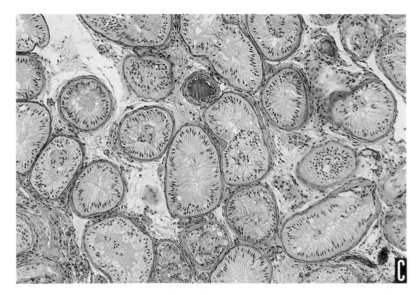

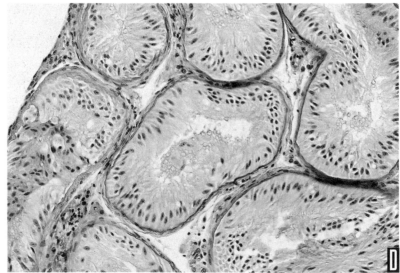

Figure 15.13 **A,** Germ cell aplasia (Sertoli cell–only syndrome) is a morphologically distinctive form of infertility. Even at this low magnification, the uniform population of tall, columnar cells lining the tubules can be seen. **B,** A higher-power view demonstrates the nuclear uniformity of the columnar Sertoli cells, in contrast with the variable nuclear features of developing germ cells.

MORPHOLOGY The microscopic appearance of the Sertoli cell–only syndrome is one of the most distinctive patterns seen in testicular biopsies. The normally complex mixture of morphologically heterogeneous cell types is absent, and the tubules are lined by a population of cytologically uniform Sertoli cells (Fig. 15.13). The cytoplasm of the columnar Sertoli cells extends into the tubular lumina in a pattern that has been likened to "windswept treetops." No germ cells in any stage of development are present, except for rare cases in which they may exist focally in a few tubules. The tubules are typically of slightly reduced diameter, but other morphologic changes are generally absent. The microscopic appearance does not suggest an underlying pathogenesis.

PERITUBULAR FIBROSIS AND HYALINIZATION

CLINICAL MANIFESTATIONS The final group of testicular biopsies for infertility is that in which the peritubular fibrous tissue shows diffuse thickening, culminating in complete tubular sclerosis. As with the other microscopic patterns, the morphology only occasionally suggests the underlying cause, which may include trauma, chronic orchitis, irradiation damage, postpubertal hypopituitarism, vascular insufficiency, alcoholism, diabetes mellitus, cystic fibrosis, varicocele, and Klinefelter's syndrome.

MORPHOLOGY Testicular tissue from any adult male frequently contains scattered tubules with peritubular fibrosis. Only when the fibrotic process becomes more generalized and affects 10% or more of tubules is fertility compromised. In this condition, a sequence of events leads to a progressive loss of germ cell function. The initial change is a subtle thickening of the tubular basement membrane (TBM), which advances to form an obvious zone of peritubular sclerosis. The increased fibrous tissue apparently inhibits nutrient or oxygen flow. The germ cells are more susceptible and disappear first; then the Sertoli cells disappear, followed by collapse of the tubular lumen and conversion into a shrunken, hyalinized core (Fig. 15.14). Peritubular elastic fibers remain if the testis had been under gonadotropin stimulation. The status of the stromal Leydig cells and the presence of stromal inflammation may provide the only other clues as to a possible cause.

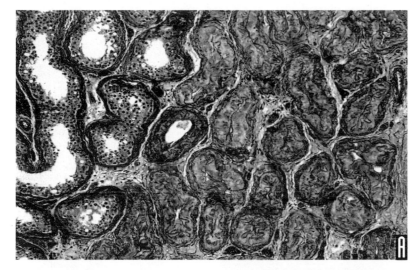

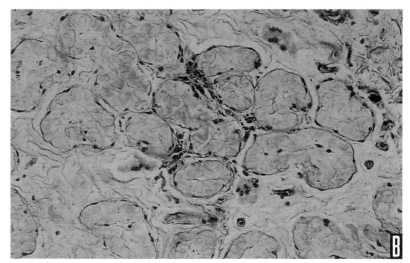

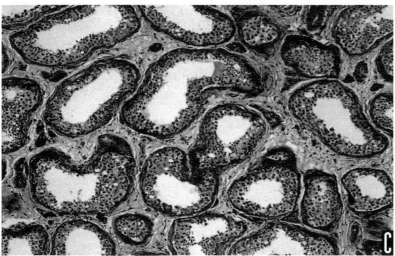

Figure 15.14 **A,** Testicular tissue from fertile males frequently contains small foci of sclerotic tubules, (right). The tubules on the left have thickened TBMs. **B,** In diffuse mild fibrosis, the earliest change is a thickening of the TBM. **C,** The seminiferous tubules in diffuse sclerosis (end-stage testis) are shrunken, sclerotic, and devoid of germ cells or Sertoli cells.

DIFFERENTIAL DIAGNOSIS *Klinefelter's syndrome* should be suspected whenever the testicular biopsy shows advanced sclerosis with associated Leydig cell hyperplasia (Fig. 15.15). In this condition, peritubular elastic tissue is absent or markedly diminished. Mosaics (XXY/XY) have less pronounced changes. *Postpubertal gonadotropin insufficiency* should be considered if Leydig cells are fewer or absent and serum-testosterone levels are correspondingly low. Feedback inhibition of pituitary function causes the same microscopic features in androgenic or estrogenic steroid excess of either an endogenous or exogenous nature. Similar changes may also be seen in *chronic orchitis* (see below).

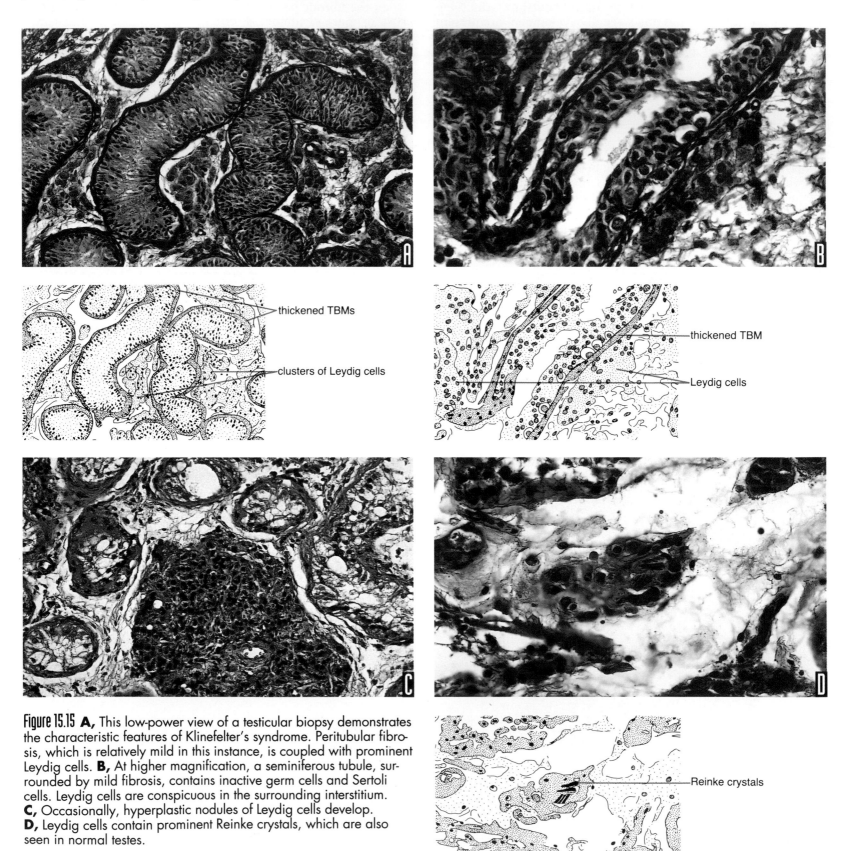

Figure 15.15 A, This low-power view of a testicular biopsy demonstrates the characteristic features of Klinefelter's syndrome. Peritubular fibrosis, which is relatively mild in this instance, is coupled with prominent Leydig cells. **B,** At higher magnification, a seminiferous tubule, surrounded by mild fibrosis, contains inactive germ cells and Sertoli cells. Leydig cells are conspicuous in the surrounding interstitium. **C,** Occasionally, hyperplastic nodules of Leydig cells develop. **D,** Leydig cells contain prominent Reinke crystals, which are also seen in normal testes.

Testicular Inflammation (Orchitis)

As Mikuz and Damjanov, as well as others, have observed, there are unique features regarding testicular anatomy and physiology that must be understood before the pathogenesis of testicular inflammation can be fully appreciated. The location of the testis in the scrotum provides the lower temperature necessary for meiosis. This lower temperature may also be important in the predilection of certain infections, particularly leprosy, to involve the testis. The location of the testis and its ductal continuity with the lower urinary tract predispose it to the retrograde spread of infection. Other modes of involvement include dissemination via lymphatic and vascular channels or along tissue planes. The germ cells are shielded from the rest of the body by a blood-testis barrier composed of TBM and Sertoli cells attached by tight junctions. This barrier may play an important role in the pathogenesis of autoimmune orchitis or in the testicular alterations occurring after the barrier is breached, such as following a vasectomy.

Numerous systems have been devised for the subclassification of testicular infections. In the sections below, the following subdivisions are considered: acute suppurative orchitis, viral orchitis, granulomatous orchitis, and vasculitis involving the testis.

Acute Suppurative Orchitis

PATHOGENESIS This form of testicular inflammation may be caused by any of a host of microorganisms, and any bacterial pathogen is potentially capable of producing a testicular infection. *Escherichia coli* is the most common agent in men over 35 years of age; *Neisseria gonorrheae* is most common in younger patients. *Streptococcus, Staphylococcus,* and other gram-positive cocci are also common causes.

CLINICAL MANIFESTATIONS There is often severe testicular pain and swelling of recent onset. Systemic symptoms, including fever and chills, are also common.

MORPHOLOGY Grossly, the testis in acute suppurative orchitis is swollen and erythematous. It may be covered with fibrinous exudate. Abscesses may be visible after transection of the specimen (Fig. 15.16). Experimental studies by Mikuz suggest that the infection begins in the interstitium, spreading to the tubules following destruction of the blood–testis barrier. Larger areas of necrosis and abscess may form. Microscopically, the abscess consists of a non-specific, fibrinopurulent exudate that replaces the testicular parenchyma. The necrosis may be due to a combination of the infection and ischemia produced by swelling within the confines of a constricting tunica vaginalis. If unresected, the parenchyma is eventually replaced by fibrous scar tissue.

Viral Orchitis

PATHOGENESIS Many viruses undoubtedly cause subclinical infections of the testis as a component of generalized viremia. Others may produce clinically symptomatic involvement, again as a component of systemic infection. Coxsackie viruses, influenza, rubella, echovirus, varicella, and vaccinia, among others, have been documented by culture or serology in patients with orchitis. Mumps virus is by far the most common cause of clinically evident viral orchitis. It is the only virus with apparent testicular tropism, at least in postpubertal individuals.

CLINICAL MANIFESTATIONS Orchitis occurs in about 20% of men with mumps infection, but it is seen in only about 1% of infected children. Bilateral clinical involvement occurs in about 16% of patients with testicular symptoms (about 3% of all infected men), and infertility due to mumps infection is, for practical purposes, limited to this small group. Viral orchitis is, nonetheless, a well documented occurrence, as is alluded to in the section above on testicular biopsy.

MORPHOLOGY Testicular biopsies are virtually never obtained during the acute phase of viral orchitis. Encounters with such infections are limited to a study of their sequelae. In about half of patients with clinical evidence of mumps orchitis, there are testicular morphologic changes, usually in the form of focal tubular sclerosis. However, only about 20% have testicular atrophy (Fig. 15.17) or azoospermia. The actual frequency of impaired fertility is difficult to determine. In addition to tubular damage, mumps may affect Leydig cells, thereby decreasing androgen secretion, leading to changes of relative estrogen excess, including gynecomastia.

Granulomatous Orchitis

This subdivision of testicular inflammatory conditions includes bacterial and fungal infections evoking a granulomatous reaction, for-

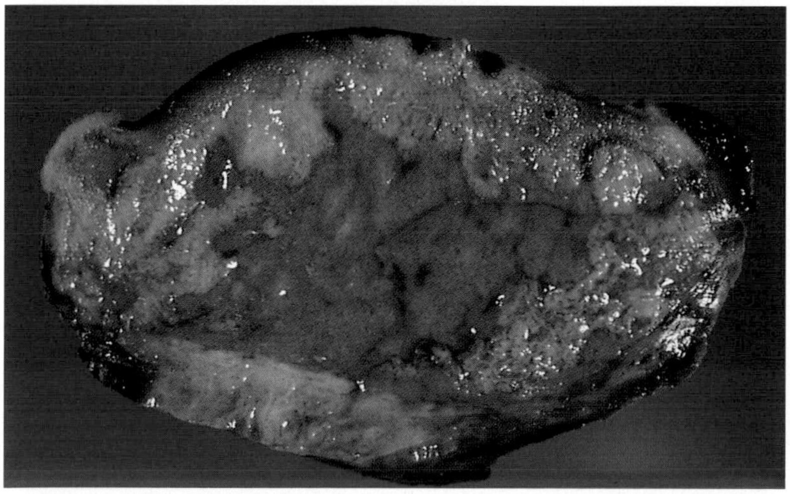

Figure 15.16 Transected testis from a patient with acute suppurative orchitis shows a large abscess cavity.

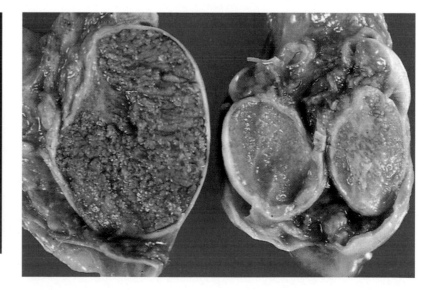

Figure 15.17 These testes from a patient with a history of clinically symptomatic mumps orchitis show marked unilateral atrophy on the right. Microscopically, the atrophic testis was identical to that seen in Figure 15.14C.

eign body granulomas, sarcoidosis, as well as idiopathic granulomas. Some forms of granulomatous orchitis may be confused grossly, and even microscopically, with testicular neoplasms. The gross image most often resembles a seminoma. The microscopic appearance may lead to confusion with lymphoma. The absence of a monomorphic population of atypical cells in granulomatous orchitis allows distinction. An even more treacherous pitfall is the misdiagnosis of a true testicular neoplasm as a granuloma. The offending tumor is invariably a seminoma with an exuberant fibroblastic, lymphoid, and giant cell reaction.

TUBERCULOSIS

Involvement of the testis in tuberculosis usually occurs in conjunction with disease elsewhere in the genitourinary tract. Spread is presumably intraductular or along lymphatics. Orchitis as a component of miliary (hematogenous) disease is uncommon. Infection typically begins in the epididymis, extending to involve the testis (Fig. 15.18).

Microscopically, well formed granulomas characteristically consist of numerous mononucleated and multinucleated histiocytes (Fig. 15.19) surrounding broad zones of central caseous necrosis. The larger granulomas are visible grossly as cheesy, white zones. Acid-fast bacilli of *Mycobacterium tuberculosis* are usually demonstrable (Fig. 15.20).

MALAKOPLAKIA

Malakoplakia of the testis is clinically and morphologically identical to its more common counterpart in the bladder and prostate (see Chapters 12, 13). This specialized form of granulomatous orchitis may produce enough testicular enlargement to be confused with a neoplasm.

The gross appearance of a cut section may mimic that of a seminoma. Microscopically, a polymorphic infiltrate of inflammatory cells is present, but the characteristic, and often predominant, cell is a large macrophage containing laminated spherules known as Michaelis–Gutmann bodies.

VASCULITIS INVOLVING THE TESTIS

The systemic vasculitides may occasionally produce testicular symptomatology. Swelling and pain lead to confusion with other processes, including infection and torsion. Periarteritis nodosa and Henoch–Schönlein purpura are the most common forms of systemic vasculitis affecting the testis.

The microscopic appearance of testicular vasculitis is identical to that seen in other sites. Periarteritis nodosa produces a segmental inflammation in the media of muscular arteries. Focal necrosis and fibrosis may result in complete obliteration of the lumen. Henoch–Schönlein purpura is a leukocytoclastic vasculitis affecting smaller vessels.

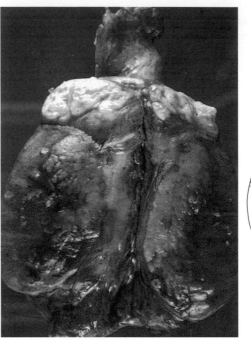
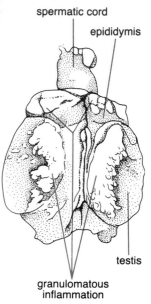

Figure 15.18 The testicular parenchyma and epididymis in testicular tuberculosis contain multiple yellow nodules corresponding to aggregates of granulomatous inflammation.

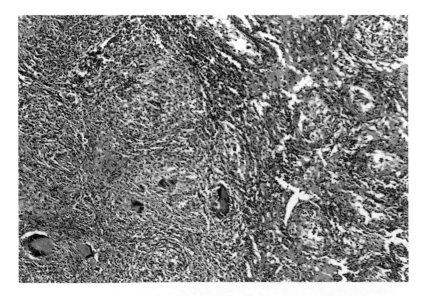

Figure 15.19 Low-power photomicrograph of testicular tuberculosis shows an inflammatory cell infiltrate with prominent giant cells replacing the testicular parenchyma. Residual seminiferous tubules are seen at the right.

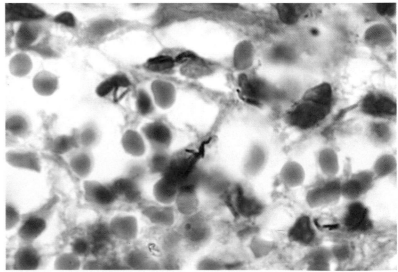

Figure 15.20 In testicular tuberculosis, rod-shaped mycobacteria stain red with acid-fast stain and are seen associated with inflammatory cells and erythrocytes.

CHAPTER 16

Testicular Neoplasms

STAGING OF TESTICULAR TUMORS

Since the clinical stage of a testicular neoplasm at the time of diagnosis affects prognosis and influences therapeutic strategies, numerous staging systems have been proposed. All of these systems consider the extent of metastatic disease, and some take into account the size and extent of the primary neoplasm. Specific classification is usually made on the basis of clinical observations, radiographic studies, and pathologic findings in both the primary tumor and, when applicable, excised lymph nodes. Lymphangiography and, more recently, computed tomography (CT) have been used increasingly in the evaluation of abdominal lymph nodes for metastases (Fig. 16.1).

One of the best known staging systems is the Walter Reed Classification system, defined as follows:

Stage IA Confinement of the tumor to the testis with no clinical or radiographic evidence of metastatic spread.

Stage IB Confinement of the tumor to the testis but with histologic evidence of metastases in iliac or para-aortic lymph nodes.

Stage II Clinical or radiographic evidence of metastases to femoral, inguinal, iliac, or para-aortic lymph nodes.

Stage III Clinical or radiographic evidence of metastases above the diaphragm or to other distant sites.

Germ Cell Neoplasms

The majority of this chapter is devoted to testicular lesions of germ cell origin. The concept that each member of this morphologically diverse family arises from germinal epithelium has been called the "holistic view" of germ cell neoplasia. Although the concept is well accepted and supported by a wide array of clinical and experimental observations, other theories were once equally popular. For example, the proposal that seminoma was a neoplasm of germ cells but that other tumors (embryonal carcinoma, teratoma, etc.) arose from blastomeres displaced during embryonic development was once favored. This concept still influences the British nomenclature, which divides testicular tumors into seminomas (germinal origin) and teratomas of varying subtype (blastomeric origin).

Most testicular germ cell tumors develop within a decade after puberty, when testosterone levels are at their peak. Some, however, develop later in life, and occasionally they appear in infants. As will be discussed, there are marked differences in the biologic behavior of germ cell tumors in prepubertal children and histologically similar tumors in young adults. With only one exception, all testicular germ cell tumors have ovarian counterparts, but there are several important differences in biologic behavior. These factors suggest that the hormonal milieu in which the tumor develops influences its growth and malignancy. There is also a tendency for different forms of germ cell neoplasia to manifest at different ages. With advancing age, seminoma in particular is more common as a pure tumor or as a component of a mixed germ cell tumor.

The development of highly effective chemotherapeutic regimens has dramatically improved the treatment of germ cell tumors in the last 15–20 years. Combined treatment with surgery, radiation, and chemotherapy now produces high cure rates even for nonseminomatous neoplasms.

At least a half dozen systems of nomenclature have been developed for classifying germ cell neoplasms. In the sections below, germ cell testicular tumors are divided into the categories of intratubular germ cell neoplasia, seminoma, embryonal carcinoma, endodermal sinus (yolk sac) tumor, teratoma, choriocarcinoma, and mixed patterns. Some of these major categories contain histologic subtypes. Although these divisions have prognostic value, the most important distinction bearing on the selection of therapy is whether the tumor contains nonseminomatous elements.

Germ cell tumors show a striking propensity to transmutate between morphologic categories. This tendency is manifested by the synchronous presence of mixed germ cell elements in up to 40% of tumors and by the development of asynchronous mixed or heterogeneous metastases. Such transformations provide further support for the holistic view of testicular neoplasia.

Intratubular Germ Cell Neoplasia

Cases of in situ or intratubular germ cell neoplasia have been repeatedly documented in recent years. Such neoplasia is most commonly seen at the edges of an invasive tumor, where it probably represents intratubular spread rather than residue of a preinvasive lesion. About 1% of testicular biopsy specimens for infertility contain intratubular proliferations of malignant germ cells without associated invasion. In such cases, many of which involve cryptorchid testes, it must be assumed that an in situ neoplasm has been intercepted prior to invasion. This assumption is supported by the results of Coffin and coworkers in which four of six patients having intratubular neoplasia in a biopsy without further therapy developed an invasive germ cell tumor from 1.3 to 4.5 years later.

Microscopically, some of the intratubular neoplastic cells resemble seminoma cells and contain abundant glycogen (Fig. 16.2). The periodic acid-Schiff (PAS) stain is valuable for highlighting these elements, since normal germ and Sertoli cells do not stain. More recently, immunocytochemical techniques have documented the presence of placental alkaline phosphatase in dysplastic or malignant intratubular cells (Fig. 16.3).

Seminoma

Seminomas are the most undifferentiated of germ cell neoplasms. By definition, they lack any evidence of maturation and consist of a proliferation of cells resembling primordial germinal epithelium. There are four morphologic subtypes of seminoma: classic, anaplastic, syncytiotrophoblastic giant cell, and spermatocytic. Seminoma with syncytiotrophoblastic giant cells and anaplastic seminoma are closely associated both clinically and morphologically with classic seminoma, although anaplastic seminoma was once considered a distinct variant. These two subtypes are discussed briefly at the end of the section on classic seminoma. Spermatocytic seminoma, which has important clinical and morphologic features distinguishing it from classic seminoma, is covered in greater depth.

Classic Seminoma

CLINICAL MANIFESTATIONS Pure seminoma is the most common type of testicular tumor, accounting for 40%–55% of germ cell neoplasms. In an additional 15% of testicular tumors, semi-

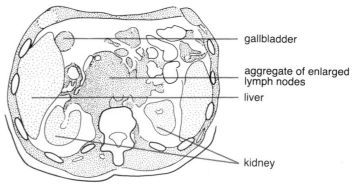

Figure 16.1 CT scan demonstrates marked enlargement of periaortic lymph nodes due to a metastatic testicular germ cell tumor. (Courtesy of T.L. Pope, Jr., MD, Charlottesville, Virginia)

gallbladder

aggregate of enlarged lymph nodes

liver

kidney

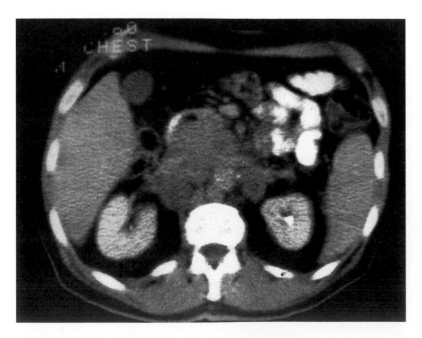

noma is one component of a mixed neoplasm. Patients are typically in their third or fourth decade of life, which is considerably older than most patients with other forms of testicular neoplasia. The lesion has a slight right-sided predilection. It arises in cryptorchid gonads in about 8% of cases. The most common complaint is of gradual increase in testicular size, sometimes with pain. In about 85% of cases, the involved testis is enlarged at the time of initial examination. It may be up to 10 times normal size but is typically much smaller. About 10% of patients have clinically demonstrable or symptomatic metastases at the time of diagnosis.

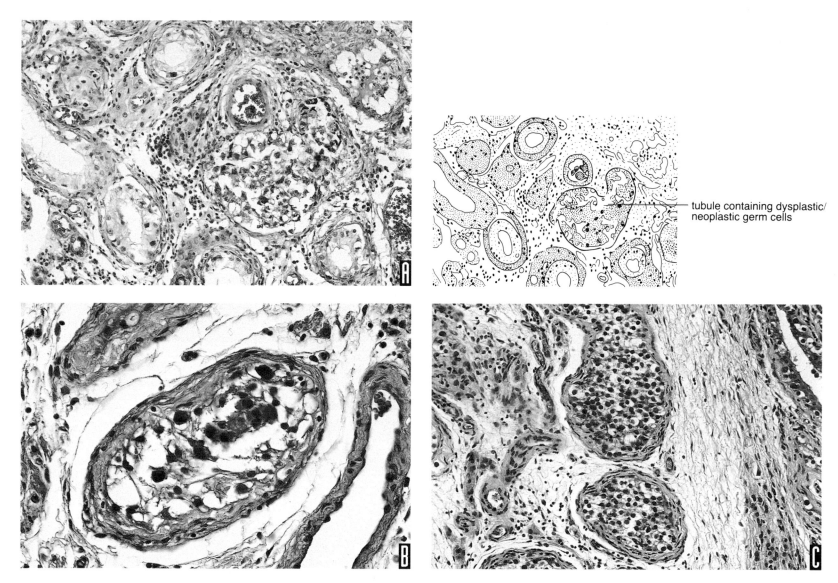

tubule containing dysplastic/neoplastic germ cells

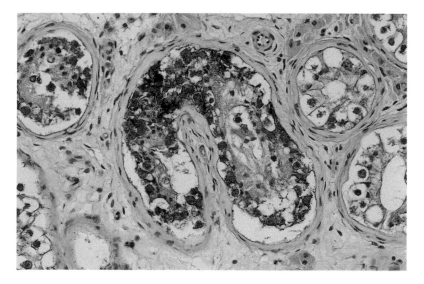

Figure 16.2 **A,** Intratubular germ cell neoplasia. The tubule just to the right of center contains a cytologically atypical population of germ cells. **B,** This seminiferous tubule in a cryptorchid testis contains a population of hyperchromatic, presumably neoplastic cells. **C,** Low-power photomicrograph of intratubular neoplasia shows tubules packed with a uniform population of cells resembling the cells of invasive seminoma.

Figure 16.3 Immunocytochemical staining for placental alkaline phosphatase demonstrates positive (brown) staining in the cytoplasm of dysplastic intratubular germ cells from a cryptorchid testis.

Approximately 8% of patients with pure, classic seminomas show elevated serum levels of human chorionic gonadotropin (β-HCG) due to the presence of scattered trophoblastic cells (see below). Alpha-fetoprotein (AFP) is always absent from pure seminoma; its presence in serum usually indicates a component of endodermal sinus tumor, embryonal carcinoma, or, possibly, immature teratoma in the primary tumor or metastases. It is worthwhile to follow these markers in seminoma patients because an increase in serum levels may document a transformation to nonseminomatous tumor in subsequent recurrences. As noted below, such transformations are associated with a more aggressive clinical course.

DIAGNOSTIC STUDIES Ultrasonography, computed tomography (CT) scanning, and magnetic resonance imaging (MRI) may sometimes help verify the existence of a space-occupying lesion involving a normal-sized testis. Percutaneous core needle biopsy is not employed for diagnosis because the tumor might seed along the needle tract. Needle aspiration cytology using small-gauge needles does not carry this risk and may be used to obtain a tentative preoperative diagnosis. However, as orchiectomy is the initial therapy for virtually all germ cell tumors, this procedure usually establishes the diagnosis.

MORPHOLOGY Grossly, seminoma forms a circumscribed, lobulated mass, which may be pink, tan, yellow, or white, and displaces the normal testicular parenchyma. Fibrous bands may exist between the lobules (see Fig. 16.4B). If the tumor is of modest size, the cut surface appears homogeneous. Larger tumors may contain areas of infarction and hemorrhage, but small hemorrhagic tumors of the testis are usually not seminomas. Tumoral extension through the testicular capsule with involvement of the epididymis, spermatic cord, or scrotum is uncommon (about 8% of cases) (Fig. 16.4).

Because the thick tunica vaginalis impedes the diffusion of formalin fixative, the testis should be carefully sectioned along its major axis before fixation. Identifying nonseminomatous elements is of utmost importance, and requires multiple microscopic sections with special attention to areas that are grossly atypical.

Microscopically, seminoma is usually readily recognized, although the degree of morphologic variation is greater than most textbooks illustrate. There are usually nests and sheets of uniform cells with distinct cell borders and clear-to-granular, eosinophilic cytoplasm. Clear cytoplasm indicates that glycogen has been removed during tissue processing (Fig. 16.5). The cell nests and sheets are separated by a fibrovascular stroma containing a prominent lymphoid infiltrate. Glandular or papillary configurations are absent. Nuclei are centrally located and have oval or round con-

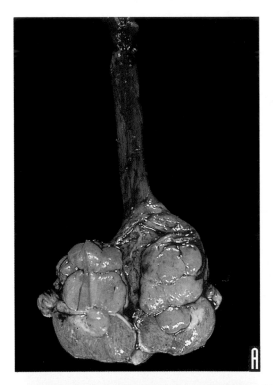
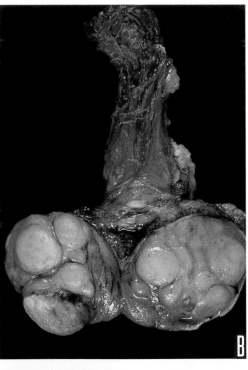

Figure 16.4 A, This seminoma, which has a uniform yellow color, extends outside the testicular parenchyma to involve the epididymis and peritesticular spermatic cord. **B,** The nodular growth pattern seen here is common with seminomas. The homogeneous, white-tan color is more common than the yellow color seen in **A.**

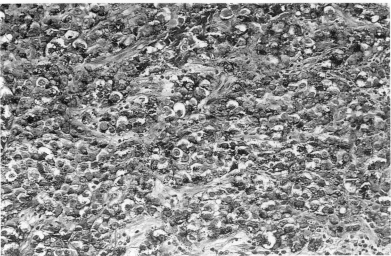

Figure 16.5 Intracytoplasmic red staining with PAS indicates the presence of glycogen. This section of seminoma was fixed in ethanol to inhibit removal of glycogen during tissue processing.

tours and evenly dispersed, granular chromatin (Fig. 16.6). Nuclear pleomorphism is usually mild but occasionally it can be quite marked (Fig. 16.7). Mitotic figures are always present and may be numerous. The stromal connective tissue varies from inconspicuous to prominent (Fig. 16.8). The lymphocytic infiltrate that is almost invariably present may contain germinal centers (Fig. 16.9). A few studies have correlated increased lymphoid infiltrate with improved survival, but this is of little value due to the overall good prognosis. Other inflammatory cells, including multinucleated histiocytes, may be seen, and granulomatous aggregates of epithelioid

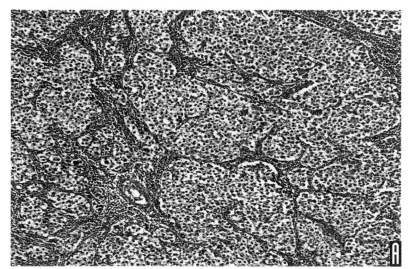

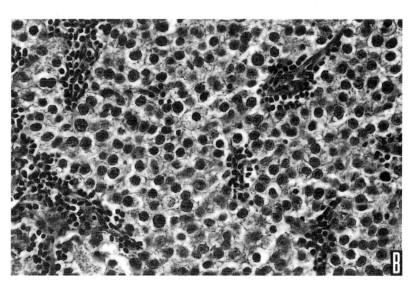

Figure 16.6 A, In this prototypical low-power view of seminoma, irregular islands of neoplastic cells are separated by a delicate fibrovascular stroma and accompanying lymphoid infiltrate. **B,** This high-power microscopic image is most commonly seen in seminoma. The nuclei have a uniform chromatin distribution, and cell borders are distinct. A small cuff of lymphocytes surrounds the capillaries.

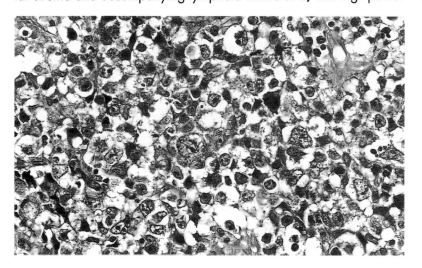

Figure 16.7 The severe nuclear pleomorphism evident in this photomicrograph, accompanied by a high mitotic rate, would place this lesion in the anaplastic seminoma category. The prognosis for this tumor is the same, stage for stage, as that of a more conventional seminoma.

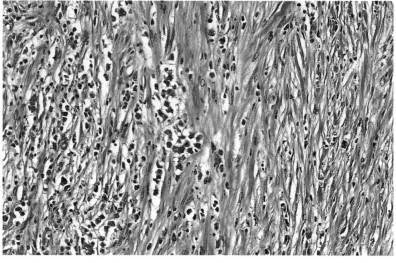

Figure 16.8 Seminomas occasionally have prominent stromal fibrosis. In such instances, the neoplastic cells are widely scattered by fibrous bands and may be overlooked.

Figure 16.9 A lymphoplasmacytic inflammatory reaction is a common component of most seminomas. Here the lymphocytes form germinal centers.

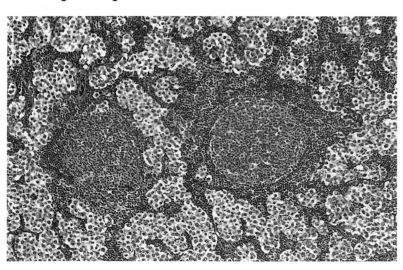

histiocytes occasionally form. Multinucleated histiocytes should not be confused with syncytiotrophoblastic cells, which occur in a morphologic variant (see below) (Fig.16.10). In rare seminomas, the degree of granulomatous response and stromal fibrosis may be so pronounced that the neoplastic cells are overlooked and the tumor may be misdiagnosed as a granulomatous orchitis.

THERAPY AND PROGNOSIS Seminoma is noted for its marked sensitivity to radiation, and therapy for stage I and II disease usually consists of orchiectomy followed by radiation therapy to pelvic and retroperitoneal lymph nodes. A nodal dissection is not performed. The prognosis for pure, classic seminoma is excellent. Most tumors are stage I at the time of diagnosis and cure rates are over 95%. Survival rates for stage II patients are equally good. Even stage III disease has a five-year survival rate of almost 70% in some studies. Metastases usually follow lymphatic drainage. Hematogenous spread is less common, developing late in the clinical course.

Autopsy findings for patients who died from the disease after having had purely seminomatous testicular primary tumors show that almost half (44%) had other forms of germ cell neoplasia in their metastases. The greater virulence of these nonseminomatous components appears to account for considerable mortality. Although nonseminomatous components in the primary lesion undoubtedly were missed in some cases due to sampling errors, other cases represent subsequent differentiation in a previously pure seminoma.

ANAPLASTIC SEMINOMA

The term *anaplastic seminoma* was originally applied to classic seminomas that had three or more mitotic figures per high-power field, along with prominent nuclear pleomorphism (see Fig. 16.17). Results of more recent studies have questioned the value of mitotic rate in this distinction, suggesting that if this criterion is maintained, the qualifying number of mitotic figures per high-power field should be raised to six or more. Some 3%–10% of seminomas fall into the anaplastic category as variously defined. The overall prognosis for anaplastic seminoma is agreed to be worse than that for classic seminoma. However, this seems to be due primarily to a tendency for patients with anaplastic seminoma to present at a

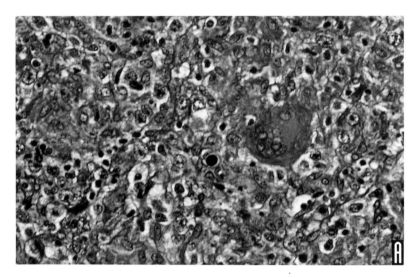

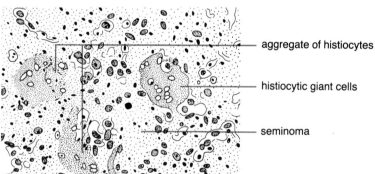

aggregate of histiocytes

histiocytic giant cells

seminoma

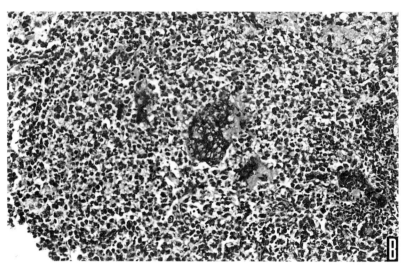

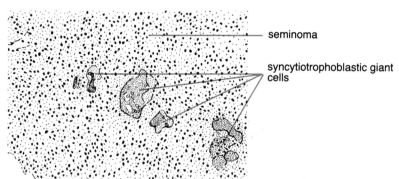

seminoma

syncytiotrophoblastic giant cells

Figure 16.10 A, Multinucleated histiocytes (giant cells) may be seen in seminomas and should not be confused with syncytiotrophoblastic cells. The nuclei of the giant cells have a uniform, vesicular appearance, which is identical to that of the mononuclear histiocytes.

B, The large, irregular giant cells in this seminoma are syncytiotrophoblastic cells resembling placental syncytial cells and producing β-HCG. In the absence of a mixture of cytotrophoblastic and syncytiotrophoblastic elements, choriocarcinoma should not be diagnosed.

more advanced stage. Stage for stage, there is no prognostic difference between the two; therefore, segregation of these neoplasms is of dubious clinical value. Occasionally, an anaplastic seminoma is so poorly differentiated that it is difficult to distinguish it from embryonal carcinoma. This should not be surprising in view of their common cellular origin.

SEMINOMA WITH SYNCYTIOTROPHOBLASTIC GIANT CELLS

Approximately 8% (range: 3%–14%) of seminomas contain scattered syncytiotrophoblastic giant cells (see Fig. 16.10B), often in association with elevated serum-HCG. Immunocytochemical staining has documented the presence of β-HCG within the cytoplasm of the giant cells. The biologic behavior of such seminomas is not entirely clear. Although some studies have suggested a slightly worse prognosis as compared with classic seminoma, the survival rate is far better than that for choriocarcinoma and the two entities must not be confused microscopically. The syncytiotrophoblasts in seminoma occur singly or in small clusters, often in close association with blood vessels. There may be small foci of hemorrhage associated with the giant cells. In contrast, choriocarcinoma contains large numbers of both cytotrophoblastic and syncytiotrophoblastic cells in close apposition (see Fig. 16.20A), along with broad zones of stromal hemorrhage.

SPERMATOCYTIC SEMINOMA

CLINICAL MANIFESTATIONS   Spermatocytic seminoma accounts for about 3.5%–7% of all seminomas. Presenting complaints are similar to those for the classic form, but the mean age at presentation is distinctly greater. Although patients as young as 30 years have been reported, most are over 50 years old (mean, 65 years). Unlike classic seminoma, the spermatocytic form is not associated with cryptorchidism and virtually always occurs in a normally descended testis. Involvement of the contralateral testis, which is usually asynchronous, occurs in about 6% of cases, as opposed to approximately 2% for classic seminoma. We are aware of only a single, well documented case of spermatocytic seminoma with associated metastases. In this example, although there was spread to para-aortic lymph nodes, the patient died of chemotherapy-related complications rather than widespread disease. Earlier reports of metastatic spermatocytic seminoma almost certainly represent testicular malignant lymphoma. There have also been rare reports of sarcomatous transformation, associated with aggressive clinical behavior, within otherwise typical spermatocytic seminomas. With these unusual exceptions, the prognosis for spermatocytic seminoma is excellent, approaching 100%. Treatment for uncomplicated cases should consist of orchiectomy without radiation therapy.

MORPHOLOGY   The gross appearance of this variant of seminoma differs from the classic form. The cut surface is typically pale gray, edematous, or mucoid. Cystic degeneration is common, but hemorrhage and necrosis are only seen in larger tumors (Fig. 16.11). The tumors vary from extremely large to only a few centimeters in size.

Microscopically, spermatocytic seminoma also differs from the classic form. It is never associated with other types of germ cell neoplasia, including classic seminoma. Syncytiotrophoblastic cells are absent. The tumor cells form sheets and nests, often widely separated by a loose, edematous stroma. Stromal inflammation, a common feature of classic seminoma, is lacking. Intratubular involvement is common at the periphery and may extend for a considerable distance from the invasive tumor.

Three main cell types, differing primarily in size, are present in spermatocytic seminoma, in contrast to the uniform cell population of classic seminoma. Most common is a *medium-sized cell* (15–20 μ) with a round nucleus and finely granular chromatin. The *small cell* (6–8 μ) has a small, round, ink-blot nucleus and a narrow rim of eosinophilic cytoplasm. The *giant cell* is large (50–100 μ), with one or

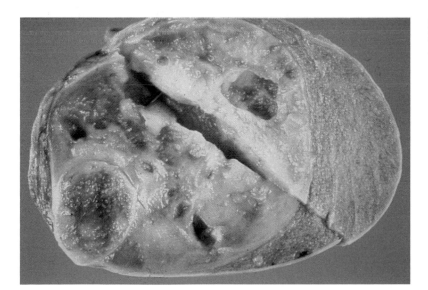

Figure 16.11 Grossly, spermatocytic seminomas typically have a mucoid, focally cystic appearance. Hemorrhage and necrosis are only seen in larger tumors. (Courtesy of A. Talerman, MD, Chicago, Illinois)

more nuclei and abundant, eosinophilic cytoplasm (Fig. 16.12). The nuclei are typically round with chromatin that varies from granular to diffusely hyperchromatic. Mitotic activity, including atypical mitotic figures, is evident, and the mitotic rate varies considerably both intra- and interlesionally. Cytoplasmic glycogen, another common finding in classic seminoma, is sparse or absent from all three cell types. Unlike other forms of germ cell neoplasia, spermatocytic seminoma is negative for placental alkaline phosphatase.

Spermatocytic seminoma is the only form of germ cell neoplasia that does not have an ovarian or extragonadal counterpart. This feature, plus the presence of small spermatid-like tumor cells, prompted speculation that spermatocytic seminoma might be a tumor composed, at least in part, of postmeiotic, haploid cells. Microspectrophotometric observations have ruled out this possibility. Most tumor cells have DNA in the hyperdiploid or peritriploid range.

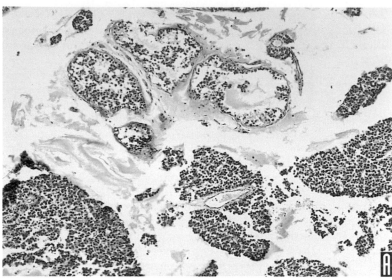

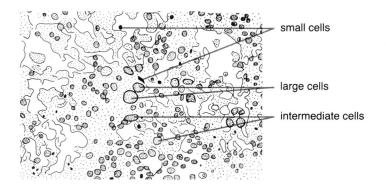

small cells

large cells

intermediate cells

Figure 16.12 **A,** Low-power photomicrograph of spermatocytic seminoma shows nests of neoplastic cells widely separated by an edematous stroma. Note the absence of an inflammatory cell infiltrate. **B,** A higher-power view shows the cytologic variability characteristic of spermatocytic seminoma. Cells with large, vesicular nuclei are present in the center of the field. Most of the cells are of intermediate size, but a few small cells with hyperchromatic nuclei are also present. (Courtesy of A. Talerman, MD, Chicago, Illinois)

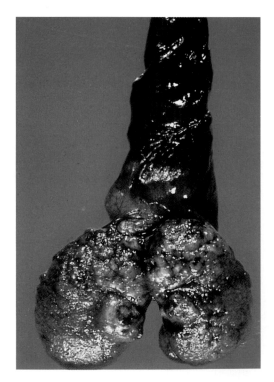

Figure 16.13 In this specimen, embyronal carcinoma is present as a small, hemorrhagic tumor at the upper pole of the testis.

Embryonal Carcinoma

Embryonal carcinoma occupies a midway position on the spectrum of differentiation between seminoma and teratoma. Its cells are highly malignant in appearance and exhibit only abortive differentiation. Maturation to a level mimicking normal embryonal tissues, as seen in an immature teratoma, is absent by definition with this terminology. The British system of nomenclature refers to embryonal carcinoma as malignant teratoma, undifferentiated. Numerous animal studies have documented the ability of embryonal carcinoma cells to progressively differentiate, forming immature and even mature teratomas. Not surprisingly, the combination of teratoma and embryonal carcinoma is common in testicular neoplasia, accounting for about 25%–30% of germ cell neoplasms. The term teratocarcinoma is sometimes applied to this mixture. Pure embryonal carcinoma, in comparison, accounts for about 10%–20% of testicular germ cell tumors.

CLINICAL MANIFESTATIONS Patients with embryonal carcinoma are a full decade younger, on average, than those with pure, classic seminoma. Most patients are between 15 and 35 years old; the lesion is uncommon in those over the age of 50. It is almost nonexistent in infants and young children, among whom endodermal sinus (yolk sac) tumor, viewed by some as a variant of embryonal carcinoma, is far more common.

Patients usually present with gradual testicular swelling. Up to one third have clinically evident metastases at the time of initial evaluation. Pure embryonal carcinoma usually produces only modest testicular enlargement, in contrast to the marked enlargement often seen with seminoma and teratoma. At least half of embryonal carcinomas are associated with elevated serum-AFP levels, probably representing foci of yolk sac differentiation. This marker is a valuable aid in following the disease's course, as elevations may herald the development of metastases before they are detected by other means. As with seminomas, embryonal carcinomas occasionally contain scattered syncytiotrophoblastic giant cells, which may be responsible for elevations in serum HCG. The levels of serum β-HCG are typically far below those seen with choriocarcinomas.

MORPHOLOGY Embryonal carcinoma is typically a small tumor with a variegated, solid, gray-white appearance and focal areas of hemorrhagic necrosis (Fig. 16.13). Extension into peritesticular structures (tunica, epididymis, spermatic cord) may be seen in up to 20% of cases.

Microscopically, embryonal carcinoma may assume a mixture of multiple patterns, in keeping with its tendency to exhibit abortive differentiation in a variety of directions (Fig. 16.14). Solid sheets of cells, glandular or acinar formations, and papillary structures may be present. With one exception, the cells do not differentiate sufficiently to clearly mimic developing embryonic or extraembryonic tissues. Lesions of the latter type are included in the spectrum of immature teratoma, endodermal sinus tumor, and choriocarcinoma. The exception involves occasional embryonal carcinomas containing small "embryoid bodies" that caricature normal embryos of

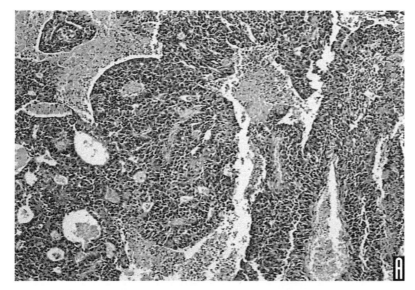

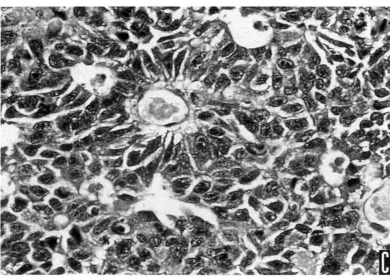

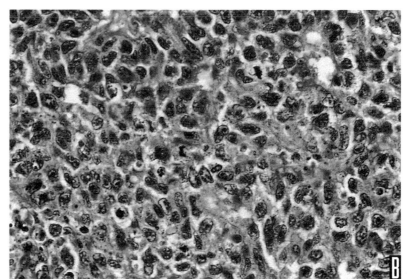

Figure 16.14 A, Low-power photomicrograph of embryonal carcinoma shows nests and cords of neoplastic cells surrounded by zones of necrosis. **B,** This high-power view shows the degree of nuclear pleomorphism, high mitotic rate, and eosinophilic cytoplasm that distinguish embryonal carcinoma from seminoma. The distinction between anaplastic seminoma and embryonal carcinoma may be difficult, however. **C,** Perivascular rosettes and irregular lumenlike structures are common in embryonal carcinoma. Many of the luminal structures probably form when central cells become necrotic and disappear.

one to two weeks' gestational age. In rare instances, germ cell neoplasms consist entirely of such embryoid bodies; the term polyembryoma has been applied to these tumors (Fig. 16.15).

Regardless of their low-power morphology, embryonal carcinomas are composed of highly pleomorphic cells, which vary tremendously in size, shape, and nuclear-chromatin staining. Many contain abundant, eosinophilic cytoplasm with indistinct cell borders. Nuclei, which are large and irregular, vary from densely hyperchromatic to vesicular with multiple prominent nucleoli (see Fig. 16.14). Mitotic figures, including grotesquely atypical forms, are common. Necrosis and hemorrhage are also prominent. The stromal component is typically small and usually lacks the lymphocytic reaction seen in seminoma. Solid areas of embryonal carcinoma may be confused with seminoma, but they can be distinguished from seminoma by the marked pleomorphism, usual absence of distinct cell borders, and lack of prominent stromal inflammation characteristic of seminoma.

As with seminoma, a small percentage of embryonal carcinomas contain scattered syncytiotrophoblastic giant cells. Their presence should not be interpreted as choriocarcinoma, a term reserved for a mixture of both cytotrophoblastic and syncytiotrophoblastic elements. Elements of true choriocarcinoma are frequently present in association with embryonal carcinoma, however, and careful gross and microscopic search of hemorrhagic areas aids in identifying these foci.

Many embryonal carcinomas also contain microscopic foci of endodermal sinus tumor. This may account for a large proportion of AFP production in tumors labeled as embryonal carcinoma. The clinical significance of focal endodermal sinus tumor is unclear, but at least one study has suggested a worsened prognosis.

THERAPY AND PROGNOSIS The treatment of embryonal carcinoma is nonstandardized. In the United States, the most common procedure is orchiectomy, followed by radiographic evaluation of retroperitoneal lymph nodes. Clinically uninvolved nodes may be treated with lymphadenectomy, and about 15%–20% contain occult metastases. Patients with clinically involved retroperitoneal lymph nodes usually receive preoperative radiation therapy and/or chemotherapy, often followed by lymphadenectomy. The role of adjuvant chemotherapy, in completely resected stage I and II disease is controversial. Recurrent disease can frequently be eradicated with newer chemotherapeutic regimens.

The survival rates for embryonal carcinoma have changed dramatically with the advent of combined surgery, radiation, and chemotherapy. Accurate five-year survival rates according to pathologic type are difficult to ascertain because of the tendency to lump all nonseminomatous germ cell tumors into one category. The 75% mortality rate quoted in the past, however, has given way to an 80%–90% overall survival rate. In fact, stage I embryonal carcinoma has a survival rate comparable with that of seminoma.

ENDODERMAL SINUS (YOLK SAC) TUMOR

This neoplasm is known by a variety of synonyms, but the favored terms—endodermal sinus tumor and yolk sac tumor—are based on the pioneering studies of Teilum, who suggested that these tumors were of germ cell derivation and mimicked the yolk sac or endodermal sinus. Even subsequent to his work, there has been confusion regarding the origin and nomenclature for these lesions. Terms such as "adenocarcinoma of infant testis" and "testicular adenocarcinoma with clear cells" have been applied, suggesting mesonephric rather than germ cell lineage. Ultrastructural studies and demonstration of AFP synthesis by both normal yolk sac and yolk sac tumors have provided additional support for Teilum's theory, which is now widely accepted.

CLINICAL MANIFESTATIONS Pure endodermal sinus tumor of the testis virtually always occurs in infants and very young children. As discussed above, it exists in postpubertal testes only as a component of mixed germ cell neoplasia. In contrast, yolk sac tumor of the ovary typically develops in adolescents and young adults.

Rapid enlargement of a normally small, prepubertal testis is readily detected and results in expeditious medical attention. The rapidity of diagnosis may account for the 50%–65% overall survival rate in studies prior to the availability of effective chemotherapy, but the testicular yolk sac tumor in infancy certainly does not carry the abysmal prognosis of its ovarian counterpart.

The histologic features of endodermal sinus tumor of the testis have not been correlated with survival, and the rarity of this tumor in its pure form has limited the understanding of its response to newer therapies. Yolk sac tumor is virtually always associated with the production of AFP, reflected in both elevated serum levels and immunohistochemical staining.

MORPHOLOGY Grossly, a yolk sac tumor looks white to yellow and is firm to soft on palpation; it may be focally hemorrhagic or cystic (Fig. 16.16). The highly variable microscopic appearance

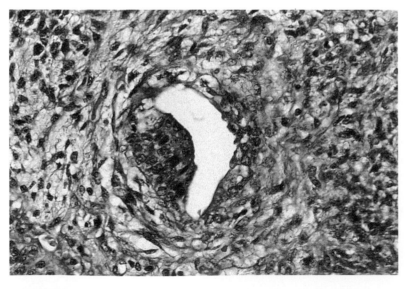

Figure 16.15 Embryoid bodies such as this abortive embryo-like structure may be found in embryonal carcinomas and immature teratomas. Tumors composed entirely of such structures are referred to as polyembryomas.

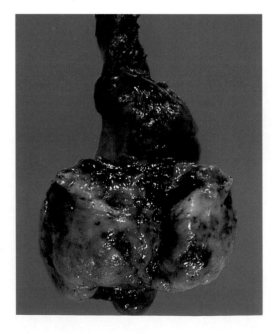

Figure 16.16 In this specimen, the testicular parenchyma is completely replaced by a fleshy yolk sac tumor with areas of hemorrhage.

reflects phases of embryologic yolk sac development (Fig. 16.17). One of the most common microscopic images is a loose reticular pattern of cells forming irregular cystic spaces in an edematous or mucinous-appearing stroma. Solid areas, papillary formations, and glandular or ductal structures may also be present. The so-called endodermal sinuses or Schiller–Duval bodies are diagnostic. They are glomeruloid structures consisting of a flattened, "parietal" layer of cells and a more conspicuous central tuft of cuboidal "visceral" cells, the latter having a fibrovascular core containing a central capillary. Unfortunately, endodermal sinuses are often absent or difficult to document convincingly.

Cytologically, yolk sac tumors often display a surprising uniformity. The pleomorphism typical of embryonal carcinoma may be lacking, and mitotic figures may be difficult to find. An important microscopic feature is the presence of intracellular and extracytoplasmic hyaline globules (see Fig. 16.17C). These globules are intensely eosinophilic, PAS positive, and diastase resistant. Immunocytochemically, they have been shown to contain both AFP and α_1-antitrypsin; other proteins may also be present. Immunocytochemical staining for AFP may help in diagnosing problematic cases presenting with metastatic disease from an occult primary tumor (Fig. 16.18).

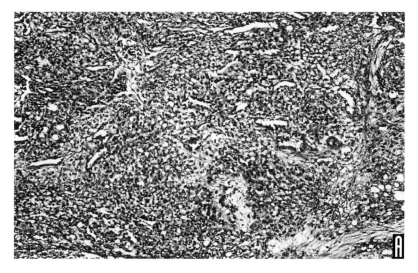
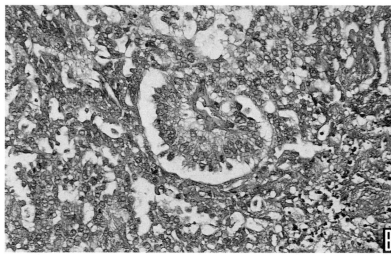

Figure 16.17 A, Low-power photomicrograph of a yolk sac tumor demonstrates irregular cystic spaces alternating with more solid areas. **B,** A small papilla with a central fibrovascular core protrudes into the lumen of the central cystic space. The resulting structure is known as a Schiller–Duval body. **C,** A high-power view demonstrates the eosinophilic globules frequently seen in yolk sac tumors. These have been shown to contain AFP and α_1-antitrypsin.

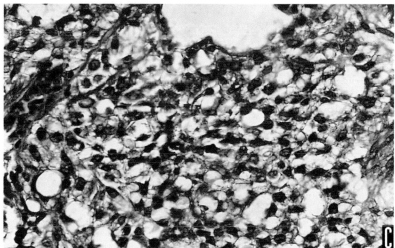

Figure 16.18 In this photomicrograph of a yolk sac tumor, the brown pigment corresponds to areas where AFP has been localized immunocytochemically (immunoperoxidase technique).

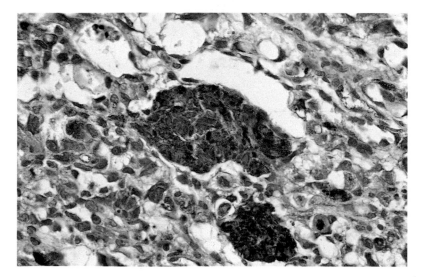

CHORIOCARCINOMA

Pure testicular choriocarcinoma is a mercifully rare neoplasm, accounting for considerably less than 1% of germ cell tumors. As a component of mixed germ cell neoplasia, however, it is much more common. Choriocarcinomas exhibit placental differentiation, manifested by the presence of both cytotrophoblastic and syncytiotrophoblastic elements. Given the angioinvasive nature of normal placental tissue, it is not surprising that choriocarcinomas are hemorrhagic tumors that metastasize hematogenously. Choriocarcinomas may also arise from ovarian germ cells, as well as from extragonadal sites, including the pineal gland and the mediastinum. All of these tumors exhibit analogous biologic behavior. In contrast, uterine or gestational choriocarcinoma, the most common form of choriocarcinoma, has a better prognosis.

CLINICAL MANIFESTATIONS Pure testicular choriocarcinoma is so rare that meaningful clinical data subsequent to the advent of effective chemotherapy are nonexistent. Most patients with pure or predominantly choriocarcinomatous tumors are in their second decade of life, although there have been rare reports of elderly men with the disease. Presenting symptoms are frequently related to metastases (hemoptysis, hepatomegaly) or to high levels of β-HCG produced by the tumor (gynecomastia). The primary tumor may be quite small and clinically unapparent. Well documented examples of regression of the primary tumor, resulting in a hemosiderin-laden scar, have been reported.

Choriocarcinoma tends to metastasize early in the clinical course of disease. Prior to the development of effective chemotherapy it was almost always fatal, but the prognosis is now identical to that for other nonseminomatous tumors when matched stage for stage. The obvious caveat is that choriocarcinomas are frequently high-stage neoplasms.

Choriocarcinoma, whether mixed or pure, invariably produces HCG. The serum levels of β-HCG may be distinctly elevated and serve as a useful marker to detect metastases before they become

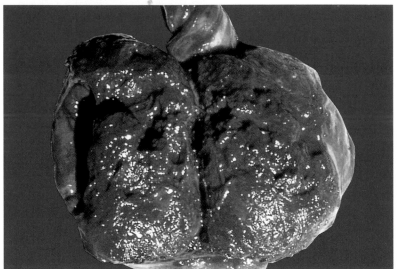

Figure 16.19 In this specimen, choriocarcinoma is present in the testicular parenchyma as a uniformly hemorrhagic mass.

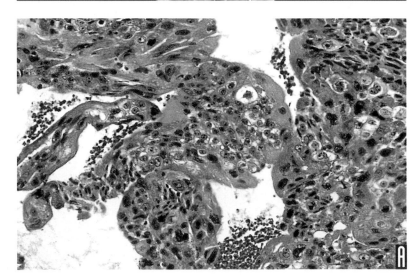

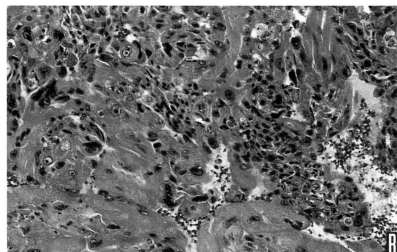

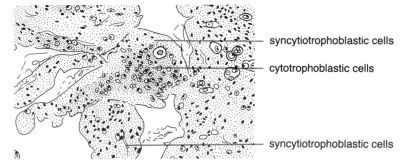

syncytiotrophoblastic cells

cytotrophoblastic cells

syncytiotrophoblastic cells

Figure 16.20 A, This medium-power view shows syncytiotrophoblastic cells with abundant eosinophilic cytoplasm surrounding central aggregates of cytotrophoblastic cells. **B,** In another medium-power view, aggregates of syncytial and cytotrophoblastic cells are associated with stromal hemorrhage.

clinically obvious. Immunocytochemical studies have demonstrated that β-HCG is present exclusively in the syncytiotrophoblastic cells.

MORPHOLOGY Pure or nearly pure choriocarcinomas appear grossly as small, markedly hemorrhagic nodules after sectioning of the testis (Fig. 16.19). The uncut testis may appear completely normal or have a somewhat tense, congested capsule. The greater the nonchorionic elements, the larger the tumor and the more prominent the surrounding rim of gray-tan, nonhemorrhagic tissue.

The microscopic diagnosis requires a mixture of syncytiotrophoblastic and cytotrophoblastic elements in proximity, usually in association with prominent stromal hemorrhage and necrosis (Fig. 16.20). Syncytiotrophoblasts are distinctive, large, multinucleated cells with prominent eosinophilic-to-amphophilic cytoplasm. The cytoplasm may be vacuolated or contain phagocytosed erythrocytes. The nuclei are typically hyperchromatic and vary tremendously in size and shape. Rims of syncytiotrophoblastic cells usually surround central aggregates of cytotrophoblasts, which have distinct cell borders and clear cytoplasm. The highly distinctive, biphasic appearance of these tumors resembles developing placenta, allowing for easy diagnosis. Immunocytochemical stains for β-HCG highlight the syncytiotrophoblastic cells but are seldom needed for diagnosis (Fig. 16.21).

TERATOMA

By definition, teratomas, wherever they occur, should exhibit differentiation toward at least two of the three germ cell layers: endoderm, mesoderm, and ectoderm. "Specialized" monodermal teratomas represent a rare exception to this rule. Conceptually, teratomas can be viewed as a spectrum of neoplasia exhibiting varying types and degrees of somatic differentiation. At their most immature, they are difficult to distinguish from embryonal carcinoma. At the other extreme are tumors composed of haphazard, disorganized arrays of otherwise normal-appearing, mature stroma and epithelium. Whereas ovarian teratomas tend to be completely mature lesions, most testicular teratomas fall in the middle ground. Testicular teratomas are frequently admixed with other germ cell elements, expecially embryonal carcinoma.

CLINICAL MANIFESTATIONS Pure teratomas account for 5%–10% of testicular germ cell neoplasms. The more common mixed cell teratocarcinoma constitutes about 25%–30% of cases. The presenting symptoms and signs are typically related to testicular enlargement, with or without pain, since teratomas tend to be among the largest testicular neoplasms (Fig. 16.22). There is a bimodal incidence curve for pure teratoma. It occurs in infants and very young children, is rare in older children, and is most common in postpubertal adolescents and young adults. The postpubertal age-incidence peak is identical to that of other nonseminomatous germ cell tumors.

In recent years, a variety of noninvasive imaging techniques such as ultrasonography, CT scanning, and MRI have been used to visualize small testicular tumors of all types. Small multicystic teratomas are easy to identify with these procedures.

There are important age-related differences in the biologic behavior and, to a lesser extent, the microscopic appearance of teratomas. Testicular teratomas in young children are typically pure tumors (no other germ cell elements), composed entirely of mature tissue. Metastatic disease has never been documented in a young child with a testicular teratoma, and orchiectomy is curative. Occasionally, teratomas in young children contain immature, usually neural, elements, but these tumors do not metastasize either. Thus, testicular teratomas occurring in infancy and early childhood are invariably benign, regardless of microscopic appearance. The tumor must be carefully sectioned, however, to exclude the presence of yolk sac differentiation. The metastatic potential of the yolk sac tumor warrants prudence.

In contrast, all postpubertal testicular teratomas, with the exception of dermoid cysts, are potentially malignant. If the entire neoplasm is carefully examined microscopically and shown to consist of uniformly mature elements, the prognosis should be excellent; it is unclear whether such tumors are capable of extratesticular spread. The great majority of adult testicular teratomas, however, do contain areas of immature elements, thus rendering them capable of metastasis. To verify the maturity of a lesion would require the examination of thousands of microscopic sections. There are well documented cases of "mature" teratomas with synchronous or metachronous metastases in which small foci of immaturity were identified only after repeat examination of the primary tumor.

Metastases from conventional testicular teratomas may consist entirely of teratoma, or they may be pure germ cell tumors of other types. More frequently, they consist of a mixture of teratomatous, embryonal, and choriocarcinomatous elements. Metastases initially tend to involve regional lymph nodes along the iliac and para-aortic chains. Vascular dissemination to liver, lung, and bone is also common. Survival figures for adults with pure testicular teratomas range from 70%–92%. Patients dying of disease usually have metastases composed of more malignant germ cell components, particularly embryonal carcinoma and choriocarcinoma.

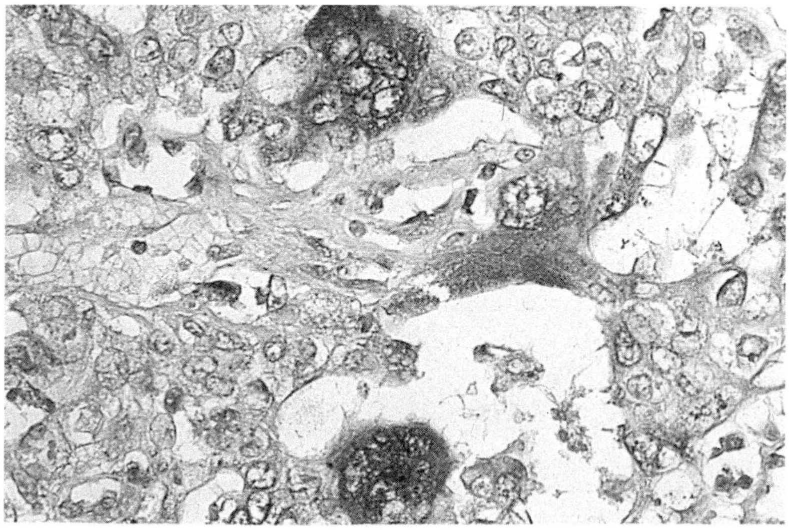

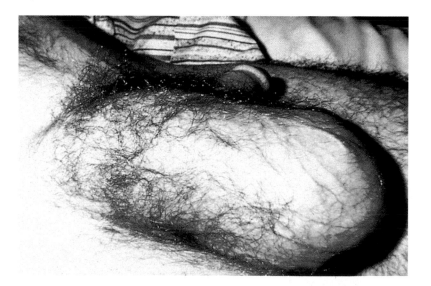

Figure 16.21 The brown pigment in this photomicrograph of choriocarcinoma corresponds to the immunocytochemical localization of β-HCG in syncytiotrophoblastic cells (immunoperoxidase technique).

Figure 16.22 The testicular enlargement seen here demonstrates the enormous size testicular teratomas may reach. (Courtesy of J.E. Fowler, Jr., MD, Chicago, Illinois)

MORPHOLOGY   The testis is often grossly enlarged and, on sectioning, the parenchyma is expanded by a variegated, focally cystic neoplasm. The appearance reflects the microscopic composition. Large areas of cartilage, which are often present, appear translucent blue (Fig. 16.23). Neural elements are soft and white. Cysts may be present, filled with serous or mucinous secretions.

The microscopic appearance is quite variable, as would be expected given the possible range of maturation and differentiation (Fig. 16.24). Immature and mature elements are often mixed haphaz-

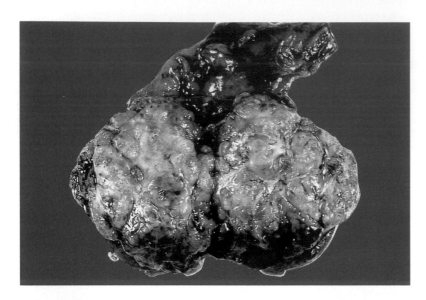

Figure 16.23 The variegated appearance of this testicular teratoma is due to the variation in microscopic constituents.

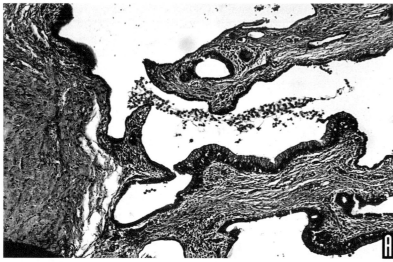

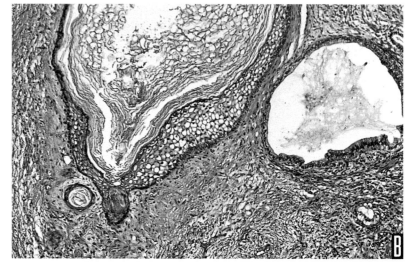

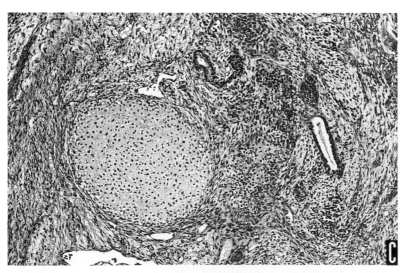

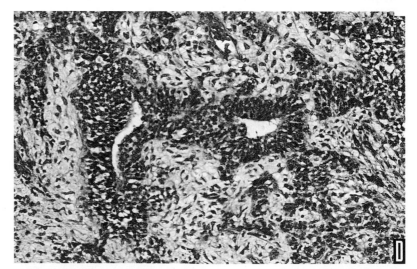

Figure 16.24 A, Low-power photomicrograph of a completely mature teratoma from a young child demonstrates that it is composed predominantly of cystic spaces lined by mucinous epithelium. **B,** Mature-appearing squamous and glandular cysts are surrounded by a fibroblastic stroma. **C,** Mature and immature elements may be intermixed. An island of mature-appering cartilage is present, but to the right of this is a zone of more hyperchromatic, immature cells. Such small foci of immaturity may be overlooked on cursory examination. **D,** This teratoma is composed of immature elements. Hyperchromatic, basaloid epithelial cells form tubular structures, probably representing primitive neural tube formations. The intervening stroma has a loose, embryonal appearance.

ardly. Cysts lined by squamous, ciliated respiratory and columnar mucinous epithelium are common. Such cysts vary tremendously in shape and size. The largest cysts may measure many centimeters in diameter; the smallest may only be visible microscopically. Neural elements are common, particularly in areas of immaturity. Abortive neural tubule structures are also common in these regions, usually in association with a highly cellular neuroepithelial background. Other neural areas may resemble more mature neuroglial tissue or complex structures such as retina. Mesenchymal elements range from immature, embryonic stroma to well formed but irregularly shaped islands of cartilage and bone. Smooth muscle and fibrous tissue are other prominent components.

VARIANTS OF TESTICULAR TERATOMA

DERMOID CYST The so-called dermoid cyst is an easily recognized, mature, benign teratoma that is common in the ovary but rare in the testis. Dermoid cysts have little or no solid component and are lined by epidermis and mature skin appendages. The cysts are filled with hair, sebaceous or keratinous debris, and frequently contain developing teeth. This is the one variant of testicular teratoma that is easily recognized as benign. Unfortunately, it is so uncommon that it accounts for only a tiny fraction of testicular tumors.

CARCINOMA AND SARCOMA ARISING IN TERATOMA Rarely, nongerm cell–type malignancies arise within teratomas. These malignancies may be of epithelial (carcinoma) or mesenchymal (sarcoma) differentiation. The World Health Organization has adopted the term teratoma with malignant transformation for this phenomenon, although this name has also been applied to ter-

atomas that metastasize as higher-grade germ cell tumors. Most often, nongerm cell neoplasms arising in teratomas are seen in recurrences after chemotherapy. It appears that destruction of the more sensitive germ cell components "unmasks" the nongerm cell elements. A recent study of 11 cases found that the nongerm cell components were most frequently sarcomas and only occasionally carcinomas. The biologic behavior did not appear to differ from that of teratomas without malignant transformation, unless the sarcoma was an embryonal rhabdomyosarcoma. (Of five patients with this sarcoma, four died of disease.)

GROWING TERATOMA SYNDROME Teratomas with focal immaturity, which are a common component of mixed germ cell neoplasms, are most frequently seen in association with embryonal carcinoma. The term growing teratoma syndrome has been applied to a clinical subgroup of patients with mixed germ cell tumors, including teratomatous elements. These patients undergo chemotherapy for residual disease or prophylactically after resection of their testicular primary tumor. During the course of treatment, they develop a stable or persistently enlarging mass, most commonly in the retroperitoneum or lungs (Fig. 16.25). The lesions's failure to regress or continued growth during chemotherapy might suggest that the high-grade germ cell neoplasm had become unresponsive to treatment—an obviously poor prognostic sign. Resection of these predominantly cystic lesions, however, reveals that they consist entirely of mature teratomatous elements (Fig. 16.26). The clinically observed enlargement is due, not to persistent neoplasia, but to the accumulation of secretion products in the cysts or to the growth of mature, benign stromal and epithelial elements.

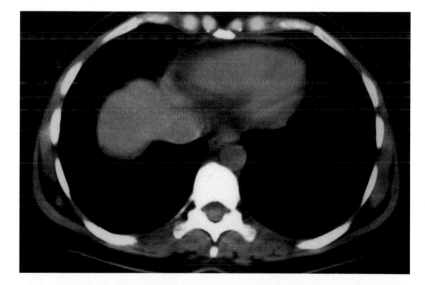

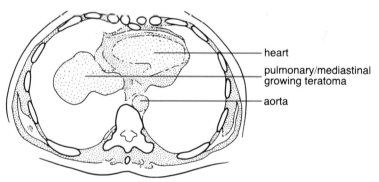

Figure 16.25 The pulmonary and mediastinal mass seen in this CT scan also represents a "growing teratoma." (Courtesy of T.L. Pope, Jr., MD, Charlottesville, Virginia)

heart

pulmonary/mediastinal growing teratoma

aorta

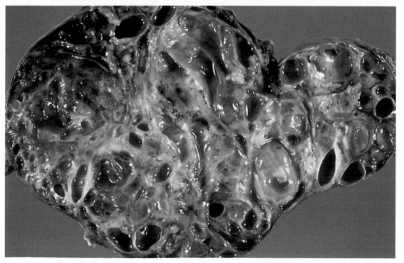

Figure 16.26 A patient with mixed embryonal carcinoma and immature teratoma had a persistently enlarging retroperitoneal mass in spite of continued chemotherapy. Excision yielded the multicystic structure seen here. Microscopically, it was composed entirely of mature elements.

Although the majority of growing masses in patients receiving chemotherapy for nonseminomatous germ cell tumors are probably malignant, the possibility of a growing teratoma should be considered. Surgical resection is the treatment of choice for the growing teratoma in order to prevent compromise of surrounding structures. In patients without residual malignancy, the survival following excision is excellent. Clinical findings favoring growing teratoma rather than persistent malignancy include cystic lesions demonstrated by CT scan or ultrasonography, normal serum markers, and a solitary lesion.

Mixed Germ Cell Neoplasia

Fully 40% of testicular germ cell tumors are composed of multiple cell types. Teratocarcinoma accounts for 25%–30% of these mixed neoplasms, while in about 6% a mixture of teratoma, seminoma, and embryonal carcinoma is seen. The incidence of embryonal carcinoma and seminoma in mixed neoplasms is 5%; that of teratoma and seminoma about 2%; and that of teratoma, embryonal carcinoma, and choriocarcinoma about 1%. In addition to these mixtures, elements of yolk sac tumor are present in up to 40% of embryonal carcinomas. Whenever mixed germ cell tumors are encountered, their constituents should be listed in order of predominance.

Gonadal Stromal Neoplasms

About 3% of testicular neoplasms arise from the specialized, nongerm cell testicular stroma. Leydig cell tumors are most common, but Sertoli cell tumors, granulosa cell tumors, mixed-pattern tumors, and less differentiated gonadal stromal tumors are also encountered.

Leydig Cell Tumors

CLINICAL MANIFESTATIONS Leydig cell tumors occur in males ranging in age from infancy to old age (average, 36 years). About 82% of patients are postpubertal. The most common complaint in postpubertal cases is testicular enlargement without endocrinologic sequelae. About 15% of these patients present with gynecomastia and an asymptomatic but clinically palpable testicular mass. Gynecomastia may also develop before the testicular lesion is detectable by palpation. Hormonal studies may demonstrate elevated estrogen levels, primarily estradiol. Testosterone levels are frequently normal or low. Prepubertal patients almost invariably develop isosexual pseudoprecocity manifested by penile enlargement, erections without ejaculation, facial and pubic hair, acne, and a growth spurt. The duration of symptoms varies from a few months to four or more years (mean, 16 months). In prepubertal individuals, serum testosterone is usually elevated and urinary levels of 17-ketosteroids may be increased. Leydig cell tumors are rarely bilateral (3%) and occur with equal frequency in both testes.

Approximately 10% of Leydig cell tumors metastasize, and there has been some controversy over whether such tumors can be identified at the time of initial diagnosis. Some investigators maintain that clinicopathologic features cannot be relied upon to predict metastases. A study by Kim and co-workers, however, noted a number of clinical and pathologic features that appeared to correlate with metastatic spread. Malignant tumors occurred in older patients (mean age, 67 years) with tumors of short clinical duration (mean, six months), no evidence of endocrine activity, and large size (mean diameter, 6.9 cm). Microscopic features associated with malignancy included an infiltrative margin (80%), necrosis (80%), vascular invasion (80%), greater than three mitotic figures per high-power field (100%), and prominent nuclear atypia (grade 2 or 3 in 80%).

MORPHOLOGY Leydig cell tumors may be as large as 10 cm in diameter, but they are usually about 3 cm. Most are yellow or brown, soft, well circumscribed nodules (Fig. 16.27), although occasionally they are firm or lobulated, and gray to tan in color. Hemorrhage, necrosis, or cystic degeneration may sometimes be seen.

The microscopic appearance of Leydig cell tumors varies, but it most often consists of sheets of cells that have prominent, eosinophilic, granular cytoplasm (Fig. 16.28). Less frequently, the stroma forms a more conspicuous component of the tumor, producing lobules of tumor cells or even thin ribbons of cells in a fibrous stroma. Kim and coworkers recognized three variants of neoplastic Leydig cells. Most common are polygonal cells with abundant eosinophilic, focally vacuolated cytoplasm, distinct cell borders, and round nuclei with a single nucleolus. The second most common cell type had more foamy cytoplasm and smaller nuclei,

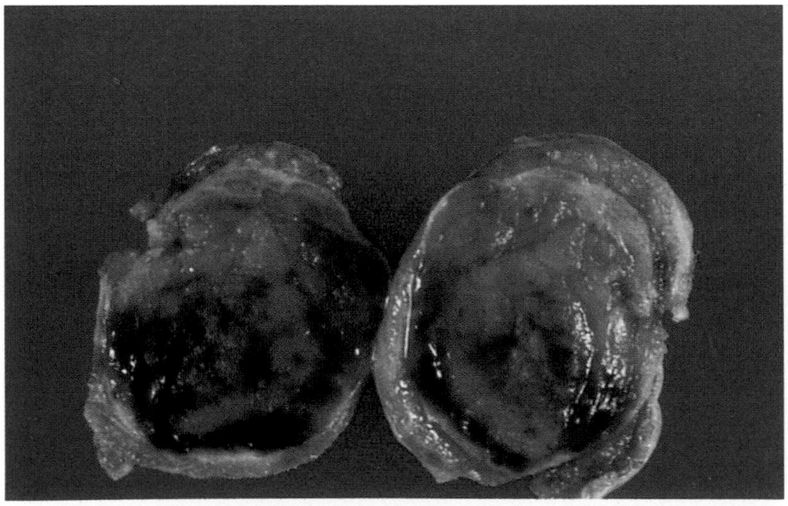

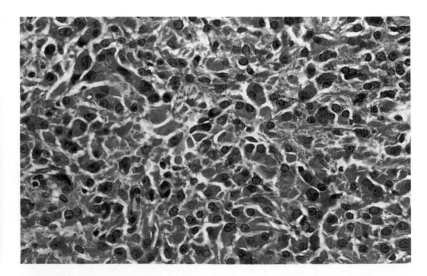

Figure 16.27 Grossly, this Leydig cell tumor is focally hemorrhagic and has replaced most of the testicular parenchyma.

Figure 16.28 Photomicrograph of a Leydig cell tumor reveals that the tumor is composed of a patternless sheet of neoplastic cells with abundant eosinophilic cytoplasm. There is moderate nuclear pleomorphism.

resembling cells of the adrenal cortex. Least common were cells with scanty cytoplasm and round hyperchromatic nuclei.

Crystalloids of Reinke, densely eosinophilic, rectangular intracytoplasmic inclusions, are present in only about 35% of tumors. They are most frequently seen in the large cells with abundant, eosinophilic cytoplasm.

Sertoli Cell Tumors

Testicular proliferations composed entirely of Sertoli cells are much less common than Leydig cell tumors. The most common Sertoli cell lesion is the presumably nonneoplastic Sertoli cell nodule seen in cryptorchid testes (see Fig. 15.7). These nodules are known by a variety of terms, including Sertoli cell hyperplasia, zones of dysgenesis, Pick's adenomas, and tubular adenomas. They are particularly common in genotypic males with the testicular feminization syndrome, in whom they may grow to several centimeters in size.

CLINICAL MANIFESTATIONS Sertoli cell neoplasms can occur at any age and are capable of metastasizing, usually to regional lymph nodes, in about 10% of cases. Some 25% to 30% of patients have clinical signs of feminizing hormonal function in the form of gynecomastia. Morphologic and clinical criteria of malignancy have not been well established.

A clinicopathologically distinctive variant of Sertoli cell tumor, probably accounting for almost half of testicular Sertoli cell neoplasms, has been recognized and termed large cell calcifying Sertoli cell tumor. This subtype tends to occur in males under 20 years of age, and is bilateral in 50% of cases. It is frequently associated with complex endocrinologic abnormalities and has also been linked with cardiac myxomas. Unlike conventional Sertoli cell tumors, this variant does not have an ovarian counterpart.

MORPHOLOGY The microscopic appearance of Sertoli cell tumors varies with the degree of differentiation, but most tumors demonstrate at least focal tubule or cord formation (Fig. 16.29). Growth within preexisting tubules, which is occasionally seen, may help distinguish Sertoli cell neoplasms from interstitially derived tumors (Fig. 16.30). Cytologically, the tumor cells have clear or eosinophilic cytoplasm and, when growing as sheets of cells, may be confused with seminoma. The large cell calcifying variant, as the name denotes, has prominent microscopic calcifications and cells with more prominent cytoplasm.

Juvenile Granulosa Cell Tumors

In a few rare cases, the testis gives rise to neoplasms that are microscopically identical to ovarian granulosa cell tumors. Most such cases have involved infants and have recapitulated the juvenile ovarian subtype. A study by Lawrence and coworkers documented 14 testicular juvenile granulosa cell tumors in young infants. All tumors behaved in a clinically benign fashion.

Grossly, the lesions in the study, ranging in size from 0.8–5 cm, were multicystic with intervening, solid, tan or yellow tissue. Microscopically, they were characterized by a mixed follicular and solid growth pattern of immature granulosa cells. Theca cells were occasionally present, forming cell layers around the follicles.

Gonadal Stromal Tumors

Although some testicular stromal tumors exhibit identifiable, unilateral differentiation, thus enabling their placement in one of the above categories, many show little or no differentiation. When stromal tumors are too poorly differentiated to be categorized or have evidence of multidirectional differentiation, they are usually labeled with the noncommittal term gonadal stromal tumor. Most often, these are proliferations of bland spindle cells without distinguishing characteristics. The rate of malignancy (metastases) in this group is difficult to ascertain, but it is probably in the range of 10%. This figure may be artificially high because of selective reporting of malignant cases.

Mixed Germ Cell–Sex Cord Stromal Neoplasms

Several microscopically and clinically distinctive lesions have been encompassed under this rubric. The unifying feature is the presence of both germ cell and sex cord stromal elements, with both presumably being neoplastic.

Gonadoblastoma

CLINICAL MANIFESTATIONS Gonadoblastomas almost always arise in individuals with developmental sexual abnormalities. They are most frequent in the second decade of life. Many are incidental findings at orchiectomy, but a few are large enough to become symptomatic. The tumor-bearing gonad may be streak or

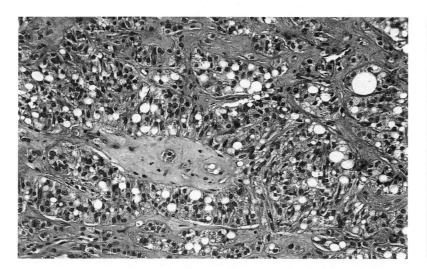

Figure 16.29 In this low-power photomicrograph of a Sertoli cell tumor, cords of cells with vacuolated cytoplasm infiltrate the testicular stroma.

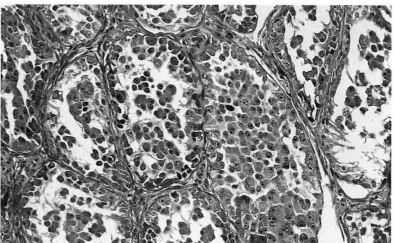

Figure 16.30 Occasionally, proliferations of intratubular Sertoli cells are present at the periphery of an infiltrative Sertoli cell tumor. In this photomicrograph of a Sertoli cell tumor in situ, the in situ cells lack cytoplasmic vacuoles and have prominent eosinophilic cytoplasm. Their intratubular location prevents confusion with Leydig cells.

dysgenetic cryptorchid. About 80% of patients are phenotypic females, usually with virilization. The remainder are phenotypic males with feminized internal sex organs. Almost all patients are genotypic males (46XY or mosaic).

The prognosis for pure gonadoblastoma is excellent, as would be expected for an in situ neoplasm. About 50% of gonadoblastomas are associated with infiltrating germ cell neoplasms, most commonly seminoma. The latter tumors presumably arise from preexisting gonadoblastomas. The prognosis in these cases is determined by the germ cell component.

MORPHOLOGY Gonadoblastoma is an intratubular neoplasm composed of cells resembling seminomalike germ cells, Sertoli cells, and granulosalike cells (Fig. 16.31). Intratubular, amorphous eosinophilic deposits are also present and typically calcify. The peritubular stroma contains prominent Leydig cells, and luteinized theca cells may also be present.

Mixed Germ Cell-Sex Cord Stromal Tumor

Tumors in this group used to be included with gonadoblastomas, but are now segregated due to important clinicopathologic differences. This variant was first described as an ovarian tumor in phenotypically and genotypically normal females during the first decade of life. It has subsequently been identified in genetically and phenotypically normal adult males, but it is extremely rare. To date, there has been no documented case of a conventional germ cell neoplasm having arisen in a mixed germ cell–sex cord stromal tumor, and all lesions have behaved benignly.

Unlike gonadoblastoma, these lesions are apparently infiltrating tumors composed of spindled sex cord cells with focal tubule formation intermixed with small numbers of germ cells (Fig. 16.32).

Miscellaneous Testicular Neoplasms

Carcinoid Tumor

There is disagreement as to whether carcinoid tumors of the testis are of germ cell origin, representing monodermal teratomas, or are derived from nongerminal, neuroendocrine cells. In some 15% of cases, carcinoid tumors of the testis are mixed with teratomatous elements, and in these instances the origin is presumably germinal.

A nongerm cell origin is also possible, and perhaps probable, although normal neuroendocrine precursors have not been demonstrated.

CLINICAL MANIFESTATIONS Whatever its derivation, testicular carcinoid tumor is uncommon, accounting for only about 0.2% of testicular tumors. Patients are typically in their fifth to sixth decade of life at the time of presentation with complaints of progressive testicular enlargement. Orchiectomy is performed for both diagnosis and treatment.

The prognosis for testicular carcinoid tumor has been excellent. Death from disease is rare, and when it does occur, it is difficult to exclude the possibility of an occult primary tumor with testicular metastasis. Indeed, the major problem related to this diagnosis is the exclusion of a metastasis. Bilateral disease is virtually always metastatic. The carcinoid syndrome, if present, indicates widely disseminated disease with testicular metastases. Statistically, primary testicular carcinoids outnumber metastatic carcinoids by approximately 3:1.

MORPHOLOGY Grossly, testicular carcinoid tumors usually consist of a solid, slightly yellow, intraparenchymal nodule (Fig. 16.33). Microscopically, the insular growth pattern typical of midgut-type carcinoid tumors is seen (Fig. 16.34). If other microscopic growth patterns are present, a metastasis should be suspected. The neuroendocrine nature of testicular carcinoid tumor can be documented by immunohistochemical stains for synaptophysin, chromogranin, or other neuroendocrine markers. Electron microscopy will demonstrate characteristic dense core granules. Unfortunately, these techniques do not allow distinction of primary from metastatic disease.

Epidermoid Cyst

As with carcinoid tumors, the origin of epidermoid cysts has been controversial, with many investigators favoring the theory that they are monodermal teratomas. There are also arguments against this interpretation. We have seen microscopic epidermoid cysts within the tunica vaginalis removed at autopsy (Fig. 16.35). In our view, most, if not all, epidermoid cysts arise from the surface mesothelium by a process of squamous metaplasia and invagination.

CLINICAL MANIFESTATIONS The uniformly benign behavior of testicular epidermoid cyst would favor clear-cut distinction from ter-

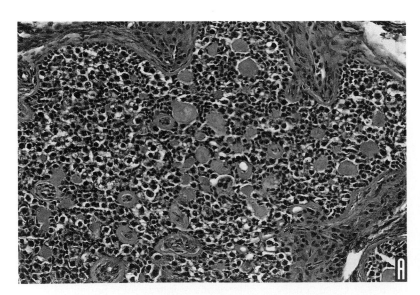
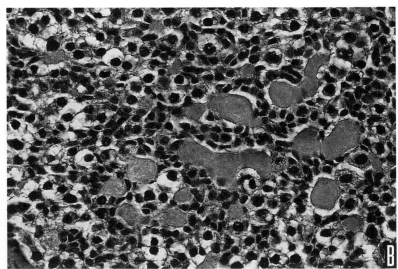

Figure 16.31 **A,** Low-power photomicrograph of a gonadoblastoma shows a seminiferous tubule from a dysgenetic testis that is expanded by a mixed cell population and acellular hyaline globules. **B,** A high-power view reveals that the tumor contains cells with clear cytoplasm resembling seminoma and a second population of smaller cells, probably representing Sertoli-like cells. The eosinophilic globules, which may calcify, are characteristic.

atoma in order to prevent unnecessary surgery. Epidermoid cysts of the testis account for only approximately 1% of testicular tumors. Most patients present in their second to fourth decade of life with gradual testicular enlargement over several years, or their tumors are

discovered during routine physical examinations. A discrete mass is typically palpable within the substance of the testis or, more frequently, just beneath the tunica vaginalis. Often, the mass bulges from the testicular surface.

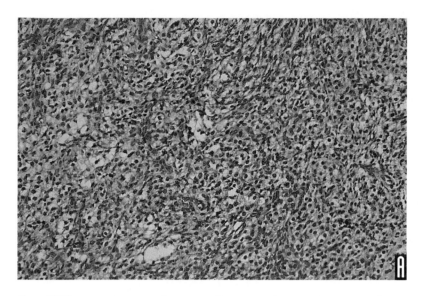

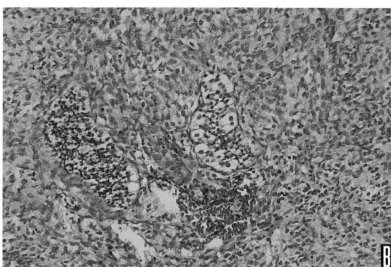

Figure 16.32 A, In this mixed germ cell–sex cord stromal tumor, cells with clear cytoplasm resembling seminoma are intermixed with spin-

dled stromal cells. **B,** Nests of cells resembling germinal cells are surrounded by a spindle cell stroma.

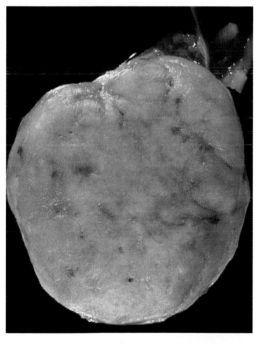

Figure 16.33 Primary testicular carcinoid tumor has replaced the testicular parenchyma in this specimen. The uniform, yellow coloration is typical of carcinoid tumors wherever they occur. (Courtesy of A.N. Walker, MD, Macon, Georgia)

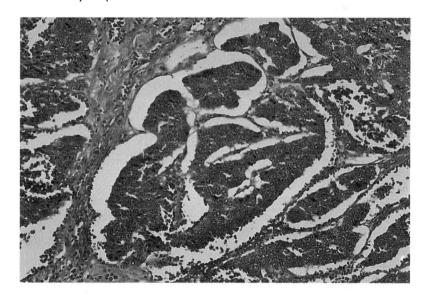

Figure 16.34 Microscopically, aggregates of cells with basophilic cytoplasm and uniform "salt and pepper" nuclei are characteristic of carcinoid tumor.

Figure 16.35 This tiny epidermoid cyst was an incidental finding within the tunica of an otherwise normal testis.

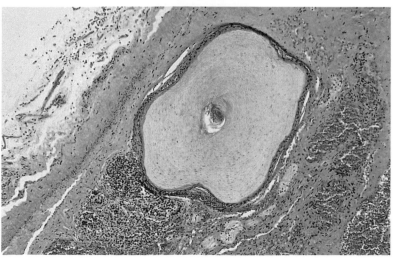

In principle, if the diagnosis is suspected and the lesion is located under the tunica vaginalis, local excision may be performed. This has been done in about 20 reported cases without recurrence of the lesion. During the procedure, the surgeon must carefully palpate the testis to confirm that the remaining parenchyma is normal. Keratinous cysts may be present as a component of testicular teratomas, and this possibility must be carefully excluded. Because epidermoid cysts may be located within the testis and may be difficult or impossible to distinguish clinically from a germ cell neoplasm, orchiectomy is often the procedure of choice.

MORPHOLOGY Grossly, epidermoid cysts are indistinguishable from their cutaneous counterparts. A sharply circumscribed, cystic structure is filled with white, flaky keratin debris (Fig. 16.36). Microscopically, the cyst is lined by mature, keratinizing squamous epithelium. Adnexal structures, as would be seen in a dermoid cyst (mature cystic teratoma), are absent (Fig. 16.37).

TESTICULAR LYMPHOMA

Non-Hodgkin's lymphomas frequently involve the testis as a component of disseminated disease. The following section, however, deals with lymphomas initially manifesting as testicular lesions.

CLINICAL MANIFESTATIONS Although testicular lymphomas account for only about 2%–5% of testicular neoplasms, they constitute from 25%–50% of testicular tumors in men over 50 years of age. The majority of patients presenting with testicular lymphoma have disseminated disease. The five-year survival for patients with localized stage I and II disease is approximately 70%. For patients with widespread dissemination, survival drops to about 20%.

There is an unusual association between testicular lymphoma and involvement of the lymphoid tissue of Waldeyer's ring. About 22% of patients with testicular lymphoma develop secondary disease in this region. Involvement of Waldeyer's ring is not necessar-

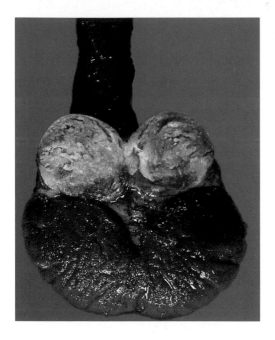

Figure 16.36 This encapsulated, keratin-filled epidermoid cyst formed at the superior pole of the testis.

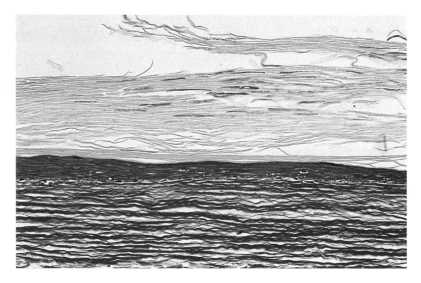

Figure 16.37 Epidermoid cysts are lined by flattened, keratinizing squamous epithelium without associated adnexal structures, as would be seen in a benign cystic teratoma (dermoid cyst). The keratin exfoliates from the surface, filling the cyst.

Figure 16.38 In testicular lymphoma, the testis is focally infiltrated by the lesion. The bulk of the tumor forms a peritesticular mass.

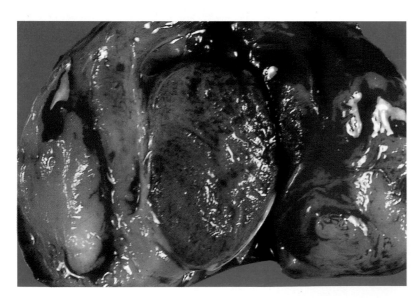

ily associated with a bad prognosis. Conversely, patients with lymphomas beginning in Waldeyer's ring have a high rate of secondary testicular disease.

MORPHOLOGY Lymphoma of the testis frequently involves the epididymis and spermatic cord in addition to the testicular parenchyma. The cut surface of the tumor, which is typically white or tan, may resemble seminoma, except that it lacks sharp circumscription (Fig. 16.38). Virtually all testicular lymphomas have a diffuse, as opposed to nodular, growth pattern. Most are scattered, large, cleaved, or noncleaved cell lymphomas. Other forms of non-Hodgkin's lymphoma, including lymphoblastic lymphoma, are also encountered, but primary testicular Hodgkin's disease is extremely rare or nonexistent.

The microscopic appearance of the lesion varies with the form of lymphoma. The most common large-cell pattern consists of sheets of cells with vesicular-to-hyperchromatic nuclei, often prominent nucleoli, and little cytoplasm. Mitotic figures are numerous and foci of necrosis are also frequent. If the tumor demonstrates immunoblastic differentiation, immature neoplastic plasmacytoid cells are present. Large-cell lymphomas may be confused with seminomas. Lymphomas have an intertubular growth pattern, whereas intratubular growth and abundant, clear, glycogen-rich cytoplasm favor seminoma. In problematic cases, immunocytochemical staining for leukocyte common antigen reliably identifies lymphoma (Fig. 16.39).

MISCELLANEOUS MESENCHYMAL TUMORS

A host of mesenchymal lesions may on rare occasions arise in the testis, presumably from nonspecialized gonadal stroma. Included in this group are lipomas, fibrous tumors, and vascular neoplasms.

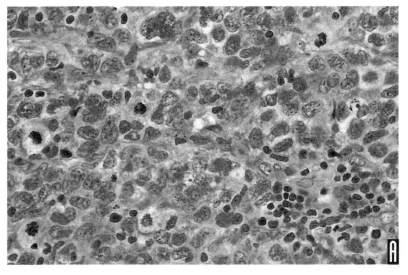

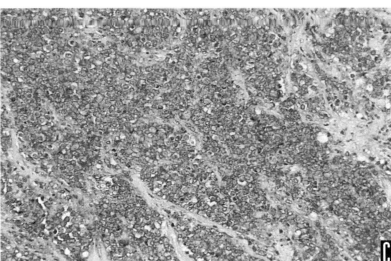

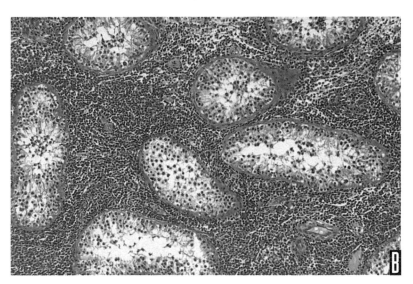

Figure 16.39 A, Most testicular lymphomas are of the diffuse large cell type, characterized by large cells with pleomorphic nuclei and a high mitotic rate. **B,** The growth of testicular lymphoma around normal seminiferous tubules may be helpful in distinguishing it from seminoma. **C,** In those instances where the distinction between lymphoma and seminoma is difficult, immunocytochemical localization of leukocyte common antigen, indicated here by the brown pigment, is extremely helpful in identifying lymphoma (immunoperoxidase technique).

Histiocytoid (epithelioid) hemangioma of the testis is a rare but histologically distinctive vascular neoplasm that also arises in the penis (see Fig. 19.15).

Metastatic Carcinoma Involving the Testis

Metastatic carcinoma only rarely presents as a clinically palpable testicular mass from an occult primary tumor. More commonly, testicular metastases are discovered incidentally in orchiectomy specimens or at autopsy. Primary tumor sites that most commonly metastasize to the testis include (in decreasing order of frequency): prostate, lung, skin (melanoma), colon, kidney, stomach, and pancreas. Carcinoid tumor metastatic to the testis is discussed above. Bilateral metastases occur in about 15% of cases.

The microscopic pattern often suggests the primary site of neoplasia (Fig. 16.40). The histologic appearance of some carcinomas may occasionally mimic a testicular primary tumor. In these instances, extensive vascular or lymphatic invasion and interstitial growth favor metastatic disease.

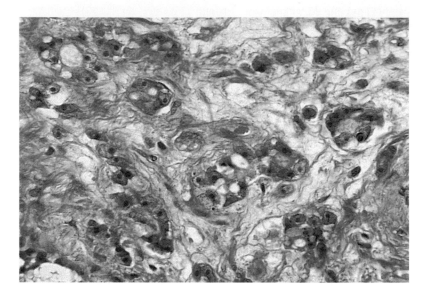

Figure 16.40 Metastatic adenocarcinoma from the prostate forms small, glandular clusters in the testicular interstitium.

CHAPTER 17

Lesions of the Tunica Vaginalis, Epididymis, Vas Deferens, and Spermatic Cord

LESIONS OF THE TUNICA VAGINALIS

HYDROCELE

Hydroceles, circumscribed collections of fluid in the tunica vaginalis or along the spermatic cord, may take several forms: the communicating hydrocele, the infantile hydrocele, and the simple or idiopathic hydrocele, which is the most common.

PATHOGENESIS As the testis descends into the scrotum during development, it acquires a peritoneal covering, the visceral portion of the tunica vaginalis. This mesothelium-lined surface is reflected off the testis to form an outer parietal portion of the tunica vaginalis, which is also lined with mesothelial cells. The visceral and parietal layers are normally in close apposition, containing only a few drops of serous fluid. During development, the virtual space between these two layers is connected to the peritoneal cavity by the funicular process, the portion of the tunica vaginalis that surrounds the spermatic cord. This opening to the peritoneum normally closes after testicular descent.

If the funicular process remains open to the abdomen, peritoneal fluid may accumulate, leading to symptomatic scrotal enlargement. Such collections of fluid, termed *communicating hydroceles,* may grow to large proportions in a patient with ascites. They can be recognized by their tendency to vary in volume with position. In the infantile form of hydrocele, the funicular process may not communicate with the abdomen but rather remains partially intact distally. The *infantile hydrocele* often disappears spontaneously as the funicular process atrophies.

The most common form is the *simple* or *idiopathic hydrocele,* in which the tunica vaginalis is normally formed, does not connect to the abdominal cavity, and is distended with fluid (Fig. 17.1). The pathogenesis is uncertain. Theories have included a posttraumatic or healed inflammatory process, a congenital defect in lymphatic drainage, and obstruction secondary to prostatic hypertrophy. Hydroceles develop following trauma, particularly herniorrhaphy, and prophylactic hydrocelectomies are usually performed whenever the scrotum is explored. The fluid in hydrocele sacs is constantly changing, so that any defect in the delicate balance of secretion versus resorption, leads to fluid accumulation.

CLINICAL MANIFESTATIONS The exact frequency of simple hydrocele is unknown, but it is present in 1% of male hospital admissions. Simple hydroceles are typically unilateral and long-lasting. Such slowly forming lesions are painless until they become large enough to stretch the spermatic cord, producing a dull pain or ache when the patient is standing. Acute hydrocele causes rapid distention of the tunica vaginalis and may be intensely painful. Acute hydrocele, which is usually secondary to an underlying process, is suspicious for infection or neoplasm evoking a secondary effusion. Hydroceles may also be seen in patients with generalized edema due to cardiovascular or renal failure. As noted above, communicating hydroceles are distinguished by their association with ascites, frequency of large size, and variation in size according to position. Infantile hydroceles are small fluid collections in newborns that typically resolve spontaneously.

Hydroceles can be easily distinguished from testicular neoplasms by palpation and transillumination. The fluid is a straw-colored transudate that readily transmits light, but if secondarily infected, it will be opaque or purulent. Distinguishing between hydrocele and inguinal hernia is usually straightforward. If a hernia is present and cannot be reduced, auscultation may demonstrate bowel sounds, and the mass should be focally tympanitic to percussion. Once an idiopathic hydrocele becomes symptomatic, treatment is usually surgical. In hydrocele secondary to infection, neoplasm, or generalized edema, the nature of the underlying condition dictates the appropriate therapy.

MORPHOLOGY The tissue removed from the hydrocele sac wall has a mesothelium-type lining, often with focal hyperplasia (Fig. 17.2). Depending on the duration and size of the hydrocele, there may be considerable fibrosis and even focal calcification. Untreated infection often resolves with the resultant inflammatory reaction leading to obliteration of the tunica vaginalis.

HEMATOCELE

CLINICAL MANIFESTATIONS A hematocele is an effusion of blood into a cavity. Injury to the testis occasionally leads to hemorrhage between the layers of the tunica vaginalis. A hematocele may also develop following traumatic needle aspiration of a hydrocele. Hematoceles do not transilluminate, and if the blood clots, they may simulate a solid testicular neoplasm (Fig. 17.3). A careful history is

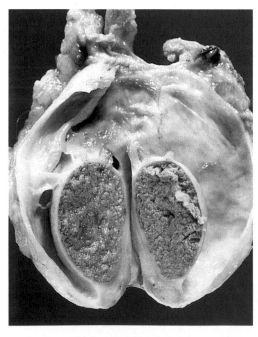
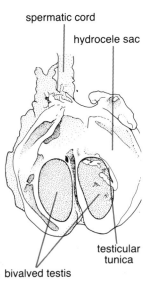

spermatic cord

hydrocele sac

testicular tunica

bivalved testis

Figure 17.1 In this specimen of a simple hydrocele, the two layers of the testicular tunica, which are normally in close apposition, have been separated by an accumulation of serous fluid. In response to the longstanding changes, the tunica has become thickened and fibrotic.

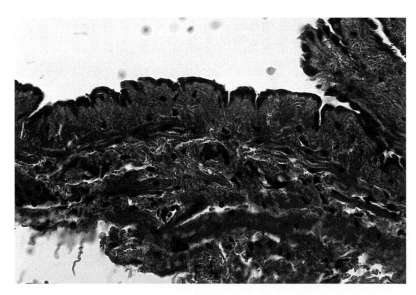

Figure 17.2 The wall of a hydrocele sac is lined by flattened-to-cuboidal mesothelial cells.

helpful and aspiration is usually diagnostic. Small hematoceles slowly resolve, but larger collections may require surgical drainage.

MORPHOLOGY Microscopically, hematoceles consist of fresh or clotted blood lying within a mesothelium-lined cavity. If the lesion is old and undergoing organization, the wall of the hematocele may contain hemosiderin-laden macrophages and foreign body-type giant cells filled with lipid or cholesterol crystals from the breakdown of the extravasated blood.

FIBROUS PERIORCHITIS In fibrous periorchitis, the normally thin wall of the tunica vaginalis is markedly thickened by multiple, firm nodules. This process presumably develops as a reaction to trauma or chronic inflammation, although the pathogenesis is

unclear. It is thought to be analogous to the fibrous mesothelial nodules more commonly encountered on the pleura. Simple excision is the treatment of choice.

Grossly, the nodules range in size from less than a millimeter to several centimeters (Fig. 17.4). Microscopically, they are composed of densely collagenized fibrous tissue with a chronic inflammatory infiltrate of varying proportions identical to that of fibrous pseudotumor (Fig. 17.5).

FIBROUS PSEUDOTUMOR

Fibrous pseudotumor represents the same fundamental process as that occurring in fibrous periorchitis—a nonneoplastic proliferation of fibrous tissue admixed with inflammation. The gross and clinical

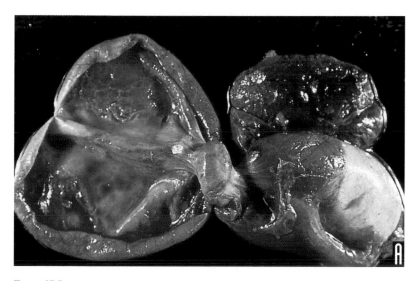

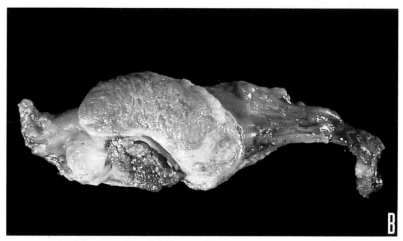

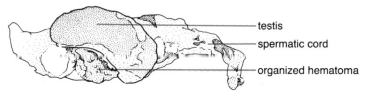
testis
spermatic cord
organized hematoma

Figure 17.3 A, Testicular trauma led to hemorrhage within a preexisting hydrocele. The hydrocele sac at the left was filled with freshly clotted blood. **B,** A large hematocele may organize to form a firm hematoma, which can mimic a testicular neoplasm.

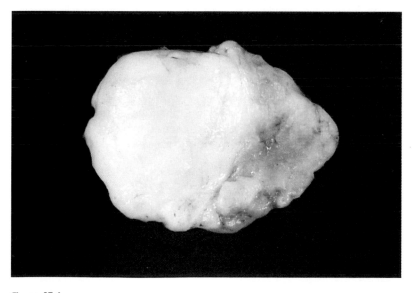

Figure 17.4 This nodule of fibrous periorchitis was one of many similar nodules covering the tunica vaginalis.

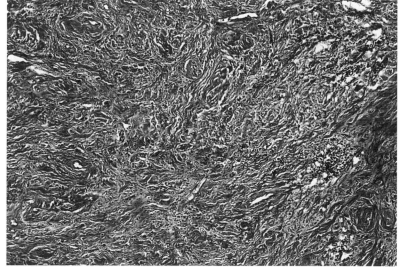

Figure 17.5 Low-power photomicrograph of fibrous periorchitis/pseudotumor shows the irregularly organized, dense collagen and scattered inflammatory cells that characterize this process.

features differ slightly, however, in that fibrous pseudotumor consists of a large dominant or single mass reaching up to 15 cm in greatest dimension (Fig. 17.6).

Microscopically, fibrous pseudotumor is indistinguishable from the smaller nodules of periorchitis (see Fig. 17.5).

NODULAR MESOTHELIAL HYPERPLASIA

In 1975, Rosai and Dehner first called attention to the fact that nodules of benign, proliferating mesothelial cells could be found in hernia sac specimens. Benign mesothelial cell aggregates may also be encountered in the tunica vaginalis.

Microscopically, these nodules consist of sheets of cells with eosinophilic cytoplasm and variably pleomorphic nuclei (Fig. 17.7). Most of the nodules lack a papillary architecture, but occasionally they may form delicate papillae with a central fibrovascular core. Laminated calcified spherules (psammoma bodies) may also be formed. Mitotic figures may be present, but atypical forms are not seen. Hemosiderin deposits and inflammatory cells are often located in the surrounding stroma. The distinction of nodular mesothelial hyperplasia from mesothelioma is based on the localized nature of the former lesion as well as its generally bland microscopic appearance.

MALIGNANT MESOTHELIOMA

CLINICAL MANIFESTATIONS Malignant mesothelioma arising from the tunica vaginalis is rare but well documented. As with mesotheliomas developing in the pleural and peritoneal cavities, there is an association with chronic exposure to asbestos fibers. The age range is broad, but most patients are at least 50 years old. Presenting signs and symptoms document a scrotal swelling or "hydrocele." Aspiration of fluid is usually followed by prompt reaccumulation, but the fluid may be used for cytologic diagnosis. Metastases typically involve regional lymph nodes, at least initially. Of 11 cases reviewed in a study by Japko and colleagues, five patients were dead of disease, one was living with metastatic disease, and the remaining five were alive and clinically disease free but had follow-up intervals of only 1.5–15 months.

MORPHOLOGY Mesotheliomas of the pleura and peritoneum may assume a bewildering array of microscopic appearances, but almost all lesions of the tunica vaginalis have had a papillary configuration. Microscopic distinction of malignant mesothelioma from papillary mesothelial hyperplasia may be difficult (Fig. 17.8). Features of malignancy include prominent nuclear pleomorphism,

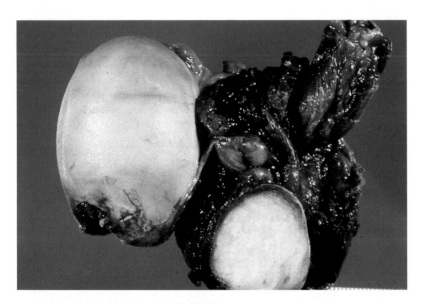

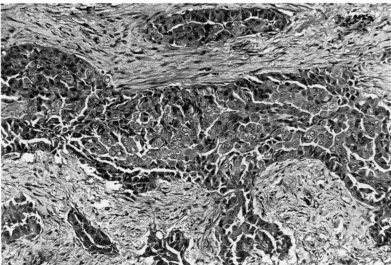

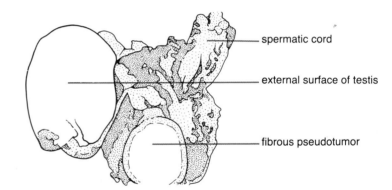

Figure 17.6 Grossly, fibrous pseudotumor consists of a single large nodule, rather than the multiple smaller nodules seen in fibrous periorchitis, although the processes are microscopically identical.

spermatic cord

external surface of testis

fibrous pseudotumor

Figure 17.7 In this low-power photomicrograph of nodular mesothelial hyperplasia, nests of proliferating mesothelial cells appear to be embedded in a fibrous stroma. This "pseudoinvasion," which is caused by sectioning parallel to the surface, may lead to confusion with malignant mesothelioma.

atypical mitotic figures, necrosis, and vascular or lymphatic invasion. A history of longstanding asbestos exposure in an older individual would also be supportive.

ADENOMATOID TUMOR

PATHOGENESIS Adenomatoid tumors are microscopically distinctive, benign neoplasms that until recently have been of uncertain histogenesis. In the past, vascular, müllerian, and mesonephric origins were proposed, but ultrastructural and immunohistochemical studies now strongly support a mesothelial derivation. Adenomatoid tumors may thus be viewed as a histologically distinctive form of benign mesothelioma. Intrascrotal adenomatoid tumors arise from the tunica vaginalis, often in the region of the epididymis. Adenomatoid tumors also, and more commonly, arise

in the myometrium of the uterus. In addition, they have been described in the fallopian tube, ovary, spermatic cord, even the adrenal gland and mesentery of the bowel.

CLINICAL MANIFESTATIONS Intrascrotal adenomatoid tumors usually affect adults over 30 years of age and present as firm, often tender intrascrotal masses. Palpation may document a close association with the epididymis, which is verified at surgery. Local excision is curative for adenomatoid tumor, and recurrences have not been documented. Large lesions may necessitate orchiectomy.

MORPHOLOGY Grossly, adenomatoid tumors are firm, white to slightly yellow nodules that are usually 2 cm or less in diameter (Fig. 17.9). Although arising outside of the testes, tumors

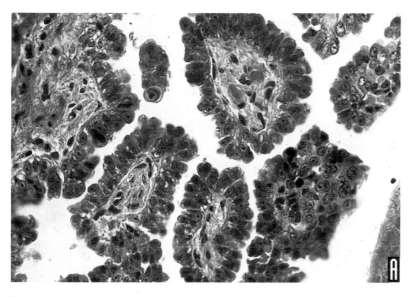
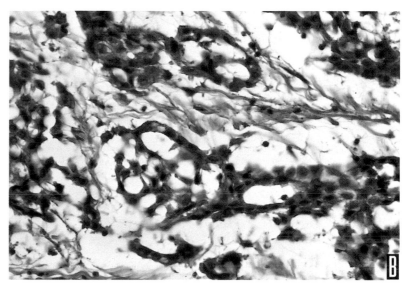

Figure 17.8 A, Malignant mesothelioma, a papillary neoplasm, may be difficult to distinguish from mesothelial hyperplasia, although the latter rarely has a papillary configuration. In this example, papillae are lined by moderately pleomorphic cells. **B,** In malignant mesothelioma, strands of neoplastic cells invade the underlying stroma.

Figure 17.9 The testis in this case of adenomatoid tumor has been bivalved to demonstrate a solid, white nodule in the wall of the tunica vaginalis.

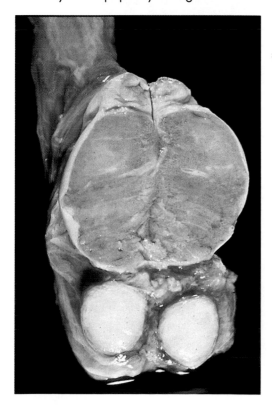
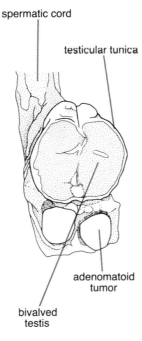

spermatic cord

testicular tunica

adenomatoid tumor

bivalved testis

occasionally invade the testicular parenchyma or, more often, replace the head of the epididymis.

The microscopic appearance of adenomatoid tumor varies. In a thorough study of histologically analogous uterine tumors, Quigley and Hart identified four characteristic patterns: adenoid, angiomatoid, solid, and cystic. Combinations of the patterns are common. The adenoid pattern is characterized by anastomosing glandlike spaces lined by cuboidal to irregularly shaped cells. Some cells contain intracytoplasmic vacuoles and resemble signet-ring cells (Fig. 17.10). The angiomatoid pattern consists of larger, pseudovascular spaces lined by flattened cells with inconspicuous cytoplasm mimicking endothelial cells. The solid pattern is typified by sheets, columns, and cords of cells, with abundant eosinophilic cytoplasm simulating epithelial cells. The cystic pattern, the least common, is characterized by large cystic cavities separated by thin fibrous septa and lined by flattened-to-cuboidal cells.

BRENNER TUMOR

PATHOGENESIS   As with adenomatoid tumors, the histogenesis of Brenner tumors has been the subject of considerable debate. A variety of origins has been proposed, but the one currently favored suggests that these tumors represent a peculiar metaplasia of mesothelium.

CLINICAL MANIFESTATIONS   In resected ovaries, Brenner tumors are relatively common incidental lesions. Their development in the peritesticular tissues is far less frequent. At least four well documented cases have been reported arising in close association with the tunica vaginalis and the epididymis. Testicular Brenner tumors have been invariably benign and, in fact, it is unclear whether they are true neoplasms. In one case, a Brenner tumor was a component of an adenomatoid tumor, but the others reported have been pure lesions.

MORPHOLOGY   Brenner tumors have a stereotypical microscopic image consisting of nests of transitional-like epithelial cells surrounded by a characteristic fibroblastic stroma (Fig. 17.11).

SEROUS NEOPLASMS OF THE TUNICA VAGINALIS

Surface neoplasms resembling ovarian serous neoplasia may occasionally arise on the tunica of the testis, probably via a "müllerian metaplasia" of lining mesothelial cells. Almost all reported examples have been proliferative, noninvasive lesions resembling serous borderline ovarian tumors. Reports of serous papillary carcinomas arising from the tunica vaginalis are rare and, to our knowledge, only one case has resulted in metastatic disease.

Microscopically, these serous neoplasms are indistinguishable from their ovarian counterparts (Fig. 17.12A,B). Neoplastic cells

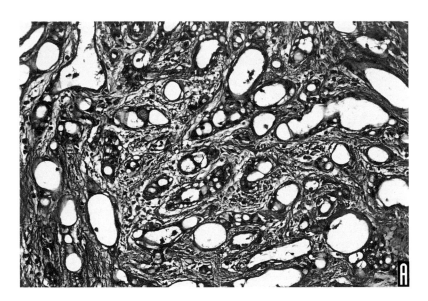

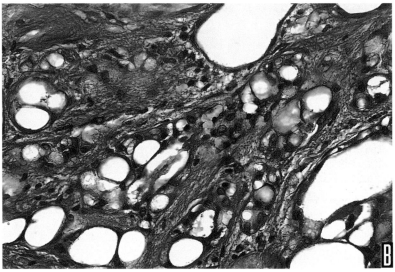

Figure 17.10 A, In this microscopic view of an adenomatoid tumor, cords of vacuolated epithelioid cells are interspersed in a fibrous stroma. The growth pattern incorrectly suggests an invasive adeno-

carcinoma. **B,** Small, intracytoplasmic vacuoles, creating signet-ring-like cells, are interspersed with larger cysts in this adenomatoid tumor.

Figure 17.11 This photomicrograph of a Brenner tumor shows the lesion's stereotypical microscopic appearance. Nests of epithelial cells (center) are surrounded by a fibroblastic stroma.

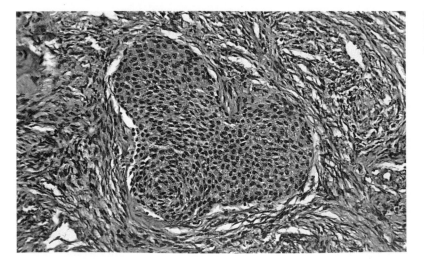

typically line fibrovascular papillae. The cells are cuboidal to columnar with prominent, eosinophilic cytoplasm (Fig. 17.12B). Ciliated cells may be easily recognized. Concentrically calcified (psammoma) bodies are typically present. Continuity with adjacent surface mesothelium may be demonstrable in appropriate sections.

Distinction of borderline serous neoplasia from malignant mesothelioma is based on the presence of tall, columnar, focally ciliated cells that do not invade the surrounding stroma. If light-microscopic features are insufficient for distinction, immunohistochemical stains for a panel of markers that usually stains serous neoplasms but not mesothelial cells may be valuable. Such panels typically include the following antibodies/antigens: B72.3, Leu M1, placental alkaline phosphatase, carcinoembryonic antigen, and Ber-EP4. Borderline serous neoplasms should also be distinguished from papillary cystadenomas of the epididymis, which often contain cells with clear cytoplasm, lack ciliated cells, and arise from the epididymis, rather than the surface mesothelium.

OTHER CYSTIC SCROTAL LESIONS

SPERMATOCELE

PATHOGENESIS Spermatoceles are cystic dilations of the efferent ductules of the rete testis. Located near the head of the epididymis, they are frequently multiple and bilateral. Their cause is unknown but is probably unrelated to obstruction, since vasectomy does not increase their frequency or result in enlargement of preexisting lesions. Careful examination of testes removed at autopsy or for surgical reasons occasionally reveals small dilatations of the efferent tubules, presumably representing early spermatocele formation.

CLINICAL MANIFESTATIONS Spermatoceles, which do not develop until after puberty, are most common in the fourth and fifth decades of life. They usually transilluminate. Palpation demonstrates a mass distinct from and displacing the testis anteriorly and caudally. Most spermatoceles are small and do not require therapy; larger lesions may be excised (Fig. 17.13).

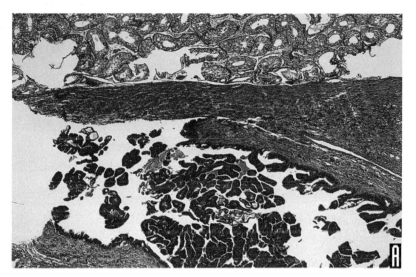

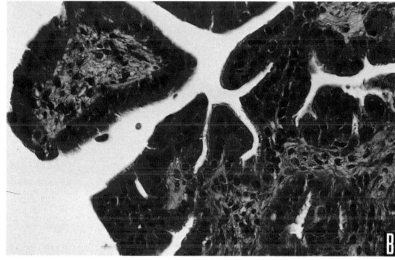

Figure 17.12 A, This "borderline" serous tumor of the tunica is a papillary, cystic neoplasm attached to the viseral tunica of the testis. There is no evidence of invasion by the neoplastic cells. **B,** At higher magnification, the cells of this borderline serous neoplasm are uniform and columnar with well formed cilia.

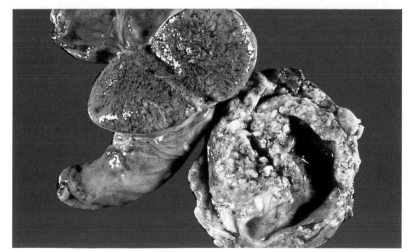

Figure 17.13 This specimen shows a large spermatocele replacing the epididymis. The cyst contained large numbers of mature spermatozoa.

MORPHOLOGY Spermatoceles are cystic structures lined by pseudostratified epithelium identical to that seen in the normal rete testis (Fig. 17.14). The cyst fluid is milky or turbid. It usually contains large numbers of mature sperm, except in elderly men who have ceased spermatogenesis.

Varicocele

Varicocele is an abnormal dilatation of the pampiniform venous plexus that drains the scrotal contents. The plexus is formed by a confluence of the anterior spermatic vein from the testis, the middle spermatic veins from the ductus deferens, and the external veins located posteriorly along the spermatic cord. This freely anastomosing venous network may serve as a countercurrent cooling system to lower the temperature of blood in the testicular artery. The association between varicocele and infertility is briefly discussed in Chapter 15.

PATHOGENESIS The pampiniform plexus merges proximally in the inguinal canal to form the spermatic vein, which drains on the right into the inferior vena cava at an oblique angle. The left sper-

matic vein enters the renal vein at a 90° angle. This anatomic difference theoretically leads to increased pressure in the left-sided venous system, perhaps accounting for the observation that fully 99% of varicoceles are left-sided lesions. Bilateral lesions are seen in the remaining 1% of patients. The sudden development of a varicocele that does not disappear on reclining or is located solely on the right side should suggest the possibility of proximal venous obstruction due to retroperitoneal disease. A complete radiographic evaluation of such patients is indicated.

CLINICAL MANIFESTATIONS The incidence of varicocele varies with the observer's definition of abnormality but probably approaches 10%. The lesion usually begins in early adulthood, and may gradually enlarge, remain stationary, or regress. Physical examination demonstrates a "bag of worms" in the proximal scrotum, often with associated blue discoloration of the overlying scrotal skin. If the varicocele is of the typical primary or idiopathic type, it is located on the left, has a gradual onset in young adulthood, and rapidly disappears when the patient reclines.

Provided that the varicocele is not associated with undesired sterility, it does not require treatment. A variety of surgical proce-

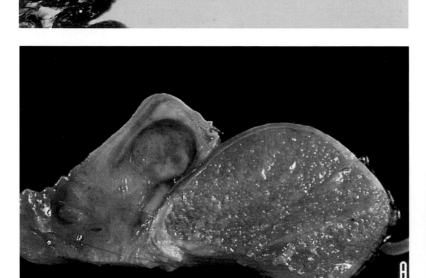

Figure 17.14 A high-power view demonstrates that the pseudostratified lining of a spermatocele resembles that of the normal rete testis. (Compare with the hydrocele sac mesothelial lining in Fig. 17.2.)

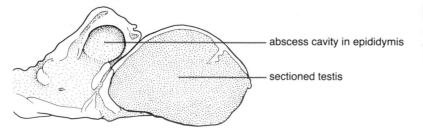

abscess cavity in epididymis

sectioned testis

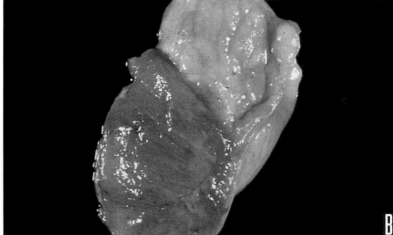

Figure 17.15 A, Gross specimen from a patient with acute epididymitis shows an enlarged epididymis containing an abscess cavity. **B,** In chronic epididymitis, the epididymis is enlarged and distorted by longstanding inflammation with resultant scarring.

dures have been advocated when treatment is desired. High ligation of the venous plexus within the inguinal canal or ligation of both veins and artery above the inguinal ring are effective. With either procedure collateral blood flow prevents testicular infarction.

MORPHOLOGY Because most varicoceles are not treated and those that are treated are ligated rather than resected, tissue is seldom submitted for microscopic examination. This is just as well; once they are removed, the previously distended venous channels tend to collapse, leaving little or no morphologic evidence of their prior pathologic state.

Epididymitis

PATHOGENESIS Most venereal infections involve the epididymis. Infection secondary to common pyogenic organisms is also common. Organisms typically reach the epididymis by retrograde flow along the vas deferens from a primary infectious focus in the bladder, urethra, prostate, or elsewhere in the genitourinary system. Hematogenous spread is much less common but does occur.

The role of trauma in the development of epididymitis is problematic, although the two appear to be related. In some instances, the trauma may be coincidental, simply serving to focus attention on a chronic, only mildly symptomatic infection. Some investigators have postulated that trauma may increase urinary reflux into the epididymis, thereby leading to more frequent infections. Epididymitis has been a common postoperative complication of urinary tract surgery. Preoperative vasectomy appears to eliminate many of these infections by blocking the normal route of spread. Improved surgical techniques, modern antibiotics, and vasectomy have lowered the rate of postoperative epididymitis to approximately 4%.

CLINICAL MANIFESTATIONS Inflammation of the epididymis is one of the most common intrascrotal abnormalities. Patients are almost exclusively postpubertal. The signs and symptoms of acute epididymitis include severe pain with swelling of recent onset, scrotal erythema, and evidence of increased testicular blood flow by ultrasonography. These findings are often accompanied by systemic changes such as fever and leukocytosis. Clinical features suggesting epididymitis in a young child more frequently represent testicular torsion or torsion of a testicular appendage.

Appropriate antibiotic therapy is usually the treatment of choice for acute epididymitis, which is seldom treated surgically. Chronic, recalcitrant disease much more often requires surgical excision.

Recurrent infections may result in tubular blockage, which leads to sterility in a high percentage of patients with bilateral disease.

MORPHOLOGY Acute epididymal inflammation, regardless of the underlying cause, consists of a polymorphonuclear leukocyte infiltrate, with or without abscess formation. Chronic epididymitis leads to fibrosis, enlargement, and distortion of the underlying architecture (Fig. 17.15).

Pseudoneoplastic and Neoplastic Lesions of the Epididymis

Pseudomalignant Change

CLINICAL MANIFESTATIONS Most pathologists have encountered bizarre, often grotesquely pleomorphic epithelial cells as an incidental finding in tissue obtained from the seminal vesicles. Cytologically similar pseudomalignant cells may be encountered in the efferent ductules or the epididymis proper. The cells are in fact benign; the changes are involutional rather than neoplastic. Generally these changes increase in frequency with advancing age, an observation supporting their involutional nature. They are of no clinical importance unless confused with carcinoma.

MORPHOLOGY Kuo and Gomez documented atypical cells in 28% of efferent ductules and 32% of epididymal tubules. The remarkable degree of nuclear pleomorphism in either location can lead to concern or confusion with an in situ carcinoma.

In the efferent ductules, the atypical cells have huge, hyperchromatic nuclei that protrude into the lumen. They appear to arise via the fusion of several smaller cells, with condensation of nuclear chromatin to form a large pyknotic nuclear mass. In the main portion of the epididymis, the atypical cells have a different appearance, showing enlarged, irregularly shaped nuclei, coarsely clumped chromatin, occasional prominent nucleoli, and frequent intranuclear cytoplasmic extensions (Fig. 17.16).

Epididymal Cyst

Exposure in utero to diethylstilbestrol has been associated with a number of abnormalities in males, the most characteristic of which are epididymal cysts. These are apparently nonneoplastic cystic dilatations of epididymal tubules, reaching several centimeters in diameter. They may be detected by the patient or on routine physical examination. There is no evidence that the cysts are premalignant.

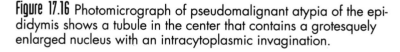
Figure 17.16 Photomicrograph of pseudomalignant atypia of the epididymis shows a tubule in the center that contains a grotesquely enlarged nucleus with an intracytoplasmic invagination.

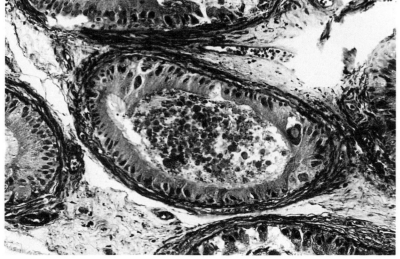

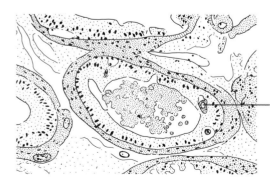
enlarged nucleus with intranuclear cytoplasmic invagination

Microscopically, the lining epithelium of the cysts is composed of cuboidal-to-columnar cells similar to those lining the normal tubules (Fig. 17.17). Epididymal cysts lack the papillations and characteristic epithelial cells of papillary cystadenoma.

Papillary Cystadenoma of the Epididymis

CLINICAL MANIFESTATIONS   Papillary cystadenomas are rare benign tumors of the epididymis. Whether they are neoplasms or unusual malformations is unclear. Unilateral lesions occur from adolescence to late adulthood. They may be discovered incidentally or may form as a scrotal mass that has been noted to be present for many years. Most are 2–5 cm in greatest dimension, originating from the head of the epididymis. Local excision is curative.

Patients with bilateral papillary cystadenomas of the epididymis should be viewed as having at least an incomplete form of Lindau's disease, which is a multifaceted neurocutaneous syndrome consisting of hemangiomas of the central nervous system, retina, or skin, plus a variety of mixed papillary and solid epithelial lesions, some of which are true neoplasms. Individual patients seldom express all of the potential manifestations. The presence of bilateral epididymal cystadenomas should lead to a careful search for epithelial and vascular tumors elsewhere in the body.

Bilateral involvement usually manifests in late adolescence or early adulthood, with most patients under 30 years of age. The clinical presentation and gross appearance are similar to those of unilateral papillary cystadenomas.

MORPHOLOGY   Gross examination of papillary cystadenoma of the epididymis usually demonstrates a multicystic and solid tumor. The cysts contain clear yellow to hemorrhagic fluid. Microscopically, the lesions are composed of complex papillary processes, ectatic ducts and microcysts, as well as fibrous stroma with inflammation (Fig. 17.18). The papillae are lined by a single to focally stratified layer of tall columnar cells with focally clear, vacuolated cytoplasm, which does not contain mucin. Nuclei, located at the base of the cells, are uniformly round to oval. The cysts contain homogeneous eosinophilic proteinaceous material, apparently secreted by the epithelium. The ectatic ducts and microcysts are lined with identical cells. Microscopically, the bilateral lesions are similar, except that they are less well circumscribed, show marked ectasia of the surrounding ducts, and have prominent microcysts and less pronounced papillations.

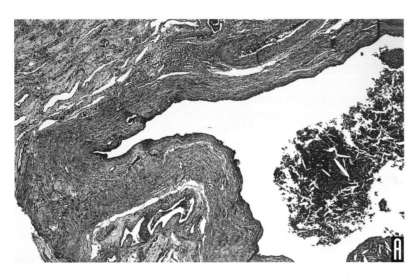

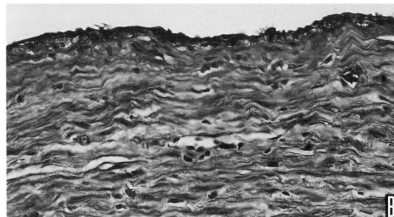

Figure 17.17 A, In the epididymal cyst, a fibrous-walled cyst is present within the epididymis, extending outward into the surrounding tissue.

B, A higher-power view demonstrates the lining of the cyst, which is composed of small cuboidal cells.

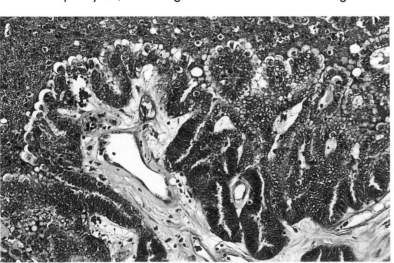

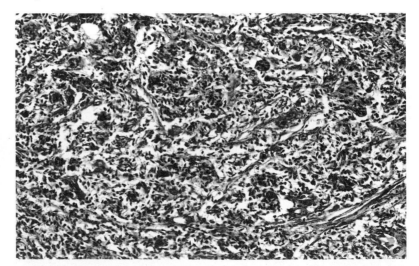

Figure 17.18 The clear cytoplasmic vacuoles within the epithelial cells lining the papillae are typical of papillary cystadenoma of the epididymis. Other cells have eosinophilic cytoplasm.

Figure 17.19 High-power photomicrograph of sperm granuloma shows extratubular collections of mature spermatozoa mixed with scattered inflammatory cells in the tissue near a transected vas deferens.

Adenocarcinoma of the Epididymis and Rete Testis

CLINICAL MANIFESTATIONS Adenocarcinomas arising in the region of the epididymis are rare. The distinction between adenocarcinoma and papillary mesothelioma may be difficult or impossible on the basis of light-microscopic examination. Some adenocarcinomas reportedly arising from this region would be better interpreted as papillary mesotheliomas or serous neoplasms of mesothelial derivation. Clinical, ultrastructural, and immunohistochemical studies may be needed for clear-cut separation.

Adenocarcinomas of the epididymis and rete testis tend to occur in older individuals. The clinical features of the rete testis lesions were recently summarized by Nochomovitz and Orenstein. Most patients are over 60 years old and present with a scrotal lump or swelling. Distant metastases and local recurrences with involvement of scrotal and perineal skin are common.

MORPHOLOGY Microscopically, these lesions are usually papillary neoplasms lacking the clear cytoplasm and nuclear uniformity of cystadenomas. Cuboidal-to-columnar cells with eosinophilic cytoplasm as well as pleomorphic nuclei line the papillae. Invasion of the intercystic stroma and surrounding soft tissue is a common feature. Adjacent tubules may show dysplastic change, a finding that supports rete testis or epididymal, rather than mesothelial, origin.

Abnormalities of the Vas Deferens Following Vasectomy

Vasectomy is a popular form of sterilization performed on an estimated 500,000 men in the United States annually. Although it is usually intended as a permanent procedure, reanastomosis via vasovasostomy is increasing in popularity. Tissue from the transected ends of the vas deferens is trimmed prior to suturing. This material frequently contains incidental microscopic abnormalities, including suture granulomas, sperm granulomas, and vasitis nodosa. More rarely, these same changes produce localized pain or a clinically detectable mass that requires excision.

Suture Granuloma

Suture granulomas, which are the least characteristic of the postvasectomy changes, are seen following any surgical suturing procedure. Suture granulomas are found in the trimmed vas deferens tissue obtained at vasovasostomy in approximately half of patients.

Microscopically, suture granulomas consist of aggregates of foreign body giant cells containing fragments of suture material.

Sperm Granuloma

A study by Taxy and co-workers identified sperm granulomas in 41% of patients undergoing vasovasostomy; they were virtually always associated with vasitis nodosa. It has been postulated that sperm granulomas play an important role in removing sperm following vasectomy and in maintaining a low-pressure state in the seminiferous tubules. There is no evidence, however, that the presence of a sperm granuloma is associated with a higher frequency of postvasovasostomy fertility.

Microscopically, sperm granulomas are nodules of inflammatory cells, particularly lymphocytes and histiocytes, admixed with extratubular spermatozoa (Fig. 17.19).

Vasitis Nodosa

Vasitis nodosa is a posttraumatic proliferation of ductal epithelium that appears to arise from the main transected lumen of the vas deferens. The most common of the postvasectomy changes, it is seen in approximately 66% of patients.

Microscopically, irregular ductal proliferations invade the surrounding smooth muscle of the vas deferens, exhibiting perineural or endoneural extension in about 16%–20% of cases (Fig. 17.20). Although neural invasion is generally associated with adenocarcinoma, it has been described in other benign epithelial proliferations in a variety of organs. Usually, the epithelium in vasitis nodosa resembles that of the normal vas deferens, but occasionally cytologic atypia in the form of vesicular nuclei, prominent nucleoli, and readily apparent mitotic figures may be present. The combination of atypia and perineural invasion, taken alone, could be confused with adenocarcinoma, but the clinical setting is likely to prevent misdiagnosis.

Neoplastic Lesions of the Spermatic Cord

The most common tumor of the spermatic cord is the benign "lipoma." Nodular proliferations of mature adipose tissue are frequently encountered and excised during inguinal herniorrhaphy. These nodules are usually labeled as lipomas, but true lipomas are encapsulated, solitary masses. Lipomas of the cord, which may reach enormous proportions, are most often encountered in middle-aged or older men.

The term fibroma has been applied to inflammatory fibrous tumors involving the spermatic cord. These are nonneoplastic proliferations best referred to as inflammatory fibrous pseudotumors. Most fibrous pseudotumors (described earlier) arise in close association with the tunica vaginalis.

After exclusion of lipomas and fibrous pseudotumors, the remainder of spermatic cord tumors are uncommon, often sarco-

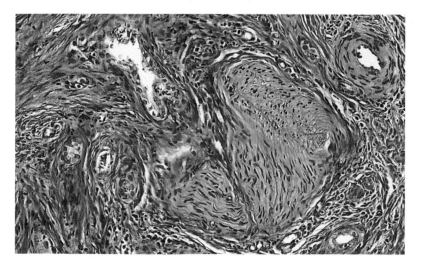

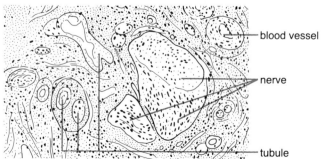

Figure 17.20 The proliferating tubules of vasitis nodosa are often closely apposed to small nerves. In many instances, intraneural or perineural growth may be seen. This finding should not be confused with carcinomatous infiltration of peripheral nerves.

blood vessel

nerve

tubule

matous, neoplasms. The frequency of the various subtypes tends to parallel that of soft tissue neoplasms in general, except for the high incidence of embryonal rhabdomyosarcoma of the spermatic cord in childhood. Leiomyomas (Figs. 17.21, 17.22), leiomyosarcomas, liposarcomas as well as others have also been reported. The histologic appearance and clinical course parallel those of analogous neoplasms arising in more conventional soft tissue locations.

EMBRYONAL RHABDOMYOSARCOMA

CLINICAL MANIFESTATIONS Embryonal rhabdomyosarcoma of the spermatic cord usually presents as a rapidly enlarging scrotal mass in a child under 15 years of age. Inguinal lymphadenopathy due to regional metastases is common at the time of diagnosis. Radical orchiectomy, radiation therapy, and adjuvant chemotherapy have dramatically improved the prognosis of this once highly fatal tumor.

MORPHOLOGY Microscopically, embryonal rhabdomyosarcomas belong to the group of childhood small cell neoplasms, including Ewing's sarcoma, lymphoma, neuroblastoma, small cell osteosarcoma, lymphoepithelioma, and others. The tumors consist of small cells with little or no visible cytoplasm and hyperchromatic, pleomorphic nuclei containing prominent mitotic figures (Fig. 17.23). Often the intercytoplasmic matrix has a delicate myxoid appearance and stains for connective tissue mucins.

Light-microscopic evidence of differentiation may be difficult or impossible to document; accurate diagnosis may require ultrastructural or immunohistochemical techniques. Ultrastructural studies suffer from their ability to sample only minute portions of the tumor, but they occasionally demonstrate convincing myofilaments and Z-bands. Immunohistochemical stains for myosin, myoglobin, rhabdomyoblast factor, desmin, or actin may be helpful. The first three stains are specific for skeletal differentiation. The last two are found in both skeletal and smooth muscle neoplasms.

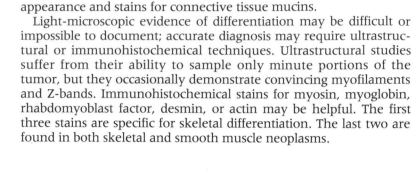

Figure 17.21 Grossly, this leiomyoma of the spermatic cord consists of a solid, tan, nodular tumor arising from the spermatic cord. It is closely apposed to the testis on the left.

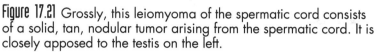

leiomyoma

testis

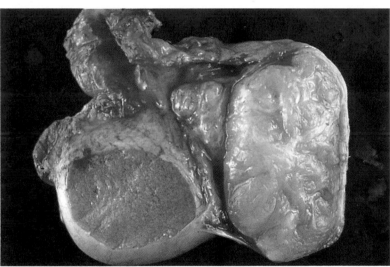

Figure 17.22 In this microscopic view, leiomyoma of spermatic cord consists of bundles of spindled cells forming sweeping fascicles. Distinction from a fibrocytic lesion may occasionally require special stains, electron microscopy, or immunocytochemistry.

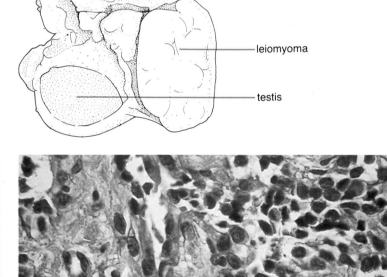

Figure 17.23 This photomicrograph of embryonal rhabdomyosarcoma shows the nests of cells with irregular, densely hyperchromatic nuclei and scant, eosinophilic cytoplasm that are typical of these poorly differentiated tumors.

Occasionally, embryonal rhabdomyosarcomas with little evidence of differentiation undergo dramatic maturation following radiation or chemotherapy (Fig. 17.24). It is unclear whether this is due to an induction of maturation or a selective destruction of undifferentiated cells. Regardless of the mechanism, the clear-cut skeletal differentiation in the treated tumor serves to confirm an often tentative initial diagnosis.

MALIGNANT FIBROUS HISTIOCYTOMA

In adults, the most common sarcoma of the spermatic cord (or elsewhere) is the malignant fibrous histiocytoma. In the past, these lesions have been categorized as pleomorphic rhabdomyosarcomas and fibrosarcomas. Clinically, they present as rapidly enlarging scrotal masses (Fig. 17.25). Metastases may

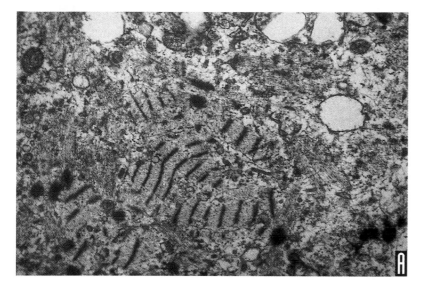

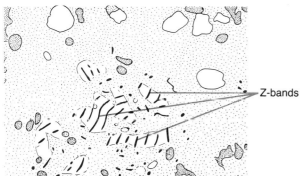

Z-bands

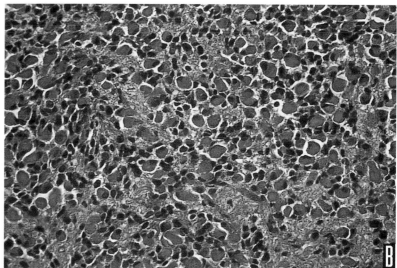

Figure 17.24 A, In this ultrastructural study of rhabdomyosarcoma, the aggregates of filaments and Z-bands in the cell cytoplasm are diagnostic of skeletal muscle differentiation. This degree of differentiation would be extremely uncommon in typical embryonal rhabdomyosarcoma. **B,** After intensive chemotherapy and radiation, the tumor has "matured." Ultrastructurally, the abundant, eosinophilic cytoplasm contains prominent skeletal muscle filaments.

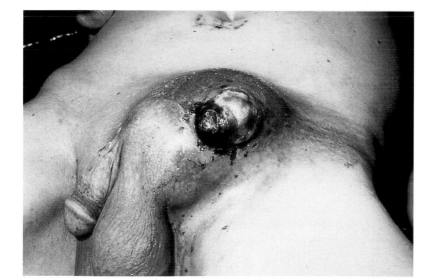

Figure 17.25 Grossly, this malignant fibrous histiocytoma of the spermatic cord is present as a large neoplasm involving the proximal portion of the spermatic cord. It has ulcerated through the scrotal skin. (Courtesy of J.E. Fowler, Jr., MD, Chicago, Illinois)

involve regional lymph nodes or disseminate hematogenously. Specific survival figures for spermatic cord lesions are unavailable, but the five-year survival rate for tumors of this type is generally about 50%.

Microscopically, malignant fibrous histiocytomas vary in appearance according to the relative predominance of spindled fibroblastic cells versus more polygonal histiocytoid cells (Fig. 17.26). A common but nondiagnostic finding is a storiform or cartwheel-shaped array of fibroblastic cells radiating outward from a central point. The presence of multinucleated tumor giant cells is helpful in distinguishing the tumor from fibrosarcoma.

VESTIGIAL INTRASCROTAL STRUCTURES, ECTOPIAS, AND APPENDAGES

APPENDIX TESTIS AND APPENDIX EPIDIDYMIS

Examining the junction between the testis and epididymis reveals an appendix testis and appendix epididymis in about one third of males. The appendix testis, also referred to as the hydatid of Morgagni, represents the most cranial portion of the vestigial müllerian duct, which forms the distal female genital tract. The appendix epididymis is derived from the mesonephric or wolffian-ductal system, which forms most of the spermatic transport ducts.

MORPHOLOGY The appendix testis arises in the groove formed by the junction of the globus major of the epididymis and the testis. Grossly, it consists of a small, 1–3 mm polyp. The appendix epi-

didymis, a saclike, polypoid structure similar in size to the appendix testis, is located on the head of the epididymis (Fig. 17.27). If both appendages are present, they are often separated by only a few millimeters.

Microscopically, the appendix testis consists of a central fibrovascular core covered by an outer layer of columnar, focally ciliated epithelium (Fig. 17.28). Occasionally, the central core may undergo dystrophic calcification. The appendix epididymis is a cystic structure whose outer surface is lined by flattened, often unapparent mesothelial cells. The internal cystic cavity is lined by columnar epithelium, which is surrounded by scattered smooth muscle cells and fibrous tissue (Fig. 17.29).

TORSION OF THE TESTICULAR APPENDAGES

Torsion of the appendix epididymis is rare (Fig. 17.30). Most appendage torsions involve the appendix testis. The clinical presentation is similar to that of testicular torsion, but the symptoms are typically less severe. The fever and constitutional complaints that often accompany testicular torsion are absent, but the pain may be intense. The age range is similar to that for testicular torsion; most patients are children. A small, tender mass may be palpable in the region of the epididymis, leading to a misdiagnosis of epididymitis. Alternately, referred pain to the abdomen may lead to confusion with appendicitis. Treatment of appendix testis torsion requires surgical excision of the small, typically gangrenous mass, followed by hydrocelectomy.

Grossly, the resected specimen is often enlarged to a centimeter or more due to edema and vascular congestion. Microscopic examination usually demonstrates unidentifiable, hemorrhagic, and infarcted tissue.

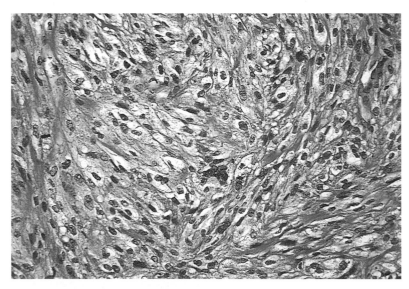

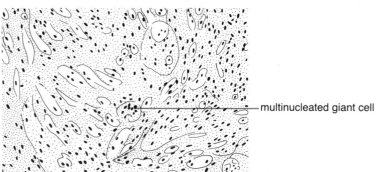
multinucleated giant cell

Figure 17.26 Microscopically, this malignant fibrous histiocytoma is composed of mononuclear, spindled fibroblast-like cells, more polygonal cells with foamy cytoplasm, and scattered multinucleated cells.

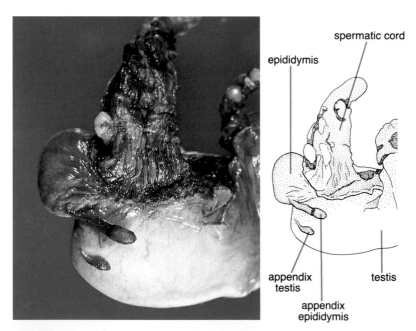

Figure 17.27 In this specimen, the smaller appendix testis, located distally, is attached to the testicular tunica. The larger appendix epididymis originates from the epididymal surface.

Other Vestigial Mesonephric Structures

There are three other vestigial structures, usually not grossly visible, that are derived from the mesonephric ducts. The cranial and caudal aberrant ductules are blind tubules usually lined by simple, ciliated, columnar epithelium. The former are located near the rete testis in the head of the epididymis, the latter near the junction of the epididymis and ductus deferens. The paradidymis or organ of Giraldes is a microscopic collection of blindly ending tubules within the spermatic cord at the level of the epididymis head. The tubules are lined by focally ciliated, columnar epithelium and form the most cephalad portion of the embryonic mesonephric duct. These mesonephric remnants have no known clinical importance.

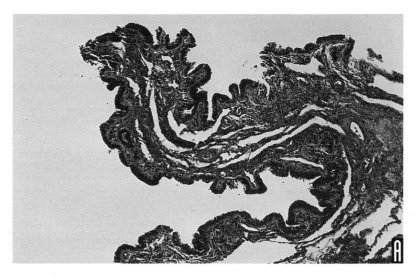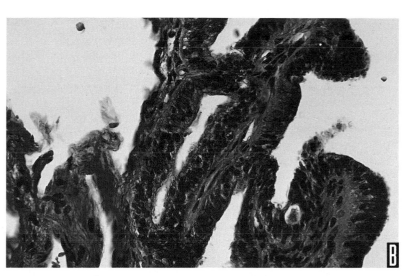

Figure 17.28 A, The appendix testis in this low-power photomicrograph has a central fibrovascular core covered by a layer of columnar epithelium. **B,** The uniform, columnar cells lining the surface of the appendix testis are seen in this high-power view.

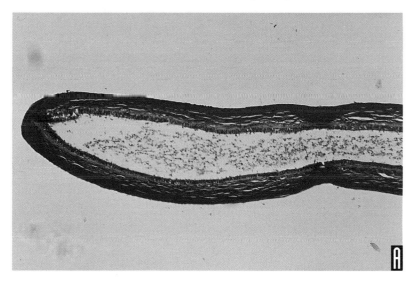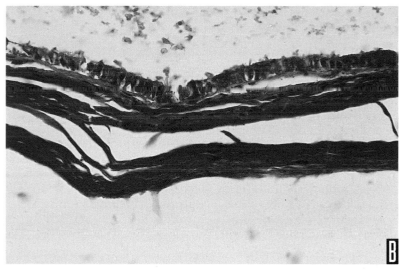

Figure 17.29 A, As shown in this low-power photomicrograph, the appendix epididymis is a cystic structure whose central cavity is lined by columnar epithelium. **B,** A high-power view demonstrates the columnar epithelium lining the cyst at the top of the field. The external surface is lined by flattened mesothelial cells, which are not visible in this photomicrograph.

Figure 17.30 Torsion of the appendix epididymis, as shown here, is much less common than torsion of the testicular appendage. The central cyst is enlarged and filled with hemorrhagic fluid.

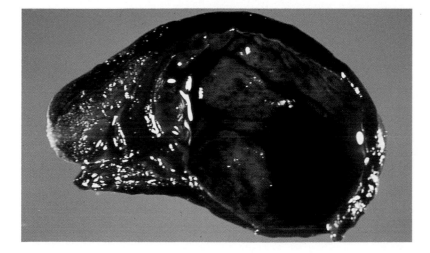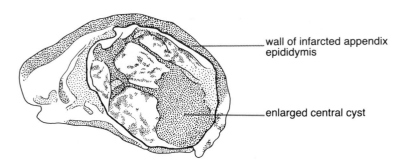

wall of infarcted appendix epididymis

enlarged central cyst

OTHER VESTIGIAL MÜLLERIAN-DUCT STRUCTURES

In males, the appendix testis and the prostatic utricle are traditionally viewed as the only remnants of the müllerian duct that persists after birth. They represent the most cranial and caudal portions of the duct, respectively. In a study of inguinal hernia sac tissue from prepubertal males, however, Walker and Mills identified tubular structures consistent with müllerian-duct remnants in 6% of specimens. Identical inclusions were also observed in spermatic cord tissue from young children. Structures of this type were not encountered in hernia sacs from postpubertal males, suggesting that they may regress with time. The only known importance of these müllerian duct vestiges is their potential for confusion, microscopically, with functional reproductive structures.

MORPHOLOGY Microscopically, these remnants consist of irregular, glandular structures surrounded by a mantle of fibrous connective tissue (Fig. 17.31). The epithelium lining the glands is composed of ciliated columnar cells with eosinophilic cytoplasm. Most specimens contain only one or two inclusions, but occasionally as many as a dozen are grouped together closely.

ADRENAL CORTICAL RESTS

Nodules of adrenal cortical tissue may be found in the region of the spermatic cord and epididymis in about 8% of male infants. The nodules vary in size from microscopic to almost a centimeter in diameter. Rare examples of functional adrenal adenomas and even cortical carcinomas have been documented arising in this aberrant tissue.

Grossly visible nodules have the distinctly yellow coloration of adrenal cortex and may appear encapsulated. Microscopically, the nodules are identical to normal adrenal cortex (Fig. 17.32). Medullary tissue is invariably absent.

SPLENOGONADAL FUSION

Nodules of ectopic splenic tissue may occasionally accompany the left testis on its embryonic descent. Association with the right testis is, as would be expected, extremely rare. These aberrant splenic nodules are usually discovered incidentally, but they are subject to the same stimuli that produce enlargement of the spleen. Under such circumstances they may become symptomatic, leading to considerable clinical confusion.

Grossly, these nodules have a deep-red to brown color, resembling nodules of ectopic splenic tissue more commonly found in the region of the splenic hilum. Their microscopic appearance mirrors that of the autologous spleen.

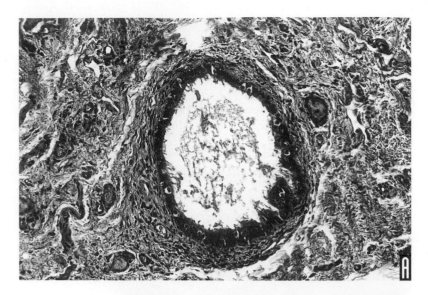

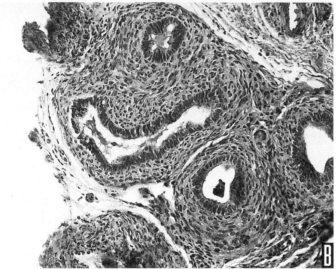

Figure 17.31 A, A single müllerian-like inclusion of ciliated columnar cells, resembling the cells of the normal fallopian tube, is present in tissue from the spermatic cord. Surrounding the glandlike inclusion is a delicate condensation of fibrous tissue. **B,** In some instances, müllerianlike inclusions may occur in small clusters. Each of the glandlike structures is encompassed by a cuff of fibrocytes.

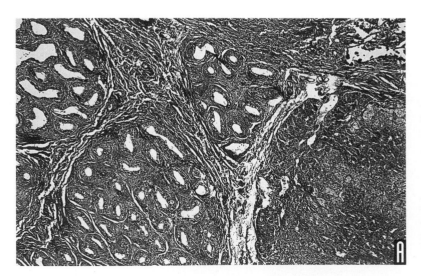

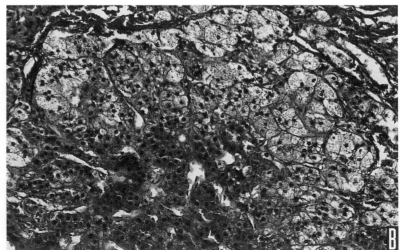

Figure 17.32 A, At low power, a nodule of adrenal cortical tissue is demonstrated at the lower right, next to tubules of the epididymis. **B,** High-power photomicroscopy shows cells of an adrenal cortical rest. They have clear, foamy-to-eosinophilic cytoplasm and are morphologically identical to the cells of the normal adrenal cortex.

SECTION VIII

Lesions of the Penis, Scrotum, and Urethra

CHAPTER 18

Nonneoplastic Lesions of the Penis, Scrotum, and Urethra

DERMATOLOGIC LESIONS WITH PREDILECTION FOR THE GENITALIA

ANGIOKERATOMA

Five clinical subtypes of angiokeratoma have been described. Angiokeratoma of Mibelli affects the dorsal surfaces of the fingers and toes. Papular angiokeratoma tends to be a solitary lesion with predilection for the legs. Angiokeratoma circumscriptum is a plaquelike growth, one or more centimeters in diameter; often present at birth, it typically involves the trunk or leg. The two remaining forms usually involve the genitalia. One type, *angiokeratoma of Fordyce*, is localized to the scrotum; the other, *angiokeratoma corporis diffusum*, or *Fabry's disease*, frequently involves the genitalia as a component of disseminated disease.

PATHOGENESIS The cause of Fordyce's angiokeratoma is unknown. Fabry's disease, one of the family of sphingolipidoses, is due to a deficiency in alpha-galactosidase, which causes ceramide trihexoside to accumulate in the body. Death usually occurs in the fourth or fifth decade of life due to renal insufficiency or myocardial infarction. Damage to dermal blood vessels because of accumulated abnormal glycosphingolipids probably accounts for the associated cutaneous lesions.

CLINICAL MANIFESTATIONS Patients with the localized scrotal form of angiokeratoma are usually middle-aged or older when first seen. Fordyce's angiokeratoma presents as multiple, red, soft, vascular papules (Fig. 18.1). With time, the papules may acquire a blue coloration and a keratotic surface.

Fabry's disease, in which angiokeratomas involve the genitalia as part of a disseminated process, typically begins in later childhood. The cutaneous eruption is often diffuse, but it has a predilection for the lower trunk, including the genitalia. Grossly, the lesions are similar to angiokeratomas of Fordyce, although they tend to be smaller (1–2 mm) and more numerous, often involving the penis (Fig. 18.2).

MORPHOLOGY The scrotal angiokeratomas of Fordyce are histologically identical to the disseminated lesions of Fabry's disease. Microscopically, the capillaries of the upper dermis are dilated to form irregular telangiectatic channels, and thrombi may exist in some vascular spaces (Fig. 18.3). The epidermis often forms elongated rete ridges between the dilated capillaries. Involvement may extend to the mid-dermis, but deeper levels are uninvolved. Angiokeratomas may be confused with cavernous hemangiomas, but they are traditionally viewed as nonneoplastic, telangiectatic lesions.

THERAPY The treatment of both localized (Fordyce's) and generalized (Fabry's) angiokeratomas is identical. Asymptomatic lesions require no specific therapy. Traumatized angiokeratomas may bleed profusely, and larger or problematic lesions may be treated by cauterization.

Pearly Penile Papules

CLINICAL MANIFESTATIONS Small fibrovascular papules occurring along the corona of the glans are seen in up to 20% of adult males and may be considered a normal variant. The pathogenesis is unknown. An example of an incidental finding is seen in

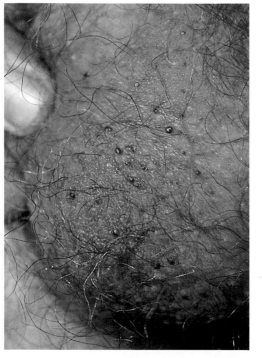

Figure 18.1 Angiokeratomas of Fordyce are multiple, red, vascular papules confined to the scrotum. (Courtesy of K.E. Greer, MD, Charlottesville, Virgina)

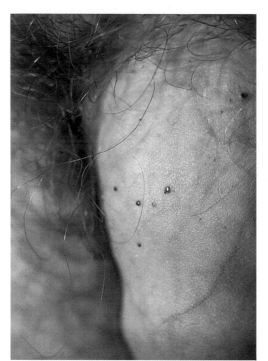

Figure 18.2 In Fabry's disease, angiokeratomas may also involve the genitalia as a component of a disseminated process. Grossly, these vascular penile papules are identical to the scrotal angiokeratomas of Fordyce. (Courtesy of K.E. Greer, MD, Charlottesville, Virginia)

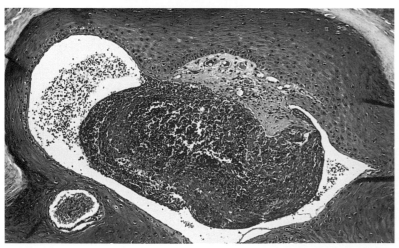

Figure 18.3 Biopsy of an angiokeratoma demonstrates dilated subepidermal vascular channels that contain erythrocytes and a fibrin thrombus that partially occludes the lumen.

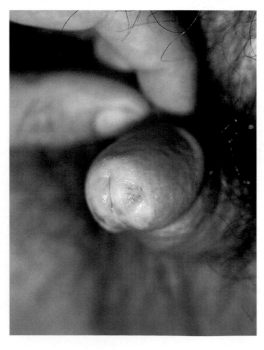

Figure 18.4 Balanitis xerotica obliterans, also known as lichen sclerosis et atrophicus, produces a pearly white, slightly elevated plaque involving the glans. (Courtesy of K.E. Greer, MD, Charlottesville, Virginia)

Figure 18.21. Lack of familiarity with this lesion may lead to confusion with condyloma acuminatum (see Fig. 18.19). Unlike condylomata, penile papules are small, uniform nodules in a linear array confined to the corona. Distinction is important to avoid labeling the patient as having a potentially infectious lesion and to prevent unnecessary treatment. Penile papules are invariably asymptomatic, requiring no therapy. They do not respond to podophyllin, a chemical often used to treat condylomata.

MORPHOLOGY   Microscopically, the papules have a rich capillary vasculature surrounded by prominent connective tissue stroma. Ackerman and Kornberg have interpreted them as small angiofibromas.

Balanitis Xerotica Obliterans

When lichen sclerosis et atrophicus involves the glans penis and prepuce, it is commonly referred to as balanitis xerotica obliterans. The pathogenesis is unknown, but a localized defect in collagen has been suggested.

CLINICAL MANIFESTATIONS   The process most often affects uncircumcised males and can result in phimosis due to contracture of the foreskin. Patients typically present with white, slightly elevated plaques (Fig. 18.4). Very few patients are prepubertal at the time of diagnosis.

There is considerable confusion regarding whether balanitis xerotica obliterans is a premalignant process. In some cases, patients with clinically similar lesions subsequently developed squamous cell carcinomas. However, we are unaware of biopsy-proven balanitis xerotica obliterans (defined by strict criteria and lacking evidence of squamous dysplasia) that was associated with carcinoma. Patients reported to have such progression may have had dysplasias that clinically mimicked balanitis xerotica obliterans.

MORPHOLOGY   There is a loss of the rete ridges with marked thinning of the epidermis, vacuolar degeneration of the basal cell layer, edema and bandlike collagenation of the upper dermis, and often a zone of inflammation in the mid-dermis (Fig. 18.5).

THERAPY   Cases of balanitis xerotica obliterans occasionally undergo spontaneous regression, but this is rare. Topical therapy with testosterone propionate in a water-soluble base produces symptomatic and clinical improvement in most patients. Intralesional injection of steroid may be necessary for patients with associated severe itching.

Lichen Nitidus

Lichen nitidus is a chronic, inflammatory dermatosis that has a predilection for the penis, lower abdomen, inner thighs, and arms. The cause of this condition is unknown. Its relationship to lichen planus (see below) is also unclear, although the absence of immunoglobulins at the dermal epidermal junction suggests that the lesions are distinct.

CLINICAL MANIFESTATIONS   Lichen nitidus is clinically characterized by asymptomatic, flat-topped papules that are typically yellow, red, or flesh-colored, and uniformly small (about 1–2 mm in diameter); they occasionally form linear arrays (Fig. 18.6). This condition may slowly progress, remain stationary, or spontaneously regress. Therapy is usually unnecessary, although topical steroids have been helpful.

MORPHOLOGY   Microscopically, a sharply circumscribed infiltrate of lymphocytes and histiocytes lies just beneath the surface epithelium, which is often flattened and shows hydropic change in the basal cell layer. At the edges of the lesion, the surrounding rete ridges extend downward to partially encompass the infiltrate (Fig. 18.7).

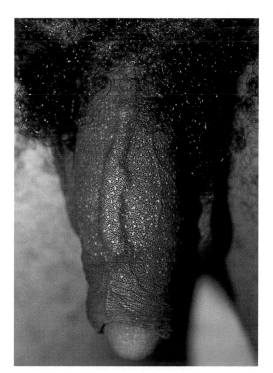

Figure 18.6 Lichen nitidus forms multiple small papules along the shaft of the penis. (Courtesy of K.E. Greer, MD, Charlottesville, Virginia)

Figure 18.5 The epithelium in balanitis xerotica obliterans is thinned, with loss of the rete ridges. The underlying dermis contains a band-like zone of edema and subepidermal collagenation. Beneath the collagen band is a zone of chronic inflammation.

LICHEN PLANUS

Lichen planus is an often intensely pruritic dermatosis that can affect any area of skin or mucous membrane, but sites of predilection include the forearms, legs, glans penis, and oral mucosa. The pathogenesis is unknown.

CLINICAL MANIFESTATIONS Lichen planus has a wide variety of clinical appearances. It usually forms polygonal, violet papules that condense to produce plaques. The plaque's surface is typically dry, shiny, or scaly, with a network of gray lines known as Wickham's striae. Penile lesions of lichen planus usually involve the glans and may have an annular configuration (Fig. 18.8). Treatment varies with the number of plaques and the severity of the associated pruritis. Intralesional steroid injection is the therapy of choice when the plaques are not too numerous.

MORPHOLOGY Microscopically, there is a bandlike infiltrate in the upper dermis mainly composed of lymphocytes. Mast cells are present, but eosinophils and plasma cells are not. The dermal border

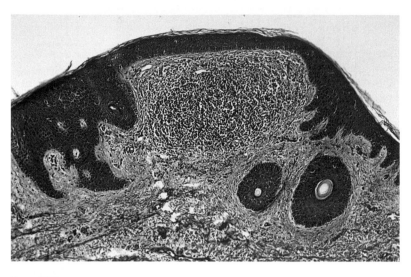

Figure 18.7 A sharply circumscribed dermal inflammatory infiltrate is typical of lichen nitidus. The surrounding rete ridges are hyperplastic and partially encompass the inflammation.

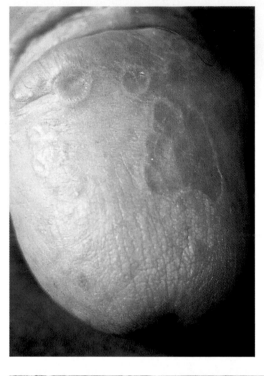

Figure 18.8 Lichen planus commonly involves the glans, often producing annular plaques. (Courtesy of K.E. Greer, MD, Charlottesville, Virginia)

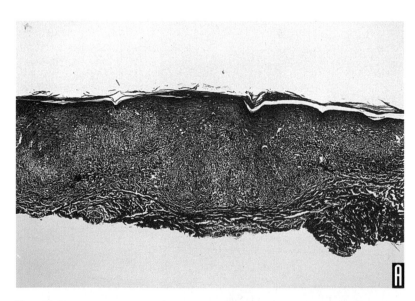

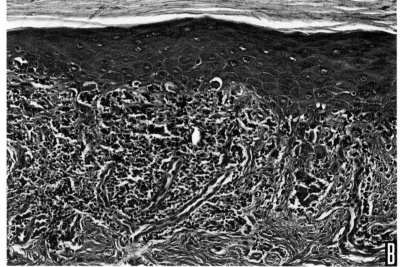

Figure 18.9 A, Bandlike inflammatory infiltrate in the upper dermis is typical of lichen planus, but not diagnostic. B, The characteristic changes in the overlying epidermis include irregular downgrowth of the rete ridges, degeneration of the basal epidermal cells, and the formation of eosinophilic colloid bodies.

keratotic layer

granular cell layer

eosinophilic colloid bodies

chronic inflammation

of the infiltrate is sharply defined. The overlying epidermis displays many changes, including hyperkeratosis, irregular downgrowth of the rete ridges, and liquifactive degeneration of the basal cell layer. The lower portion of the epidermis frequently contains eosinophilic colloid bodies formed from degenerating keratinocytes (Fig 18.9).

Reiter's Syndrome

PATHOGENESIS Reiter's syndrome occurs predominantly in genetically predisposed males of histocompatibility genotype HLA-B27 and appears to represent an abnormal host response to infection by a variety of agents. *Chlamydia trachomatis* has been implicated in some patients, but Reiter's syndrome may also develop in patients with bacterial gastrointestinal lesions.

CLINICAL MANIFESTATIONS Reiter's syndrome is defined as the triad of urethritis, conjunctivitis, and arthritis. Cutaneous lesions are a common feature. Penile involvement is common in the form of a circinate balanitis consisting of a brown-red to pustular patch with central clearing (Fig. 18.10). Associated lesions elsewhere on the body tend to be predominantly pustular.

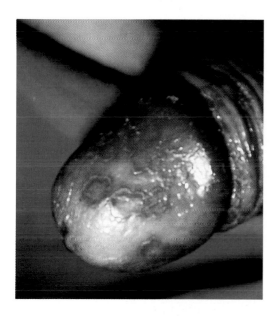

Figure 18.10 Circinate balanitis, a common feature of Reiter's syndrome, consists of red, often pustular patches with central clearing. (Courtesy of K.E. Greer, MD, Charlottesville, Virginia)

MORPHOLOGY Nonspecific changes vary with the lesion's age. Spongiosis, hyperkeratosis, acanthosis, and pustule formation are described (Fig. 18.11). Organisms are not demonstrable.

THERAPY The mucocutaneous lesions of Reiter's syndrome are self-limited, usually clearing within a few months. Nonsteroidal anti-inflammatory agents are the first line of therapy. Recalcitrant lesions may be treated with long-acting intramuscular steroids or even methotrexate.

Venereal and Nonvenereal Infections of the Genitalia

Syphilis

Infection with *Treponema pallidum* may produce a myriad of clinical manifestations. This section deals with two of the more common syphilitic lesions: the genital *chancre* of primary syphilis and the *condyloma latum* of secondary disease.

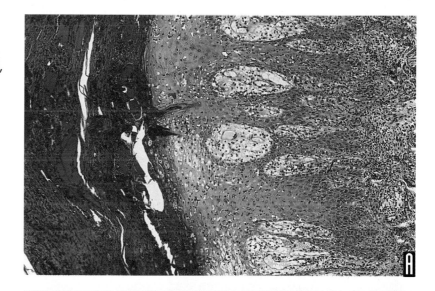

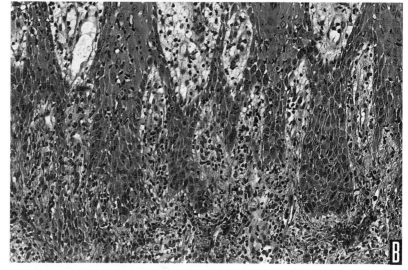

Figure 18.11 A, The microscopic features of cutaneous Reiter's syndrome are nonspecific. This advanced lesion has marked parakeratosis with intraepithelial pustules. There is also prominent, irregular downgrowth of the rete ridges. **B,** Prominent dermal inflammation and epithelial hyperplasia are frequent findings in Reiter's syndrome. Organisms are not present.

CLINICAL MANIFESTATIONS The genital chancre is the first cutaneous lesion of syphilis, appearing a little less than 3 weeks after inoculation. It is usually a single, nontender lesion. In men, it typically occurs in the coronal sulcus, but it is infrequently seen in women because of its predilection for the vaginal wall or cervix. Initially, a small red papule forms. Over a period of several weeks, it enlarges and becomes centrally eroded (Fig. 18.12). On palpation, the surrounding tissue is indurated to an extremely firm consistency. Occasionally, the primary chancre develops within the urethra, often near the meatus. The associated induration may be palpable; there may be a bloodtinged discharge.

Condyloma latum is a hypertrophic, papular lesion of secondary syphilis that usually develops on or around the genitals or in moist intertriginous zones. Grossly, it has an erythematous-to-white surface, and may actively weep serous fluid (Fig. 18.13). Condyloma latum may have a lobular surface, but it invariably lacks the villiform or verrucous surface characterizing the unrelated viral lesion of condyloma acuminatum.

MORPHOLOGY The superficial portion of the primary chancre consists of a nonspecific ulcer with a fibrinopurulent exudate overlying granulation tissue. More characteristic features are found at the edges of the ulcer and in the deeper, underlying tissue. Primary syphilis is associated with marked reactive changes in endothelial cells. Proliferating capillaries with reactive, enlarged endothelial cells are surrounded by cuffs of lymphocytes and prominent plasma cells (Fig. 18.14). Toward the lesion's center, the inflammatory infiltrate becomes confluent, and its perivascular configuration is less apparent. Spirochetes can be seen around capillaries with a Warthin-Starry silver stain, but care must be taken to differentiate organisms from reticulin fibers and dendritic melanocytes, which also stain.

The secondary syphilitic lesion of condyloma latum is microscopically similar to the primary chancre. A perivascular inflammatory cell infiltrate, prominent plasma cells, and reactive endothelial cells are also typical. However, confluence of inflammation and prominent ulceration with granulation tissue are not typical in condyloma latum, whereas the overlying epithelium usually shows marked epithelial hyperplasia (Fig. 18.15). Immunofluorescence and immunoperoxidase staining techniques using antisera directed against specific *T. pallidum antigens* have become increasingly valuable in diagnosing syphilis at the primary and secondary stages because of their high sensitivity and specificity as compared with other morphologic methods.

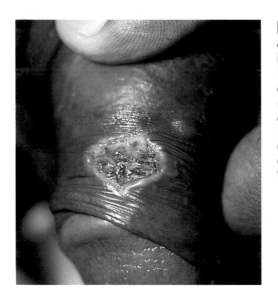

Figure 18.12 The genital chancre is the primary lesion of syphilis and is usually solitary. The central ulcer is surrounded by a zone of firm induration. (Courtesy of K.E. Greer, MD, Charlottesville, Virginia)

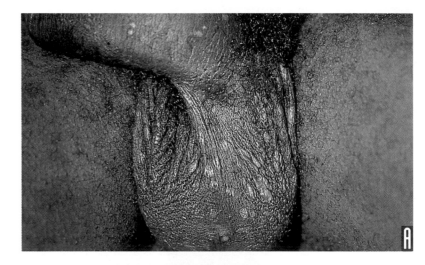

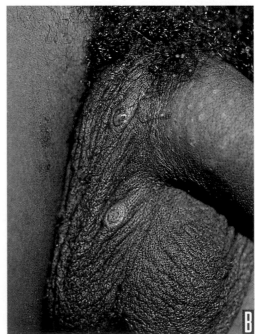

Figure 18.13
A, Secondary syphilis produces multiple hypertrophic papules referred to as condylomata lata. **B,** The lesions may have a keratotic surface (lower lesion), or they may be erythematous and weep serous fluid (upper lesion). (Courtesy of K.E. Greer, MD, Charlottesville, Virginia)

Chancroid

This venereal infection, which is uncommon in the United States, is due to *Hemophilus ducreyi*. The disease typically begins on the glans or prepuce as a single pustule that rapidly ruptures to form an ulcer with soft margins, lacking the induration of a syphilitic chancre (Fig. 18.16). Multiple lesions may subsequently develop due to autoinfection. Inguinal lymphadenopathy is often present.

Culturing the organism is difficult and requires freshly clotted human blood as the culture medium. Smears from the edges of the ulcers contain recognizable organisms in only about 50% of cases. The following criteria have been suggested for diagnosis: (1) one or multiple penile ulcers, (2) negative microscopic studies for *T. pallidum*, (3) negative serologic tests for syphilis, (4) negative Wright's stain for Donovan bodies, and (5) gram-negative rods on smear preparations. Various antibiotics are effective in treating chancroid.

Granuloma Inguinale

A primarily genital infection, granuloma inguinale is rare in the United States; only about 100 new cases are reported each year. It is far more common in tropical and subtropical climates.

PATHOGENESIS *Calymmatobacterium granulomatis*, a gram-negative, encapsulated bacillus, is the causative organism. Although the method of transmission is unclear, sexual contact is probably important, but nonsexual spread also occurs. The disease is only mildly contagious; chronic exposure may be necessary to develop clinically obvious lesions. The incubation time is unknown, but may be as short as 8 days.

CLINICAL MANIFESTATIONS The condition begins as subcutaneous nodules around the genitalia. The nodules erode through the skin to produce beefy-red, hypertrophic granulation tissue with

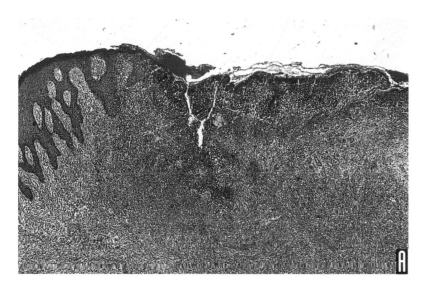

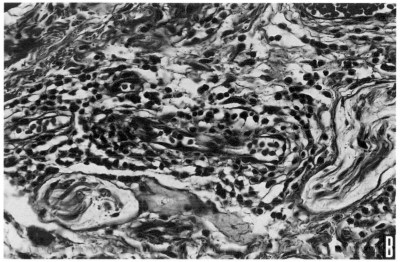

Figure 18.14 A, A primary chancre of syphilis shows surface ulceration. The inflammatory infiltrate extends laterally (left), producing the associated induration. **B,** More characteristic features of primary syphilis

include lymphocytes and prominent plasma cells that rim a group of capillaries with reactive, enlarged endothelial cells.

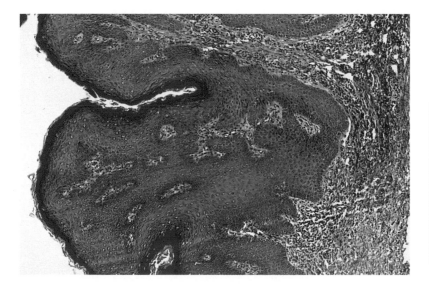

Figure 18.15 In contrast with the ulcer of a primary chancre, the lesion of condyloma latum often has a hypertrophic surface epithelium overlying the characteristic perivascular inflammation.

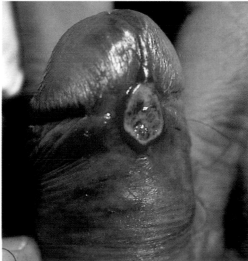

Figure 18.16 The ulcer of chancroid is similar to that of syphilis except that it typically lacks the surrounding induration. (Courtesy of K.E. Greer, MD, Charlottesville, Virginia)

focal zones of fibrinopurulent exudate (Fig. 18.17). Lymphadeno-pathy is usually absent, at least until advanced disease develops. The progression of the disease is slow and the lesions are typically not painful. Antibiotic therapy with various agents, including tetra-cycline, ampicillin, and trimethoprim-sulfamethoxazole, has been effective. Longstanding, untreated disease may result in sinus tracts, hypertrophic scars, lymphedema due to obstruction of proximal lymphatics, and hematogenous dissemination. Clinically, the hypertrophic scars may be confused with squamous cell carcinoma, and carcinoma may arise within them in rare cases.

MORPHOLOGY Large portions of the epidermis are ulcerated and replaced by exuberant granulation tissue. Marked epithelial hyperplasia at the edges of the lesions may be confused with squa-mous carcinoma. The stroma contains an intense inflammatory reaction, predominantly with lymphocytes and plasma cells, as well as granulomatous aggregates of histiocytes. Macrophages with pale-staining cytoplasm filled with large numbers of *C. granulomatis* are also present. The bacteria are easiest to demonstrate in Wright- or Giemsa-stained smears obtained from the exudate. Macrophages containing clusters of blue-to-black organisms with characteristic bipolar staining (Donovan bodies) are diagnostic.

DIFFERENTIAL DIAGNOSIS Granuloma inguinale must be differ-entiated from other ulcerating genital lesions, including carcinoma. Distinction from syphilis and lymphogranuloma venereum is based on negative syphilis serology and negative Frei test, respectively. In contrast with granuloma inguinale, lymphogranuloma venereum usually produces lymphadenopathy early in the clinical course. It should be remembered that multiple genital infections may coexist.

Fournier's Gangrene

Fournier's gangrene is a severe, necrotizing infection of the penis and/or scrotum that often extends into the fascia of the abdominal wall (Fig. 18.18). The mortality rate is approximately 35%. Predisposing factors include diabetes, trauma, paraphimosis, local infection, and recent surgery. The lesions begin as a focal area of swelling and crepitus due to the growth of gas-forming anaerobes. Deep-violet or black gangrenous areas rapidly develop and spread into the surrounding tissues. Cultures typically contain anaerobes mixed with colonic flora (*Escherichia coli*, as well as *Klebsiella* and *Enterobacter* organisms). Therapy consists of extensive incision and drainage with debridement, coupled with high-dose intravenous antibiotics.

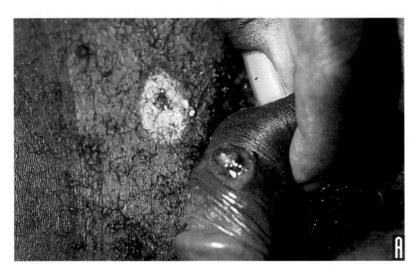

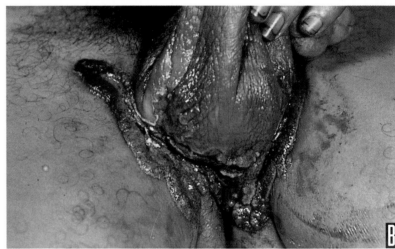

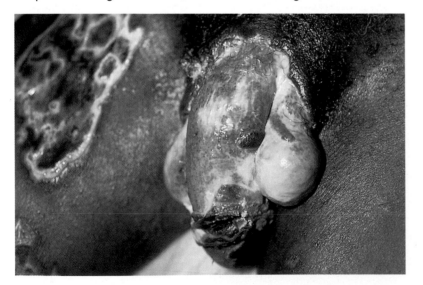

Figure 18.17 A, Nodules of early granuloma inguinale are located on the penis and inguinal skin. **B,** In more extensive granuloma

inguinale, there are broad zones of scrotal and periscrotal hyper-trophic tissue. (Courtesy of K.E. Greer, MD, Charlottesville, Virginia)

Figure 18.18 Extensive necrosis and sloughing of skin from the penis and scrotum are typical of Fournier's gangrene. (Courtesy of K.E. Greer, MD, Charlottesville, Virginia).

CONDYLOMA ACUMINATUM

Human papilloma virus (HPV) is known to be the causative agent of condyloma acuminatum, but understanding of HPV has been hampered by the lack of an in-vitro culture medium. Sophisticated techniques, including DNA hybridization, have identified dozens of HPV subtypes. Most genital condylomata appear to be due to HPV-6 and HPV-11. The theoretical importance of subtyping HPV relates to its apparent role in the development of squamous cell carcinoma in genital sites, particularly the cervix. Some forms of the virus, such as HPV-16 and HPV-18, are strongly associated with the development of carcinoma, whereas other forms, including HPV-6 and HPV-11, are less commonly associated with neoplasia. Although several studies have suggested an etiologic role for HPV in the development of genital carcinomas in males, particularly squamous cell carcinoma of the penis, such work has not been nearly as extensive as that done for cervical carcinoma. Other factors, including circumcision, must also be involved.

CLINICAL MANIFESTATIONS Genital warts usually grow as papillary, cauliflowerlike proliferations, in contrast with the verrucoid growth associated with extragenital lesions. This difference may be due both to the location and to the subtype of virus involved. The most frequent sites of involvement in males (usually uncircumcised) are the glans and foreskin, but all of the external genitalia may be involved in extensive disease (Fig. 18.19). In females, the lesions have a predilection for the vulva, perineum, or perianal regions. Transmission occurs by direct, usually sexual, contact. When the asymptomatic sexual partners of women with clinically apparent condylomata are carefully examined, a small urethral condyloma is often found just inside the meatus.

MORPHOLOGY Microscopically, condylomata exhibit marked epithelial hyperplasia with prominent papillomatosis, and are characterized by the presence of epithelial cells with koilocytotic atypia: a clearing of the perinuclear cytoplasm and hyperchromatic

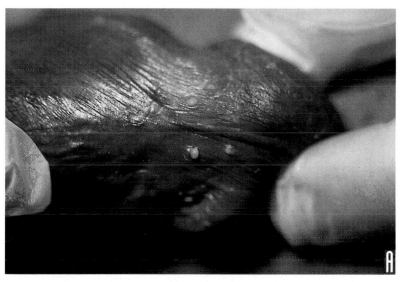

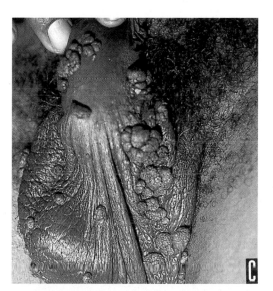

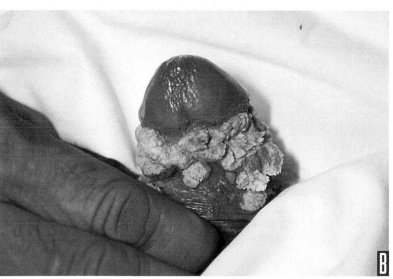

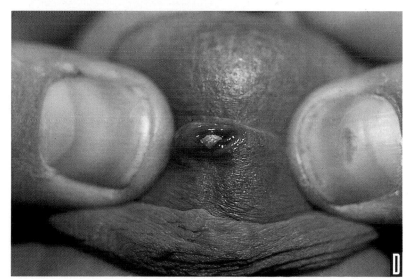

Figure 18.19 **A,** In this case of condyloma acuminatum, small genital warts are located adjacent to the frenulum. **B,** In a more extensive case, the condyloma involve the periglanular area. The white appearance is due to the moist keratin surface of the condylomata in this uncircumcised patient. **C,** The lesions may also involve the scrotum. **D,** When the urethral meatus is involved, the lesions may escape clinical detection unless the meatus is manually everted. (Courtesy of K.E. Greer, MD, Charlottesville, Virginia).

nuclei with borders that appear folded or crumpled (Fig. 18.20). The cytoplasmic clearing is not due to glycogen deposition, as is the case with normal mucosal clear cells, but results from the virally induced destruction of cytoplasmic organelles. Immunocytochemical stains have demonstrated viral antigens in the koilocytotic cells, and crystalline arrays of viral particles may be seen ultrastructurally.

THERAPY Many treatments have been applied to genital condylomata, although the frequently spontaneous regression of these lesions has made treatment protocols difficult to assess. Topical podophyllin is a common, effective treatment for most genital condylomata. Cryotherapy, electrodessication, ultrasound, and topical formalin have also been used with some success. For large, recalcitrant lesions, carefully controlled laser excision has been highly effective, producing excellent cosmetic results.

Herpes Simplex

The genital region is a common site for primary infection with *Herpesvirus hominis* type 2. The incidence of genital herpes has increased dramatically in the United States in the last decade, and it is currently one of the most common genital infections. Initial lesions are usually acquired through sexual contact. Recurrent disease, representing activation of latent virus, does not require exogenous exposure and is often related to trauma or emotional stress. The possible role of herpesvirus in the development of geni-

tal carcinoma was once a subject of considerable debate. Although formerly viewed as a prime suspect in carcinogenesis, that role has been adopted in recent years by the human papilloma virus.

CLINICAL MANIFESTATIONS From 3 to 14 days (mean, 5 days) following initial exposure, painful vesicles begin to develop. Favored sites in males include the glans, prepuce, and shaft (Fig. 18.21). In females, vesicles usually arise on the labia, vulva, clitoris, or cervix. Eruption of the vesicles may be associated with generalized symptoms of malaise. Within several days the vesicles rupture to form shallow, nonindurated ulcers. Healing of the ulcers typically occurs in 8 to 14 days.

MORPHOLOGY Herpetic lesions are usually not biopsied because they are relatively easily recognized on clinical examination. When obtained, biopsy specimens demonstrate intraepidermal vesicle formation with acantholysis and prominent ballooning degeneration of epithelial cells. The upper dermis and vesicle show a variable inflammatory infiltrate. Intranuclear inclusion bodies are characteristic but are not always demonstrable. The inclusions are brightly eosinophilic, approximately the diameter of a red blood cell, and are usually surrounded by a halo (Fig. 18.22). Ultrastructurally, inclusion bodies indicate the site of viral replication, but the intact viral particles may no longer be present.

THERAPY The lesions of genital herpes are self-limited but often recurrent and extremely painful. Supportive measures and anal-

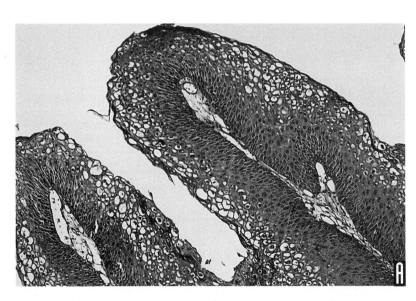

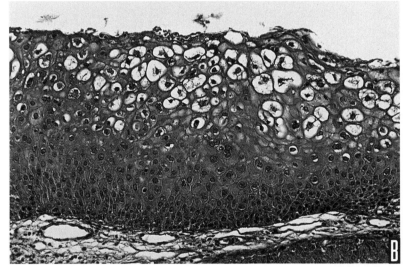

Figure 18.20 A, Condyloma acuminatum forms papillary fronds lined by squamous cells with prominent cytoplasmic clearing. **B,** The nuclei

also typically appear crinkled or folded. These changes are referred to as koilocytitic atypia.

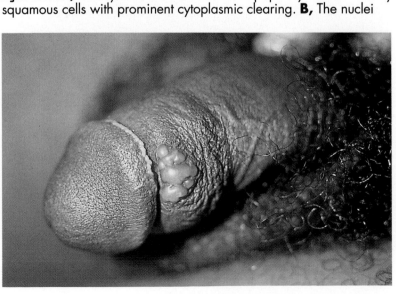

Figure 18.21 This clinical photograph shows coalescing vesicles of herpes simplex. Pearly penile papules, an unrelated finding, are also present along the corona. (Courtesy of K.E. Greer, MD, Charlottesville, Virginia)

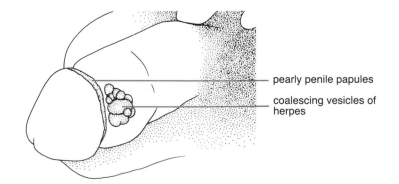

pearly penile papules

coalescing vesicles of herpes

gesics have been the traditional mode of treatment. Antiviral agents, including acyclovir and interferon, have also been demonstrated to decrease the duration and severity of recurrent disease.

Miscellaneous Congenital and Acquired Anomalies
Epispadias and Hypospadias

Defects in the formation of the urethral groove lead to epispadias and hypospadias. Epispadias is an abnormal urethral opening on the dorsal surface of the penis and is usually associated with exstro-

phy of the bladder, incomplete formation of the external sphincter, and incontinence (Fig. 18.23). It occurs in only about 1 in 50,000 newborns. A female counterpart to male epispadias associated with a bifid clitoris is about one fourth as common.

Hypospadias is far more prevalent, occurring in approximately 1 in 500 births, and represents an abnormal urethral meatus on the ventral aspect of the genitalia (Fig. 18.24). In most cases, hypospadias is a minor defect in which the urethral orifice is just proximal to its normal location on the glans (glanular hypospadias). More severe defects lead to more proximal urethral openings, referred to as *penile* hypospadias when the orifice occurs on the ventral surface of the shaft, and *scrotal* hypospadias when the opening is in the

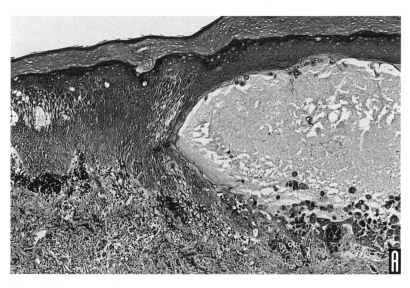

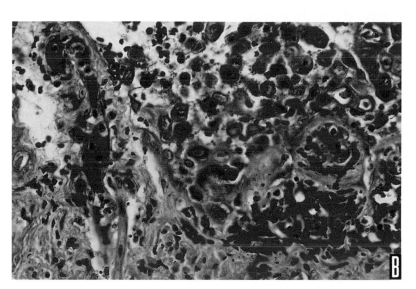

Figure 18.22 **A,** An intraepidermal vesicle of herpes simplex contains proteinaceous fluid and acantholytic epithelial cells. **B,** The exfoliated epithelial cells within the vesicle contain the characteristic intranuclear eosinophilic inclusions of herpes simplex.

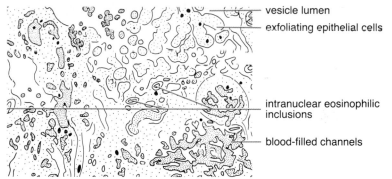

vesicle lumen
exfoliating epithelial cells

intranuclear eosinophilic inclusions

blood-filled channels

Figure 18.23 This clinical photograph of a newborn infant demonstrates the often combined conditions of exstrophy of the bladder and a malformed penis with epispadias. (Courtesy of S.S. Howards, MD, Charlottesville, Virginia)

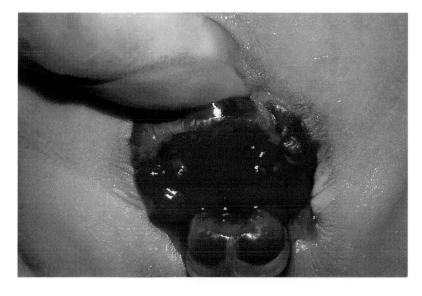

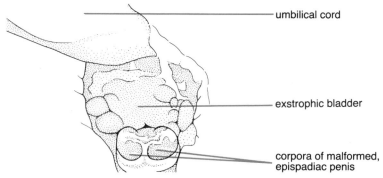

umbilical cord

exstrophic bladder

corpora of malformed, epispadiac penis

midline of the scrotum. Hypospadias, which may reflect a degree of feminization, is often associated with other defects, including cryptorchidism, hypogonadism, hyperplasia of the prostatic utricle, and hypoplasia of the prostate.

URETHRAL CARUNCLE

CLINICAL MANIFESTATIONS   These nonneoplastic proliferations may be indistinguishable from urethral carcinoma and are virtually confined to females, most of whom are postmenopausal. The pathogenesis is unknown. Urethral caruncles may be asymptomatic, but complaints of dysuria, hematuria, or bloody discharge are typical. They generally arise from the lower lip of the urethral meatus and are usually less than a centimeter in maximum dimen-

sion. They may be pedunculated or sessile, usually have an erythematous, vascular appearance, and are sensitive to the touch (Fig. 18.25). There is considerable variation in appearance, however, leading to confusion with condyloma, papilloma, and carcinoma. Symptomatic lesions are usually treated with local excision, often with cauterization of the underlying vasculature.

MORPHOLOGY   Urethral caruncles also exhibit variation in microscopic appearance. Some lesions show marked stromal inflammation; others are highly vascular or fibrous. In general, any swelling of the distal urethra may be viewed as a urethral caruncle if there is some degree of stromal inflammation, edema, increased vascularity, or fibrosis, and the lesion is covered by squamous or transitional epithelium with reactive hyperplasia (Fig. 18.26).

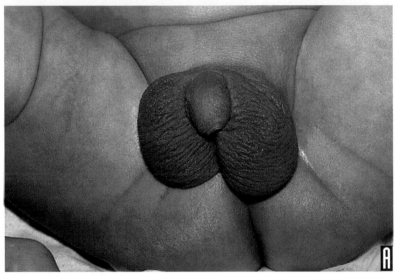

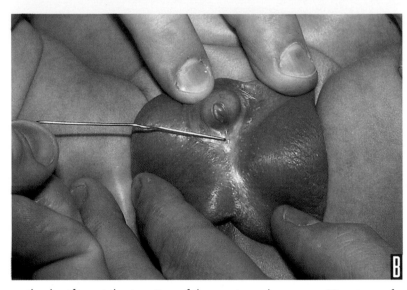

Figure 18.24 A, The dorsal surface of a penoscrotal hypospadias appears normal except for the suggestion of abnormal downward curvature. **B,** Reflecting the penis, however, reveals the abnormal

urethral orifice at the junction of the penis and scrotum. (Courtesy of S.S. Howards, MD, Charlottesville, Virginia)

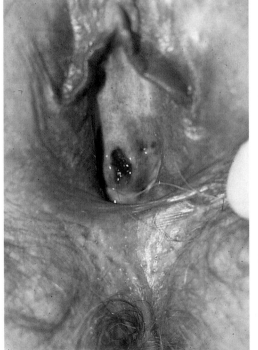

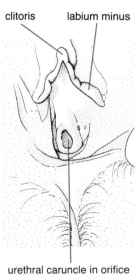

clitoris   labium minus

urethral caruncle in orifice

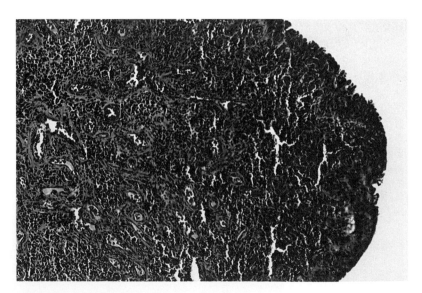

Figure 18.26 In this case of urethral caruncle, the lesion is composed predominantly of granulation tissue with proliferating capillaries and intense inflammation.

Figure 18.25 A urethral caruncle forms a vascular, polypoid mass at the urethral orifice.

Phimosis

The congenital or acquired presence of an abnormally stenotic prepuce that cannot be retracted over the glans penis is termed a phimosis. If the congenital form is not surgically corrected soon after birth, fibrous adhesions may develop between the glans and the foreskin. In rare cases, the phimosis may be so marked as to lead to urinary retention. If forcibly retracted, a phimotic prepuce may become swollen due to vascular obstruction and produce secondary vascular compromise of the glans. The retention of the swollen foreskin is known as a paraphimosis.

Urethral Diverticula

Urethral diverticula are abnormal outpouchings of the urethra, which are most commonly congenital but also may be acquired. Congenital diverticula usually arise from the ventral aspect of the anterior penile urethra. Defects in the periurethral glands or the corpus spongiosum have been postulated as causative. Acquired diverticula may be due to trauma, infection, or obstruction, and typically develop more proximally. The symptoms are the same for both the congenital and the acquired forms. Most often, the patient describes the development of a urethral mass during micturition with subsequent leakage of urine and resolution of the mass. Surgical excision with urethral reconstruction is the treatment of choice. The resected specimen typically consists of a pouch lined by squamous or transitional epithelium with variable stromal inflammation.

Peyronie's Disease

Also referred to as plastic induration of the penis, Peyronie's disease is a fibromatosis involving Buck's fascia and the fascia surrounding the corpora. The cause is unknown, although inflammatory processes and genetic predispositions have been suggested.

CLINICAL MANIFESTATIONS Patients develop penile curvature, with the fibromatosis located on the concave side. Most patients are over 55 years of age, and the lesion may have slowly enlarged over many years. Pain associated with erection is invariably present and, as the lesion progresses, difficulty in urination may develop. In the absence of therapy, lesions may progress, remain stationary, or even regress. Local excision is probably the optimal treatment, but a variety of nonsurgical techniques have been employed.

MORPHOLOGY This process is microscopically identical to Dupuytren's contracture of the hand; about 25% of patients with penile fibromatosis also have palmar disease. The histologic appearance varies, perhaps in relation to the lesion's age. Initially, there appears to be a prominent inflammatory component that with time is replaced by cellular and, ultimately, hyalinized fibrous tissue. The fibrous component may assume a nodular configuration (Fig. 18.27).

Idiopathic Scrotal Calcinosis

Most patients with calcinosis cutis have underlying, often mild, connective tissue disease. Calcinosis associated with Raynaud's phenomenon, sclerodactyly, and telangiectasia, the so-called CRST syndrome, is well recognized. The minority of patients who have cutaneous calcinosis without underlying connective tissue disease generally fall into two groups: those with the often familial tumoral calcinosis and those with idiopathic scrotal calcinosis.

CLINICAL MANIFESTATIONS Scrotal calcinosis consists of multiple rock-hard nodules in the scrotal skin that first appear in childhood or early adulthood. The lesions slowly increase in size and number. They may erode through the overlying skin and extrude innumerable chalklike fragments, but they are otherwise asymptomatic (Fig. 18.28).

MORPHOLOGY In scrotal calcinosis, amorphous aggregates of calcium phosphate are located in the dermis. Microscopically, they are surrounded by varying degrees of inflammation and foreign

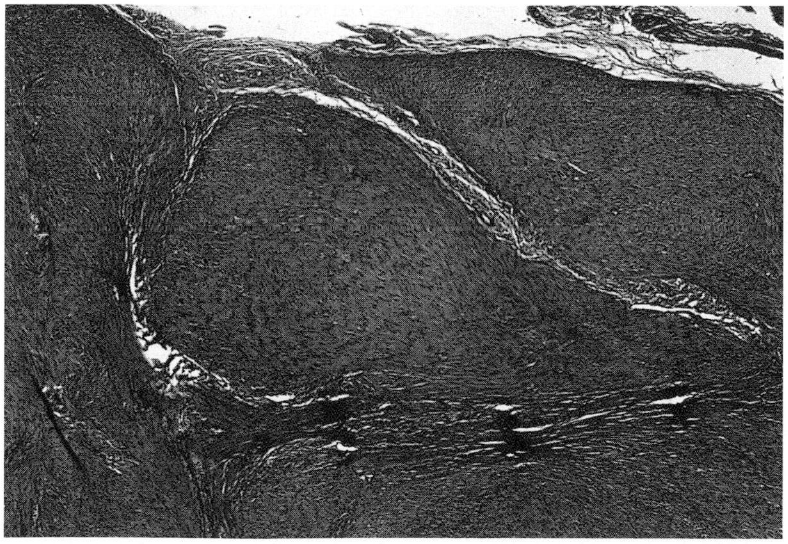

Figure 18.27 Penile fibromatosis (Peyronie's disease) is characterized by nodular proliferation of fibrous tissue.

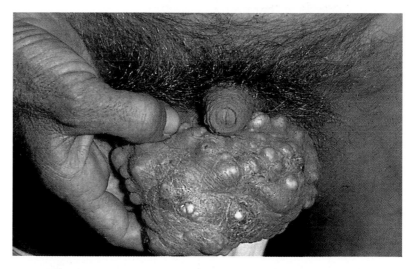

Figure 18.28 Scrotal calcinosis is characterized by multiple rock-hard subcutaneous nodules. Several nodules are exuding chalky white material. (Courtesy of K.E. Greer, MD, Charlottesville, Virginia)

body giant cell reaction (Fig. 18.29). The overlying dermis may be thinned or focally ulcerated due to the enlarging mass.

DIFFERENTIAL DIAGNOSIS Scrotal calcinosis should be differentiated from epidermal cysts of the scrotum, which also produce multiple subcutaneous masses (Fig. 18.30). Distinction is usually possible on clinical examination. Epidermal cysts are firm to palpation, but lack the rock-hard consistency of calcinosis. Microscopically, epidermal cysts are keratinous masses lined by squamous epithelium, an appearance quite distinct from that of calcinosis.

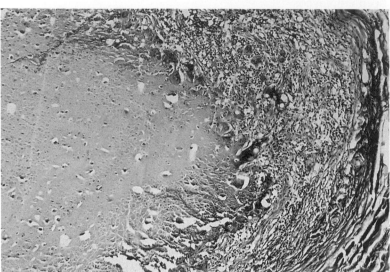

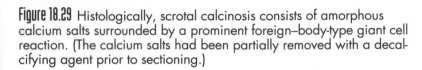

Figure 18.29 Histologically, scrotal calcinosis consists of amorphous calcium salts surrounded by a prominent foreign–body-type giant cell reaction. (The calcium salts had been partially removed with a decalcifying agent prior to sectioning.)

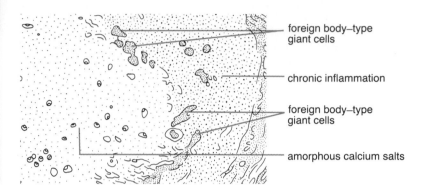

foreign body–type giant cells

chronic inflammation

foreign body–type giant cells

amorphous calcium salts

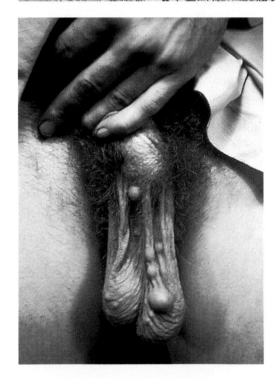

Figure 18.30 Epidermal cysts of the scotum may clinically resemble scrotal calcinosis. (Courtesy of K.E. Greer, MD, Charlottesville, Virginia)

CHAPTER 19

Neoplastic Lesions of the Penis, Scrotum, and Urethra

NEOPLASTIC LESIONS OF THE PENIS

CARCINOMA IN SITU

Intraepithelial carcinoma of the penis is known by a variety of eponyms, including Bowen's disease and erythroplasia of Queyrat. The former term describes in situ lesions involving penile skin; the latter applies to mucosal lesions of the glans and prepuce. It was once thought necessary to differentiate these variants because Bowen's disease was associated with other malignancies of the skin and viscera, a finding that may have been related to the development of multiple carcinomas in patients who chronically ingested arsenical solutions. Since this practice has been discontinued, the relationship of Bowen's disease to other malignancies has been less clear-cut. Most authors now prefer to combine these microscopically identical lesions under the general rubric of carcinoma in situ.

PATHOGENESIS A growing body of literature has incriminated specific subtypes of human papilloma virus (HPV) in the development of squamous cell carcinoma of the male and female genitalia. The evidence is most extensive for cervical carcinomas, but the role of HPV in the development of genital lesions in males has also been documented. Other factors implicated in the development of squamous cell carcinoma of the male genitalia include: (1) lack of circumcision, with the associated carcinogenic effect of smegma; and (2) exposure to other chemical carcinogens. The development of scrotal squamous cell carcinomas in chimney sweeps is a well known example of the latter phenomenon.

CLINICAL MANIFESTATIONS Carcinoma in situ of the penis most commonly involves the glans, coronal sulcus, and prepuce; in these locations it always occurs in uncircumcised men. Less frequently, the scrotum or perigenital skin may be involved. Most patients are over 40 years of age. Grossly, there is typically a single, erythematous patch, which varies in size from a few millimeters to several centimeters. The patch's surface is usually scaly or crusted, but it may be papillary, verrucous, or focally eroded. Although the margins may be irregular in contour, they are sharply circumscribed. Hyperkeratosis and underlying inflammation may produce slight thickening, but a nodular consistency suggests focal invasion (Fig. 19.1).

MORPHOLOGY The microscopic appearance of squamous cell carcinoma in situ of the penis is identical to that of analogous lesions involving the vulva or nongenital skin. It differs somewhat from the appearance of carcinoma in situ of the uterine cervix.

The epithelium usually shows acanthotic change with elongated rete ridges. The epithelial architecture is completely disorganized, with the exception of the focal zones of keratosis or parakeratosis on the surface of the lesions. Nuclei exhibit marked degrees of pleomorphism, with mitotic figures, including atypical forms, present at all levels. Dyskeratotic cells are usually prominent. Typical bowenoid cells with cytoplasmic clearing and bizarre, often multiple nuclei that have numerous atypical mitotic figures are characteristic (Fig. 19.2). The dysplastic cells may extend into the surrounding hair follicles, but seldom involve the sweat ducts.

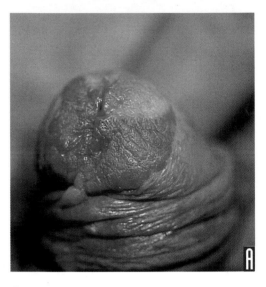
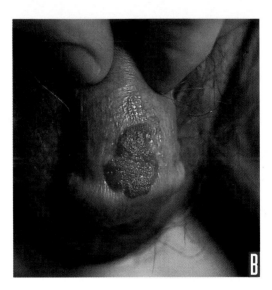
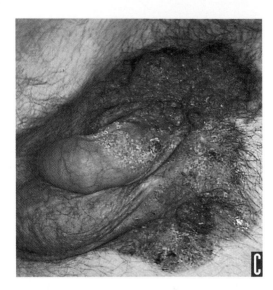

Figure 19.1 A, Carcinoma in situ of the glans presents clinically as a well demarcated, slightly elevated erythematous plaque. **B,** In this case involving the coronal sulcus, note the sharply circumscribed borders and uniformly erythematous appearance. **C,** Extensive carcinoma in situ may involve the proximal penis, scrotum, and perigenital skin. The surface irregularity suggests the possibility of progression to invasive disease. (Courtesy of K.E. Greer, MD, Charlottesville, Virginia)

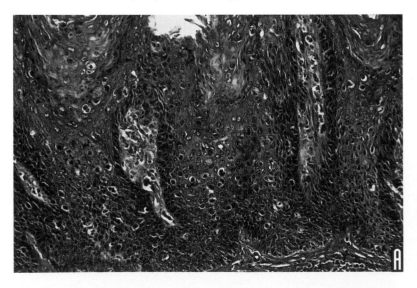
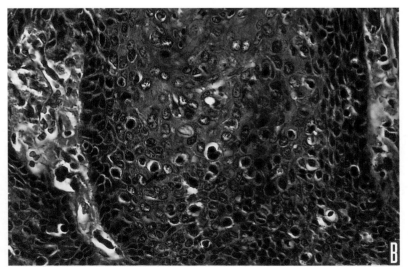

Figure 19.2 A, Medium-power view reveals the marked epithelial cell disorganization and nuclear pleomorphism that typify carcinoma in situ of the penis. **B,** Mitotic figures, including markedly atypical forms, are present throughout the epithelium in this higher-power view. Note the cells with bizarre nuclei and cytoplasmic clearing (bowenoid cells) typical of this condition.

THERAPY AND PROGNOSIS Carcinoma in situ progresses to invasive disease in only a few patients and usually only after many years (Fig. 19.3). The percentage of patients whose lesions progress to invasive disease varies from 11% to almost none. Patients who present with invasive squamous cell carcinoma must also have had in situ lesions, but the duration of the in situ component may be relatively brief. Thus, there may be two patient populations: those who have longstanding in situ disease and present as such, and those who rapidly progress, presenting with invasive carcinoma.

As long as the carcinoma remains in situ and does not breach the underlying basement membrane, there can be no metastatic spread. Once invasion does occur in longstanding bowenoid-type carcinoma in situ, the prognosis changes dramatically. Metastases in this setting develop in about 33% of patients, a much higher rate than for invasive carcinoma arising in actinically damaged skin.

Simple excision, when possible, is the best therapy. Larger lesions have been successfully treated with topical antineoplastic agents (5-fluorouracil) or sensitizing agents (dinitrochlorobenzene).

BOWENOID PAPULOSIS

Bowenoid papulosis has been said to be histologically identical to carcinoma in situ (Bowen's disease), but it differs in subtle histologic features and important clinical aspects. It has only recently been recognized as a frequently occurring genital lesion that is often associated with prior condylomata.

CLINICAL MANIFESTATIONS Bowenoid papulosis typically develops in young adults, almost always under 40 years of age, producing multiple red-brown papules approximately 7 mm in diameter (Fig. 19.4). The surface of the papules may be verrucoid; the clinician is likely to interpret them as genital warts. Solitary lesions may be seen, but multiple lesions are usual, affecting the shaft, glans, or both, in decreasing order of frequency. Many patients with lesions of the glans were circumcised in childhood. Individual lesions may remain stable for many years, regress, or be replaced by successive waves of new papules.

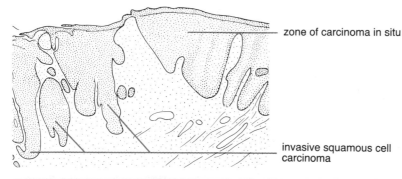

zone of carcinoma in situ

invasive squamous cell carcinoma

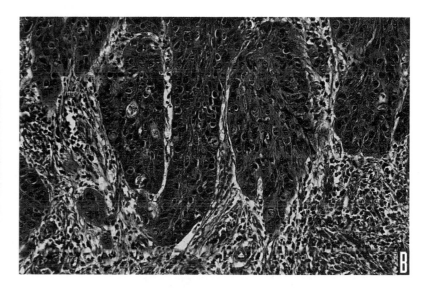

Figure 19.3 A, Superficially invasive penile squamous cell carcinoma is present immediately adjacent to carcinoma in situ. **B,** A higher power view demonstrates the irregular nests of invasive carcinoma.

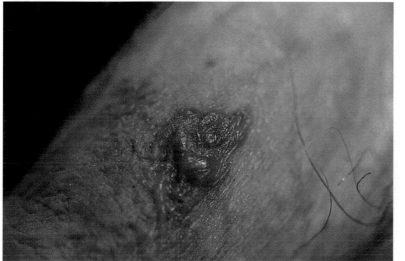

Figure 19.4 Bowenoid papulosis produces two closely approximated erythematous papules with irregular margins. (Courtesy of K.E. Greer, MD, Charlottesville, Virginia)

MORPHOLOGY Although initial descriptions of bowenoid papulosis equated its microscopic appearance with that of Bowen's disease, Ulbright, Patterson, and their coworkers have suggested that this entity can be distinguished microscopically from carcinoma in situ by its more uniform appearance, the absence of hair-follicle involvement, as well as the frequent presence of sweat-duct extension (Fig. 19.5). Podophyllin applied to a typical condyloma acuminatum may produce transient microscopic changes that potentially mimic carcinoma in situ or bowenoid papulosis.

THERAPY AND PROGNOSIS Invasive carcinoma has not been convincingly demonstrated to develop in bowenoid papulosis, but there is at least one example of progression to plaquelike carcinoma in situ (DeVillez and Stevens). Treatment of bowenoid papulosis should be conservative. Any locally destructive procedure that would be adequate for ordinary condylomata is sufficient. Resection margins do not need to be evaluated for the presence of disease, as this does not correlate with the risk of recurrence.

Squamous Cell Carcinoma

Invasive squamous cell carcinoma of the penis accounts for only about 1%–2% of malignancies developing in males in the United States and appears to be decreasing in frequency. In other countries, however, it represents up to 12% of carcinomas in males.

Although its pathogenesis is unclear, circumcision in childhood conveys nearly complete protection against its development.

CLINICAL MANIFESTATIONS The lesions almost always begin on the glans, sulcus, or prepuce in an uncircumcised individual. Most patients are over 50 years of age. Many present with advanced disease, presumably due to a reluctance to seek medical therapy. The tumors form nodular, ulcerated, often secondarily infected masses. Small carcinomas may be hidden under a redundant or phimotic foreskin (Fig. 19.6). Invasion into the corpora and urethra may produce urinary obstruction or fistula formation. Inguinal lymph nodes are frequently enlarged, sometimes due to metastatic involvement, but most commonly because of infection (58% of cases).

The Jackson staging system is usually applied to penile carcinomas:
Stage I   Confinement of the tumor to the glans and/or prepuce.
Stage II   Invasion of the shaft or corpora, but without metastases.
Stage III Confinement of the tumor to the shaft with histologically proven regional lymph node metastases.
Stage IV   Invasion of the shaft with inoperable regional and/or distant metastases.

MORPHOLOGY Most of these neoplasms are well or moderately differentiated, keratinizing carcinomas that pose no diagnostic difficulty. Unlike verrucous carcinoma (see below), they exhibit considerable nuclear pleomorphism with large vesicular-to-hyperchromatic

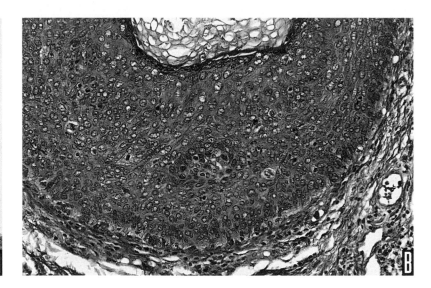

Figure 19.5 **A,** Low-power photomicrograph of bowenoid papulosis shows its typical papular configuration. **B,** On a higher-power view, the epithelial disorganization, bowenoid clear cells, and numerous mitotic figures are consistent with carcinoma in situ.

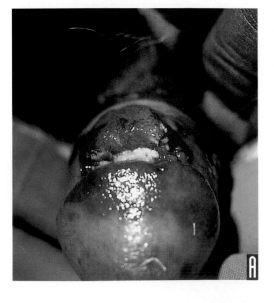
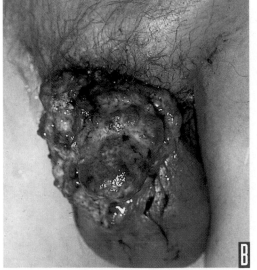

Figure 19.6 **A,** In this case of invasive squamous cell carcinoma of the penis, a relatively small lesion is localized to the region of the coronal sulcus. **B,** Unfortunately, many patients present with highly advanced lesions that totally destroy the penis, extending into the scrotum or perigenital skin. Note the inguinal lymphadenopathy on the patient's left.

nuclei and numerous, often atypical, mitotic figures (Fig. 19.7). Abrupt keratinization of invasive cells with keratin "pearl" formation is a common finding.

Two histologic variants of squamous cell carcinoma, which are probably not clinically significant, may cause diagnostic difficulty. Spindle cell carcinoma is known by a variety of terms, including pseudosarcomatous carcinoma, carcinoma with sarcomalike stroma, and carcinosarcoma (Fig 19.8). Tumors of this type are more common in other areas of the body, particularly the head and neck. The nature of the spindle cells is controversial. Theories have suggested that they are reactive stromal cells, a second population of malignant stromal cells (collision tumor), malignant stromal cells arising from the associated carcinoma (stromal metaplasia), or malignant epithelial cells superficially resembling stromal cells. Battifora has presented ultrastructural evidence to support the stromal-metaplasia theory. Regardless of their exact nature, spindle cell carcinomas of the penis, as elsewhere, tend to behave more like conventional squamous cell carcinomas than like sarcomas. Their distinction from the very rare sarcomas of the penis, therefore, is essential and is usually based on careful light-microscopic examination. Spindle cell carcinomas often contain small nests of more conventional squamous cell carcinoma that may be detected with thorough sectioning. In problematic cases, electron microscopy or immunocytochemistry for epithelial cell markers may be helpful.

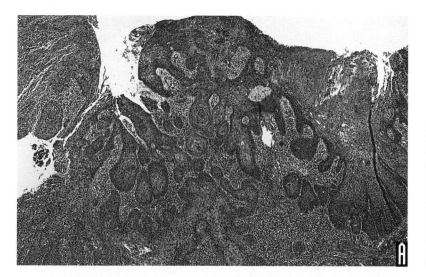

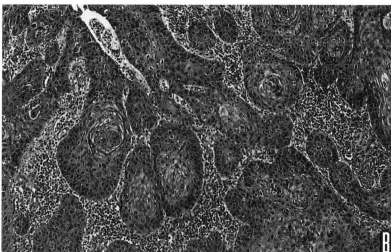

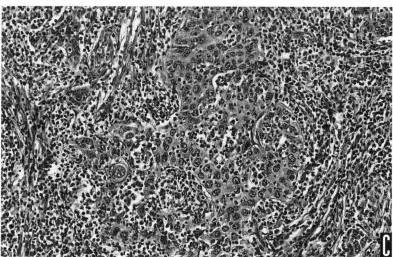

Figure 19.7 A, Irregular nests of squamous cell carcinoma invade the underlying tissue. **B,** A higher-power view of infiltrating squamous cell carcinoma demonstrates focal keratinization. **C,** At the point of deepest invasion, the squamous carcinoma cells are nonkeratinizing and exhibit considerable pleomorphism with large vesicular nuclei. Note the associated intense inflammation often seen in invasive carcinoma.

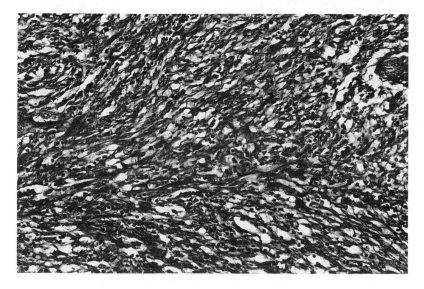

Figure 19.8 The spindle-cell variant of squamous carcinoma may be confused with a sarcoma. In microscopic fields such as this, the distinction is not possible with a standard hematoxylin and eosin-stained section. In other areas, this tumor exhibited the typical appearance of squamous cell carcinoma. Immunocytochemical markers for epithelial cells or electron microscopy may be required in problematic cases.

Adenoid squamous cell carcinoma, also known as acantholytic squamous cell carcinoma, is a microscopically distinctive variant in which the squamous cells form glandlike spaces that superficially resemble an adenocarcinoma (Fig. 19.9). Unlike the latter, however, the spaces are lined by squamous, often randomly oriented cells.

THERAPY AND PROGNOSIS   Surgical resection has been the therapeutic mainstay in the treatment of penile carcinoma (Fig. 19.10). Regional lymphadenectomy is also typically performed, even for patients with stage I disease, because of the high incidence (20%–30%) of clinically occult nodal involvement. Radiation therapy, which has also been advocated for small stage I lesions, has yielded promising results. Patients with advanced disease may partially respond to chemotherapy, but complete remissions have not been achieved. Three-year survival rates according to stage, as reported by deKernion and colleagues, are: Stage I, 95%; Stage II, 67%; Stage III, 29%; and Stage IV, 0%. Most patients dying of the disease develop intractable pelvic involvement with erosion of bones and large blood vessels. Distant hematogenous spread is an uncommon, usually preterminal, event.

VERRUCOUS CARCINOMA

Verrucous carcinoma occurs in a patient population similar to that of conventional squamous carcinoma, but the tumors differ in important biologic and microscopic aspects. The so-called *giant condyloma of Buschke and Löwenstein* is identical to verrucous carcinoma in all respects; this confusing eponym should be abandoned.

CLINICAL MANIFESTATIONS   The papillary or wartlike lesions characteristic of verrucous carcinoma mimic the typical condyloma acuminatum in their surface appearance and consistency, but differ from genital warts in their large size and destructive nature (Fig. 19.11).

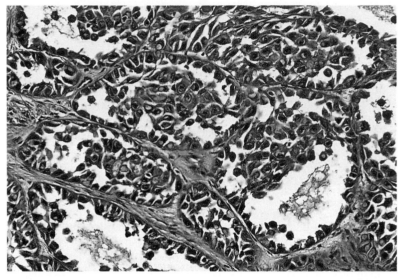

Figure 19.9 Acantholytic or adenoid squamous cell carcinoma somewhat resembles the glands of adenocarcinoma. The squamous nature of the cells is evident, however.

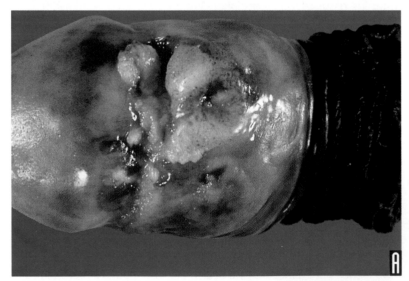

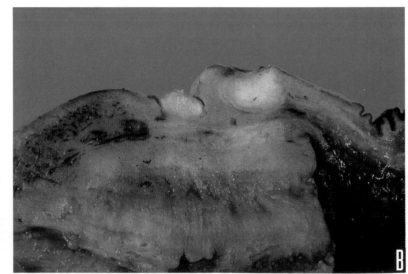

Figure 19.10 A, Resected penile specimen shows a small squamous cell carcinoma arising in the coronal sulcus. **B,** Cut section from the specimen demonstrates two small nodules of invasive carcinoma.

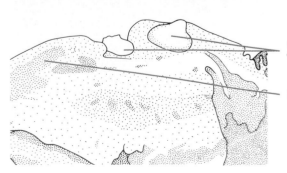

nests of squamous cell carcinoma

glans of penis

MORPHOLOGY Microscopically, verrucous carcinoma consists of papillomatous proliferations of mature, apparently normal, or minimally atypical keratinocytes. Cytologic features of malignancy are absent by definition. The distinction from condyloma acuminatum may be difficult or impossible on superficial biopsy. The diagnosis can be made histologically only when there is invasion of the underlying stroma by nests of bland squamous cells (Fig. 19.12). Careful search should be made for foci of conventional squamous cell carcinoma. Mixed conventional squamous and verrucous carcinomas are common; these mixed lesions may metastasize.

THERAPY AND PROGNOSIS If the tumor is carefully defined morphologically, it is a nonmetastasizing neoplasm with an excellent prognosis. Regional lymph nodes may be enlarged, but this is invariably due to associated infection. Treatment is usually local excision, which may be extensive for large, destructive lesions.

EXTRAMAMMARY PAGET'S DISEASE

Paget first described this lesion and compared it to histologically similar lesions of the breast in 1874. Since then, very few additional examples of penile Paget's disease have been reported, in contrast with its far more common occurrence in the female external genitalia.

Paget's disease is a distinctive, epidermotropic adenocarcinoma that may occur in situ or may be associated with an underlying invasive carcinoma of sweat-gland type. The origin of the intraepidermal cells is controversial, but they probably arise in situ from basal epithelial cells.

CLINICAL MANIFESTATIONS Paget's disease of the penis produces erythematous, crusted, and indurated lesions that are typically intensely pruritic. The associated scratching may lead to exco-

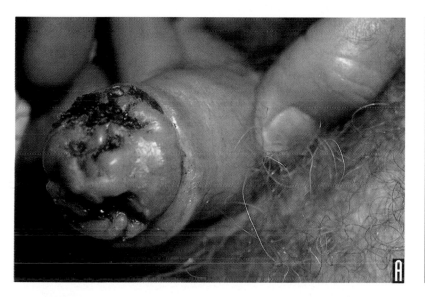

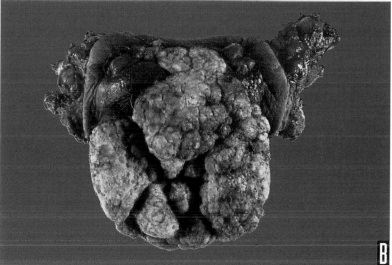

Figure 19.11 A, In verrucous carcinoma of the penis, infiltration can extensively deform the glans. The verrucous surface of the tumor is covered with eschar. **B,** The destructive nature of untreated verrucous carcinoma is amply demonstrated in this resected specimen. A cauli-

flowerlike mass has replaced the penis and scrotal contents. Attached inguinal lymph nodes are enlarged due to lymphoid hyperplasia, not metastases. (**A:** Courtesy of J.E. Fowler, Jr., MD, Chicago, Illinois)

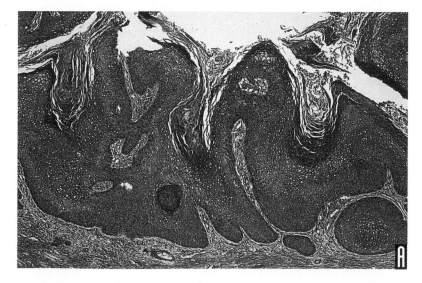

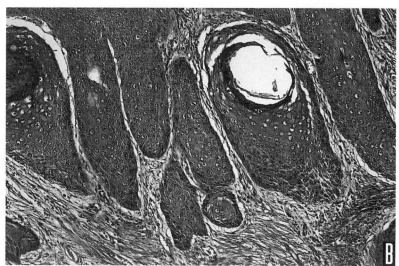

Figure 19.12 A, Verrucous carcinoma invades the underlying stroma as large nests and bulbous protrusions of squamous cells that appear cytologically benign. **B,** Nests of invasive verrucous carcinoma cells

are composed of cytologically uniform cells lacking the conventional morphologic features of carcinoma (see Figure 19.7B,C).

riations and secondary infection. The clinical appearance of penile Paget's disease is identical to that of its more common vulvar counterpart (Fig. 19.13).

MORPHOLOGY Nests of Paget's cells with abundant pale eosinophilic or vacuolated cytoplasm, large pleomorphic nuclei, and often prominent nucleoli cluster in the basal layer of the epithelium, migrating into the more superficial epidermis as single cells. Diastase-resistant, periodic acid-Schiff (PAS)–positive material in the cytoplasm aids in distinguishing these cells from melanocytes or unusual squamous cells (Fig. 19.14).

THERAPY AND PROGNOSIS The lesion is treated by wide excision. Paget's cells are often seen in specimen margins that appear clinically uninvolved. Not surprisingly, recurrences are frequent, but metastases do not occur if there is no invasive carcinoma. Once invasion develops, even if only superficially, the rate of metastatic disease is high and the prognosis is correspondingly poor.

Miscellaneous Penile Neoplasms

Stromal neoplasms of the penis are extremely rare. Virtually every form of stromal neoplasia occurring in soft tissues may involve the penis, but vascular tumors are the most frequent.

Histiocytoid (Epithelioid) Hemangioma

This benign vascular neoplasm is known by a variety of other terms, including angiolymphoid hyperplasia with eosinophilia and epithelioid hemangioma. Clinically, it presents as one or more indurated subcutaneous nodules. Microscopically, it consists of proliferating vascular channels lined by endothelial cells with prominent eosinophilic cytoplasm (Fig. 19.15). The surrounding stroma often contains abundant eosinophils. There may be a spectrum of cytologic pleomorphism, ranging from obviously benign lesions to more pleomorphic tumors. Lesions of the latter type have been termed epithelioid hemangioendotheliomas.

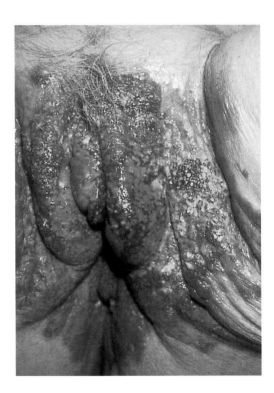

Figure 19.13 Paget's disease of the vulva is clinically identical to its far less common penile counterpart. Raised erythematous plaques with crusting secondary to excoriation are typical. The clinical circumscription is deceptive; grossly uninvolved margins often contain neoplastic cells. (Courtesy of W.A. Andersen, MD, Charlottesville, Virginia)

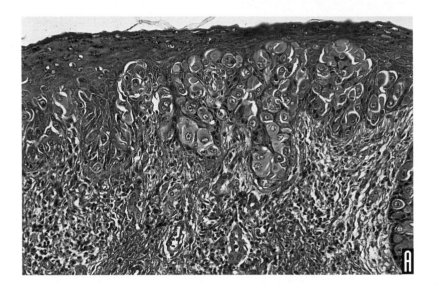

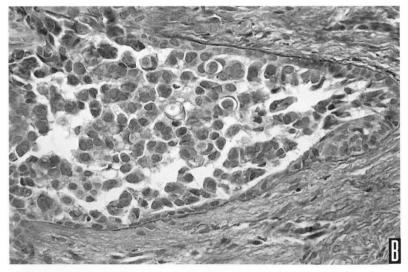

Figure 19.14 A, Paget's disease, an intraepithelial adenocarcinoma, is characterized by large neoplastic cells with vesicular nuclei and abundant eosinophilic cytoplasm located within the surface epithelium. **B,** PAS stain with diastase predigestion demonstrates intracytoplasmic mucopolysaccharides (mucin), staining pink to red, within the cells of Paget's disease.

Angiosarcoma

The penis may also be the site of conventional angiosarcoma (Fig. 19.16). It has been suggested that sarcomas of all types, including angiosarcoma, are slightly less aggressive when they involve the penis. Although this may be statistically true, they are still full-fledged sarcomas capable of metastasizing (Fig. 19.17).

Carcinoma of the Scrotum

Carcinoma of the scrotum is now rare in the United States, and usually occurs without obvious predisposing factors. The tumor remains slightly more common in Great Britain. Squamous cell carcinoma of the scrotum is particularly rare in American blacks.

PATHOGENESIS Squamous cell carcinoma of the scrotum was one of the first occupationally related neoplasms to be recognized. Potts is generally credited with first linking this tumor to chimney sweeps. Groups at increased risk include paraffin and shale oil workers, machinery operators involved in metal cutting, as well as other workers who are exposed to large amounts of petroleum oils, soots, and tars. Protective measures have markedly reduced the frequency of industry-related scrotal carcinoma.

CLINICAL MANIFESTATIONS Squamous cell carcinoma of the scrotum often develops on the anterolateral aspect. Most patients are at least 50 years of age. A solitary, nodular, often ulcerated lesion is found on examination. Inguinal lymphadenopathy exists in about 50% of patients, but it is often reactive and responds to antibiotics.

MORPHOLOGY Scrotal squamous cell carcinomas are microscopically identical to their penile counterparts (see Fig. 19.7). Most tumors are moderately differentiated and focally keratinizing, posing no diagnostic difficulty. Basal cell carcinoma of the scrotum is far less common than squamous neoplasia. It is microscopically and biologically identical to basal cell carcinomas occurring elsewhere in the skin.

THERAPY AND PROGNOSIS Wide local excision, with skin grafting if necessary, is the treatment of choice. Patients with lateral lesions may undergo ipsilateral lymph node resection and biopsy of the contralateral sentinel node. If the latter is positive, bilateral lymph node resection is mandatory. Survival rates for scrotal squamous cell carcinoma are analogous to those for penile carcinoma of equivalent stage. About 70% of patients with disease confined to the scrotum will survive. Regional lymph node metastases diminish survival by a factor of two.

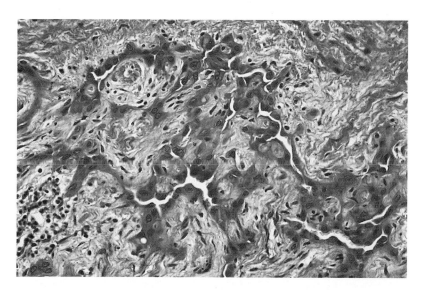

Figure 19.15 Irregular vascular spaces lined by plump endothelial cells with prominent eosinophilic cytoplasm are typical of histiocytoid (epithelioid) hemangioma, a low-grade vascular neoplasm known by numerous synonyms.

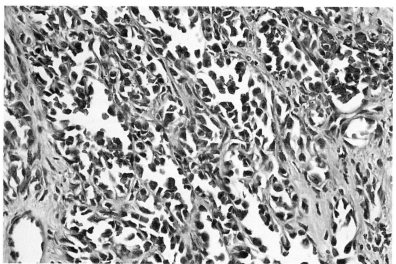

Figure 19.16 Angiosarcoma, in contrast with histiocytoid (epithelioid) hemangioma, is a cytologically pleomorphic tumor. Hobnail-shaped endothelial cells with prominent, hyperchromatic nuclei protrude into the complex vascular lumina.

Figure 19.17 In this resected specimen of a soft tissue metastasis from a penile angiosarcoma, the red-brown appearance suggests a highly vascular tumor.

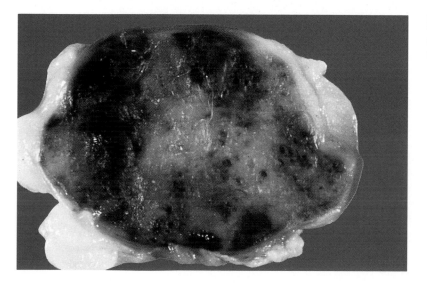

Neoplastic Lesions of the Urethra

Carcinoma of the Urethra

Even though the male urethra has approximately four times as much epithelium at risk, carcinoma of the urethra in males is only about half as common as in females. Regardless of sex, squamous cell carcinoma is the most common type involving the urethra, accounting for about 78% of cases in males and 70% of cases in females. The remainder of urethral carcinomas are either transitional cell carcinoma or adenocarcinoma.

CLINICAL MANIFESTATIONS   Clinical presentation varies with the tumor's size and location. Carcinomas of the prostatic urethra may produce symptoms of outlet obstruction, leading to confusion with nodular prostatic hyperplasia, or they may produce hematuria. More distal lesions involving the urethra in males or females may produce dysuria, hematuria, a palpable mass, or partial obstruction. Neglected urethral carcinomas invade surrounding structures, leading to fistula formation (Fig. 19.18). Different clinical staging systems have been developed for male and female patients with urethral carcinomas.

MORPHOLOGY   Squamous cell carcinoma of the urethra is usually a moderately differentiated, focally keratinizing neoplasm (Fig. 19.19). Transitional cell carcinomas of the urethra are histologically identical to their counterparts in the urinary bladder (Fig. 19.20).

Adenocarcinomas of the urethra, the least common form of urethral carcinoma, assume a variety of histologic appearances. Tumors involving the prostatic urethra in males may resemble endometrial carcinomas of the uterus, but they have been shown immunohistochemically to be variants of prostatic carcinoma (see Chapter 14). There have been reports of clear cell carcinomas involving the urethra in females that are similar by light-microscopy to müllerian-type carcinomas of the female genital tract. Ultrastructurally, these tumors differ from genital clear cell carcinomas and are suspected to be of mesonephric origin. Mucinous as well as papillary adenocarcinomas of the male urethra may arise in the periurethral glands. Because of their apparent origin in the surrounding glandular tissue, these adenocarcinomas can be extremely difficult to biopsy transurethrally, in spite of clinically obvious tumor.

THERAPY AND PROGNOSIS   Surgical excision is the treatment of choice for urethral carcinomas of all histologic types. Large lesions may require extensive surgery, with its associated high morbidity. Radiation therapy is a valuable adjuvant in selected cases. The prognosis for urethral carcinoma is more closely related to the location and extent of the lesion than to histologic type or degree of differentiation. Distal lesions in both male and female patients have a better prognosis than more proximal disease. Five-year survival rates for distal lesions are approximately 50%–70%, but only about 5%–10% for more proximal tumors.

Malignant Melanoma

Malignant melanoma may involve the meatus or fossa navicularis in the male or the distal urethral orifice in the female. The distal female urethra and periurethral vulva are the most common sites for genitourinary melanoma, although it is rare in comparison with carcinoma. As with mucosal melanomas arising from other sites, urethral melanomas may assume a variety of cytologic images, leading to potential diagnostic problems. Junctional change may not be demonstrable, but its presence is diagnostic. The presence of melanin pigment in tumor cells is also helpful, but some malignant melanomas are completely amelanotic (Fig. 19.21). Wide local excision, which is the treatment of choice, usually achieves local control. As with malignant melanomas involving other mucosal surfaces, the prognosis is poor; most patients develop lymphatic and hematogenous metastases.

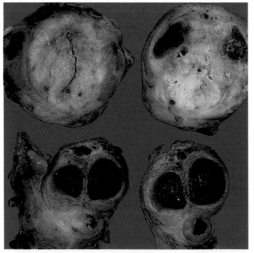
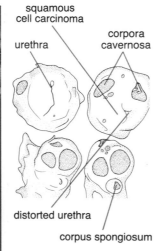

squamous cell carcinoma

urethra

corpora cavernosa

distorted urethra

corpus spongiosum

Figure 19.18 Resected penile specimen demonstrates an extensively infiltrating squamous cell carcinoma of the distal urethra. The corpus spongiosum is completely replaced by tumor in several sections. (Courtesy of P.S. Feldman, MD, Charlottesville, Virginia)

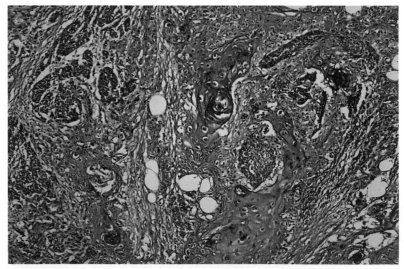

Figure 19.19 Squamous cell carcinoma of the urethra invades the periurethral stroma as nests of pleomorphic, focally keratinizing cells.

Benign Urethral Neoplasms

A variety of benign, presumably neoplastic, processes may involve the urethra. Some show a marked male predilection or exclusivity.

Nephrogenic Adenoma

Although it is more common in the bladder, this lesion may involve the urethra. In the latter location, it is more frequent in men, but occasionally occurs in women, particularly after childbirth. Whether these lesions are true neoplasms is unclear, but evidence favors a metaplastic and hyperplastic process. In the urethra, nephrogenic adenomas typically form polypoid masses. The microscopic features of these lesions are discussed in Chapters 12 and 14.

Prostatic-Type Polyps

A spectrum of lesions of the male urethra may be included under this heading. Some are reactive eversions of normal-appearing prostatic ductal epithelium into the urethral lumen, whereas others are more cellular and adenomatous. The microscopic features are described in Chapter 14.

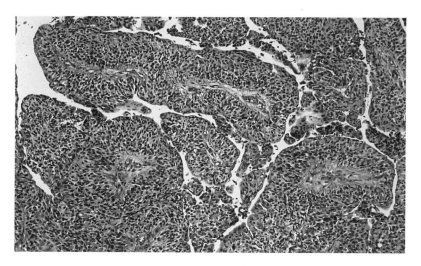

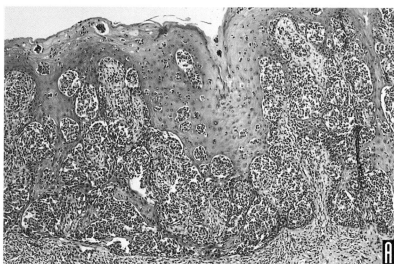
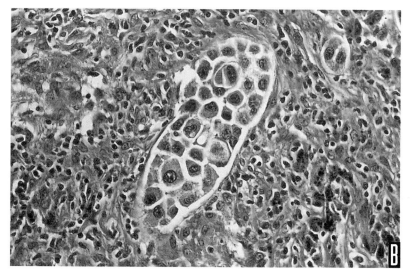

Figure 19.20 Transitional cell carcinoma of the urethra may have a papillary configuration. Such tumors are far more common in the bladder and ureters.

Figure 19.21 A, In malignant melanoma, which may arise from the periurethral mucosa in both males and females, nests or theques of tumor cells are seen at the dermal-epidermal junction. This junctional growth is characteristic of primary melanoma. **B,** The cells of malignant melanoma may assume an almost endless variety of cytologic appearances. The dark-brown pigment is melanin, and its presence is a helpful diagnostic feature.

SECTION IX

Lesions of the Adrenal Gland

CHAPTER 20

Adrenal Gland Tumors

Neoplasms of the Adrenal Cortex

Adrenal gland cortical tissue may undergo a variety of nonneoplastic alterations, including diffuse hyperplasia, nodular hyperplasia, primary pigmented nodular adrenocortical disease, and nodular (nonhyperplastic) transformation. The last is a relatively common autopsy finding that has been associated with hypertension. It has been postulated that abnormal adrenal steroid synthesis does not cause the hypertension. Instead, it is the hypertensive vascular changes that cause adrenal nodularity.

The clinical, functional, genetic, and pathologic variations of these nonneoplastic adrenal lesions are complex and beyond the scope of this text. For a detailed review of nonneoplastic adrenal disease and adrenal pathology in general, the reader is referred to the recent text edited by Lack.

Adrenal Cortical Adenoma

CLINICAL MANIFESTATIONS The distinction of an adrenal cortical nodule from a cortical adenoma is somewhat arbitrary, but if one requires evidence of autonomous endocrine function for diagnosis, then cortical adenomas are relatively uncommon lesions. Most functional cortical adenomas produce only a single steroidal hormone and are associated with a corresponding clinical syndrome. Hyperaldosteronism (Conn's syndrome) is most frequent, followed closely by Cushing's syndrome. Virilization is less common; feminizing signs are distinctly rare. Mixed endocrine features, virilization and, particularly, feminization, are worrisome features for adrenal cortical carcinoma. Rare, virilizing "cortical adenomas" with Leydig cell differentiation and Reinke crystals have been reported by Pollock et al.

Although aldosterone secretion is the most common endocrine manifestation of cortical adenomas, the frequency of Conn's syndrome as a cause of hypertension is unclear. Ranges from 0.5%–20% have been reported. The latter figure probably reflects confusion with adrenal cortical nodules noted as an apparently secondary change in hypertensive patients. Adrenal cortical adenomas show a predilection for women. They probably occur with equal frequency in the left and right adrenal glands.

MORPHOLOGY Adrenal cortical adenomas are typically solitary, small neoplasms with grossly well circumscribed or encapsulated margins. Most weigh between 10–40 g. Adenomas weighing over 50 g are distinctly uncommon. It should be noted, however, that although increasing weight is one criterion for distinguishing cortical adenomas from cortical carcinomas (see below), adenomas weighing in excess of 100 g do occur. On cut section, most cortical adenomas have a yellow to light-brown color (Fig. 20.1). Rarely, cortical adenomas will be dark brown or black due to the deposition of large amounts of lipofuscin pigment. The term "black adenoma" has been applied to such lesions. There is no evidence, however, that these lesions have distinctive clinical features, thus there is no reason to segregate them from more conventionally-colored neoplasms. Areas of hemorrhage or necrosis are uncommon in cortical adenomas; if present, they should strongly suggest the possibility of carcinoma.

Although minor light-microscopic differences have been described for cortical adenomas according to their hormonal product, there is considerable overlap. A capsule may be seen microscopically, separating the adenoma from the surrounding cortex. More often, there is a sharp, but unencapsulated margin. The neoplastic cells have prominent, clear to eosinophilic cytoplasm arranged in nests, cords, and sheets (Fig. 20.2). Variable amounts of intracytoplasmic lipofuscin pigment with a golden brown coloration may be seen and is present in large amounts in so-called "black adenomas." Nuclei in cortical adenomas are typically uniform, small, and round with small nucleoli. Nuclear pleomorphism, if present at all, is usually focal and of moderate degree. However, occasional cortical adenomas may show foci of remarkable nuclear variation, as do other endocrine adenomas (Fig. 20.3). Bizarre nuclear pleomorphism as an isolated finding, therefore, is not a helpful criterion for malignancy. Mitotic figures are rare in cortical adenomas. Atypical forms are virtually never seen.

In Cushing's syndrome, the adrenal cortex surrounding the adenoma and in the contralateral gland is atrophic. In Conn's syndrome, however, there is often hyperplasia of the zona glomerulosa just beneath the adrenal capsule. For almost thirty years, it has been noted that patients receiving spironolactone for the treatment of hyperaldosteronism develop intracytoplasmic, laminated eosinophilic bodies within the cytoplasm of the adrenal cortical cells in the zona glomerulosa. Subsequently, Shrago and colleagues found these structures in aldosterone-secreting adenomas. They have been referred to as "spironolactone bodies." Immunohisto-chemical studies have confirmed the presence of aldosterone within these structures.

Adrenal Cortical Carcinoma

Adrenal cortical carcinomas are rare neoplasms. Approximately 100 new cases are reported yearly in the United States. There is a bimodal age distribution, with peaks in childhood and in older adults. There is no obvious sex predilection. Presenting signs and symptoms are usually related to an abdominal mass with associated pain. Traditionally, from 25%–50% of patients have had demonstrable metastatic disease at presentation. This figure may decrease with the advent of more sensitive radiographic modalities.

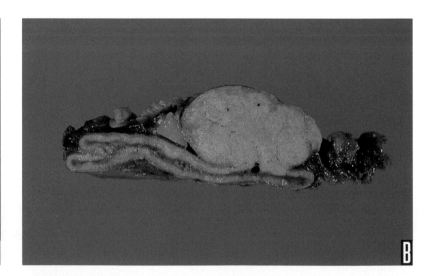

Figure 20.1 A, This cortical adenoma from a patient with Cushing's syndrome exhibits a characteristic uniform yellow coloration and sharp circumscription. **B,** A cortical adenoma from a patient with Conn's syndrome is also a sharply demarcated yellow nodule. The prominence of the normal adrenal cortex suggests the possibility of associated hyperplasia of the zona glomerulosa.

Although a high percentage of adrenal cortical carcinomas can be shown to produce hormones, clinical features of excess hormone production are usually confined to those with very large tumors or metastases. Cushing's syndrome is most common and, in contrast to cortical adenomas, there is often evidence of mixed hormone production. Adrenal cortical carcinomas may show a slight predilection for the left adrenal gland. Most are large neoplasms weighing approximately 700–1000 g.

In most studies of adrenal cortical carcinomas, childhood cases are lumped with the more common adult tumors, obscuring any distinctive features in this age group. Subsequent studies specifically examining adrenal cortical tumors in childhood (adenomas and carcinomas) have shown an up to 3:1 female to male ratio, with most cases occurring in infants under four years of age. The remainder primarily develop in adolescents. Unlike adults, almost all children with adrenal cortical neoplasia, whether benign or malignant, present with endocrine abnormalities, often having "mixed" features. Adrenal cortical neoplasms in childhood have been associated with hemihypertrophy, the Li–Fraumeni/Lynch cancer family syndrome, the Beckwith–Wiedemann syndrome, and, possibly, neurofibromatosis. Lack et al. noted that the Li–Fraumeni syndrome accounted for 10% of their childhood adrenal neoplasms.

MORPHOLOGY The cut surface of an adrenal cortical carcinoma typically demonstrates a large, nodular mass, often with areas of

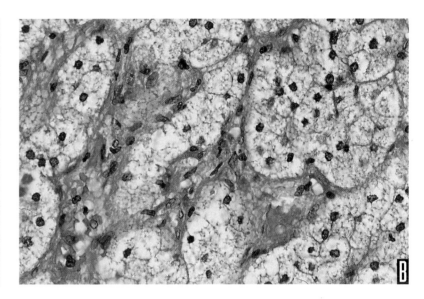

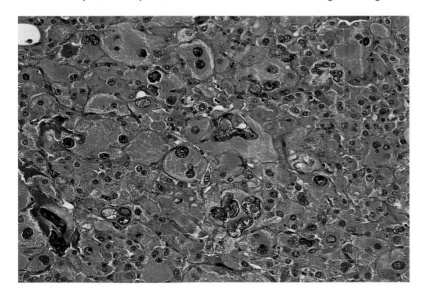

Figure 20.2 A, Adrenal cortical adenomas characteristically consist of nests of uniform cells with clear, finely vacuolated cytoplasm. The cell nests are separated by a fibrovascular stroma. **B,** At higher magnification, the clear cells of this adrenal cortical adenoma have small, uniform nuclei devoid of mitotic activity.

Figure 20.3 Occasional adrenal adenomas exhibit microscopic foci of cells with overtly bizarre nuclei. In the absence of mitotic figures and other features of malignancy, this finding is insufficient for a diagnosis of carcinoma.

grossly obvious necrosis (Fig. 20.4). Areas of hemorrhage and secondary cystic change are also common. Nonnecrotic tumor typically has a yellow-to-brown color, much like that of a cortical adenoma (see Fig. 20.4A).

Microscopically, the neoplastic cells may grow in nests, sheets, or trabeculae (Fig. 20.5). The last pattern is particularly characteristic. Typically, the trabeculae of carcinoma are separated by prominent or ectatic vascular channels. Lack and colleagues note that this pattern is so typical of adrenal cortical carcinoma that its presence demands a cautious approach to making an unequivocally benign diagnosis. The amount of fibrous tissue present is highly variable and, in some instances, there may be broad fibrous bands. Rarely, adrenal cortical carcinomas may exhibit "pseudoglandular" growth, usually as a focal change within an otherwise typical neoplasm. Tang and associates have shown that cortical carcinomas may also display a "chordoid" pattern, with strands of neoplastic cells separated by a prominent myxoid stroma.

The neoplastic cells of adrenal cortical carcinoma typically contain less cytoplasmic lipid than their adenomatous counterparts. Most cells have finely or nonvacuolated eosinophilic cytoplasm. Although cytoplasmic eosinophilic hyaline globules are more typical of pheochromocytomas, they may rarely be encountered in cor-

tical carcinomas. Necrosis, although variable in extent, is usually present in all but the smallest cortical carcinomas (see Fig. 20.5B,D). It ranges from small foci of individual cell necrosis to more typical, broad zones of infarctlike "geographic" necrosis.

The degree of nuclear pleomorphism in adrenal cortical carcinomas is often diffusely greater than in adenomas but, as noted above, adenomas may have overtly bizarre nuclei. Lack and colleagues noted that the background small cells in cortical carcinoma have enlarged nuclei and a correspondingly higher nuclear-to-cytoplasmic ratio when compared to similar cells in cortical adenomas (see Fig. 20.5A). Mitotic figures are often numerous in cortical carcinomas and, as discussed below, this is a helpful feature for establishing a diagnosis of malignancy, as is the presence of atypical division figures (see Fig. 20.5B). Other microscopic features of malignancy include capsular invasion, invasion of adjacent structures, and vascular invasion.

DISTINGUISHING CARCINOMA FROM ADENOMA In most instances, the distinction of cortical adenoma from carcinoma is straightforward. Adenomas are typically small, cytologically uniform lesions with a clinical presentation dominated by endocrine dysfunction. Cortical carcinomas are much less common, typically presenting as

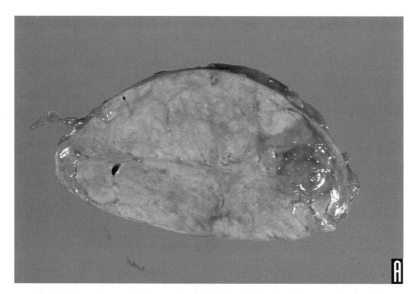
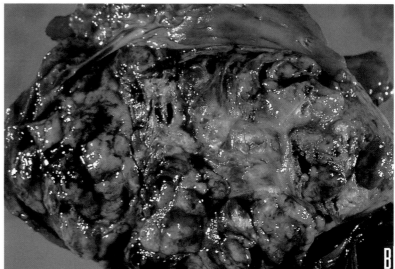
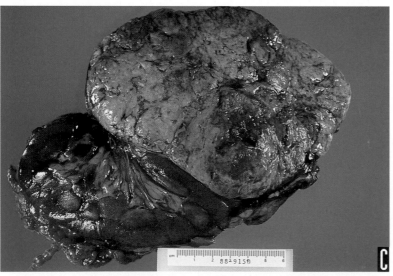

Figure 20.4 Adrenal cortical carcinomas show considerable variation in their gross appearances. **A,** This relatively small carcinoma has a deceptively uniform cut surface. **B,** Areas of obvious hemorrhage and necrosis are seen in this larger carcinoma. **C,** A distinctly yellow col-

oration characterizes this large adrenal cortical carcinoma, which compresses the upper pole of the kidney. **D,** Adrenal cortical carcinomas may develop central liquifactive necrosis with pseudocyst formation.

large, space-occupying lesions with absent or less apparent endocrine abnormalities. Up to 50% have demonstrable metastases at presentation, resulting in an obvious diagnosis of carcinoma. Yet, criteria for distinguishing "grey zone" or "borderline" lesions have been the subject of numerous publications, with some variation in results.

No single criterion can reliably distinguish adrenal adenoma from carcinoma, but a series of features can allow distinction of the great majority of problematic lesions. Hough et al. analyzed a series of metastasizing and nonmetastasizing adrenal cortical tumors. Histologic features found to have statistically predictive value for metastasis included (in decreasing order of value): broad fibrous bands, diffuse growth pattern, vascular invasion, widespread tumor necrosis, > 10 mitotic figures per 100 HPF, cellular pleomorphism, and capsular invasion. Gross tumor weight over 100 g was also of predictive value.

Weiss reviewed 43 adrenal cortical tumors, noting that nine histologic criteria were predictive of malignant behavior (metastasis). These nine features were: high nuclear grade, mitotic rate > 5 per 50 HPF, atypical mitotic figures, eosinophilic cytoplasm in > 75% of tumor cells, diffuse architecture, necrosis, venous invasion, sinusoidal invasion, and capsular invasion. A mitotic rate > 5 per 50 HPF,

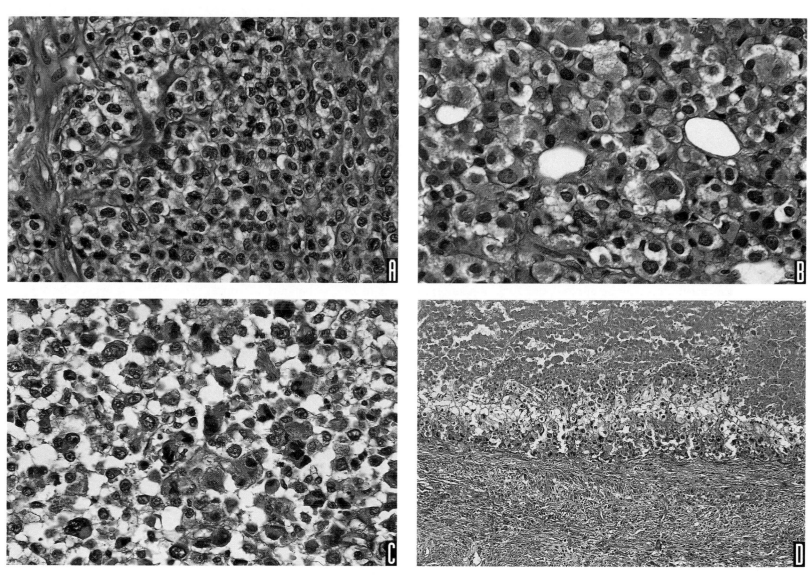

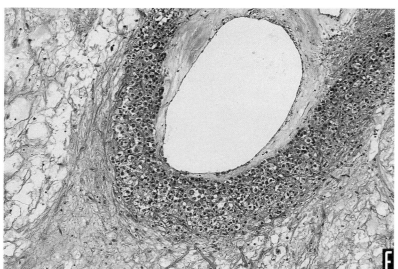

Figure 20.5 **A,** Adrenal cortical carcinomas typically consist of cells with larger nuclei and a correspondingly higher nuclear-to-cytoplasmic ratio than is encountered in cortical adenomas. **B,** This adrenal cortical carcinoma contains a tripolar mitotic figure in the center of the field. **C,** Cells exhibiting marked nuclear pleomorphism compose this adrenal cortical carcinoma. **D,** Areas of extensive necrosis (top) may be present in adrenal cortical carcinomas, with only a thin rim of recognizable neoplasm. This image may superficially resemble a hemorrhagic vascular cyst. **E,** In some adrenal cortical carcinomas, the recognizable tumor forms distinct perivascular cuffs.

atypical mitotic figures, and venous invasion were found only in malignant tumors. Eighteen of 19 carcinomas possessed 4 or more of these features. All 24 adenomas had two or fewer features.

Yet a third, similar system has been proposed by Van Slooten and colleagues. As Medeiros and Weiss noted in a recent review, all three systems are useful in anticipating the behavior of cortical neoplasms, and all have excellent predictive value. Of the features evaluated to date, mitotic rate appears to be the single most important predictor of malignancy.

Several immunohistochemical studies have assessed the value of antigen–antibody recognition for the distinction of carcinoma from adenoma. Although trends are evident, it is doubtful that this technique will supplant the more traditional methods discussed above. Nonneoplastic adrenal cortex regularly expresses cytokeratins in formalin-fixed, paraffin-embedded tissue. Although Gaffey et al. have shown that adrenal cortical carcinomas have low levels of cytokeratin on frozen section and Western immunoblot analysis, they are almost invariably cytokeratin negative in routinely processed tissues. Adrenal adenomas display keratin staining to a degree intermediate between normal cortex and cortical carcinoma. Vimentin expression in normal, benign, and carcinomatous cortical cells tends to be the inverse of cytokeratin. Normal adrenal cortex is vimentin negative, whereas over 50% of cortical carcinomas express vimentin. Adrenal adenomas occasionally express low levels of vimentin.

The role of DNA ploidy analysis in distinguishing cortical adenomas from carcinomas has been assessed by multiple studies. Although early works predicted superiority over histologic assessment, more recent studies are much less encouraging. DNA aneuploidy does correlate with histologic features of malignancy but, in individual cases, it is not a reliable criterion for malignancy. Up to 30% of cortical carcinomas may be euploid and 20% of adenomas may be aneuploid.

Whether the above features clearly predict malignant behavior for childhood adrenal cortical neoplasms is even less clear. Cagle et al. noted a tendency to overdiagnose malignancy in childhood and believed that tumor size (> 500 g) was the only criterion predictive of malignant outcome. Lack and colleagues, in a review of 30 pediatric adrenal cortical neoplasms, also noted a tendency for the overdiagnosis of carcinoma, as well as the presence of considerable cellular pleomorphism in clinically benign tumors. Factors in their study that correlated with metastatic behavior included increased mitotic rate, extensive tumor necrosis (> 25%), and vascular invasion. It should be noted that the mean mitotic rate in their group of clinically benign lesions was 16 per 50 HPF, with a range of 1–61 per 50 HPF and atypical forms in 15% of cases. A sizable percentage of such tumors would have exceeded the Weiss criteria for adrenal malignancy, which was based primarily on tumors occurring in adults. Additional refinement of malignancy criteria in this age group is needed. Many large tumors with some worrisome features may currently have to be considered to be of indeterminate biologic behavior.

DIFFERENTIAL DIAGNOSIS The distinction between adrenal cortical neoplasia and pheochromocytoma, although typically straightforward, may sometimes be quite vexing. Pheochromocytomas may produce ACTH, creating a Cushing's syndrome with adrenal hyperplasia that leads to a clinical diagnosis of cortical neoplasm. To further the confusion, pheochromocytomas may exhibit prominent cytoplasmic clearing due to "lipid degeneration." Staining for neuroendocrine markers such as chromogranin, argentaffin stains, or electron microscopy documenting appropriate granules should allow ready distinction in problematic cases.

Adrenal cortical neoplasms (benign or malignant) must be distinguished from tumors metastatic to the adrenal gland. Hepatocellular and renal carcinoma may be easily confused with adrenal neoplasia. Both hepatocellular and renal cell carcinomas frequently express cytokeratin and epithelial membrane antigen, in contrast to adrenal cortical carcinomas. Occasionally, metastatic malignant melanoma may be confused with a cortical neoplasm. The latter tumors can be easily identified by staining for S-100 protein or with the highly melanoma-specific antibody, HMB-45. The latter should be used in addition to antibodies to S-100 protein, as S-100–positive adrenal cortical carcinomas have been described.

PROGNOSIS Once a patient has been determined to have an adrenal cortical carcinoma, the prognosis can be expected to be poor. As summarized by Medeiros and Weiss, the mean or median survival in several large series ranges from 4–30 months. Overall mortality has ranged from 70%–92%.

Metastases follow both hematogenous and lymphatic routes of spread with liver and lung being the most common sites of distant disease. Involvement of the opposite adrenal gland may be seen in about 25% of patients at autopsy. There have, however, been long-term survivors and apparent cures following surgical excision. A variety of clinical and pathologic features have been analyzed for their prognostic significance. Factors that may be important include: clinical stage, mitotic activity, nuclear grade/differentiation, tumor size, resectability, and endocrine functional status. Among pediatric patients with *bone fide* adrenal cortical carcinoma, survival in adolescent patients seems to be considerably worse than in infantile cases (17% vs. 53%).

NEOPLASMS OF THE ADRENAL MEDULLA
PHEOCHROMOCYTOMA

Pheochromocytoma (intra-adrenal paraganglioma) is a rare tumor of the adrenal medulla. Most cases are sporadic, typically manifesting between the third and fourth decades of life; there is no sex predilection.

Familial pheochromocytomas, which comprise 5%–10% of cases, are most often diagnosed within the first two decades of life.

Inherited as an autosomal dominant trait with high penetrance, they are usually bilateral and multicentric (compared to 0%–5% bilaterality in sporadic cases). Syndromes associated with familial pheochromocytomas can be divided into two major groups: multiple endocrine neoplasia (MEN) and neurocutaneous phacomatosis (Fig. 20.6). Pheochromocytomas, which occur in up to 70% of patients with MEN types II and III, may be the first clinical manifestation of the syndrome. Pheochromocytomas occur less frequently (0.5%–5%) with phacomatoses.

CLINICAL MANIFESTATIONS Clinical manifestations are highly variable, but signs and symptoms are typically related to hypersecretion of catecholamines. Hypertension is the major finding. Patients may have sustained hypertension with or without episodes of paroxysmal hypertension (about 67% of cases), only paroxysmal hypertension (25%), or essential hypertension (10%). Occasional patients, particularly those with small tumors, may be normotensive. Severe throbbing headache, diaphoresis, weakness, palpitations with or without tachycardia, and often severe anxiety are more common in patients with paroxysmal hypertension. Pallor and flushing of the face and upper body are also frequent. Complications secondary to the hypertension include cerebrovascular accidents, myocardial infarcts or a peculiar cardiomyopathy, as well as benign or malignant nephrosclerosis with renal failure.

Epinephrine comprises 85%–95% of the catecholamine secretion from the normal medulla, but pheochromocytomas, except for those associated with MEN Type II syndrome, secrete more norepinephrine than epinephrine. Measuring urinary VMA and metanephrines is useful for screening patients and will detect 80%–90% of cases. Catecholamine measurements have the highest sensitivity for diagnosing pheochromocytomas, permitting the determination of norepinephrine to epinephrine ratios, but may require histamine stimulation for a positive test.

High morbidity or mortality during surgery has been attributable to the effects of catecholamines, which include cardiac arrhythmias, hypertensive crises, and vascular shock. Preoperative management should include α-adrenergic blocking agents, particularly phenoxybenzamine, to control hypertension.

Figure 20.6
Familial Pheochromocytoma Syndromes

Multiple Endocrine Neoplasia (MEN) Syndromes

Type II (or IIA):
    C-cell hyperplasia/medullary thyroid carcinoma
    Adrenal medullary hyperplasia/ pheochromocytoma
    Parathyroid hyperplasia/adenoma

Type III (or IIB):
    C-cell hyperplasia/medullary thyroid carcinoma
    Adrenal medullary hyperplasia/ pheochromocytoma
    Corneal, mucocutaneous, and GI ganglioneuromatosis
    Marfanoid habitus

Neurocutaneous Phacomatosis Syndromes

von Hippel-Lindau Disease:
    Retinal angiomatosis
    Cerebellar hemangioblastoma
    Renal, pancreatic, epididymal cysts
    Renal cell carcinoma
    Pheochromocytoma

von Recklinghausen's Disease:
    Neurofibromas, café-au-lait spots
    Schwannoma
    Meningioma
    Glioma
    Pheochromocytoma

Sturge-Weber Syndrome:
    Cavernous hemangiomas of face and CNS
    Pheochromocytoma

Beta-adrenergic blockers also may be needed if cardiac arrhythmias and hypotension develop.

MORPHOLOGY Nonfamilial pheochromocytomas, which more commonly arise in the right adrenal gland, occur as single, ovoid-to-spherical, grey–pink-to-tan masses (Fig. 20.7). They can weigh up to 3600 g, but the majority are 3–5 cm in diameter with a mean weight of 100 g. Large tumors, which may have a pseudocapsule containing a compressed rim of adrenal cortex as well as fibrous tissue, show areas of hemorrhage, necrosis, cyst formation, and calci-

fication (Fig. 20.8). Prolonged exposure to air and bright light oxidizes endogenous catecholamines, resulting in the production of dark brown adrenochrome pigment from epinephrine.

In contrast to the unilobular appearance of sporadic pheochromocytomas, resected adrenals from patients with familial syndromes are characteristically multilobular with nodules that vary from several mm up to 10 cm in diameter (Fig 20.9). The intervening medulla may also show hyperplasia that is diffuse as well as nodular, which is felt to be the precursor of pheochromocytoma in MEN type II syndrome.

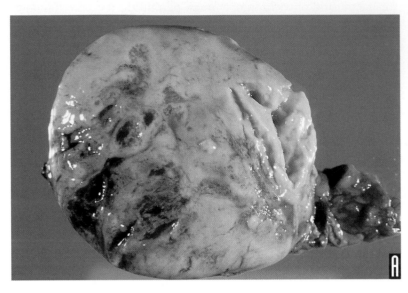

Figure 20.7 **A,** This pheochromocytoma, which has a typical grey-pink cut surface, shows focal congestion and hemorrhage. A remnant of uninvolved adrenal gland is seen on the right. **B,** The tan-brown appearance of this tumor is probably due to adrenochrome pigment produced by the oxidation of epinephrine.

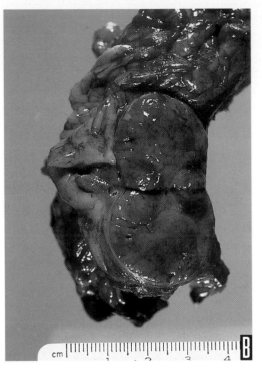

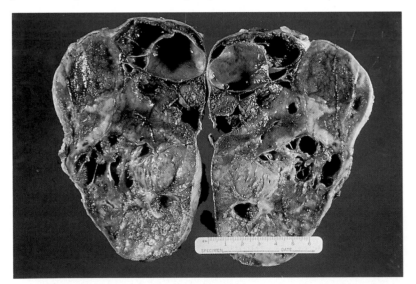

Figure 20.8 Large pheochromocytomas, such as this 12-cm-in-diameter tumor, commonly show hemorrhage, cyst formation, and necrosis, which are not reliable signs of malignancy.

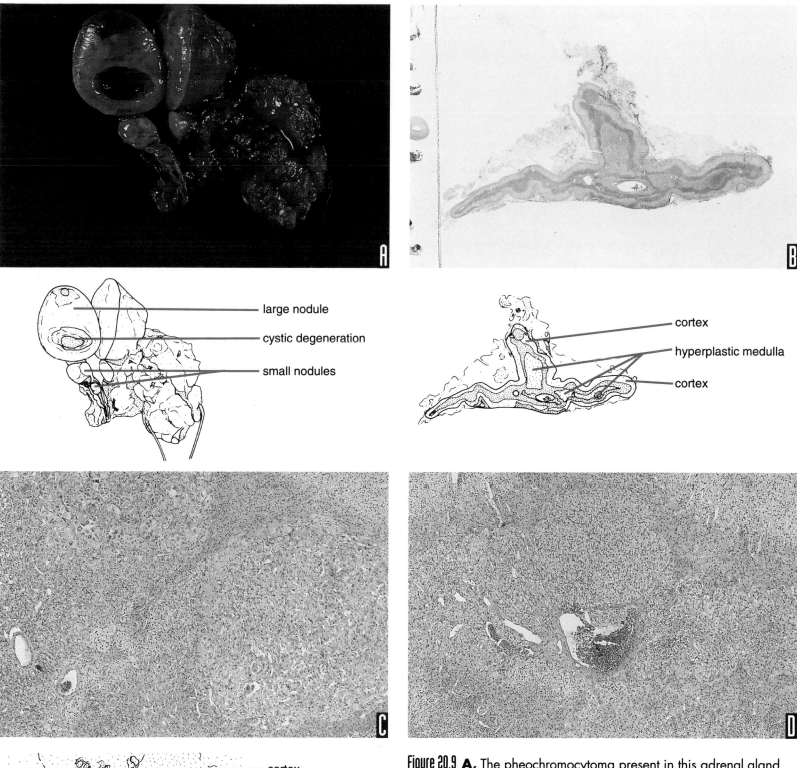

large nodule

cystic degeneration

small nodules

cortex

hyperplastic medulla

cortex

cortex

pleomorphic nuclei

hyperplastic medulla

Figure 20.9 A, The pheochromocytoma present in this adrenal gland from a 40-year-old asymptomatic man with MEN-Type II, has a characteristic multilobular appearance. The larger nodule shows cystic degeneration. **B,** Whole-mount histologic section shows medullary hyperplasia in the crest and right alar regions. **C,** Microscopically, the hyperplastic medulla appears nodular and shows nuclear pleomorphism. **D,** An adjacent area in the alar region shows "invasion" of a medullary vein (center).

Both sporadic and familial pheochromocytomas have similar histologic features. Most resemble normal adrenal medulla (Fig. 20.10). In the classic pattern, described as "Zellballen," alveolar nests and cords of polyhedral cells (pheochromocytes) are separated by a reticulin-rich fibrovascular stroma (Fig. 20.11). Trabecular and diffuse patterns are also common (Fig. 20.12). Cytoplasm is eosinophilic-to-basophilic and finely granular. Numerous PAS+ hyaline globules may be present, as may extensive cytoplasmic vacuolization. Although pleomorphism may be marked, nuclei are generally round-to-oval with vesicular, coarsely clumped chromatin

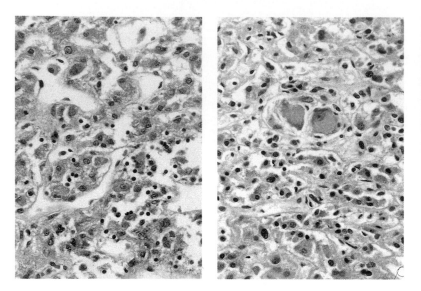

Figure 20.10 The adrenal medulla contains nests of pheochromocytes, which have finely granular basophilic or eosinophilic cytoplasm and are surrounded by capillaries. Lymphocytes and ganglion cells (right panel) are a normal finding.

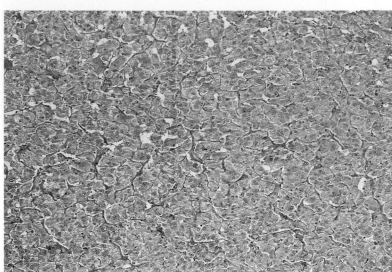

Figure 20.11 The small nesting (alveolar) arrangement with prominent endocrine-type microvasculature in this pheochromocytoma characterizes the classic organoid (Zellballen) pattern.

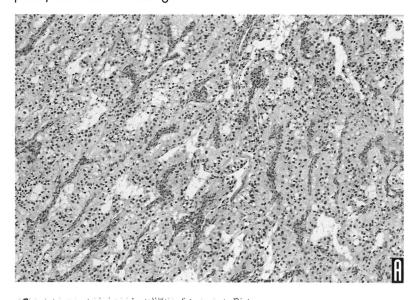

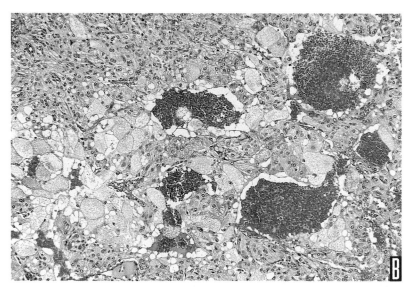

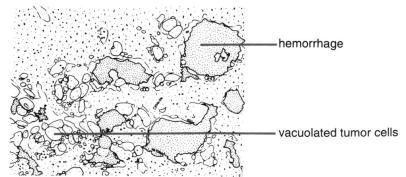

Figure 20.12 A, This clinically malignant pheochromocytoma has a trabecular pattern. Vascular channels are lined by hyperplastic endothelial cells, giving the tumor an angiomatous appearance. **B,** This pheochromocytoma has a more solid or diffuse growth pattern, with pseudoglandular spaces containing blood. Although many tumor cells have fine-to-coarse cytoplasmic vacuoles, others have a more typical granular amphophilic cytoplasm. The appearance should not be mistaken for an adrenal cortical neoplasm.

and a distinct nucleolus (Fig. 20.13). Nuclear pseudoinclusions, produced by cytoplasmic invaginations, are common.

Ultrastructurally, catecholamines appear as large (mean, 270 nm), pleomorphic, membrane-bound, partially empty, dense core secretory granules (Fig. 20.14). The catecholamine content can be demonstrated by the chromaffin reaction to chromate-containing fixatives, but this technique has limited sensitivity since the pigments are highly soluble. Immunohistochemically, cells are positive for neurofilament proteins, chromogranin, and NSE, as well as a variety of neuropeptides, including somatostatin, leu- and metenkephalin, in addition to neurotensin (Fig. 20.15).

Occasional pheochromocytomas contain small cells with hyperchromatic, round-to-oval nuclei, and scant, faintly eosinophilic cytoplasm (pheochromoblasts). Spindle cell variants comprise less than 5% of pheochromocytomas. Degenerative changes, which are common in large tumors, may produce a

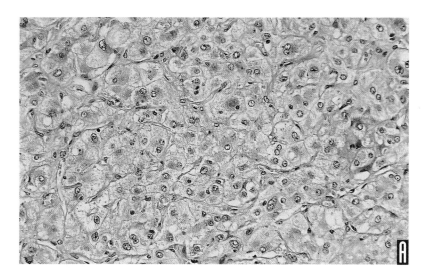
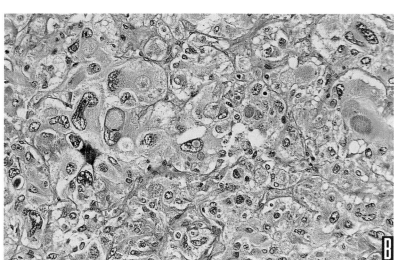

Figure 20.13 A, The large, polygonal tumor cells in this pheochromocytoma have moderate amounts of lightly eosinophilic cytoplasm and relatively uniform, round-to-oval nuclei with vesicular chromatin and a distinct central or eccentric nucleolus. Several small eosinophilic intra- cytoplasmic hyaline globules are present. **B,** This benign pheochromocytoma shows marked nuclear pleomorphism. Intranuclear cytoplasmic invaginations and nuclear pseudoinclusions are present as well as occasional intracytoplasmic hyaline globules.

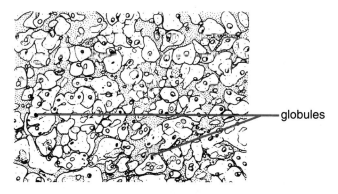
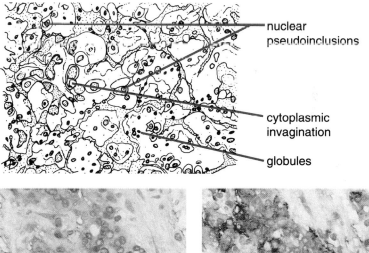

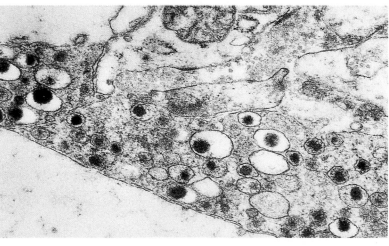
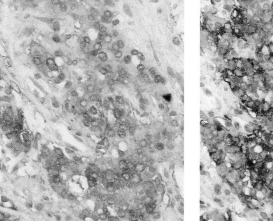
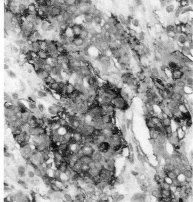

Figure 20.14 Ultrastructurally, the dense core neurosecretory granules in pheochromocytomas are large and pleomorphic. The correlation of morphology with catecholamine content may be difficult. Many of these granules have a prominent, eccentric electron luscent space adjacent to the dense core characteristic of "norepinephrine-type" granules.

Figure 20.15 Pheochromocytomas frequently show immunoreactivity for NSE (left panel) and chromogranin proteins (right panel).

pseudoglandular or angioma-like pattern and are frequently associated with clusters of lymphocytes (Fig. 20.16). Ganglion-type cells may be present. Examples of biphasic tumors that contain large numbers of ganglion cells embedded in a matrix of Schwann cells (ganglioneuroma) have been reported in association with the Verner–Morrison syndrome (i.e., watery diarrhea plus hypokalemia secondary to vasoactive intestinal polypeptide [VIP] secretion). Pheochromocytomas may also secrete calcitonin and ACTH.

Nuclear atypia, capsular and vascular invasion, as well as mitotic activity, are of little value in predicting the behavior of adrenal pheochromocytomas. Large numbers of mitoses, however, should be regarded as suspicious for malignancy; an increased risk for local recurrence or metastases may be indicated. Less than 5% of pheochromocytomas are malignant. Medeiros et al. found that malignant pheochromocytomas were usually larger (mean weights, 759 g vs. 156 g), had extensive areas of necrosis, and were composed of small tumor cells. Nevertheless, there are no reliable gross or microscopic features for distinguishing benign from malignant pheochromocytomas. The only reliable criterion for malignancy is the presence of metastases, which most commonly involve the liver, lymph nodes, and bone.

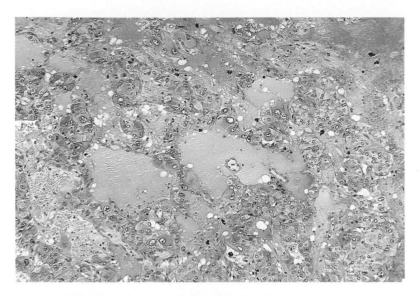

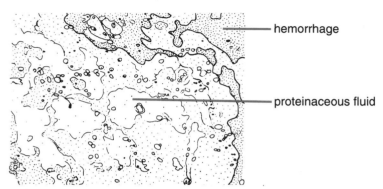

Figure 20.16 Hemorrhage and proteinaceous fluid within pseudo-acini represent degenerative changes in this pheochromocytoma.

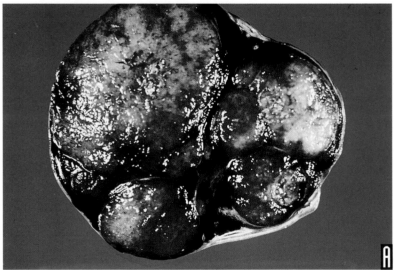

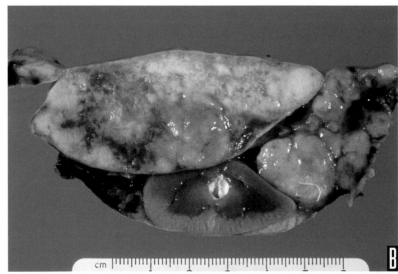

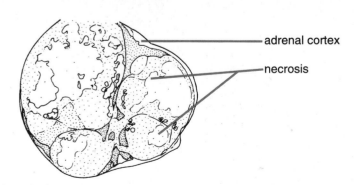

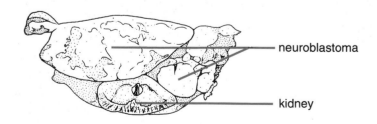

Figure 20.17 A, This neuroblastoma has coarse, bulging lobulations and shows extensive hemorrhage with foci of necrosis; viable tumor appears white. It is sharply circumscribed with residual adrenal gland stretched over its surface. **B,** Neuroblastoma in this example has extended beyond the adrenal gland. Multiple, discrete, and confluent gray-pink masses in the peri-renal adipose tissue impinge upon but do not invade the kidney.

NEUROBLASTOMA

Neuroblastoma is a highly malignant neoplasm that arises from primitive neural crest elements in the adrenal medulla and sympathetic ganglia. It is the most common solid extracranial neoplasm of infancy and childhood. The majority arise within the abdomen, either as an adrenal (36% of cases) or extra-adrenal (18%) malignancy. Approximately 70% of neuroblastomas become clinically manifest before the age of 4 years. Less than 20% occur between 7–19 years of age; they are rare in adults. There is no sex predilection.

CLINICAL MANIFESTATIONS Neuroblastomas most commonly present as an abdominal mass, particularly in children under 2 years of age. Other signs and symptoms relate to the primary site of origin as well as the extent of disease at presentation. A variety of developmental defects have been associated with neuroblastomas, particularly congenital heart defects. Most patients excrete increased levels of catecholamines and their metabolites in the urine. Excretory levels of vanillylmandelic acid (VMA), in addition to homovanillic acid, are useful for diagnosis as well as for monitoring the course of disease after therapy.

MORPHOLOGY Microscopic nodules of immature neural crest cells are present in 100% of fetuses, having a peak number and size at 17–20 weeks gestation. They are regarded by some authorities as stages of normal adrenal morphogenesis. However, it has been suggested that nodules greater than 2000 μm in diameter represent precursor or latent forms of neuroblastoma. In autopsy studies of infants less than 3 months of age, these so-called in situ neuroblastomas have been identified in 1:39–1:259 cases. This is a much higher frequency than clinically manifest neuroblastomas (9.6 cases/million children), suggesting that many of these microscopic nodules regress, either by degeneration or maturation.

Neuroblastomas are soft, extremely friable, white-to-gray–pink, and sharply circumscribed (Fig. 20.17). Necrosis, hemorrhage, cyst formation, and calcifications are common even in small tumors. Adrenal tumors tend to form multiple, discrete, or confluent masses that grow toward the midline. Invasion of the contralateral adrenal gland is common. Depending upon the site of origin, the kidney, pancreas, liver, or vertebral bodies may also be directly invaded.

Microscopically, the least differentiated forms of neuroblastoma are composed of sheets of cells with small, round, or occasionally triangular, hyperchromatic nuclei, inconspicuous nucleoli, and scant cytoplasm. Mitoses are typically prominent. The often loosely cohesive cells are arranged in lobules separated by thin fibrovascular septa, which are often infiltrated by lymphocytes or other mononuclear cells (Fig. 20.18). A finely fibrillar eosinophilic matrix composed of unmyelinated axons is frequently associated. Neoplastic cells will tend to grow in a streaming fashion. Homer Wright rosettes (pseudorosettes), a characteristic feature, are

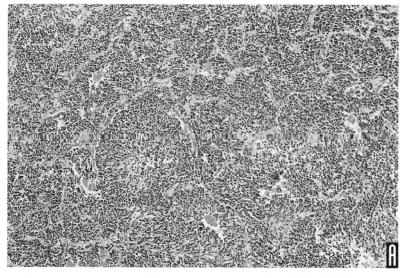

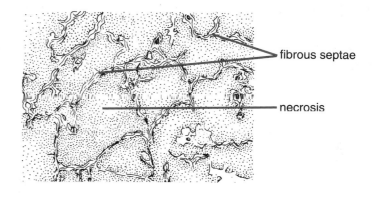

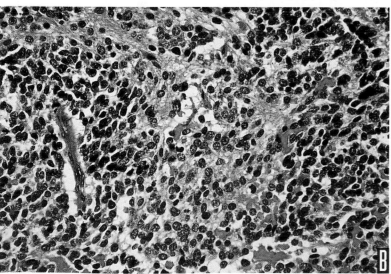

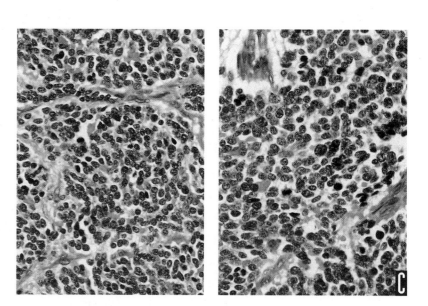

Figure 20.18 A, This neuroblastoma is composed of sheets of loosely cohesive, small, round cells that form indistinct lobules separated by thin, fibrous septa. Necrosis is focally present. B, A typical neurofibrillary matrix (neuropil) can be seen in the upper portion of this field.

C, The primitive tumor cells have scant cytoplasm and small, round or triangular, hyperchromatic nuclei with stippled chromatin and inconspicuous nucleoli. Mitoses are easily identified.

prominent in only about 30% of cases and are composed of 1–2 layers of neuroblasts arranged around a central tangle of neurofibrillary processes (Fig. 20.19). Cellular features indicative of maturation to ganglion cells are the development of abundant eosinophilic cytoplasm in addition to large, vesicular nuclei with coarsely clumped chromatin and prominent nucleoli.

Electron microscopic findings of diagnostic importance are the presence of dendritic-type cell processes that contain 10 nm in diameter intermediate filaments, bundles of microtubules that are 20–30 nm in diameter, 80–150 nm neurosecretory granules, and clear vesicles. Immunohistochemically, neuroblastoma cells mark for NSE and 68kd neurofilament proteins.

PROGNOSIS Neuroblastomas are highly invasive, tending to metastasize via lymphatics and blood vessels to the lymph nodes, bone, and liver. *Hutchinson's syndrome* refers to the development of massive skeletal metastases, particularly in the skull. The occurrence of massive hepatomegaly secondary to tumor invasion has been termed *Pepper's syndrome.*

Prognosis is in part related to the tumor stage:

Stage I   Tumor confined to the structure or organ of origin.

Stage II   Local invasion confined to one side, with or without involvement of ipsilateral lymph nodes.

Stage III Extension beyond the midline, with or without lymph node involvement.

Stage IV   Metastases to noncontiguous organs or distant lymph nodes.

Stage IVS Metastases to skin, bone marrow, and liver in patients who otherwise have Stage I or II disease.

Multiple factors, however, have been shown to influence prognosis, including histologic grade, i.e., percent of differentiating elements (I > 50%; II 5–50%; III < 5%; IV 0%), sex, site of primary tumor, and age at diagnosis. Age appears to be the single most important prognostic indicator; survival is significantly increased if the tumor is diagnosed before 1 year of age. Amplification of N-myc oncogene and absence of DNA aneuploidy have been associated with a poor prognosis. Although neuroblastomas may spontaneously mature, maturation into a ganglioneuroma is infrequent.

Prognosis may be related to the amount of intercellular stroma and mitotic activity. In the Shimada classification, tumors are divided into stroma-poor (i.e., classic neuroblastoma) and stroma-rich (corresponding to ganglioneuroblastoma). Differentiation in

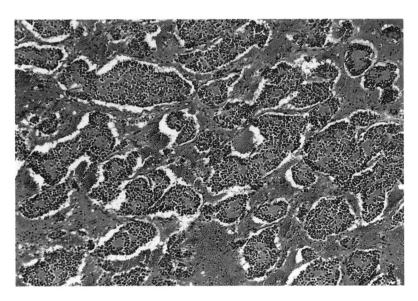

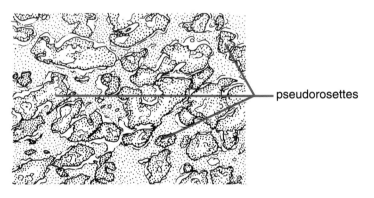

Figure 20.19 Marked hemorrhage in this neuroblastoma accentuates the numerous Homer Wright pseudorosettes, which appear as circular areas formed by one or more cells with a central, pale-staining fibrillary matrix composed of a tangle of neuritic cell processes.

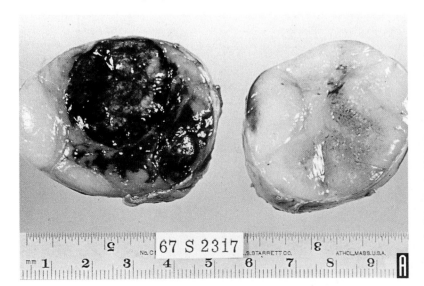

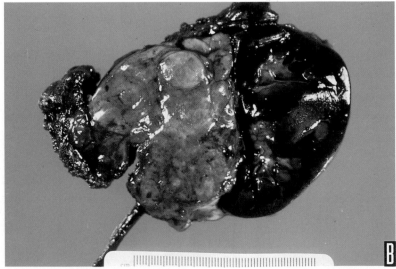

Figure 20.20 A, This small ganglioneuroblastoma is confined to the adrenal gland. Areas of hemorrhage with punctate yellow-white calcifications (left) provide gross evidence of neuroblastic foci.

B, The extra-adrenal ganglioneuroblastoma in this example (left) compresses the renal hilum. The absence of distinct ganglioneuromatous foci is consistent with a "maturing" or imperfect type of tumor.

stroma-poor tumors, as evidenced by cells with nuclear enlargement, moderate amounts of eosinophilic cytoplasm, and cell processes, had a significant impact on survival—72% for differentiating tumors (> 5% differentiating elements) vs. 36% for undifferentiated tumors (< 5% differentiating elements). Shimada et al. also calculated a mitosis–karyorrhexis index (MKI) per 5000 tumor cells, categorized as low (< 100), intermediate (100–200), and high (> 200). These prognostic indicators seemed especially useful in patients less than 1.5 years of age—83% survival with MKI < 200 vs. 9% survival with MKI > 200, regardless of tumor differentiation. For patients 1.5–5 years old, there was a 94% survival with differentiating tumors having an MKI < 100, vs. 0% survival with an MKI > 100. Independent of the MKI, survival was 5% for patients 1.5–5 years old with undifferentiated tumors and 0% for patients with tumors diagnosed after age 5.

GANGLIONEUROBLASTOMA

Ganglioneuroblastomas are tumors that are composed of neuroblastic elements in addition to benign foci of ganglioneuroma. They are most frequent in children under 10 years of age and show no sex predilection. The majority (65%) occur in the retroperitoneum, while remaining cases are equally distributed in the neck, mediastinum, and adrenal gland. Symptoms are typically related to the presence of a mass lesion.

MORPHOLOGY Adrenal ganglioneuroblastomas tend to be smaller than extra-adrenal tumors. They often appear encapsulated. The cut surface has a variable appearance, depending upon the proportion of differentiated elements (Fig. 20.20). Ganglioneuromatous foci are glistening, pink-tan, and fibrous, while primitive neuroblastic foci are nodular and soft with hemorrhage, necrosis, and frequent calcification.

Microscopically, the degree of differentiation varies widely. Tumors are composed of a mixture of neuroblasts and ganglion cells, with a large number of cells intermediate between the two (Fig. 20.21). The key histologic feature is the presence of (sympathetic) ganglion cells, which have abundant cytoplasm containing Nissl's substance and neuromelanin, large vesicular nuclei, plus a prominent nucleolus.

Ganglioneuroblastomas can be classified as *imperfect* or *composite*. The imperfect type, also referred to as "maturing" neuroblastoma, has a diffuse pattern, with neuroblastic cells showing varying degrees of differentiation throughout the tumor. The composite (or immature) type resembles mature ganglioneuroma, but contains discrete nodular collections of neuroblastoma. In both types, ganglion cells may be multinucleated or appear immature.

Ganglionic and neuroblastic elements are NSE- as well as neurofilament protein-positive, while Schwann cells mark for S100 protein. Ganglioneuromatous foci have a neurofibrillary-rich eosinophilic matrix, which ultrastructurally consists predominantly of abundant neuritic processes surrounded by Schwann cells.

PROGNOSIS Ganglioneuroblastoma is a malignant tumor that behaves unpredictably. Complete local excision of well encapsulated tumors is generally curative. However, tumors may show extensive local invasion, regional nodal metastases, or distant metastases. The staging system for neuroblastomas is applicable.

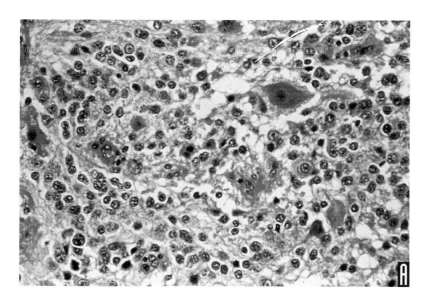
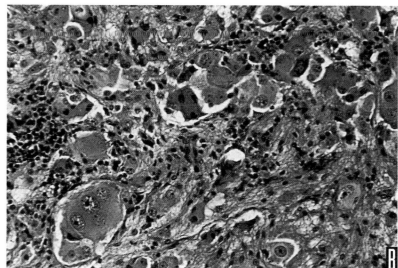

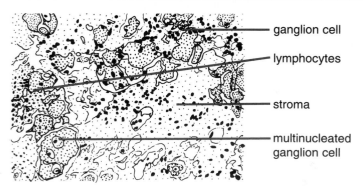

ganglion cell

lymphocytes

stroma

multinucleated ganglion cell

Figure 20.21 A, The imperfect type of ganglioneuroblastoma has a diffuse pattern. Neuroblastic cells show varying degrees of differentiation, and there is a neurofibrillary rich eosinophilic matrix. A mature-appearing ganglion cell is present. **B,** This area contains mature and immature ganglion cells, one of which is multinucleated. The stroma contains scattered spindled Schwann cells and a lymphocytic infiltrate.

These stroma-rich tumors have been classified by Shimada et al. into three categories based upon differentiation, which correlates with survival: well differentiated (100%), intermixed (92%), and nodular (18%). The nodular type corresponds to the composite ganglioneuroblastoma, which has a greater risk for metastases than the imperfect type (65% vs. 18%).

GANGLIONEUROMA

Ganglioneuromas are benign tumors composed of mature ganglion cells, neurites with variable numbers of Schwann cells, and collagen. They most commonly occur along the sympathetic chain and, like ganglioneuroblastomas, they more frequently arise in the mediastinum or retroperitoneum (56%) than in the adrenal gland (13%–30%).

Adrenal tumors tend to occur in patients 20–40 years of age. They are typically small, asymptomatic, and may be an incidental autopsy finding. Because of the high frequency of calcification, they may be discovered on plain films of the abdomen. Tumors producing VIP may cause the Verner–Morrison syndrome of hypertension, watery diarrhea, and hypokalemia.

MORPHOLOGY Adrenal ganglioneuromas are sharply demarcated from the adjacent medulla, but are not encapsulated. They are typically pale gray and firm, with a leiomyoma-like appearance (Fig. 20.22). Fingerlike projections of tumor resembling thickened nerve bundles may extend into the adjacent medulla.

Microscopically, variable numbers of ganglion cells are typically aggregated into small clusters (Fig. 20.23). They have round, somewhat eccentric vesicular nuclei with a single prominent nucleolus;

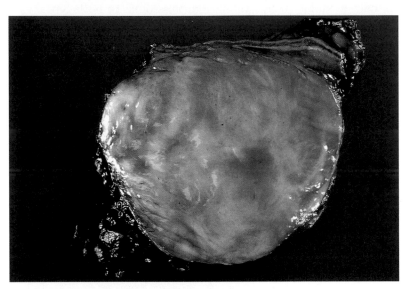

Figure 20.22 This ganglioneuroma has a typical gray-white, dense, fibrous appearance and is surrounded by a compressed rim of yellow adrenal cortical tissue.

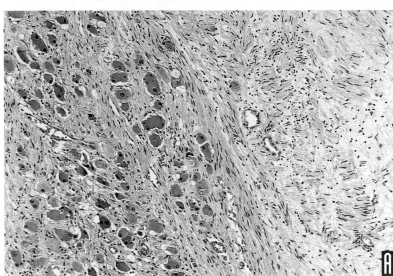

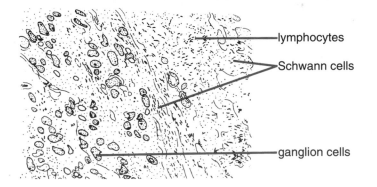

lymphocytes

Schwann cells

ganglion cells

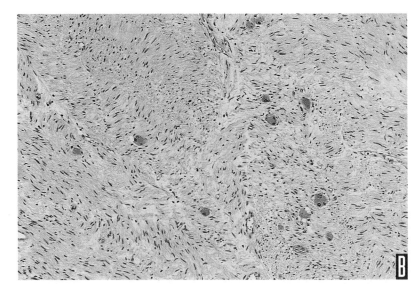

Figure 20.23 A, Clusters of mature ganglion cells and an abundant spindle cell (Schwannian) matrix are typical of ganglioneuroma. The focally edematous stroma contains lymphocytes, which should not be mistaken for primitive neuroblasts. **B,** In this area, which contains few scattered ganglion cells, the stroma is more compact and arranged in interlacing fascicles.

binucleated or multinucleated forms may be present. The cytoplasm has well developed Nissl's substance as well as neuromelanin granules. The stroma, which may appear edematous or compact, contains spindle-shaped Schwann cells separated by variable amounts of collagen, arranged in interlacing bundles or fascicles. Numerous neurofibrils are present throughout the tumor. Variable numbers of mature lymphocytes may be present.

Ultrastructurally, the stroma contains masses of unmyelinated nerve bundles and large numbers of mature Schwann cells, which are completely surrounded by well formed basal lamina. Neuritic processes contain neurofilaments and neurotubules, as well as clear and cored vesicles.

Miscellaneous Tumors of the Adrenal Gland

Myelolipoma

Myelolipomas are uncommon, benign, tumorlike lesions that usually occur in the fifth to seventh decades of life. They have a 0.08%–0.4% incidence at autopsy. Development of these lesions has been associated with various types of endocrine dysfunction (e.g., in adrenal cortical hyperplasia associated with Cushing's disease). Most experts favor an origin in metaplasia of adrenocortical cells resulting from stimulation of a common precursor cell within the cortical stroma by ACTH and/or cortisol.

CLINICAL MANIFESTATIONS Because most myelolipomas are small (< 4 cm diameter), they are frequently asymptomatic and an incidental finding. Large tumors may cause abdominal discomfort or flank pain, produce a palpable mass, or rarely rupture, causing spontaneous retroperitoneal hemorrhage. Radiographically, they appear either as a hyperlucent mass that may displace the kidney (IVP), an avascular mass (arteriography), or as a solid mass that may resemble an adrenal metastasis (ultrasound).

MORPHOLOGY Myelolipomas are unencapsulated, bright yellow, with pink-to-red–brown foci representing hematopoietic components (Fig. 20.24). They can be multiple or bilateral. Larger lesions may appear lobulated.

Microscopically, lesions are composed of mature fat and proliferating hematopoietic elements in different stages of maturation (Fig. 20.25). Adrenal cortical tissue is usually displaced, but may be admixed. Bizarre adrenal cortical cells occur in association with excess ACTH production. Foci of myelolipomatous change have been observed within cortical adenomas and hyperplasias.

Vascular Adrenal Cysts

Nonneoplastic "cysts" of the adrenal gland have been traditionally divided into endothelial, hemorrhagic (pseudocystic), parasitic, and epithelial types. The last two are extremely rare, but the first two are more common and may cause diagnostic problems, both clini-

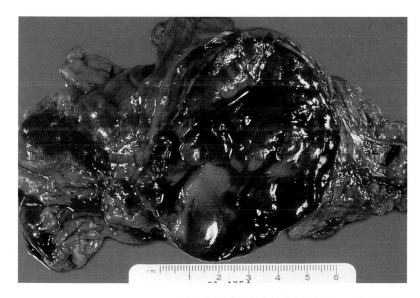

Figure 20.24 The cut surface of this adrenal myelolipoma shows yellow fatty areas and dark red areas composed of hematopoietic tissue.

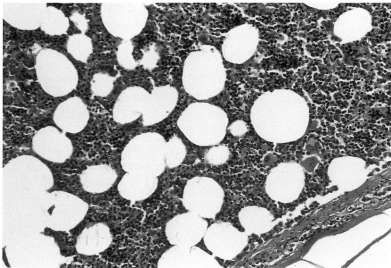

Figure 20.25 Microscopically, myelolipomas contain mature fat and a variable amount of admixed hematopoietic elements. This example shows myeloid cells, darkly staining clusters of eyrthroid cells, and

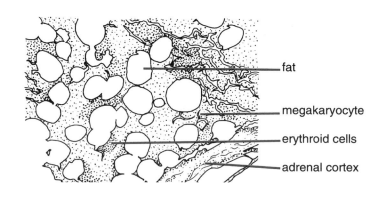

megakaryoctyes. A compressed rim of displaced adrenal cortex is present at the periphery.

cally and microscopically. Endothelial and hemorrhagic cysts, which are closely related, will be considered together here as vascular adrenal cysts. Both probably represent a vascular anomaly with (hemorrhagic) or without (endothelial) associated hemorrhage.

CLINICAL MANIFESTATIONS Patients are typically adults, but vary greatly in age. There is no sex predilection. The right and left glands are involved with equal frequency. Patients typically complain of abdominal pain or mass of several months' duration. Radiographic studies invariably disclose a mass that is solid, or solid and cystic, occasionally with calcifications (Fig. 20.26). Clinical diagnoses usually include various neoplastic considerations.

MORPHOLOGY Grossly, vascular adrenal cysts are often large, thin-walled cysts filled with clear fluid, hemorrhagic fluid, or clotted blood (Fig. 20.27). The cysts average about 13 cm in greatest dimension. Attenuated adrenal cortical tissue can often be identifed grossly in the cyst wall.

Microscopically, the cysts have a thin-to-thick fibrous wall, with or without an identifiable endothelial cell lining (Fig. 20.28). The hemorrhagic cysts cause the greatest diagnostic difficulty due to secondary changes. Islands of cortical cells may be present within organizing hemorrhage (Fig. 20.29A). The cyst's large size coupled with misinterpreting the cortical islands in organizing thrombus as necrotic neoplasm, can lead to a diagnosis of cortical carcinoma. The key to the dis-

tinction lies in considering the possibility of a vascular (hemorrhagic) cyst, recognizing the normal appearance of the cortical islands, and distinguishing organizing thrombus from necrotic neoplasm.

Hemorrhagic adrenal cysts may also contain papillary endothelial hyperplasia as a component of the organizing thrombus (Fig. 20.29B). Such areas have occasionally been misinterpreted as angiosarcoma of the adrenal gland, obviously a critical misdiagnosis. Vascular adrenal cysts have also been associated with metastatic carcinoma, intracystic fat, and myelolipomatous metaplasia.

METASTATIC CANCER OF THE ADRENAL GLAND

The adrenal gland is the fourth most common site of hematogenously disseminated malignancy, following the lung, liver, and bone marrow. Per unit weight, the adrenal glands show the highest affinity for metastatic disease. The reasons for this striking predilection are unclear. The high vascularity of the glands is an insufficient explanation. Lung and breast are the most common primary sites of adrenal metastases (Fig. 20.30A), followed by a variety of other neoplasms, including GI tract adenocarcinomas, germ cell tumors of the gonad, malignant melanoma, transitional cell carcinoma of the GU tract, and sarcomas of varying subtype (Fig. 20.30B). In spite of their proximity, only about 6% of renal cell carcinomas have metastasized to the adjacent adrenal gland at the time of nephrectomy. A higher percentage will have adrenal metastases at

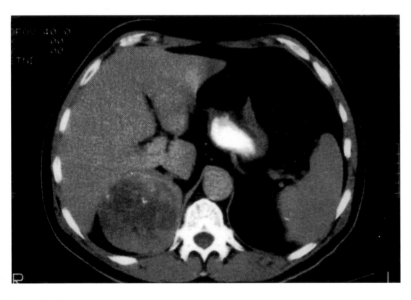

Figure 20.26 Large vascular adrenal cysts are easily detected on CT scan as mixed solid and cystic masses in the paravertebral region.

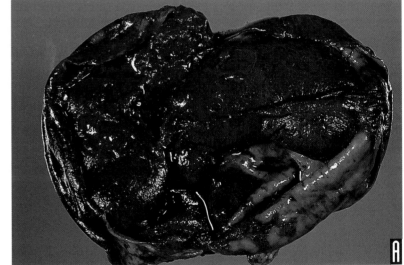

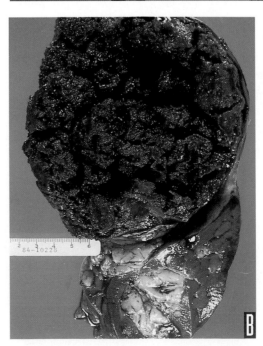

Figure 20.27 A, Fluid filled this vascular adrenal cyst of endothelial subtype. The cyst has a uniform, hemosiderin-colored wall. **B,** This vascular adrenal cyst of pseudocystic subtype appeared clinically as a large hematoma, which compressed and distorted the attached kidney.

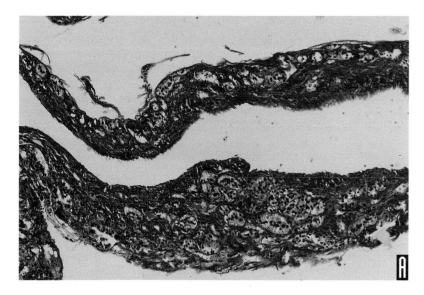 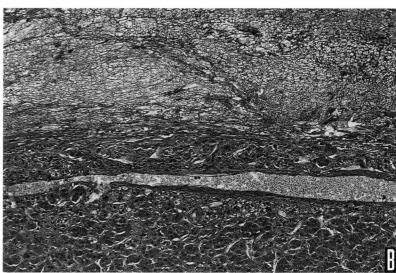

Figure 20.28 **A,** Endothelial vascular cysts consist of a fibrous wall lined by attenuated, often inapparent endothelial cells. In this example, adrenal cortical nests are embedded in the cyst wall. **B,** A hemorrhagic adrenal cyst consists of a rim of adrenal cortex (bottom) with an overlying area of organizing hematoma that may be confused with necrosis (see Fig. 20.5D). Note the large blood vessel in the adrenal cortex.

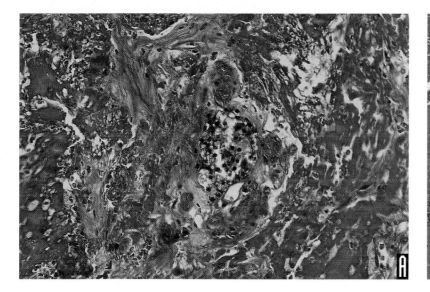 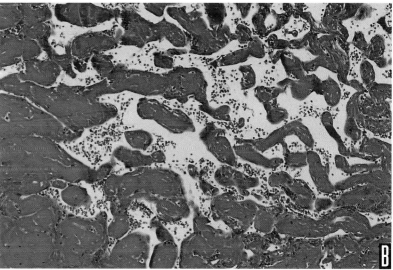

Figure 20.29 **A,** Small islands of normal cortical cells may become entrapped in the organizing hematoma of a hemorrhagic cyst. These should not be confused with a necrotic cortical neoplasm. **B,** The organizing hematoma of a hemorrhagic cyst may contain areas of papillary endothelial hyperplasia. This is a normal reactive change that must not be mistaken for angiosarcoma.

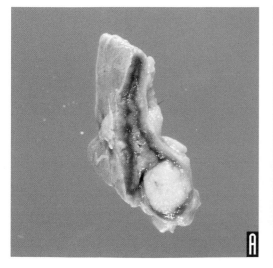 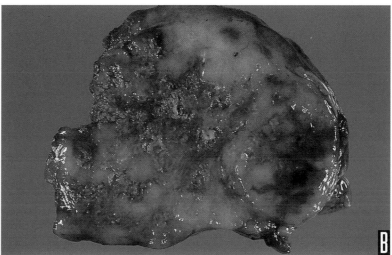

Figure 20.30 **A,** This patient with pulmonary adenocarcinoma had a small adrenal metastasis at the time of autopsy. **B,** Metastatic alveolar rhabdomyosarcoma completely replaced this adrenal gland from a six-year-old.

autopsy (Fig. 20.31). Renal cell carcinomas may also present with contralateral or bilateral adrenal involvement.

Although metastases to the adrenal gland are very common, adrenal insufficiency due to metastatic disease is rarely reported, apparently due to the great functional reserve of adrenal cortical tissue. Adrenal cortical insufficiency may be underdiagnosed, however, due to the clinically distracting, attendant problems of disseminated carcinoma. This is unfortunate, because adrenal insufficiency can be easily corrected, preventing premature death.

The microscopic diagnosis of adrenal metastatic disease is typically straightforward, due to usually obvious clinical features. As discussed above, however, renal cell carcinoma, hepatocellular carcinoma, and malignant melanoma, as well as large cell undifferentiated pulmonary carcinoma, may occasionally be confused with primary adrenal neoplasia. Travis and colleagues also noted that metastatic islet cell tumor to the adrenal gland could mimic a primary adrenal pheochromocytoma. The immunohistochemical distinction of primary adrenal carcinoma from metastastic disease is discussed briefly under the former heading.

Rare Primary Adrenal Tumors

There have been isolated reports of apparently primary adrenal malignant melanomas. Criteria for distinction from metastatic disease, although admittedly arbitrary, include: unilateral adrenal involvement; no prior or current skin, mucosal, or ocular lesions; and failure to detect an extra-adrenal primary at autopsy. Adrenal gland involvement by malignant lymphoma is almost invariably in the setting of disseminated disease, but rare, apparently primary, adrenal lymphomas have been reported. Intra-vascular lymphomatosis, a unique form of lymphoma once mistakenly considered to represent an endothelial neoplasm (malignant angioendotheliomatosis), commonly involves the adrenal gland (Fig. 20.32). Small leiomyomas of the adrenal gland may be encountered rarely at autopsy and probably arise from the adrenal vein. Rare examples of adenomatoid tumor of the adrenal gland, a benign tumor with mesothelial differentiation, more commonly seen in the epididymis, have also been described.

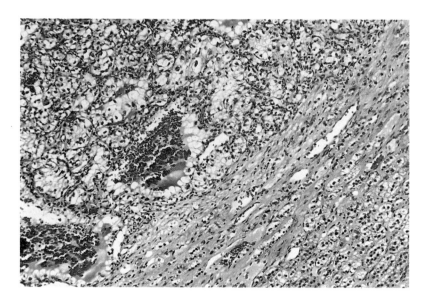

Figure 20.31 Metastatic renal cell carcinoma involving the adrenal gland is a relatively uncommon occurrence. This clear cell carcinoma (left) may be confused with a primary adrenal neoplasm. In problematic cases, immunohistochemical stains will aid in this distinction.

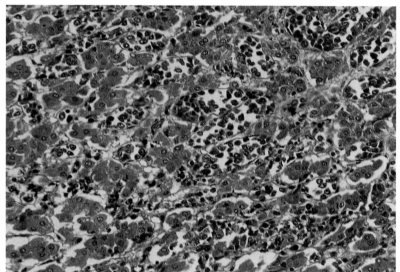

Figure 20.32 Intravascular lymphomatosis, an unusual intravascular variant of lymphoma, often involves the adrenal gland. The neoplastic lymphoid cells fill and distend the adrenal vessels.

References and Further Readings

Section 1: Cystic and Dysplastic Lesions of the Kidney

Bernstein J: The classification of renal cysts. Nephron 11:91–100, 1973.

Gardner KD: Cystic Diseases of the Kidney. AUA Update Series, Lesson 19, Vol. IV. American Urological Assn, Houston, 1985.

Gardner KD (ed.): Cystic Diseases of the Kidney. John Wiley & Sons Inc, New York, 1976.

Kissane J: Congenital malformations. In Heptinstall RH (ed.) Pathology of the Kidney. Little Brown & Co, Boston, 1974.

Osathanondh V, Potter E: Pathogenesis of polycystic kidneys. Arch Path 77:459–465, 1964.

Chapter 1: Hereditary Cystic Diseases

Bernstein J: Hereditary renal disease. In Churg J, Spargo BH, Mostofi FK (eds.) Kidney Disease: Present Status. International Academy of Pathology Monograph. Williams & Wilkins Co, Baltimore, 1979.

Bernstein J: Hereditary disorders of the kidney: Part I. Parenchymal defects and malformations. In Bolande RP, Rosenberg H (eds.) Perspectives in Pediatric Pathology, vol. 1. Year Book Medical Publishers Inc, Chicago, 1973.

Gardner KD: Evolution of clinical signs in adult-onset cystic disease of the renal medulla. Ann Intern Med 74:47–54, 1971.

Lieberman E, Salinas-Madrigal L, Gwinn JL, et al: Infantile polycystic disease of the kidneys and liver: Clinical, pathological and radiological correlations and comparison with congenital hepatic fibrosis. Medicine 50:277–318, 1971.

Ross DG, Travers H: Infantile presentation of adult-type polycystic disease in a large kindred. J Pediatr 87:760–763, 1975.

Schechterman L: Lindau's disease: Report of an unusual case and two additional cases in a Negro family. Med Ann District of Columbia 30:64–76, 1961.

Chapter 2: Developmental Cystic Diseases

Bernstein J: Developmental abnormalities of the renal parenchyma: Renal hypoplasia and dysplasia. In Sommers SC (ed.) Pathology Annual. Appleton-Century-Crofts, New York, 1968.

Bernstein J: The morphogenesis of renal parenchymal maldevelopment (renal dysplasia). Pediatr Clin North Am 18:395–407, 1971.

Bernstein J, Brough AJ, McAdams AJ: The Renal Lesion in Syndromes of Multiple Congenital Malformations: Cerebrohepatorenal Syndrome; Jeune Asphyxiating Thoracic Dystrophy; Tuberous Sclerosis; Meckel Syndrome. In 5th Conference on the Clinical Delineation of Birth Defects. Birth Defects: Original Article Series, vol. X 4:35–43. The National Foundation, New York, 1974.

Spence HM, Singleton R: What is sponge kidney disease and where does it fit in the spectrum of cystic disorders? J Urol 107:176–183, 1972.

Yow RM, Bunts RC: Calyceal diverticulum. J Urol 73:663–670, 1955.

Chapter 3: Acquired Cystic Diseases

Dunnill MS, Millard PR, Oliver D: Acquired cystic disease of the kidneys: A hazard of long-term intermittent maintenance hemodialysis. J Clin Pathol 30:868–877, 1977.

Hughson MD, Hennigar RR, McManus JFA: Atypical cysts, acquired renal cystic disease, and renal cell tumors in end stage dialysis kidneys. Lab Invest 42:475–480, 1980.

Khorsand D: Carcinoma within solitary renal cysts. J Urol 93:440–444, 1965.

Section II: Anomalies of the Urinary Tract
Chapter 4: Anomalies of the Kidney

Abeshouse BS: Aneurysm of renal artery: Report of 2 cases and review of literature. Urol & Cutan Rev 55:451–463, 1951.

Abeshouse BS, Bhisitkul I: Crossed renal ectopia with and without fusion. Urol Int 9:63–91, 1959.

Arant BS Jr, Sotelo-Avila C, Bernstein J: Segmental "hypoplasia" of the kidney (Ask-Upmark). J Pediatr 95:931–939, 1979.

Ashley DJB, Mostofi FK: Renal agenesis and dysgenesis. J Urol 83:211–230, 1960.

Bain AD, Scott JS: Renal agenesis and severe urinary tract dysplasia: A review of 50 cases with particular reference to the associated anomalies. Br Med 1:841–846, 1960.

Bernstein J: Developmental abnormalities of the renal parenchyma: Renal hypoplasia and dysplasia. Patho Annu 3:213–247, 1968.

Boatman DL, Culp DA Jr, Culp DA, et al: Crossed renal ectopia. J Urol 108:30–31, 1972.

Boatman DL, Kolln CP, Flocks RH: Congenital anomalies associated with horseshoe kidney. J Urol 107:205–207, 1972.

Cho KJ, Stanley JC: Non-neoplastic congenital and acquired renal arteriovenous malformations and fistulas. Radiology 129:333–343, 1978.

Collins DC: Congenital unilateral renal agenesis. Ann Surg 95:715–726, 1932.

Doroshow LW, Abeshouse BS: Congenital unilateral solitary kidney: Report of 37 cases and a review of the literature. Urol Survey 11:219–229, 1961.

Elfenbein IB, Baluarte HJ, Gruskin AB: Renal hypoplasia with oligomeganephronia: Light, electron, fluorescent microscopic and quantitative studies. Arch Pathol 97: 143–149, 1973.

Geisinger JF: Supernumerary kidney. J Urol 38:331–356, 1937.

Gray SW, Skandalakis JE: Embryology for Surgeons. WB Saunders Co, Philadelphia, 1972.

Hageman JH, Smith RF, Szilagyi DE, et al: Aneurysms of the renal artery: Problems of prognosis and surgical management. Surgery 84:563–571, 1978.

Kissane JM: Congenital malformations. In Heptinstall RH (ed.) Pathology of the Kidney, 3rd ed. Little Brown & Co, Boston, 1983.

Kolln CP, Boatman DL, Schmidt JD, et al: Horseshoe kidney: A review of 105 patients. J Urol 107:203–204, 1972.

Longo VJ, Thompson GJ: Congenital solitary kidney. J Urol 68:63–68, 1952.

Malek RS, Kelalis PP, Burke EC: Ectopic kidney in children and frequency of association with other malformations. Mayo Clin Proc 46:461–467, 1971.

Mauer SM, Dobrin RS, Vernier RL: Unilateral and bilateral renal agenesis in monoamniotic twins. J Pediatr 84:236–238, 1974.

N'Guessan G, Stephens FD: Supernumerary kidney. J Urol 130:649–653, 1983.

Perlmutter AD, Retik AB, Bauer SB: Anomalies of the upper urinary tract. In Walsh PC, Gittes RF, Perlmutter AD, et al. (eds.) Campbell's Urology, 5th ed. WB Saunders Co, Philadelphia, 1986.

Potter EL: Bilateral absence of ureters and kidneys: A report of 50 cases. Obstet Gynecol 25:3–12, 1965.

Potter EL: Bilateral renal agenesis. J Pediatr 29:68–76, 1946.

Potter EL: Facial characteristics in infants with bilateral renal agenesis. Am J Obstet Gynecol 51:885–888, 1946.

Thompson GJ, Pace JM: Ectopic kidney: A review of 97 cases. Surg Gynecol Obstet 64:935–943, 1937.

Van Acker KJ, Vincke H, Quatacker J, et al: Congenital oligonephronic renal hypoplasia with hypertrophy of nephrons (oligonephronia). Arch Dis Child 46:321–326, 1971.

Weyrauch HM Jr: Anomalies of renal rotation. Surg Gynecol Obstet 69:183–199, 1939.

Chapter 5: Ureteral and Bladder Anomalies

Bauer SB, Retik AB: Bladder diverticula in infants and children. Urology 3:712–715, 1974.

Blichert-Toft M, Nielsen OV: Congenital patent urachus and acquired variants. Diagnosis and treatment. Review of the literature and report of five cases. Acta Chir Scand 137:807–814, 1971.

Burger RH: A theory on the nature of the transmission of congenital vesicoureteral reflux. J Urol 108:249–254, 1972.

Cook WA, King LR: Vesicoureteral reflux. In Harrison JH, Gittes RF, Perlmutter AD, et al. (eds.) Campbell's Urology, 4th ed. WB Saunders Co, Philadelphia, 1979

Culp OS: Ureteral diverticulum: Classification of the literature and report of an authentic case. J Urol 58:309–321, 1947.

Dwoskin JY: Sibling uropathology. J Urol 115:726–727, 1976.

Dwoskin JY, Perlmutter AD: Vesicoureteral reflux in children: A computerized review. J Urol 109:888–890, 1973.

Engel RM, Wilkinson HA: Bladder exstrophy. J Urol 104:699–704, 1970.

Ezell WW, Carlson HE: A realistic look at exstrophy of the bladder. Br J Urol 42:197–202, 1970.

Forsythe IW, Smith BT: Diverticulum of the bladder in children: A study of 13 cases. Pediatrics 24:322–329, 1959

Hawthorne AB: The embryologic and clinical aspect of double ureter. JAMA 106:189–193,1936.

Hinman F Jr: Surgical disorders of the bladder and umbilicus of urachal origin. Surg Gynecol Obstet 113:605–614, 1961.

Johnson JH, Penn IA: Exstrophy of the cloaca. Br J Urol 38:302–307, 1966.

Lyon RP, Marshall S, Tanagho EA: The ureteral orifice: Its configuration and competency. J Urol 102:504–509, 1969.

Mackie GG, Stephens FD: Duplex kidneys: A correlation of renal dysplasia with position of the ureteral orifice. Urol 114:274–280, 1975.

Malek RS, Kelalis PP, Burke EC, et al: Simple and ectopic ureterocele in infancy and childhood. Surg Gyneco J Obstet 134:611–616, 1972.

Marshall VF, Muecke EC: Variations in exstrophy of the bladder. J Urol 88:766–796, 1962.

Muecke EC: The embryology of the urinary system. In Harrison JH, Gittes RF, Perlmutter AD, et al. (eds.) Campbell's Urology, 4th ed. WB Saunders Co, Philadelphia, 1979.

Muecke EC: The role of the cloacal membrane in exstrophy: The first successful experimental study. J Urol 92:659–667, 1964.

Nation EF: Duplication of the kidney and ureter: A statistical study of 230 new cases. J Urol 51:456–465, 1944

Norman CH Jr, Dubowy J: Multiple ureteral diverticula J Urol 96:152–154, 1966.

Nunn LL: Urachal cysts and their complications. Am J Surg 84:252–255, 1952.

Perlmutter AD, Retik AB, Bauer SB: Anomalies of the upper urinary tract. In Walsh PC, Gittes RF, Perlmutter AD, et al. (eds.)

Campbell's Urology, 5th ed. WB Saunders Co, Philadelphia, 1986.

Privett JTJ, Jeans WD, Roylance J: The incidence and importance of renal duplication. Clin Radiol 27:521–530, 1976.

Rank WB, Mellinger GT, Spiro E: Ureteral diverticula: Etiologic considerations. J Urol 83:566–569, 1960.

Schmidt JD, Hawtrey CE, Flocks RH, et al: Vesicoureteral reflux: An inherited lesion. JAMA 220:821–824, 1972.

Stephens D: Caecoureterocele and concepts on the embryology and aetiology of ureteroceles. Aust NZ J Surg 40:239–248, 1971.

Tank ES, Lindenauer SM: Principles of management of exstrophy of the cloaca. Am J Surg 119:95–98, 1970.

Timothy RP, Decter A, Perlmutter AD: Ureteral duplication: Clinical findings and therapy in 46 children. J Urol 105:445–451, 1971.

Section III: Obstructive Uropathy

Chapter 6: Hydronephrosis and Urolithiasis

Brock WA, Nachtscheim DA, Kaplan GW, et al: Congenital giant hydroureteronephrosis. Urol Radiol 1:67–75, 1979.

Crooks KK, Hendren WH, Pfister RC: Giant hydronephrosis in children. J Pediatr Surg 14:844–850, 1979.

Heptinstall RH: Pathology of the Kidney, 3rd ed., vol. 3. Little Brown & Co, Boston, 1983, pp. 1583–1585, 1599–1627.

Lalli A: Renal parenchymal calcifications. Semin Roentgenol 17:101–112, 1982.

Mathieu H: Urinary infection and the pathology of interstitial tissue. In Royer P, Habib R, Mathieu H, Broyer A (eds.) Major Problems in Clinical Pediatrics: Pediatric Nephrology, vol. II. WB Saunders Co, Philadelphia, 1974, pp. 183–192, 193–204.

Robbins SL, Cotran RS, Kumar V: Pathologic Basis of Disease, 3rd ed. WB Saunders Co, Philadelphia, 1984, pp. 1038–1039, 1051–1053.

Warshaw BL, Hymes LC, Woodward JR: Long term outcome of patients with obstructive uropathy. Symposium on pediatric nephrology. Pediatr Clin North Am 29:815–826, 1982.

Chapter 7: Ureteropelvic Junction Obstruction

Addonizio JC, Patel RC: Innocent aberrant renal vessels producing ureteropelvic junction obstruction. Urology 16:176–180, 1980.

Antonakopoulas GN, Fuggle WJ, Neuman J, et al: Idiopathic hydronephrosis: Light microscopic features and pathogenesis. Arch Pathol Lab Med 109:1097–1101, 1985.

Bejjani B, Belman B: Ureteropelvic junction obstruction in newborns and infants. J Urol 128:770–773, 1982.

Das S, Amar AD: Ureteropelvic junction obstruction with associated renal anomalies. J Urol 131:872–874, 1984.

Hanna MK, Jeffs RD, Sturgess JM, et al: Ureteral structure and ultrastructure: Part II. Congenital ureteropelvic junction obstruction and primary obstructive megaureter. J Urol 116:725–730, 1976.

Jiminez-Mariscal JL, Flah LM: Ureteropelvic junction obstruction secondary to vesicoureteral reflux: Later complication after successful vesicoureteral reimplant. Urology 18:203–206, 1981.

Kench P: A morphometric study of the pelvi-ureteric junction and review of the pathogenesis of the upper ureteric obstruction. Pathology 14:309–312, 1982.

Lowe FC, Marshall FF: Ureteropelvic junction obstruction in adults. Urology 23:331–335, 1984.

Marshall FF, Jeffs RD, Smolev JK: Neonatal bilateral ureteropelvic junction obstruction. J Urol 123:107–109, 1980.

Perlberg S, Pfau A: Management of ureteropelvic junction obstruction associated with lower polar vessels. Urology 23:13–18, 1984.

Snyder HM, Lebowitz RL, Colodny AH, et al: Ureteropelvic junction obstruction in children. Urol Clin North Am 7:273–290, 1980.

Stephens FD: Ureterovascular hydronephrosis and the "aberrant" renal vessels. J Urol 128:984–987, 1982.

Wadsworth DE, McClennan BL: Benign causes of acquired ureteropelvic junction obstruction: A uroradiologic spectrum. Urol Radiol 5:77–82, 1983.

White JM, Kaplan GW, Brock WA: Ureteropelvic junction obstruction in children. Am Fam Physician 29:211–216, 1984.

Chapter 8: Urinary Tract Obstruction

Aaronson IA: Posterior urethral valves: A review of 120 cases. S Afr Med J 65:418–422, 1984.

Dallemand S, Kutcher R, McPherson H, et al: Endometriosis with ureteric involvement. NY State J Med 79(pt 1):382–383, 1979.

Fer MF, McKinney TD, Richardson RL, et al: Cancer and the kidney: Renal complications of neoplasms. Am J Med 71:704–718, 1981.

Fitzer PM: Congenital ureteral valve. Pediatr Radiol 8:54–55, 1979.

Fletcher CDM, Jarrett PEM: Variable symptomatology in idiopathic retroperitoneal fibrosis. J R Soc Med 76:1023–1025, 1983.

Frohneberg D, Walz PH, Hohenfellner R: Primary mega ureter in adults. Eur Urol 9:321–328, 1983.

Glassberg KI: Current issues regarding posterior urethral valves. Urol Clin North Am 12:175–185, 1985.

Heptinstall RH: Pathology of the Kidney, 3rd ed., vol. 3. Little Brown & Co, Boston, 1983; 1226–1238, pp. 1426–1430.

Krinsky S, Zieverink SE, Peterson GH, et al: Computerized tomographic diagnosis of retroperitoneal fibrosis. South Med J 76:517–519,1983.

Lockhart JL, Singer AM, Glenn JF: Congenital megaureter. J Urol 122:310–314, 1979.

Meyers MA: Uriniferous peri-renal pseudocyst: New observations. Diagn Radiol 117:539–546, 1975.

Miles RM, Brock J, Martin C: Idiopathic retroperitoneal fibrosis: A sometimes surgical problem. Am Surg 50:76–84, 1984.

Minford JE, Davies P: The urographic appearances in acute and chronic retroperitoneal fibrosis. Clin Radiol 35:51–57, 1984.

Norman RW, Mack FG, Awad SA, et al: Acute renal failure secondary to bilateral ureteric obstruction: Review of 50 cases. Can Med Assoc J 127:601–604, 1982.

Pujari BR, Moss WD: Adynamic ureteral segment: Primary megaureter. W Va Med J 77:27–31, 1981.

Rault R, Kapoor W, Kam W: Peri-aneurysmal fibrosis and ureteric obstruction: Case report and review of the literature. Clin Nephrol 18:159–162, 1982.

Reiner I, Yachia D, Nissum F, et al: Retroperitoneal fibrosis with urothelial tumor. J Urol 132:115–116, 1984.

Sauls CL, Nesbit RM: Pararenal pseudocysts: A report of four cases. J Urol 87:288–296, 1962.

Spriggs AI: Perinephric cysts. J Urol 67:414–432, 1952.

Stewart TS, Friberg TR: Idiopathic retroperitoneal fibrosis with diffuse involvement: Further evidence of systemic idiopathic fibrosis. South Med J 77:1185–1187, 1984.

Tokunaka S, Gotoh T, Koyanagi T, et al: Muscle dysplasia in megaureters. J Urol 131:383–390, 1984.

Tokunaka S, Koyanagi T: Morphological study of primary nonreflux megaureters with particular emphasis on the role of ureteral sheath and ureteral dysplasia. J Urol 128:399–402, 1982.

Tokunaka S, Koyanagi T, Tsuji I, et al: Histopathology of the nonrefluxing megaloureter: A clue to its pathogenesis. J Urol 127:238–244, 1982.

Waldron JA, Newcomer LN, Kotz ME, et al: Sclerosing variants of follicular center cell lymphomas presenting in the retroperitoneum. Cancer 52:712–720, 1983.

Section IV: Urinary Tract Infection and Inflammatory Lesions

Chapter 9: Pyelonephritis and Inflammatory Lesions of the Kidney

Abraham E, Brenner BE, Simon RR: Cystitis and pyelonephritis (collective review). Ann Emerg Med 12:228–234, 1983.

Barens JL, Osgood RW, Lee JC, et al: Host-parasite interactions in the pathogenesis of experimental renal candidiasis. Lab Invest 49:460–470, 1983.

Bathena DB, Holland NH, Weiss JH, et al: Morphology of coarse renal scars in reflux associated nephropathy in man. In Hodson J, Kincaid-Smith P (eds.) Reflux Nephropathy. Masson Publishing USA Inc, New York, 1979.

Beckman EN, Busby JD, Brannon W: Hematopoietic tumor of the renal hilus. J Urol 126:403–405, 1981.

Davides KC, Johnson SH, Marshall M, et al: Plasma cell granuloma of the renal pelvis. J Urol 107:938–939, 1972.

Fisch AE, Brodey PA: Plasma cell granuloma of kidney. Urology 8:89–91, 1976.

Gardner KD, Castellino RA, Kempson R, et al: Primary amyloidosis of the renal pelvis. N Engl J Med 284:1196–1198, 1971.

Habib R: Pathology of renal segmental corticopapillary scarring in children with hypertension: The concept of segmental hypoplasia. In Hodson J, Kincaid-Smith P (eds.) Reflux Nephropathy. Masson Publishing USA Inc, New York, 1979.

Hellman RN, Hinrichs J, Sicard G, et al: Cryptococcal pyelonephritis and disseminated cryptococcosis in a renal transplant recipient. Arch Intern Med 141:128–130, 1981.

Heptinstall RH: Pyelonephritis: Pathologic features. In Heptinstall RH (ed.) Pathology of the Kidney, 3rd ed., vol. 3. Little Brown & Co, Boston, 1983.

Heptinstall RH: Urinary tract infection, reflux and pyelonephritis. In Heptinstall RH (ed.) Pathology of the Kidney, 3rd ed., vol. 3. Little Brown & Co, Boston, 1983.

Itoh H, Namiki M, Yoshioka T, et al: Plasma cell granuloma of the renal pelvis. J Urol 127:1177–1178, 1982.

Khan MY: Anuria from Candida pyelonephritis and obstructing fungus balls. Urology 21:421–423, 1983.

Kincaid-Smith P: Glomerular lesions in atrophic pyelonephritis (RN). In Hodson J, Kincaid-Smith P (eds.) Reflux Nephropathy. Masson Publishing USA Inc, New York, 1979.

Kunin CM: Does kidney function cause renal failure? Annu Rev Med 36:165–176, 1985.

Malek RS, Greene LF, DeWeerd JH, et al: Xanthogranulomatous pyelonephritis. Br J Urol 44:296–308, 1972.

Mathieu H: Urinary infection and the pathology of interstitial tissue. In Royer P, Habib R, Mathieu H, Broyer A (eds.) Major Problems in Clinical Pediatrics: Pediatric Nephrology, vol. 11. WB Saunders Co, Philadelphia, 1974, pp. 131–146, 147–159.

Michaeli J, Mogle P, Perlberg S, et al: Emphysematous pyelonephritis (review article). J Urol 131:203–208, 1984.

Ravel R: Megalocytic interstitial nephritis: An entity probably related to malakoplakia. Am J Clin Pathol 47:781–789, 1967.

Robbins SL, Cotran RS, Kumar V: The kidney. In Robbins SL, Cotran RS, Kumar V (eds.) Pathologic Basis of Disease. WB Saunders Co, Philadelphia, 1984.

Roberts JA: Etiology and Pathophysiology of pyelonephritis (in-depth review). Am J Dis XVII:1–9, 1991.

Schneiderman C, Simon MA: Malakoplakia of the urinary tract. J Urol 100:694–698, 1968.

Senekjian HI, Suki WN: Vesicoureteral reflux and reflux nephropathy. Am J Nephrol 2:245–250, 1982.

Tolkoff-Rubin NE, Rubin RH: Urinary tract infection. In Contemporary Issues in Nephrology. Churchill Livingstone Inc, New York, 1983.

Tripathi VNP, Desautels RE: Primary amyloidosis of the urogenital system: A study of 16 cases and brief review. J Urol 102:96–101, 1969.

Winberg J, Bollgren I, Kallenius G, et al: Clinical pyelonephritis and focal renal scarring: A selected review of pathogenesis, prevention and prognosis. Pediatr Clin North Am 29:801–814, 1982.

Chapter 10: Inflammatory, Proliferative, and Metaplastic Lesions of the Bladder

Aabech HS, Lien EN: Cystitis cystica in childhood: Clinical findings and treatment procedures. Acta Paediatr Scand 71:247–252, 1982.

Albores-Saavedra J, Manivel C, Essenfeld H, et al: Pseudosarcomatous myofibroblastic proliferations in the urinary bladder of children. Cancer 66:1234–1241, 1990.

Devine P, Ucci AA, Krain H, et al: Nephrogenic adenoma and embryonic kidney tubules share PNA receptor sites. Am J Clin Pathol 81:728–732, 1984.

Droller MJ, Erozan YS: Thiotepa effects on urinary cytology in the interpretation of transitional cell cancer. J Urol 134:671–674, 1985.

Ehrlich RM, Freedman A, Goldsobel AB, et al: The use of sodium 2-mercaptoethane sulfonate to prevent cyclophosphamide cystitis. J Urol 131:960–962, 1984.

Forni AM, Koss LG, Geller W: Cytological study of the effect of cyclophosphamide on the epithelium of the urinary bladder in man. Cancer 17:1348–1355, 1964.

Fujihara S, Glenner GG: Primary localized amyloidosis of the genitourinary tract: Immunohistochemical study on eleven cases. Lab Invest 44:55–60, 1981.

Goldberg ID, Garnick MB, Bloomer WD: Urinary tract toxic effects of cancer therapy (review article). J Urol 132:1–6, 1984.

Ito N, Hirose M, Shirai T, et al: Lesions of the urinary bladder epithelium in 125 autopsy cases. Acta Pathol Jpn 31:545–557, 1981.

Johansson SL: Light microscopic findings in bladders of patients with interstitial cystitis. In Staskin D, Hannu P, Wein A (eds.) Interstitial Cystitis. Springer-Verlag, New York, 1988.

Klein FA, Smith MJV: Urinary complications of cyclophosphamide therapy: Etiology, prevention and management. South Med J 76:1413–1416, 1983.

Koss LG: A light and electron microscopic study of the effects of a single dose of cyclophosphamide on various organs in the rat: I. The urinary bladder. Lab Inves 16:44–65, 1967.

Lage JM, Bauer WC, Kelley DR, et al: Histological parameters and pitfalls in the interpretation of bladder biopsies in bacillus Calmette-Guerin treatment of superficial bladder cancer. J Urol 135:916–919, 1986.

Lamm DL: Bacillus Calmette-Guerin immunotherapy for bladder cancer. J Urol 134:40–46, 1985.

Larsen S, Thompson SA, Hald T, et al: Mast cells in interstitial cystitis. Br J Urol 54:283–286, 1982.

Littleton RH, Farah RN, Cerny J: Eosinophilic cystitis: An uncommon form of cystitis. J Urol 127:132–133, 1982.

McClurg FV, D'Agostino AN, Martin JH, et al: Ultra structural demonstration of intracellular bacteria in three cases of malakoplakia of the bladder. Am J Clin Pathol 60:780–788, 1973.

Malek RS, Greene LF, Farrow GM: Amyloidosis of the urinary bladder. Br J Urol 43:189–200, 1971.

Marshall FF, Middleton AW: Eosinophilic cystitis. J Urol 112:335–337, 1974.

Mattila J, Linder E: Immunoglobulin deposits in bladder epithelium and vessels in interstitial cystitis: Possible relationship to circulating anti-intermediate filament autoantibodies. Clin Immunol Immunopathol 32:81–89, 1984.

Mostofi FK, Davis CJ: Epithelial abnormalities of urinary bladder. In Kuss R, Khoury S, Denis L, Murphy GP, Karr JP (eds.)

Progress in Clinical and Biological Research, vol. 162A. Bladder Cancer, Part A: Pathology, Diagnosis, and Surgery. Alan R Liss Inc, New York, 1984.

Murphy WM, Soloway MS, Finebaum PJ: Pathological changes associated with topical chemotherapy for superficial bladder cancer. J Urol 126:461–464, 1981.

Nochomovitz LE, Orenstein JM: Inflammatory pseudotumor of the urinary bladder: Possible relationship to nodular fasciitis. Am J Surg Pathol 9:366–373, 1985.

Parivar F, Bradbrook RA: Interstitial cystitis (review). Br J Urol 58:239–244, 1986.

Peterson NE: Eosinophilic cystitis. Urology 26:167–169, 1985.

Pinkert TC, Catlow CE, Strauss R: Endometriosis of the urinary bladder in a man with a prostatic carcinoma. Cancer 43:1562–1567, 1979.

Reece RW, Koontz WW: Leukoplakia of the urinary tract: A review. J Urol 114:165–171, 1975.

Ro JY, Ayala AG, Ordonez NG, et al: Pseudosarcomatous fibromyxoid tumor of the urinary bladder. Am J Clin Pathol 86:583–590, 1986.

Rubin P, Casarett GW: Clinical Radiation Pathology, vol 1. WB Saunders Co, Philadelphia, 1968.

Schneiderman C, Simon MA: Malacoplakia of the urinary tract. J Urol 100:694–698, 1968.

Smith BH: Malacoplakia of the urinary tract: A study of 24 cases. Am J Clin Pathol 43:409–417, 1965.

Spagnolo DV, Waring PM: Bladder granulomata after surgery. Am J Clin Pathol 86:430–437, 1986.

Wells M, Anderson K: Mucin histochemistry of cystitis glandularis and primary adenocarcinoma of the urinary bladder. Arch Pathol Lab Med 109:59–61, 1985.

Widran J, Sanchez R, Gruhn J: Squamous metaplasia of the bladder: A study of 450 patients. J Urol 112:479–482, 1974.

Young RH, Scully RE: Nephrogenic adenoma: A report of 15 cases, review of the literature and comparison with clear cell adenocarcinoma of the urinary tract. Am J Surg Pathol 10:268–275, 1986.

Section V: Neoplasms of the Urinary Tract
Chapter 11: Neoplasms of the Kidney, Renal Pelvis, and Ureter

Akhtar M, Kott E, Brooks B: Extrarenal Wilms' tumor: Report of a case and review of the literature. Cancer 40:3087–3091, 1977.

Babaian RJ, Skinner DG, Waisman J: Wilms' tumor in the adult patient: Diagnosis, management and review of the world medical literature. Cancer 45:1713–1719, 1980.

Barajas L, Bennett CM, Connor G, et al: Structure of a juxtaglomerular cell tumor: The presence of a neural component. A light and electron microscopic study. Lab Invest 37:357–368, 1977.

Barnes CA, Beckman EN: Renal oncocytoma and its congeners. Am J Clin Pathol 79:312–318, 1983.

Batata M, Grabstald H: Upper urinary tract urothelial tumors. Urol Clin North Am 3:79–86, 1976.

Beckwith JB: Wilms' tumor and other renal tumors of childhood: A selective review from the National Wilms' Tumor Study Pathology Center. Hum Pathol 14:481–492, 1983.

Beckwith JB, Kiviat NB, Bonadio JF: Nephrogenic rests, nephroblastomatosis, and the pathogenesis of Wilms' tumor. Pediat Pathol 10:1–36, 1990.

Bennington JL: Cancer of the kidney: Etiology, epidemiology and pathology. Cancer 32:1017–1029, 1973.

Bennington JL, Beckwith JB: Tumors of the kidney, renal pelvis and ureter. In Firminger HI (ed.) Atlas of Tumor Pathology, 2nd series, fascicle 12. Armed Forces Institute of Pathology, Washington DC, 1975.

Bernstein J, Evan AP, Gardner KD Jr: Epithelial hyperplasia in polycystic kidney disease. Its role in pathogenesis and risk of neoplasia. Am J Pathol 129:92–101, 1987.

Bonsib SM, Lager DJ: Chromophobe cell carcinoma: Analysis of five cases. Am J Surg Pathol 14:260–267, 1990.

Bonsib SM, Fischer J, Plattner S, et al: Sarcomatoid renal tumors: Clinicopathologic correlation of three cases. Cancer 59:527–532, 1987.

Bove KE, McAdams AJ: The nephroblastomatosis complex and its relationship to Wilms' tumor: A clinicopathologic treatise. In Rosenberg HS, Bolande RP (eds.) Perspectives in Pediatric Pathology, vol. 3. Year Book Medical Publishers Inc, Chicago, 1976.

Buck BE, Bove KE: Wilms' tumor. In Henson DE, Albores-Saavedra J (eds.) Pathology of Incipient Neoplasia. WB Saunders Co, Philadelphia, 1986, pp. 345–353.

Case records of the Massachusetts General Hospital. N Engl J Med 313:1596–1603, 1985.

Cohen AJ, Li FP, Berg S, et al: Hereditary renal cell carcinoma associated with a chromosomal translocation. N Engl J Med 301:592–595, 1979.

Daly JJ: Carcinoma in situ of the urothelium. Urol Clin North Am 3:87–105, 1976.

Eble JN, Hull MT: Morphologic features of renal oncocytoma: A light and electron microscopic study. Hum Pathol 15:1054–1061, 1984.

Farrow GM, Harrison EG, Utz DC: Sarcomas and sarcomatoid and mixed malignant tumors of the kidney in adults. Cancer 22:545–563, 1968.

Farrow GM, Harrison EG, Utz DC, et al: Renal angiomyolipoma: A clinicopathologic study of 32 cases. Cancer 22:564–570, 1968.

Ferry JA, Malt RA, Young RH: Renal angiomyolipoma with sarcomatous transformation and pulmonary metastases. Am J Surg Pathol 15:1083–1088, 1991.

Fleming S, Lewi HJE: Collecting duct carcinoma of the kidney. Histopathology 10:1131–1141, 1986.

Fuhrman SA, Lasky LC, Limas C: Prognostic significance of morphologic parameters in renal cell carcinoma. Am J Surg Pathol 6:655–663, 1982.

Gonzalez-Crussi F, Hsueh W, Ugarte N: Rhabdomyogenesis in renal neoplasia of childhood. Am J Surg Pathol 5:525–532, 1981.

Gonzalez-Crussi F, Sotelo-Auila C, Kidd JM: Mesenchymal renal tumors in infancy: A reappraisal. Hum Pathol 12:78–85, 1981.

Haas JE, Bonadio JF, Beckwith JB: Clear cell sarcoma of the kidney with emphasis on ultrastructural studies. Cancer 54:2978–2987, 1984.

Haas JE, Palmer NF, Weinberg AG, et al: Ultrastructure of malignant rhabdoid tumor of the kidney: A distinctive renal tumor of children. Hum Pathol 12:646–657, 1981.

Hartwick RJW, Srigley J, Shaw P: Uncommon histologic patterns mimicking malignancy in angiomyolipoma. Lab Invest 60:39A, 1990.

Holthofer H, Miettinen A, Paasivuo R, et al: Cellular origin and differentiation of renal carcinoma: A fluorescence microscopic study with kidney-specific antibodies, anti-intermediate filament antibodies, and lectins. Lab Invest 49:317–326, 1983.

Ibrahim RD, Weinberg DS, Weidner N: Atypical cysts and carcinomas of the kidney in the phacomatoses. A quantitative DNA study using static and flow cytometry. Cancer 63:148–157, 1989.

Joshi VV, Beckwith JB: Multilocular cyst of the kidney (cystic nephroma) and cystic, partially differentiated nephroblastoma. Terminology and criteria for diagnosis. Cancer 64:466–479, 1989.

Joshi VV, Beckwith JB: Pathologic delineation of the papillonodular type of cystic partially differentiated nephroblastoma. A review of 11 cases. Cancer 66:1568–1577, 1990.

Joshi VV, Kasznica J., Walters TR: Atypical mesoblastic nephroma: Pathologic characterization of a potentially aggressive variant of conventional congenital mesoblastic nephroma. Arch Pathol Lab Med 110:100–106, 1986.

Kandel LB, Harrison LH, Woodruff RD, et al: Renal plasmacytoma: A case report and summary of reported cases. J Urol 132:1167–1169, 1984.

Kovacs G, Welter C, Wilkens L, et al: Renal oncocytoma. A phenotypic and genotypic entity of renal parenchymal tumors. Am J Pathol 134:967–971, 1989.

Lack EE, Cassady JR, Sallan SE: Renal cell carcinoma in childhood and adolescence: A clinical and pathological study of 17 cases. J Urol 133:822–828, 1985.

Ljunberg B, Stenling R, Roos G: DNA content and prognosis in renal cell carcinoma. Cancer 57:2346–2350, 1986.

McCarron JP, Chasko SB, Gray GF: Systematic mapping of nephroureterectomy specimens removed for urothelial cancer: Pathological findings and clinical correlations. J Urol 128:243–246, 1982.

Mahoney JP, Saffos RO: Fetal rhabdomyomatous nephroblastoma with a renal pelvic mass simulating sarcoma botryoides. Am J Surg Pathol 5:297–306, 1981.

Mishriki Y, D'Amore J, Harris M, et al: Bilateral adult Wilms' tumor. Cancer 59:1210–1213, 1987.

Mukai M, Torikata C, Hisami I, et al: Crystalloids in angiomyolipoma. A previously unnoticed phenomenon of renal angiomyolipoma occurring at a high frequency. Am J Surg Pathol 16:1–10, 1992.

Murphy WM, Zambroni BR, Emerson LD, et al: Aspiration biopsy of the kidney: Simultaneous collection of cytologic and histologic specimens. Cancer 56:200–205, 1985.

Pathak S, Strong LC, Ferrell RE, Trindale A: Familial renal cell carcinoma with a 3:11 chromosome translocation limited to tumor cells. Science 217:939–941, 1982.

Pettinato G, Manivel JC, Wick MR, Dehner LP: Classical and cellular (atypical) congenital mesoblastic nephroma. A clinocopathologic ultrastructural, immunohistochemical and flow cytometric study. Hum Pathol 20:682–690, 1989.

Pritchett TR, Lieskovsky G, Skinner DG: Extension of renal cell carcinoma into the vena cava: Clinical review and surgical approach. J Urol 135:460–464, 1986.

Ro JY, Ayala AG, Sella A, et al: Sarcomatoid renal cell carcinoma: Clinicopathologic. A study of 42 cases. Cancer 59:516–526, 1987.

Rumpelt HJ, Storkel S, Moll R, et al: Bellini duct carcinoma: further evidence for this rare variant of renal cell carcinoma. Histopathol 18:115–122, 1991.

Schmidt D, Harms D, Evers KG, et al: Bone metastasizing renal tumor (clear cell sarcoma) of childhood with epithelioid elements. Cancer 56:609–613, 1985.

Schumann GB, Weiss MA: Atlas of Renal and Urinary Tract Cytology and Its Histopathologic Bases. JB Lippincott Co, Philadelphia, 1981.

Seizinger BR, Rouleau GA, Ozelius LJ, et al: Von Hippel-Lindau disease maps to the region of chromosome 3 associated with renal cell carcinoma. Nature 332:268–269, 1988.

Skinner DG, Colvin RB, Vermillion CD, et al: Diagnosis and management of renal cell carcinoma: A clinical and pathologic study of 309 cases. Cancer 28:1165–1177, 1971.

Sotelo-Avila C, Gonzalez-Crussi F, Sadowinski S, et al: Clear cell sarcoma of the kidney: A clinicopathologic study of 21 patients with long-term follow-up evaluation. Hum Pathol 16:1219–1230, 1986.

Squires JP, Ulbright TM, DeSchryver-Kecskemeti K, et al: Juxtaglomerular cell tumor of the kidney. Cancer 53:516–523, 1984.

Strong DW, Pearse HD: Recurrent urothelial tumors following surgery for transitional cell carcinoma of the upper urinary tract. Cancer 38:2178–2183, 1976.

Thoenes W, Storkel ST, Rumpelt HJ, et al: Chromophobe renal cell carcinoma and its variants—a report on 32 cases. J Pathol 155:277–287, 1988.

Tsuneyoshi M, Daimaru Y, Hashimoto H, et al: Malignant soft tissue neoplasms with histologic features of renal rhabdoid tumors: An ultrastructural and immunohistochemical study. Hum Pathol 16:1235–1242, 1985.

Ugarte N, Gonzalez-Crussi F, Hsueh W: Wilms' tumor: Its morphology in patients under one year of age. Cancer 48:346–353, 1981.

von Schreeb T, Franzen S, Ljungquist A: Renal adenocarcinoma. Evaluation of malignancy on a cytologic basis: A comparative cytologic and histologic study. Scand J Urol Nephrol 1:265–269, 1967.

Weiss MA, Saleba KP, Henderson KS: Fine needle aspiration cytology of renal masses. American Society of Clinical Pathologists Check Sample (C84-6), vol. 12, no. 6, 1984.

Chapter 12: Bladder Neoplasms

Anderstrom C, Johannson SL, von Schultz L: Primary adenocarcinoma of the urinary bladder: A clinicopathologic and prognostic study. Cancer 52:1273–1280, 1983.

Bessette PL, Abell MR, Herwig KR: A clinicopathologic study of squamous cell carcinoma of the bladder. J Urol 112:66–67, 1974.

Boon ME, Blomjous ECM, Zwartendijk J, et al: Carcinoma in situ of the urinary bladder: clinical presentations, cytologic pattern, and stromal changes. Acta Cytol 30:360–366, 1986.

Bouffioux CRA: Epidemiology of bladder cancer. In Kuss R, Khoury S, Denis L, et al. (eds.) Bladder Cancer Part A: Pathology, Diagnosis and Surgery. Progress in Clinical and Biological Research, vol. 162A. Alan R Liss Inc, New York, 1984, pp. 11–25.

Chin JL, Huben RP, Nava E, et al: Flow cytometric analysis of DNA content in human bladder tumors and irrigation fluids. Cancer 56:1677–1681, 1985.

Choi H, Lamb S, Pintar K, et al: Primary signet-ring cell carcinoma of the urinary bladder. Cancer 53:1985–1990, 1984.

Coon JS, McCall A, Miller AW, et al: Expression of blood group-related antigens in carcinoma in situ of the urinary bladder. Cancer 56:797–804, 1985.

Coon JS, Schwartz D, Summers JL, et al: Flow cytometric analysis of deparaffinized nuclei in urinary bladder cancer: Comparison with cytogenetic analysis. Cancer 57:1594–1601, 1986.

Coon JS, Weinstein RS, Summers JL: Blood group precursor T-antigen expression in human urinary bladder carcinoma. Am J Clin Pathol 77:692–699, 1982.

Cummings KB: Carcinoma of the bladder: Predictors. Cancer 45:1849–1855, 1980.

Cummings KB: Classification of patients with bladder cancer: Clinical versus pathologic staging. In Kuss R, Khoury S, Denis L, et al. (eds.) Bladder Cancer Part A: Pathology, Diagnosis and Surgery. Progress in Clinical and Biological Research, vol. 162A. Alan R Liss Inc, New York, 1984, pp. 33–54.

Dalesio O, Schulman CC, Sylvester R, et al: Prognostic factors in superficial bladder tumors. A study of the European Organization for Research on Treatment of Cancer: Genitourinary Tract Cancer Cooperative Group. J Urol 129:730–733, 1983.

Farrow GM: Urine cytology of transitional cell carcinoma: Diagnostic efficacy. In Weid CL, Koss LG, Reagan JW (eds.) Compendium on Diagnostic Cytology, 5th ed. Tutorials of Cytology, Chicago, 1983, pp. 428–435.

Hofstadter F, Delgado R, Jakse G, et al: Urothelial dysplasia and carcinoma in situ of the bladder. Cancer 57:356–361, 1986.

Johnson DE, Schoenwald MB, Ayala AG, et al: Squamous cell carcinoma of the bladder. J Urol 115:542–544, 1976.

Knoll LD, Segura JW, Scheithauer BW: Leiomyoma of the bladder. J Urol 136:906–908, 1986.

Koss LG: Evaluation of patients with carcinoma in situ of the bladder. In Sommers SC, Rosen PP (eds.) Pathology Annual, vol. 17, pt. 2. Appleton–Century-Crofts, Norwalk, 1982, pp. 353–359.

Koss LG: Mapping of the urinary bladder: Its impact on the concept of bladder cancer. Hum Pathol 10:533–538, 1979.

Koss LG: Tumors of the urinary bladder. In Firminger HI (ed.) Atlas of Tumor Pathology, 2nd series, fascicle 11. Armed Forces Institute of Pathology, Washington DC, 1975.

Kunze E, Schauer A, Schmitt M: Histology and histogenesis of two different types of inverted urothelial papillomas. Cancer 51:348–358, 1983.

Leestma JE, Price EB: Paraganglioma of the urinary bladder. Cancer 28:1063–1073, 1971.

Limas C, Lange F: T-antigen in normal and neoplastic urothelium. Cancer 58:1236–1245, 1986.

Limas C, Lange PH: Tissue blood group-associated antigens in urothelial neoplasia: Theory and clinical application. In Platt NR (ed.) Pathology Update Series, vol. 1, lesson 40. Continuing Professional Education Center, Inc, Princeton, 1984.

Mahadevia PS, Alexander JE, Rojas-Corona R, Koss LG: Pseudosarcomatous stromal reaction in primary and metastatic urothelial carcinoma. A source of diagnostic difficulty. Am J Surg Pathol 13:782–790, 1989.

Mahadevia PS, Koss LG, Tar IJ: Prostate involvement in bladder cancer: Prostate mapping in 20 cytoprostatectomy specimens. Cancer 58:2096–2102, 1986.

Miller DC, Gang DL, Gavris V, et al: Villous adenoma of the urinary bladder: A morphologic or biologic entity. Am J Clin Pathol 79:728–731, 1983.

Mills SE, Wolfe JT, Weiss MA, et al: Small cell undifferentiated carcinoma of the urinary bladder: A light microscopic, immunocytochemical, and ultrastructural study of 12 cases. Am J Surg Pathol (in press).

Mincione GP: Primary malignant lymphoma of the urinary bladder with a positive cytology report. Acta Cytol 26:69–72, 1982.

Mostofi FK, Sesterhenn IA: Pathology of epithelial tumors and carcinoma in situ of bladder. In Kuss R, Khoury S, Denis L, et al. (eds.) Bladder Cancer Part A. Pathology, Diagnosis and Surgery. Progress in Clinical and Biological Research, vol. 162A. Alan R Liss Inc, New York, 1984, pp. 55–74.

Murphy WM, Soloway MS: Developing carcinoma (dysplasia) of the urinary bladder. In Sommers SC, Rosen PP (eds.) Pathology Annual, vol. 17, pt. 1. Appleton-Century-Crofts, Norwalk, 1982, pp. 197–217.

Murphy WM, Soloway MS: Urothelial dysplasia. J Urol 127:849–854, 1982.

Murphy WM, Soloway MS, Jukkola AF, et al: Urinary cytology and bladder cancer: The cellular features of transitional cell neoplasms. Cancer 53:1555–1565, 1984.

Nagy GK, Frable WJ, Murphy WM: Classification of premalignant urothelial abnormalities: A Delphi study of the National Bladder Cancer Collaborative Group A. In Sommers SC, Rosen PP (eds) Pathology Annual, vol. 17, pt. 1. Appleton-Century-Crofts, Norwalk, 1982, pp. 219–233.

Obe JA, Rosen N, Koss LG: Primary choriocarcinoma of the urinary bladder: Report of a case with probable epthelial origin. Cancer 52:1405–1409, 1982.

Prout GR: Classification and staging of bladder carcinoma. Semin Oncol 6:189–197, 1979.

Richie JP, Waisman J, Skinner DG, et al: Squamous cell carcinoma of the bladder: Treatment by radical cystectomy. J Urol 115:670–672, 1976.

Schroeder LE, Weiss MA, Hughes C: Squamous cell carcinoma of bladder: An increased incidence in blacks. Urology 28:288–291, 1986.

Schuman GB, Weiss MA: Atlas of Renal and Urinary Tract Cytology and Its Histopathologic Bases. JB Lippincott Co, Philadelphia, 1981.

Shenoy VA, Colby TV, Schumann GB: Reliability of urinary cytodiagnosis in urothelial neoplasms. Cancer 56:2041–2045, 1985.

Soloway MS: Overview of treatment of superficial bladder cancer. Urology 26(suppl):18–26, 1985.

Soloway MS, Bicknell L: Role of selected mucosal biopsies in the evaluation of patients with bladder cancer. In Kuss R, Khoury S, Denis L, et al. (eds.) Bladder Cancer Part A: Pathology, Diagnosis and Surgery. Progress in Clinical and Biological Research, vol. 162A. Alan R Liss Inc, New York, pp. 275–281, 1984.

Weiss MA: Urinary cytology of transitional cell neoplasms of the bladder, p. 245. In Young R (ed.): Pathology of the Urinary Bladder. Churchill Livingstone, New York, 1989.

Young RH: Carcinosarcoma of the urinary bladder. Cancer 59:1333–1339, 1987.

Young RH, Proppe KH, Dickerson R, et al: Myxoid leiomyosarcoma of the urinary bladder. Arch Pathol Lab Med 111:359–362, 1987.

Zincke H, Utz DC, Farrow GM: Review of Mayo Clinic experience with carcinoma in situ. Urology 26(suppl): 39–46, 1985.

Young RH, Wick MR: Transitional cell carcinoma of the urinary bladder with pseudosarcomatous stroma. Am J Clin Pathol 89:216–219, 1988.

Section VI: Lesions of the Prostate and Seminal Vesicles

Chapter 13: Nonneoplastic Lesions of the Prostate and Seminal Vesicles

Arias-Stella J, Takano-Moron J: Atypical epithelial changes in the seminal vesicle. Arch Pathol 66:761–766, 1958.

Ayala AG, Srigley JR, Ro JY, et al: Clear cell cribriform hyperplasia of prostate. Report of 10 cases. Am J Clin Pathol 10:665–671, 1986.

Beckman EN, Leonard GL, Pintado SO, et al: Endometriosis of the prostate. Am J Surg Pathol 9:374–379, 1985.

Bryan RL, Newman J, Campbell A, et al: Granulomatous prostatitis: A clinicopathological study. Histopathology 19:453–457, 1991.

Cleary KR, Choi HY, Ayala AG: Basal cell hyperplasia of the prostate. Am J Clin Pathol 80:850–854, 1983.

Cramer SF: Benign glandular inclusions in prostatic nerve. Am J Clin Pathol 75:854–855, 1981.

Drach GW, Kohnen PW: Prostatitis. In Tannenbaum M (ed.) Urologic Pathology: The Prostate. Lea & Febiger, Philadelphia, 1977.

Drach GW, Meares EM, Fair WR, et al: Classification of benign diseases associated with prostatic pain: Prostatitis or prostatodynia? (letter). J Urol 120:266, 1978.

Epstein JI, Hutchins GM: Granulomatous prostatitis: Distinction among allergic, nonspecific, and posttransurethral resection lesions. Hum Pathol 15:818–825, 1984.

Epstein JI, Cho KR, Quinn BD: Relationship of severe dysplasia to Stage A (incidental) adenocarcinoma of the prostate. Cancer 65:2321–2327, 1990.

Eykyn S, Bultitude MI, Mayo ME, et al: Prostatic calculi as a source of recurrent bacteriuria in the male. Br J Urol 46:527–532, 1974.

Fair WR, Couch J, Wehner N: Prostatic antibacterial factor: Identity and significance. Urology 7:169–177, 1976.

Frauenhoffer EE, Ro JY, El-Naggar AK, et al: Clear cell cribriform hyperplasia of the prostate. Immunohistochemical and DNA flow cytometric study. Am J Clin Pathol 95:446–453, 1991.

Gleason DF: Atypical hyperplasia, benign hyperplasia, and well-differentiated adenocarcinoma of the prostate. Am J Surg Pathol 9:53–67, 1985.

Kelalis PP, Greene LF, Harrison EG Jr: Granulomatous prostatitis: A mimic of carcinoma of the prostate. JAMA 191:287–289, 1965.

Kost LV, Evans GW: Occurrence and significance of striated muscle within the prostate. J Urol 92:703–704, 1964.

Krieger JN: Prostatitis, epididymitis, and orchitis. In Mandell GL, Douglas RG Jr, Bennett JE (eds.) Principles and Practice of Infectious Diseases, 2nd ed. John Wiley & Sons Inc, New York, 1985.

Kuo T-T, Gomez LG: Monstrous epithelial cells in human epididymis and seminal vesicles: A pseudomalignant change. Am J Surg Pathol 5:483–490, 1981.

Lager DJ, Goeken JA, Kemp JD, Robinson RA: Squamous metaplasia of the prostate. An immunohistochemical report. Am J Clin Pathol 90:597–601, 1988.

McNeal JE: Origin and development of carcinoma in the prostate. Cancer 23:24–34, 1969.

McNeal JE, Bostwick DG: Intraductal dysplasia: A premalignant lesion of the prostate. Hum Pathol 17:64–71, 1986.

McNeal JE, Villers A, Redwine EA, et al: Microcarcinoma of the prostate: Its association with duct-acinar dysplasia. Hum Pathol 22:644–652, 1991.

Meares EM Jr: Influence of infections of the male accessory glands on secretory function, sperm viability and fertility. In Spring-Mills E, Hafez ESE (eds.) Accessory Glands of the Male Reproductive Tract. Ann Arbor Science, Ann Arbor, 1979.

Meares EM, Stamey TA: Bacteriologic localization patterns in bacterial prostatitis and urethritis. Invest Urol 5:492–518, 1968.

Melicow MM: Allergic granulomas of the prostate gland. J Urol 65:288–296, 1951.

Mies C, Balogh K, Stadecker M: Palisading prostate granulomas following surgery. Am J Surg Pathol 8:217–221, 1984.

Mostofi FK, Morse WH: Epithelial metaplasia in "prostatic infarction." Arch Pathol 51:340–345, 1951.

Pieterse AS, Aarons I, Jose JS: Focal prostatic granulomas rheumatoidlike—probably iatrogenic in origin. Pathology 16:174–177, 1984.

Price MJ, Lewis EL, Carmalt JE: Coccidioidomycosis of prostate gland. Urology 19:653–655, 1982.

Quinn BD, Cho KR, Epstein JI: Relationship of severe dysplasia to stage B adenocarcinoma of the prostate. Cancer 65:2328–2337, 1990.

Proppe KH, Scully RE, Rosai J: Postoperative spindle cell nodules of genitourinary tract resembling sarcomas: A report of eight cases. Am J Surg Pathol 8:101–108, 1984.

Randall A: Surgical Pathology of Prostatic Obstructions. Williams & Wilkins Co, Baltimore, 1931.

Schwarz J: Mycotic prostatitis. Urology 19:1–5, 1982.

Simon HB, Weinstein AJ, Pasternack MS: Genitourinary tuberculosis: Clinical features in a general hospital population. Am J Med 63:410–420, 1977.

Walsh PC: Benign prostatic hyperplasia. In Harrison JH, Gittes RF, Perlmutter AD, et al. (eds.) Campbell's Urology, 4th ed. WB Saunders Co, Philadelphia, 1979.

Chapter 14: Neoplastic Lesions of the Prostate and Seminal Vesicles

Accetta PA, Gardner WA Jr: Squamous metastases from prostatic adenocarcinoma (abstract). Lab Invest 46:2A, 1982.

Almagro UA: Argyrophilic prostatic carcinoma: Case report with literature review on prostatic carcinoid and "carcinoid-like" prostatic carcinoma. Cancer 55:608–614, 1985.

Azumi N, Shibuya H, Ishikura M: Primary prostatic carcinoid tumor with intracytoplasmic prostatic acid phosphatase and prostatic-specific antigen. Am J Surg Pathol 8:545–550, 1984.

Azumi N, Traweek ST, Battifora H: Prostatic acid phosphatase in carcinoid tumors. Immunohistochemical and immunoblot studies. Am J Surg Pathol 15:785–790, 1991.

Azzopardi JG, Evans DJ: Argentaffin cells in prostatic carcinoma: Differentiation from lipofuscin and melanin in prostatic epithelium. J Pathol 104:247–251, 1970.

Babaian RJ, Camps JL: The role of prostate-specific antigen as part of the diagnostic triad and as a guide when to perform a biopsy. Cancer 68:2060–2063, 1991.

Bain GO, Koch M, Hanson J: Feasibility of grading prostatic carcinomas. Arch Pathol Lab Med 106:265–267, 1982.

Bhagavan BS, Tiamson EM, Wenk RE, et al: Nephrogenic adenoma of the urinary bladder and urethra. Hum Pathol 12:907–916, 1981.

Bostwick DG, Brawer MK: Prostatic intra-epithelial neoplasia and early invasion in prostate cancer. Cancer 59:788–794, 1987.

Bostwick DG, Kindrachuk RW, Rouse RV: Prostatic adenocarcinoma with endometrioid features: Clinical, pathologic, and ultrastructural findings. Am J Surg Pathol 9:595–609, 1985.

Bostwick DG, Mann RB: Malignant lymphomas involving the prostate: A study of 13 cases. Cancer 56:2932–2938, 1985.

Cho KR, Epstein JI: Metastatic prostatic carcinoma to supradiaphragmatic lymph nodes. A clinicopathologic and immunohistochemical study. Am J Surg Pathol 11:457–463, 1987.

diSant' Agnese PA, de Mesy Jensen KL: Endocrine-paracrine cells of the prostate and prostatic urethra: An ultrastructural study. Hum Pathol 15:1034–1041, 1984.

diSant' Agnese PA, de Mesy Jensen KL: Neuroendocrine differentiation in prostatic carcinoma. Hum Pathol 18:849–856, 1987.

Epstein JI, Lieberman PH: Mucinous adenocarcinoma of the prostate gland. Am J Surg Pathol 9:299–308, 1985.

Epstein JI, Woodruff JM: Adenocarcinoma of the prostate with endometrioid features: A light microscopic and immunohistochemical study of ten cases. Cancer 57: 111–119, 1986.

Frankel K, Craig JR: Adenoid cystic carcinoma of the prostate: Report of a case. Am J Clin Pathol 62:639–645, 1974.

Franks LM: Etiology and epidemiology of human prostatic disorders. In Tannenbaum M (ed.) Urologic Pathology: The Prostate. Lea & Febiger, Philadelphia, 1977.

Franks LM: Etiology, epidemiology and pathology of prostatic cancer. Cancer 32:1092–1095, 1973.

Glancy RJ, Gaman AJ, Rippey JJ: Polyps and papillary lesions of the prostatic urethra. Pathology 15:153–157, 1983.

Gleason DF: Histologic grading and clinical staging of prostatic carcinoma. In Tannenbaum M (ed.) Urologic Pathology: The Prostate. Lea & Febiger, Philadelphia, 1977.

Gleason DF, Mellinger GT: Veterans Administration Cooperative Urologic Research Group: Prediction of prognosis for prostatic adenocarcinoma and combined histologic grading and clinical staging. J Urol 111:58–64, 1974.

Gray GF Jr, Marshall VF: Squamous carcinoma of the prostate. J Urol 113:736–738, 1975.

Grignon DJ, Ro JY, Ordonez NG, et al: Basal cell hyperplasia, adenoid basal cell tumor, and adenoid cystic carcinoma of the prostate gland. An immunohistochemical study. Hum Pathol 19:1425–1433, 1988.

Hedrick L, Epstein JI: Use of keratin 903 as an adjunct in the diagnosis of prostate carcinoma. Am J Surg Pathol 13:389–396, 1989.

Holmes EJ: Crystalloids of prostatic carcinoma: Relationship to Bence-Jones crystals. Cancer 39:2073–2080, 1973.

Johnson DE, Hogan JM, Ayala AG: Transitional cell carcinoma of the prostate: A clinical morphological study. Cancer 29:287–293, 1972.

Kafandaris PM, Polyzonis MB: Fibroadenoma-like foci in human prostatic nodular hyperplasia. Prostate 4:33–36, 1983.

Kamoshida S, Tsutsumi Y: Extraprostatic localization of prostatic specific acid phosphatase and prostate-specific antigen: Distribution in cloacogenic glandular epithelium and sex-dependent expression in human anal gland. Hum Pathol 21:1108–1111, 1990.

Kuhajda FP, Mann RB: Adenoid cystic carcinoma of the prostate: A case report with immunoperoxidase staining for prostatic-specific acid phosphatase and prostate-specific antigen. Am J Clin Pathol 81:257–260, 1984.

Manivel C, Shenoy BV, Wick MR, et al: Cystosarcoma phyllodes of the prostate: A pathologic and immunohistochemical study. Arch Pathol Lab Med 110: 534–538, 1986.

Martin SA, Santa Cruz DJ: Adenomatoid metaplasia of the prostatic urethra. Am J Clin Pathol 75:185–189, 1981.

McNeal JE, Reese JH, Redwine EA, et al: Cribriform adenocarcinoma of the prostate. Cancer 58:1714–1719, 1986.

McNeal JE, Alroy J, Villers A, et al: Mucinous differentiation in prostatic adenocarcinoma. Hum Pathol 22:979–988, 1991.

Melicow MM, Pachter MR: Endometrial carcinoma of the prostatic utricle (uterus masculinus). Cancer 20:1715–1722, 1967.

Melicow MM, Tannenbaum M: Endometrial carcinoma of the uterus masculinus (prostatic utricle): Report of six cases. J Urol 106:892–902, 1971.

Moore GH, Lawshe B, Murphy G: Diagnosis of adenocarcinoma in transurethral resectates of the prostate gland. Am J Surg Pathol 10:165–169, 1986.

Moyana TN: Adenosquamous carcinoma of the prostate. Am J Surg Pathol 11:403–407, 1987.

Murphy GP, Whitmore WF Jr: A report of the workshops on the current status of the histologic grading of prostate cancer. Cancer 44:1490–1494, 1979.

Murphy WM, Dean PJ, Brasfield JA, et al: Incidental carcinoma of the prostate: How much sampling is adequate? Am J Surg Pathol 10:170–174, 1986.

Nadji M, Tabei SZ, Castro A, et al: Prostatic origin of tumors: An immunohistochemical study. Am J Clin Pathol 73:735–739, 1980.

Nadji M, Tabei SZ, Castro A, et al: Prostatic-specific antigen: An immunohistologic marker for prostatic neoplasms. Cancer 48:1229–1232, 1981.

Nowels K, Kent E, Rinsho K, Oyasu R: Prostate specific antigen and acid phosphatase-reactive cells in cystitis cystica and glandularis. Arch Pathol Lab Med 112:734–737, 1988.

Reed RJ: Consultation case (adenoid basal-cell tumor). Am J Surg Pathol 8:699–704, 1984.

Remick DG Jr, Kumar NB: Benign polyps with prostatic-type epithelium of the urethra and the urinary bladder: A suggestion of histogenesis based on histologic and immunohistochemical studies. Am J Surg Pathol 8:833–839, 1984.

Rhamy RK, Buchanan RD, Spalding MJ: Intraductal carcinoma of the prostate gland. J Urol 109:457–463, 1973.

Ro JY, Ayala AG, Ordonez NG, et al: Intraluminal crystalloids in prostatic adenocarcinoma: Immunohistochemical, electron microscopic, and X-ray microanalytic studies. Cancer 57:2397–2407, 1986.

Ro JY, Tetu B, Ayala AG, Ordonez NG: Small cell carcinoma of the prostate. II. Immunohistochemical electron microscopic studies in 18 cases. Cancer 59:977–982, 1987.

Ro JY, El-Naggar A, Ayala AG, et al: Signet-ring-cell carcinoma of the prostate. Electron-microscopic and immunohistochemical studies of eight cases. Am J Surg Pathol 12:453–460, 1988.

Ro JY, Grignon DJ, Ayala AG, et al: Mucinous adenocarcinoma of the prostate. Histochemical and immunohistochemical studies. Hum Pathol 21:593–600, 1990.

Rubenstein AB, Rubnitz ME: Transitional cell carcinoma of the prostate. Cancer 24:543–546, 1969.

Saito R, Davis BK, Ollapally EP: Adenosquamous carcinoma of the prostate. Hum Pathol 15:87–89, 1984.

Schron DS, Gipson T, Mendelsohn G: The histogenesis of small cell carcinoma of the prostate: An immunohistochemical study. Cancer 53:2478–2480, 1984.

Stein BS, Vangore S, Peterson RO, et al: Immunoperoxidase localization of prostatic-specific antigen. Am J Surg Pathol 6:553–557, 1982.

Taylor NS: Histochemistry in the diagnosis of early prostatic carcinoma. Hum Pathol 10:513–520, 1979.

Tetu B, Ro JY, Ayal AG, et al: Small cell carcinoma of the prostate. Part I. A clinicopathologic study of 20 cases. Cancer 59:1803–1809, 1987.

Turbat-Herrera EA, Herrera GA, Gore I, et al: Neuroendocrine differentiation in prostatic carcinomas. A retrospective autopsy study. Arch Pathol Lab Med 112:1100–1105, 1988.

Vollmer RT: Prostate cancer and chip specimens: Complete versus partial sampling. Hum Pathol 17:285–290, 1986.

Walker AN, Mills SE, Fechner RE, et al: "Endometrial" adenocarcinoma of the prostatic urethra arising in a villous polyp: A light microscopic and immunoperoxidase study. Arch Pathol Lab Med 106:624–627, 1982.

Walker AN, Mills SE, Fechner RE, et al: Epithelial polyps of the prostatic urethra: A light microscopic and immunohistochemical study. Am J Surg Pathol 7:351–356, 1983.

Waring PM, Newland RC: Prostatic embryonal rhabdomyosarcoma in adults. A clinicopathologic review. Cancer 69:755–762, 1992.

Wenk RE, Bhagavan BS, Levy R, et al: Ectopic ACTH, prostatic oat cell carcinoma, and marked hypernatremia. Cancer 40:773–778, 1977.

Young RH, Fierson HF Jr, Mills SE, et al: Adenoid cystic-like tumor of the prostate gland. A report of two cases and review of the literature on "adenoid cystic carcinoma" of the prostate. Am J Clin Pathol 89:49–56, 1988.

Young RH, Scully RE: Clear cell adenocarcinoma of the bladder and urethra: A report of three cases and review of the literature. Am J Surg Pathol 9:816–826, 1985.

Zaloudek C, Williams JW, Kempson RL: "Endometrial" adenocarcinoma of the prostate: A distinctive tumor of probable prostatic duct origin. Cancer 37:2255–2262, 1976.

Section VII: Lesions of the Testis and Associated Structures

Chapter 15: Nonneoplastic Lesions of the Testis

Allen TD: Disorders of sexual differentiation. Urology 7:1–32, 1976.

Craig JM: The pathology of infertility. Pathol Annu 10:299–328, 1975.

Levin HS: Testicular biopsy in the study of male infertility: Its current usefulness, histologic techniques, and prospects for the future. Hum Pathol 5:569–584, 1979.

Jones EC, Clement PB, Young RH: Sclerosing adenosis of the prostate gland. A clinicopathologic and immunohistochemical study of 11 cases. Am J Surg Pathol 15:1171–1180, 1991.

MacLeod J: Human male infertility. Obstet Gynecol Surv 26:335–351, 1971.

Mikuz G, Damjanov I: Inflammation of the testis, epididymis, peritesticular membranes and scrotum. Pathol Annu 17:101–128, 1982.

Morris JM, Mahesh VB: Further observations on the syndrome of "testicular feminization." Am J Obstet Gynecol 87:731–745, 1963.

Nistal M, Paniagua R, Diez-Pardo JA: Histologic classification of undescended testes. Hum Pathol 11:666–674, 1980.

Robboy SJ, Miller T, Donahoe PK, et al: Dysgenesis of testicular and streak gonads in the syndrome of mixed gonadal dysgenesis: Perspective derived from a clinicopathologic analysis of twenty-one cases. Hum Pathol 13:700–716, 1982.

Ronnett BM, Epstein JI: A case showing sclerosing adenosis and an unusual form of basal cell hyperplasia of the prostate. Am J Surg Pathol 13:866–872, 1989.

Rutgers JL, Young RH, Scully RE: The testicular "tumor" of the adrenogenital syndrome. A report of six cases and review of the literature on testicular masses in patients with adrenocortical disorder. Am J Surg Pathol 12:503–513, 1988.

Sakamoto N, Tsuneyoshi M, Enjoji M: Sclerosing adenosis of the prostate. Histopathologic and immunohistochemical analysis. Am J Surg Pathol 15:660–667, 1991.

Scorer CG: The descent of the testis. Arch Dis Child 39:605–609, 1964.

Smith SP, King LR: Torsion of the testis: Techniques of assessment. Urol Clin North Am 6(2):429–443, 1979.

Sohval AR: Hermaphroditism with "atypical" or "mixed" gonadal dysgenesis. Am J Med 36:281–292, 1964.

Sudmann E: The undescended testis: A clinical and histological study. Acta Chir Scand 137:815–822, 1971.

van Niekerk WA: True hermaphroditism: An analytical review with a report of 3 new cases. Am J Obstet Gynecol 126:890–907, 1976.

Wheeler JE, Rudy FR: The testis, paratesticular structures, and male external genitalia. In Silverberg SG (ed.) Principles and Practice of Surgical Pathology. John Wiley & Sons Inc, New York, pp. 1147–1188, 1983.

Williams JD, Hodgson NB: Another look at torsion of the testis. Urology 14:36–38, 1979.

Wong T-W, Straus FH II, Warner NE: Testicular biopsy in the study of male infertility: I. Testicular causes of infertility. Arch Pathol 95:151–159, 1973.

Wong T-W, Straus FH II, Warner NE: Testicular biopsy in the study of male infertility: II. Posttesticular causes of infertility. Arch Pathol 95:160–164,1973.

CHAPTER 16: TESTICULAR NEOPLASMS

Babaian RJ, Johnson DE: Management of stages I and II nonseminomatous germ cell tumors of the testis. Cancer 45:1775–1781, 1980.

Banks ER, Mills SE: Histiocytoid (epithelioid) hemangioma. The so-called vascular variant of "anenomatoid tumor." Am J Surg Pathol 14:584–589, 1990.

Bell DA, Flotte TJ, Bhan AK: Immunohistochemical characterization of seminoma and its inflammatory cell infiltrate. Hum Pathol 18:511–520, 1987.

Berdjis CC, Mostofi FK: Carcinoid tumors of the testes. J Urol 118:777–782, 1977.

Bolen JW: Mixed germ cell–sex cord stromal tumor: A gonadal tumor distinct from gonadoblastoma. Am J Clin Pathol 75:565–573, 1981.

Bredeal JJ, Vugrin D, Whitmore WF Jr: Autopsy findings in 154 patients with germ cell tumors of the testis. Cancer 50:548–551, 1982.

Burke AP, Mostofi FK: Placental alkaline phosphatase immunohistochemistry of intratubular malignant germ cells and associated testicular germ cell tumors. Hum Pathol 19:663–670, 1988.

Cockburn AG, Vugrin D, Batata M, et al: Poorly differentiated (anaplastic) seminoma of the testis. Cancer 53:1991–1994, 1984.

Coffin CM, Ewing S, Dehner LP: Frequency of intratubular germ cell neoplasia with invasive testicular germ cell tumors. Arch Pathol Lab Med 109:555–559, 1985.

Dehner LP: Gonadal and extragonadal germ cell neoplasia of childhood. Hum Pathol 14:493–511, 1983.

Duncan PR, Checa F, Gowing NFC, et al: Extranodal non-Hodgkin's lymphoma presenting in the testicle: A clinical and pathologic study of 24 cases. Cancer 45:1578–1584, 1980.

Epstein BE, Order SE, Zinreich ES: Staging, treatment, and results in testicular seminoma. A 12-year report. Cancer 65:405–411, 1990.

Floyd C, Ayala AG, Logothetis CJ, Silva EG: Spermatocytic seminoma with associated sarcoma of the testis. Cancer 61:409–414, 1988.

Goldstein AMB, Mendez R, Vargas A, et al: Epidermoid cysts of testis. Urology 15:186–189, 1980.

Haupt HM, Mann RB, Trump DL, et al: Metastatic carcinoma involving the testis: Clinical and pathologic distinction from primary testicular neoplasms. Cancer 54:709–714, 1984.

Hedinger Chr, von Hochstetter AR, Egloff B: Seminoma with syncytiotrophoblastic giant cells: A special form of seminoma. Virchows Arch Pathol Anat 383:59–67, 1979.

Hopkins GB, Parry HD: Metastasizing Sertoli cell tumor (androblastoma). Cancer 23:463–467, 1969.

Jacobs EM, Muggia FM: Testicular cancer: Risk factors and the role of adjuvant chemotherapy. Cancer 45:1782–1790, 1980.

Jacobsen GK, Henriksen OB, Der Masse HV: Carcinoma in situ of testicular tissue adjacent to malignant germ cell tumors. Cancer 47:2660–2662, 1981.

Jacobsen GK, Jacobsen M, Clausen PP: Distribution of tumor-associated antigens in the various histologic components of germ cell tumors of the testis. Am J Surg Pathol 5:257–266, 1981.

Javadpour N: The role of biologic tumor markers in testicular cancer. Cancer 45:1755–1761, 1980.

Javadpour N, McIntire KR, Waldman TA: Human chorionic gonadotropin (HCG) and alpha-fetoprotein (AFP) in sera and tumor cells of patients with testicular seminoma. Cancer 42:2768–2772, 1978.

Kim I, Young RH, Scully RE: Leydig cell tumors of the testis: A clinicopathological analysis of 40 cases and review of the literature. Am J Surg Pathol 9:177–192, 1985.

Koide O, Iwai S, Baba K, Iri H: Identification of testicular atypical germ cells by an immunohistochemical technique for placental alkaline phosphatase. Cancer 60:1325–1330, 1987.

Loftus BM, Gilmartin LG, O'Brien MJ, Carney DN, Dervan PA: Intratubular germ cell neoplasia of the testis: Identification of placental alkaline phosphatase immunostaining and argyrophilic nucleolar organizer region quantification. Hum Pathol 21:941–948, 1990.

Logothetis CJ, Samuels ML, Trindade A, et al: The growing teratoma syndrome. Cancer 50:1629–1635, 1982.

Manivel JC, Jessurun J, Wick MR, Dehner LR: Placental alkaline phosphatase immunoreactivity in testicular germ-cell neoplasms. Am J Surg Pathol 11:21–29, 1987.

Manivel JC, Reinberg Y, Niehans GA, Fraley EE: Intratubular germ cell neoplasia in testicular teratomas and epidermoid cysts. Correlation with prognosis and possible biologic significance. Cancer 64:715–720, 1989.

Matoska J, Ondrus D, Hornak M: Metastatic spermatocytic seminoma. A case report with light microscopic, ultrastructural, and immunohistochemical findings. Cancer 62:1197–1201, 1988.

Mostofi FK: Pathology of germ cell tumors of testis: A progress report. Cancer 45:1735–1754, 1980.

Mostofi FK: Testicular tumors: Epidemiologic, etiologic, and pathologic features. Cancer 32:1186–1201,1973.

Mostofi FK, Price EB Jr: Tumors of the Male Genital System. Armed Forces Institute of Pathology, Washington, DC, 1973.

Niehans GA, Manivel JC, Copland GT, et al: Immunohistochemistry of germ cell and trophoblastic neoplasms. Cancer 62:1113–1123, 1988.

Nochomovitz LE, Rosai J: Current concepts in the histogenesis, pathology and immunochemistry of germ cell tumors of the testis. Pathol Annu 13:327–362, 1978.

Paladug VPP, Bearman RM, Rappaport H: Malignant lymphoma with primary manifestation in the gonad. Cancer 45:561–571, 1980.

Proppe KH, Scully RE: Large-cell calcifying Sertoli cell tumor of the testis. Am J Clin Pathol 74:607–619, 1980.

Pugh RCB (ed.) Pathology of the Testis. Blackwell Scientific Publications Inc, Oxford, 1976.

Shah KH, Maxted WC, Chun B: Epidermoid cysts of the testis: A report of three cases and an analysis of 141 cases from the world literature. Cancer 47:577–582, 1981.

Skakkebaek NE: Carcinoma in situ of the testis: Frequency and relationship to invasive germ cell tumours in infertile men. Histopathology 2:157–170, 1978.

Talerman A: A distinctive gonadal neoplasm related to gonadoblastoma. Cancer 30:1219–1224, 1972.

Talerman A: Germ cell tumors of the testis: In Fenoglio CM, Wolff M (eds.) Progress in Surgical Pathology, vol. 1. Masson Publishing USA Inc, New York, 1980;175–204.

Talerman A: Spermatocytic seminoma: Clinicopathologic study of 22 cases. Cancer 45:2169–2176, l980.

Talerman A, Fu YS, Okagaki T: Spermatocytic seminoma: Ultrastructural and microspectrophotometric observations. Lab Invest 51:343–349, 1984.

Tiffany P, Morse MJ, Bosl G, et al: Sequential excision of residual thoracic and retroperitoneal masses after chemotherapy for Stage II germ cell tumors. Cancer 57:978–983, 1986.

True LD, Otis CN, Delprado W, Scully RE, Rosai J: Spermatocytic seminoma of testis with sarcomatous transformation. A report of five cases. Am J Surg Pathol 12:75–82, 1988.

Turner RR, Colby TV, MacKintosh FR: Testicular lymphomas: A clinicopathologic study of 35 cases. Cancer 48:2095–2102, 1981.

Ulbright TM, Loehrer PJ, Roth LM, et al: The development of non-germ cell malignancies within germ cell tumors: A clinicopathologic study of 11 cases. Cancer 54:1824–1833, 1984.

Wick MR, Swanson PE, Manivel JC: Placental-like alkaline phosphatase reactivity in human tumors: An immunohistochemical study of 520 cases. Hum Pathol 18:946–954, 1987.

Zukerberg LR, Young RH, Scully RE: Sclerosing Sertoli cell tumor of the testis. A report of 10 cases. Am J Surg Pathol 15:829–834, 1991.

Chapter 17: Lesions of the Tunica Vaginalis, Epididymis, Vas Deferens, and Spermatic Cord

Arlen M, Grabstald H, Whitmore WF Jr: Malignant tumors of the spermatic cord. Cancer 23:525–532, 1969.

Axiotis CA: Intratesticular serous papillary cystadenoma of low malignant potential: An ultrastructural and immunohistochemical study suggesting müllerian differentiation. Am J Surg Pathol 12:56–63, 1988.

Balogh K, Travis WD: The frequency of perineural ductules in vasitis nodosa. Am J Clin Pathol 82:710–713, 1984.

Barbera V, Rubino M: Papillary mesothelioma of the tunica vaginalis. Cancer 10:183–189, 1957.

Barwick KW, Madri JA: An immunohistochemical study of adenomatoid tumors utilizing keratin and factor VIII antibodies: Evidence for a mesothelial origin. Lab Invest 47:276–280, 1982.

Benisch B, Peison B, Sobel HJ, et al: Fibrous mesotheliomas (pseudofibroma) of the scrotal sac: A light and ultrastructural study. Cancer 47:731–735, 1981.

Blumberg HM, Hendrix LE: Serous papillary adenocarcinoma of the tunica vaginalis testis with metastasis. Cancer 67:1450–1453, 1991.

Crisp-Lindgren N, Travers H, Well MM, Cawley LP: Papillary adenocarcinoma of rete testis. Autopsy findings, histochemistry, immunohistochemistry, ultrastructure, and clinical correlations. Am J Surg Pathol 12:492–501, 1988.

Feldman AE, Rosenthal RS, Shaw JL: Aberrant adrenal tissue: An incidental finding during orchiopexy. J Urol 113:706–708, 1975.

Gill WB, Schumacher GFB, Bibbo M: Pathological semen and anatomical abnormalities of the genital tract in human male subjects exposed to diethylstilbestrol in utero. J Urol 117:477–480, 1977.

Goldman R: A Brenner tumor of the testis. Cancer 26:853–856, 1970.

Goldman RL, Azzopardi JG: Benign neural invasion in vasitis nodosa. Histopathology 6:309–315, 1982.

Halvorsen JE, Stray O: Splenogonadal fusion. Acta Paediatr Scand 67:379–381, 1978.

Japko L, Horta AA, Schreiber K, et al: Malignant mesothelioma of the tunica vaginalis testis: Report of first case with preoperative diagnosis. Cancer 49:119–127, 1982.

Kragel PJ, Pestaner J, Travis WD, Linehan WM, Filling-Katz MR: Papillary cystadenoma of the epididymis. A report of three cases with lectin histochemistry. Arch Pathol Lab Med 114:672–675, 1990.

Kuo T-T, Gomez LG: Monstrous epithelial cells in human epididymis and seminal vesicles: A pseudomalignant change. Am J Surg Pathol 5:483–490, 1981.

Nochomovitz LE, Orenstein JM: Adenocarcinoma of the rete testis: Case report, ultrastructural observations, and clinicopathologic correlates. Am J Surg Pathol 8:625–634, 1984.

Nogales FF Jr, Matilla A, Ortega I, et al: Mixed Brenner and adenomatoid tumor of the testis: An ultrastructural study and histogenetic considerations. Cancer 43:539–543, 1979.

Price EB Jr: Papillary cystadenoma of the epididymis: A clinicopathologic analysis of 20 cases. Arch Pathol 91:456–470, 1971.

Quigley JC, Hart WR: Adenomatoid tumors of the uterus. Am J Clin Pathol 76:627–635, 1981.

Ricketts RR, Majmudarr B: Epididymal melanotic neuroectodermal tumor of infancy. Hum Pathol 16:416–420, 1985.

Rosai J, Dehner LP: Nodular mesothelial hyperplasia in hernia sacs: A benign reactive condition simulating a neoplastic process. Cancer 35:165–175, 1975.

Simon HB, Larkin PC: Torsion of the appendix testis: Report of 13 cases. JAMA 202:140–141, 1967.

Skoglund RW, McRoberts JW, Ragde H: Torsion of testicular appendages: Presentation of 43 new cases and a collective review. J Urol 104:598–600, 1970.

Taxy JB, Marshall FF, Erlichman RJ: Vasectomy: Subclinical pathologic changes. Am J Surg Pathol 5:767–772, 1981.

Thompson GJ: Tumors of the spermatic cord, epididymis, and testicular tunics. Surg Gynecol Obstet 62:712–728, 1936.

Tsuda H, Fukushima S, Takahashi M, et al: Familial bilateral papillary cystadenoma of the epididymis: Report of three cases in siblings. Cancer 37:1831–1839, 1976.

Visscher DW, Talerman A, Rivera LR, Mazur MT: Adenocarcinoma of the rete testis with a spindle cell component. A possible metaplastic carcinoma. Cancer 64:770–775, 1989.

Young RH, Scully RE: Testicular and paratesticular tumors and tumor-like lesions of ovarian common epithelial and müllerian types. A report of four cases and review of the literature. Am J Clin Pathol 86:146–152, 1986.

Walker AN, Mills SE: Glandular inclusions in inguinal hernial sacs and spermatic cords: Müllerian-like remnants confused with functional reproductive structures. Am J Clin Pathol 82:85–89, 1984.

Walker AN, Mills SE, Jones PF, Stanley CM III: Borderline serous cystadenoma of the tunica vaginalis testis. Surg Pathol 1:431–436, 1988.

Wick MR, Rife CC: Paratesticular accessory spleen. Mayo Clin Proc 56:455–456, 1981.

Zimmerman KG, Johnson PC, Paplanus SH: Nerve invasion by proliferating ductules in vasitis nodosa. Cancer 51:2066–2069, 1983.

Section VIII: Lesions of the Penis, Scrotum, and Urethra

Chapter 18: Nonneoplastic Lesions of the Penis, Scrotum, and Urethra

Ackerman AB, Kornberg R: Pearly penile papules: Acral angiofibromas. Arch Dermatol 108:673–675, 1973.

Crum CP, Ikenberg H, Richart R, et al: Human papillomavirus type 16 and early cervical neoplasia. N Engl J Med 310:880–883, 1984.

Domonkos AN, Arnold HL Jr, Odom RB: Andrews' Diseases of the Skin: Clinical Dermatology, 7th ed. WB Saunders Co, Philadelphia, 1982.

Gissman L, Wolnick L, Ikenberg H, et al: Human papillomavirus types 6 and 11, DNA sequences in genital and laryngeal papillomas and in some cervical cancers. Proc Natl Acad Sci (USA) 80:560–563, 1983.

Lever WF, Schaumburg-Lever G: Histopathology of the Skin, 6th ed. JB Lippincott Co, Philadelpha, 1983.

Mandell GL, Douglas RG, Bennett JE: Principles and Practice of Infectious Diseases, 2nd ed. John Wiley & Sons Inc, New York, 1985.

Marshall FC, Uson AC, Melicow MM: Neoplasms and caruncles of the female urethra. Surg Gynecol Obstet 110:723–733, 1960.

Smith BH: Peyronie's disease, Am J Clin Pathol 45: 670–678, 1966.

Chapter 19: Neoplastic Lesions of the Penis, Scrotum, and Urethra

Battifora H: Spindle cell carcinoma: Ultrastructural evidence of squamous origin and collagen production by tumor cells. Cancer 37:2275–2282, 1976.

Dehner LP, Smith BH: Soft tissue tumors of the penis: A clinicopathologic study of 46 cases. Cancer 25:1431–1447, 1970.

deKernion JB, Tynberg P, Persky L, et al: Carcinoma of the penis. Cancer 32:1256–1262, 1973.

DeVillez RL, Stevens CS: Bowenoid papules of the genitalia: A case progressing to Bowen's disease. J Am Acad Dermatol 3:149–152, 1980.

Fraley EE, Zhang G, Sazama R, et al: Cancer of the penis: Prognosis and treatment plans. Cancer 55:1618–1624, 1985.

Grabstad H: Tumors of the urethra in men and women. Cancer 32:1236–1255, 1973.

Hanash KA, Furlow WL, Utz DC, et al: Carcinoma of the penis: A clinicopathologic study. J Urol 104: 291–297, 1970.

Higgins GD, Uzelin DM, Phillips GE, et al: Differing prevalence of human papillomavirus RNA in penile dysplasias and carcinomas may reflect differing etiologies. Am J Clin Pathol 97:272–278, 1992.

Levine RL: Urethral cancer. Cancer 45:1965–1972, 1980.

Lowe FC: Squamous cell carcinoma of the scrotum. J Urol 130:423–427, 1983.

Manglani KS, Manaligod JR, Ray B: Spindle cell carcinoma of the glans penis: A light and electron microscopic study. Cancer 46:2266–2272, 1980.

McDonald MW: Carcinoma of scrotum. Urology 19:269–274, 1982.

McKee PH, Lowe D, Haigh RJ: Penile verrucous carcinoma. Histopathology 7:897–906, 1983.

Merrin CE: Cancer of the penis. Cancer 45:1973–1979, 1980.

Mitsudo S, Nakanishi I, Koss LG: Paget's disease of the penis and adjacent skin. Arch Pathol Lab Med 105:518–520, 1981.

Narayana AS, Olney LE, Loening SA, et al: Carcinoma of the penis: Analysis of 219 cases. Cancer 49:2185–2191, 1982.

Oldbring J, Mikulowski P: Malignant melanoma of the penis and male urethra. Report of nine cases and review of the literature. Cancer 59:581–587, 1987.

Patterson JW, Kao GF, Graham JH, et al: Bowenoid papulosis: A clinicopathologic study with ultrastructural observations. Cancer 57:823–836, 1986.

Perez MA, LaRossa DD, Tomaszewski JE: Paget's disease primarily involving the scrotum. Cancer 63:970–975, 1989.

Sprigley JR, Ayala AG, Ordonez NG, et al: Epithelioid hemangioma of the penis: A rare and distinctive vascular lesion. Arch Pathol Lab Med 109:51–54, 1985.

Ulbright TM, Stehman FB, Roth LM, et al: Bowenoid dysplasia of the vulva. Cancer 50:2910–2919, 1982.

Varma VA, Sanchez-Lanier M, Unger ER, et al: Association of human papillomavirus with penile carcinoma: A study using polymerase chain reaction and in-situ hybridization. Hum Pathol 22:908–913, 1991.

Wade TR, Kopf AW, Ackerman AB: Bowenoid papulosis of the penis. Cancer 42:1890–1903, 1978.

Section IX: Lesions of the Adrenal Gland

Chapter 20: Adrenal Gland Tumors

Bennett B, McKenna TJ, Hough AJ, et al: Adrenal myelolipoma associated with Cushing's disease. Am J Clin Pathol 73:443–447, 1980.

Bolande RP: Developmental pathology. Am J Pathol 94. 627–683, 1979.

Breslow N, McCann B: Statistical estimation of prognosis for children with neuroblastoma. Cancer Research 31, 2098–2103, 1971.

Cagle PT, Hough AJ, Pysher TJ, et al: Comparison of adrenal cortical tumors in children and adults. Cancer 57:2235-2237, 1986.

Carney JA, Sizemore GW, Sheps SG: Adrenal medullary disease in multiple endocrine neoplasia type 2. Am J Clin Pathol 66:279–290, 1976.

Carstens PHB, Kuhns JG, Ghazi C: Primary malignant melanomas of the lung and adrenal. Hum Pathol 15:910-914, 1984.

Cibas EE, Medeiros LJ, Weinberg DS, et al: Cellular DNA profiles of benign and malignant adrenocortical tumors. Am J Surg Pathol 14:948-955, 1990.

DeLellis RA, Stephenson RA: Diseases of the adrenal glands. In Murphy Wm (ed.) Urological Pathology, WB Saunders, Philadelphia 1989, p 525.

DeLellis RA, Wolfe HJ, Gagel RF, Feldman ZT, et al: Adrenal medullary hyperplasia. Am J Patho 83: 177–196, 1976.

Delorimer AA, Bragg AB, Linden G: Neuroblastoma in childhood. Am J Dis Child 118:441–450, 1969.

Dluhy RG, Gittes RF: The adrenals. In Walsh PC, Gittes RF, Perlmutter AD, Stamey TA (eds.) Campbell's Urology, 5th ed. WB Saunders, Philadelphia, 1986, Ch. 85.

Gaffey MJ, Mills SE, Fechner RE, et al: Vascular adrenal cysts. A clinicopathologic and immunohistochemical study of endothelial and hemorrhagic (pseudocystic) variants. Am J Surg Pathol 13:740–747, 1989.

Gaffey MJ, Mills SE, Medeiros LJ, Weiss LM: Unusual variants of adrenal pseudocysts with intracystic fat, myelolipomatous metaplasia, and metastatic carcinoma. Am J Clin Pathol 94:706–713, 1990.

Gaffey MJ, Traweek ST, Mills SE, et al: Cytokeratin expression in adrenocortical neoplasia: An immunohistochemical and biochemical study with implications for the differential diagnosis of adrenocortical, hepatocellular, and renal cell carcinoma. Hum Pathol 23:144–153, 1992.

Gerson JM, Koop CE: Neuroblastoma. Seminars In Oncology 1:35–46, 1974.

Gould VE, Sommers SC: Adrenal medulla and paraganglia. In Bloodworth JMB (ed.) Endocrine Pathology. Williams and Wilkins, Baltimore, 1982, 473–510.

Hough AJ, Hollifield JW, Page DL, Hartmann WH: Prognostic factors in adrenal cortical tumors. A mathematical analysis of clinical and morphologic data. Am J Clin Pathol 72:390–399, 1979.

Joshi VV, Chatten J, Sather HN, Shimada H: Evaluation of the Shimada classification in advanced neuroblastoma with a special reference to the mitosis-karyorrhexis index: A report from the Childrens Cancer Study Group. Mod Pathol 4:139–147, 1991.

Lack EE, Travis WD, Oertel JE: Adrenal cortical neoplasms. In Lack EE (ed.) Pathology of the Adrenal Glands. Churchill Livingstone, New York, 1990.

Lack EE, Mulvihill JJ, Travis WD, Kozakewich HPW: Adrenal cortical neoplasms in the pediatric and adolescent age group. Clinicopathologic study of 30 cases with emphasis on epidemiologic and prognostic factors. Pathol Annu 27(1):1–53, 1992.

Lack EE: Adrenal medullary hyperplasia and pheochromacytoma. In Lack EE (ed.) Pathology of the Adrenal Glands, Churchill Livingstone, New York, 1990, 173–235.

Lack EE, Kozakewich HPW: Adrenal neuroblastoma, ganglio-neuroblastoma, and related tumors. In Lack EE (ed.): Pathology of the Adrenal Glands Churchill-Livingstone, New York, 1990, 277–309.

Medeiros LJ, Weiss LM: New developments in the pathologic diagnosis of adrenal cortical neoplasms. A review. Am J Clin Pathol 97:73–83, 1992.

Medeiros, LJ, Wolf BC, Balogh K, Federman M: Adrenal Pheochromocytoma: A clinicopathologic review of 60 cases. Hum Pathol, 16:580–589, 1985.

Miettinen M: Neuroendocrine differentiation in adrenocortical carcinoma. New immunohistochemical findings supported by electron microscopy. Lab Invest 66:169–174, 1992.

Miettinen M, Lehto V-P, Virtanen I: Immunofluorescence microscopic evaluation of the intermediate filament expression of the adrenal cortex and medulla and their tumors. Am J Pathol 118:360–366, 1985.

Mukai, M, Torikata C, Iri H, et al: Expression of neurofilament triplet proteins in human neural tumors. An immunohistochemical study of paragangliomas, ganglioneuroma, ganglioneuroblastoma, and neuroblastoma. Am J Pathol 122:28–35, 1986.

Neville AM: The adrenal medulla. In Symington T (ed.) Functional Pathology of the Human Adrenal Gland. Williams and Wilkins, Baltimore, 1969, 217–324.

O'Brien WM, Lynch JH: Adrenal metastases by renal cell carcinoma. Incidence at nephrectomy. Urology 29:605–607, 1987.

Page DL, DeLellis RA, Hough AJ: Tumors of the Adrenal. Atlas of Tumor Pathology, second series, fasicle 23. Armed Forces Institute of Pathology, Washington, D.C. 1985.

Pollock WJ, McConnell CF, Hilton C, Lavine RL: Virilizing Leydig cell adenoma of adrenal gland. Am J Surg Pathol 10:816–822, 1986.

Ramsay JA, Asa SL, van Nostrand AWP, et al: Lipid degeneration in pheochromocytomas mimicking adrenal cortical tumors. Am J Surg Pathol 11:480–486, 1987.

Redman BG, Pazdur R, Zingas AP, Loredo R: Prospective evaluation of adrenal insufficiency in patients with adrenal metastasis. Cancer 60:103-107, 1987.

Remine WH, Chong GC, van Heerden JA, Sheps SG, et al: Current management of pheochromocytoma. Ann Surg 179:740–748, 1974.

Shimada H, Chatten J, Newton WA, et al: Histopathologic prognostic factors in neuroblastic tumors: Definition of subtypes of ganglioneuroblastoma and an age-linked classification of neuroblastomas. J Natl Cancer Inst 73:405–416, 1984.

Shrago SS, Weisman J, Cooper PH: Spironolactone bodies in adrenal adenoma. Arch Pathol Lab Med 99:416–420, 1975.

Slooten HV, Schaberg A, Smeenk D, Moolenaar AJ: Morphologic characteristics of benign and malignant adrenocortical tumors. Cancer 55:766–773, 1985.

Stout AP: Ganglioneuroma of the sympathetic nervous system. Surg Gynecol Obstet 84:101–110, 1947.

Tang CK, Gray GF: Adrenocortical neoplasms. Prognosis and morphology. Urology 5:691–695, 1975.

Tang CK, Harriman BB, Toker C: Myxoid adrenal cortical carcinoma. A light and electron microscopic study. Arch Pathol Lab Med 103:635–638, 1979.

Tannenbaum M: Ultrastructural pathology of adrenal medullary tumors. In Sommers SC (ed.) Pathology Annual. Appleton-Century-Crofts, New York, 1970, 145–171.

Taylor SR, Locker J: A comparative analysis of nuclear DNA content and N-myc gene amplification in neuroblastoma. Cancer 65: 1360–1366, 1990.

Travis WD, Oertel JE, Lack EE: Miscellaneous tumors and tumefactive lesions of the adrenal gland. In Lack EE (ed.) Pathology of the Adrenal Glands. Churchill Livingstone, New York, 1990.

Weiss LM, Medeiros LJ, Vickery AL Jr: Pathologic features of prognostic significance in adrenocortical carcinoma. Am J Surg Pathol 13:202–206, 1989.

Weiss LM: Comparative histologic study of 43 metastasizing and nonmetastasizing adrenocortical tumors. Am J Surg Pathol 8:163–169, 1984.

Wick MR, Cherwitz DL, McGlennen RC, Dehner LP: Adrenocortical carcinoma. An immunohistochemical comparison with renal cell carcinoma. Am J Pathol 122:343–352, 1986.

Index

Note: Numbers in **bold** refer to figure numbers.

A

Acquired renal cystic disease of dialysis (ARCD), 3.4–3.5
  clinical manifestations, 3.4
  complications, associated, 3.4–3.5
  morphology, 3.5, **3.10–3.12**
  pathogenesis, 3.4
Actinomyces, and acute pyelonephritis, 9.2
Adenocarcinoma, bladder, 12.16–12.18
  clinical manifestations, 12.16
  morphology, 12.17–12.18, **12.40–12.45**
Adenocarcinoma, prostate
  adenoid basal cell tumor, 14.14
    morphology, **13.21,** 14.14, **14.23**
  adenosquamous and squamous cell carcinoma, **13.24,**
    14.16–14.17, **14.29**
  "carcinoid tumor," 14.14–14.15
    morphology, 14.15, **14.24**
  "endometrioid" adenocarcinoma, prostatic urethra
    and ducts, 14.3
      clinical manifestations, 14.3
      morphology, 14.3, **14.3**
      pathogenesis, 14.3
  mucinous, 14.13–14.14
    morphology, 14.13–14.14, **14.21, 14.22**
  small cell, 14.15
    morphology, 14.15, **14.25**
  transitional cell, 14.15–14.16
    clinical manifestations, 14.15
    morphology, 14.15–14.16, **14.26–14.28**
  typical (acinar), 14.3–14.13
    clinical manifestations, 14.4, **14.4, 14.5**
    morphology, **13.16,** 14.5–14.12, **14.6–14.9**
      detection of clinically latent carcinoma, 14.8
      grading, 14.9–14.12
        Gleason grade 1, 14.9, **14.10**
        Gleason grade 2, 14.9, **14.11**
        Gleason grade 3, 14.9–14.11, **14.12, 14.13**
        Gleason grade 4, 14.11, **14.14, 14.15**
        Gleason grade 5, 14.11–14.12, **14.16–14.18**
      immunocytochemical markers for prostatic
      carcinoma, 14.12, **14.19, 14.20**
    pathogenesis, 14.3–14.4
    prognosis, 14.12–14.13
    staging, 14.4–14.5
Adenomas
  cortical, 11.1–11.2
    morphology, 11.2, **11.1–11.4**
    relationship to renal cell carcinoma, 11.1–11.2
  nephrogenic, 10.19–10.20
    clinical manifestations, 10.19
    morphology, 10.19–10.20, **10.41, 10.42**
    pathogenesis, 10.19

Adenomatoid tumor, 17.5–17.6
  clinical manifestations, 17.5
  morphology, 17.5–17.6, **17.9, 17.10**
  pathogenesis, 17.5
Adrenal gland tumors, 20.1–20.20
  metastatic cancer, 20.18–20.20, **20.30, 20.31**
  myelolipoma, 20.17
    clinical manifestations, 20.17
    morphology, 20.17, **20.24, 20.25**
  neoplasms of the adrenal cortex, 20.1–20.6
    adrenal cortical adenoma, 20.1–20.2
      clinical manifestations, 20.1–20.2
      morphology, 20.2, **20.1–20.3**
    adrenal cortical carcinoma, 20.2–20.6
      differential diagnosis, 20.6
      morphology, 20.2–20.6, **20.4, 20.5**
      prognosis, 20.6
  neoplasms of the adrenal medulla, 20.6–20.17
    ganglioneuroblastoma, 20.15–20.16
      morphology, 20.15, **20.20, 20.21**
      prognosis, 20.15–20.16
    ganglioneuroma, 20.16–20.17
      morphology, 20.16–20.17, **20.22, 20.23**
    neuroblastoma, 20.13–20.15
      clinical manifestations, 20.13
      morphology, 20.13–20.14, **20.17, 20.19**
      prognosis, 20.14–20.15
    pheochromocytoma, 20.6–20.12, **20.6**
      clinical manifestations, 20.7–20.8
      morphology, 20.8–20.12, **20.7–20.16**
  rare primary tumors, 20.20, **20.32**
  vascular adrenal cysts, 20.17–20.18
    clinical manifestations, 20.18, **20.26**
    morphology, 20.18, **20.27–20.29**
Adult polycystic kidney disease (APKD), 1.1–1.4 , 3.1
  associated anomalies and complications, 1.3–1.4, **1.6, 1.7**
  clinical manifestations, 1.2
  morphology, 1.3, **1.1–1.5**
  pathogenesis, 1.1
Aerobacter, and acute pyelonephritis, 9.3
Amyloidosis, bladder, 10.22
  clinical manifestations, 10.22
  morphology, 10.22, **10.44**
  pathogenesis, 10.22
Angiokeratoma, 18.1–18.2
  clinical manifestations, 18.2, **18.1, 18.2**
  morphology, 18.2, **18.3**
  pathogenesis, 18.1
  therapy, 18.2
Angiomyolipoma, 11.24–11.26
  clinical manifestations, 11.24–11.25
  morphology, 11.25–11.26, **11.48–11.52**
Angiosarcoma, penile, 19.9, **19.16, 19.17**
Aortic aneurysm with perianeurysmal fibrosis, 8.8
  clinical manifestations, 8.8
  morphology, 8.8–8.9
  pathogenesis, 8.8

clinical manifestations, 6.2–6.3, **6.1**
  giant, 6.4, **6.8**
  morphology, 6.3–6.4, **6.2–6.7**
  pathogenesis, 6.1–6.2
Hydroureteronephrosis, 6.4, **6.9**
Hypospermatogenesis, 15.9
  clinical manifestations, 15.9
  morphology, 15.9, **15.11**

I

Idiopathic retroperitoneal fibrosis (IRF), 8.7–8.8
  clinical manifestations, 8.7, **8.10**
  morphology, 8.7–8.8, **8.11–8.13**
  pathogenesis, 8.7
Idiopathic scrotal calcinosis, 18.13–18.14
  clinical manifestations, 18.13, **18.28**
  differential diagnosis, 18.14, **18.30**
  morphology, 18.13–18.14, **18.29**
Infantile polycystic kidney disease-congenital hepatic fibrosis
  (IPKD-CHF), 1.4–1.7
  clinical manifestations, 1.5, **1.8**
  morphology, 1.5–1.7, **1.9–1.17**
  pathogenesis, 1.5
Infertility, testicular, 15.7–15.12
  germ cell aplasia (Sertoli cell-only syndrome), 15.10–15.11
    clinical manifestations, 15.10
    morphology, 15.11, **15.13**
  histology, normal, 15.7–15.8
    clinical manifestations, 15.7
    morphology, 15.7–15.8, **15.9**
  hypospermatogenesis, 15.9
    clinical manifestations, 15.9
    morphology, 15.9, **15.11**
  maturation arrest, 15.9–15.10
    clinical manifestations, 15.9–15.10
    morphology, 15.10, **15.12**
  peritubular fibrosis and hyalinization, 15.11–15.12
    clinical manifestations, 15.11
    differential diagnosis, 15.12, **15.15**
    morphology, 15.11, **15.14**
  sloughing of germ cells, 15.9, **15.10**
  testicular immaturity, 15.8–15.9, **15.1**
Inflammatory pseudotumors of the bladder (IPTB), 10.20–10.22
  clinical manifestations, 10.20
  morphology, 10.21–10.22, **10.43**
Intersexuality, 15.4–15.7
  female pseudohermaphrodism, 15.6–15.7
  gonadal dysgenesis, 15.7, **15.8**
  male pseudohermaphrodism, 15.4–15.6
    clinical manifestations, 15.4–15.5
    morphology, 15.5–15.6, **15.5–15.7**
  mixed gonadal dysgenesis, 15.7
  true hermaphrodism, 15.4, **15.4**
Intestinal metaplasia, morphology, 10.18–10.19, **10.39, 10.40**
Intravenous pyelogram (IVP), 7.2, **7.2, 7.3**
Inverted papilloma, bladder, 12.2
  morphology, 12.2, **12.2**
IPKD-CHF. *See* Infantile polycystic kidney disease-congenital hepat-
  ic fibrosis
IPTB. *See* Inflammatory pseudotumors of the bladder
IRF. *See* Idiopathic retroperitoneal fibrosis
IVP. *See* Intravenous pyelogram

J

Jeune's syndrome, 2.5
JGCT. *See* Juxtaglomerular cell tumor

Juxtaglomerular cell tumor (JGCT), 11.26–11.27
  clinical manifestations, 11.27
  morphology, 11.27, **11.55**

K

Kidneys, anomalies, **4.1**
Klebsiella
  and acute bacterial prostatitis, 13.1
  and acute pyelonephritis, 9.3
  and urinary tract infection, 9.1

L

Leiomyoma, 12.22, **12.52**
Leiomyosarcomas, 11.28, **11.57**
  morphology, **10.43,** 12.24–12.25, **12.56–12.58**
Leukemia, kidney, 11.34, **11.67**
Leydig cell tumors, 16.16–16.17
  clinical manifestations, 16.16
  morphology, 16.16–16.17, **16.27, 16.28**
Lichen nitidus, 18.3
  clinical manifestations, 18.3, **18.6**
  morphology, 18.3, **18.7**
Lichen planus, 18.4–18.5
  clinical manifestations, 18.4, **18.8**
  morphology, 18.4–18.5, **18.9**
Li-Fraumen/Lynch syndrome, 20.3
Lindau's disease, 1.8
Liposarcomas, 11.29
Lymphangiomas, renal, 11.28
Lymphomas
  malignant, 8.12–8.14
    clinical manifestations, 8.12
    morphology, 8.12–8.14, **8.24–8.26**
  primary, 12.26
  secondary, 11.34
    clinical, 11.34, **11.68**
    morphology, 11.34, **11.69, 11.70**
  testicular, 16.20–16.21
    clinical manifestations, 16.20–16.21
    morphology, 16.21, **16.38, 16.39**

M

Malakoplakia, 9.15, 10.8–10.10
  clinical manifestations, 9.15, 10.9
  morphology, 9.15, **9.23,** 10.9–10.10, **10.16, 10.17**
  pathogenesis, 10.8–10.9
  testicle, 15.14
Malignant epithelial neoplasms, 12.2–12.20, **12.3**
Malignant mesothelioma, 17.4–17.5
  clinical manifestations, 17.4
  morphology, 17.4–17.5, **17.8**
Malignant rhabdoid tumor, kidney (MRTK), 11.23–11.24
  clinical manifestations, 11.23
  morphology, 11.23–11.24, **11.45–11.47**
MCD-FJN. *See* Medullary cystic disease-familial juvenile
  nephronophthisis complex
Meckel's syndrome, 2.5
Medullary cystic disease-familial juvenile nephronophthisis complex (MCD-FJN), 1.7–1.8
  clinical manifestations, 1.7
  morphology, 1.7–1.8, **1.18, 1.19**
  pathogenesis, 1.7
Medullary sponge kidney (MSK), 2.5–2.7
  clinical manifestations, 2.5–2.6, **2.8**
  morphology, 2.6–2.7, **2.9, 2.10**